*A VETERINARY BOOK FOR DAIRY FARMERS*

# A VETERINARY BOOK FOR DAIRY FARMERS

R. W. BLOWEY, BSc., BVSc., FRCVS

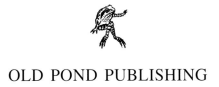

OLD POND PUBLISHING

First published 1985
Second edition 1988
Reprinted 1990, 1993, 1996, 1998
Third edition 1999
Reprinted 2006

**Published by Old Pond Publishing**
Dencora Business Centre
36 Whitehouse Road
Ipswich
IP1 5LT
United Kingdom

www.oldpond.com


Distributed in North America
by Diamond Farm Enterprises
Box 537, Bailey Settlement Road,
Alexandria Bay, NY13607, USA.


A catalogue record for this book is available from the British Library.


ISBN 1-905523-29-7


Illustrations by Jane Upton
Cover design by Isobel Boreham
Origination by TSS Digital, Margate, Kent
Printed in Hong Kong through World Print Ltd

# CONTENTS

end of milking; liner and other rubberware; overmilking. Milking the mastitic cow. Post milking teat disinfection: potential disadvantages of post milking teat disinfection. Dry cow therapy. The environment and mastitis. Treatment of mastitis: choice of antibiotic; taking a milk sample for bacteriology; antibiotic sensitivity testing; factors affecting treatment efficacy; inserting an intramammary tube; other mastitis treatments. Mastitis records and targets. Somatic cell counts. Total bacterial count of milk. Antibiotic residues in milk. Summer mastitis. Uncommon causes of mastitis: Corynebacterium bovis, Staphylococcus epidermidis and micrococci; mycoplasma; yeasts; leptospira hardjo; pseudomonas, klebsiella, bacillus species; gangrenous mastitis. Disorders of the teat and udder: milking machine damage; blackspot; cut teats; udder oedema and necrotic dermatitis; pseudocowpox; bovine herpes mamillitis; udder impetigo; teat warts; teat chaps; milk let-down failure; blind quarters; blood in milk; pea in teat.

## 8  FERTILITY AND ITS CONTROL 231

Costs of a missed heat: extended calving intervals. The components of the calving interval. The oestrus cycle: physical changes; hormonal changes; recognition of pregnancy detection; action of fertility cycle drugs; embryo transfer; cystic ovaries; failure to cycle. Pregnancy detection: milk progesterone tests; ultrasound scanning; bovine pregnancy associated glycoprotein; rectal palpatation; oestrone sulphate. Heat detection: measurement of heat detection. Synchronisation of oestrus: prostaglandin; progesterone releasing devices; effective synchronisation. Conception rates. Causes of low conception rates: poor embryo recognition, serving too soon after calving; poor heat detection, timing of insemination, endometritis; fatty liver; genital and other infections; stress; poor handling facilities; operator technique; semen quality; nutrition. The repeat breeder cow: adhesions; use of GnRH; use of embryos; dosing individual cows. Abortion. Stillborn calves. Preventive medicine and herd facility management: the costs of disease; use of records.

## 9  LAMENESS AND FOOT TRIMMING 279

The structure of the foot: the hoof, the corium, the bones. Correct weightbearing. Hoof overgrowth: effects of overgrowth. Foot trimming: lifting the foot; equipment used; trimming technique. Sole ulcers and white line disease: coriosis; sole ulcers; heel and toe ulcers; white line diseases; causes and controlo of sole ulcers and white line diseases. Other causes of foot lameness: foreign body penetration of the sole; slurry heel; haematoma in the heel; vertical fissures; hardship lines; horizontal fissures; interdigital necrobacillosis; digital dermatitis; interdigital skin hyperplasia; mud fever; fracture of the pedal bone; pedal bone tip necrosis; pedal arthritis. Nursing, footbaths, dressings and blocks: nursing; footbaths; foot dressings and blocks. Lameness due to leg disorders: knocked down pin bone; split H-bones; dislocated hip; fractures; spinal abscess and osteomyelitis; arthritis and stifle ligament rupture; capped knee and hocks, cellulitis; radial nerve paralysis; spastic paresis; contracted tendons.

## 10 DISEASES OF THE SKIN 329

Parasitic causes: ringworm; lice; mange; warble fly; fly strike. Infectious causes: lumpy jaw; wooden tongue; jaw abscesses; malignant oedema; warts; skin tumours, skin TB. Toxic causes: photosensitisation, urticaria, septicaemia, scouring, poorly mixed milk substitute, alopecia. Traumatic injuries: haematomas, bursitis, abscesses, sterile abscesses; cellulitis, ingrowing horns, burns, tail injuries.

## 11 NOTIFIABLE DISEASES, SALMONELLOSIS AND ZOONOSES 347

Notifiable diseases: anthrax; foot-and-mouth disease; brucellosis; warble flies, enzootic bovine leucosis (EBL); tuberculosis (TB); bovine spongiform encephalopathy (BSE); salmonellosis; zoonoses.

# ACKNOWLEDGEMENTS

Thanks must go the farmers around Gloucester who have given me my experience and training over the past thirty years and especially to those who have had to pause while I photographed various cases. In particular, I am grateful to R.S. and J.M. Musson of Hill Court Farm, Forthampton, Gloucester, for the front cover photograph of their four year old home-bred Holstein cow Threelimes Agnes 21. I would like to thank my many colleagues who have been pestered for photographs, tables, drawings and information generally and I am grateful to Mrs Catherine Girdler for typing and proof-reading. Thanks are also due to Kate Bazeley, James Booth, James Greenwood, Diane Powell and George Chancellor, all of whom commented on the initial script for the first edition. Finally I must acknowledge and apologise to my wife Norma and to my family for the many hours that I have had to spend locked away from them during the preparation of this book.

**Dedicated to my children and grandchildren. They have given me enormous pleasure.**

# PREFACE TO THE THIRD EDITION

It was 11 years ago that the Second Edition was published and I find it gratifying that I have been able to include so much new material in this Third Edition. It demonstrates how my own knowledge has moved forward, which presumably in turn reflects the general increase in our understanding of farm livestock. Whether that increased knowledge has led to an improvement in the incidence of disease remains open to question, but if we have been able at least to maintain disease within reasonable bounds, whilst at the same time increasing both the level and intensity of production (milk yields and number of cows per herd have both risen), then presumably we have achieved something.

During the past eleven years, I have had three other books published, namely *Cattle Lameness and Hoofcare*, *Mastitis Control in Dairy Herds* and *A Colour Atlas of Diseases and Disorders of Cattle*. One of the difficulties in writing this third edition has been knowing where to condense and precis material. On the one hand I needed to make the book sufficiently brief to keep it to a reasonable size and cost, and on the other hand I had to maintain sufficient depth and description to keep it useful for the increasingly knowledgeable reader.

The major changes in this third edition are the inclusion of colour photographs throughout and a considerable increase in detail. The use of colour photographs is clearly a major investment. It makes the book much more useful and I hope readers will consider the extra cost worthwhile. The book contains considerably more detail than previous editions and will hopefully now be of value to farmer and veterinarian alike. There will be times when additional information is needed and to meet this need I have included a list of suggested further reading. I hope that the book will continue to be used. One of my greatest pleasures is to see an obviously well-worn copy lying open at the relevant page when I arrive on a farm. Improvements in animal health must surely be founded upon a thorough understanding of the nature of disease, and this should be a goal for all of us.

There will be no further new edition until we are well into the 21st century. By that stage BSE will be history. What other changes will then be facing us? Only time can answer that question, but I look forward to the challenge.

Minsterworth, Gloucester                                                          Roger W. Blowey
July 1999


# FURTHER READING

*Bovine Medicine* (1992). Ed. A,H. Andrews, R.W. Blowey, H. Boyd & R.G. Eddy. Published by Blackwells Scientific Publications, Oxford.

*Feeding the Dairy Cow* (1996) by Tom Chamberlain & Mike Wilkinson, published by Chalcombe Publications, Welton, Lincs.

*Mastitis Control in Dairy Herds* (1995) by Roger Blowey and Peter Edmondson, published by Farming Press.

*Cattle Lameness and Hoofcare* (1993) by Roger Blowey, published by Farming Press.

*Understanding the Dairy Cow* (1993) by John Webster, published by Blackwell Scientific Publications, Oxford.

ARC (1980) *The nutrient requirements of Farm Livestock*, Commonwealth Agricultural Bureau, Slough.

*Footcare in Cattle* [video] (1992) written and presented by Roger Blowey, released by Farming Press.

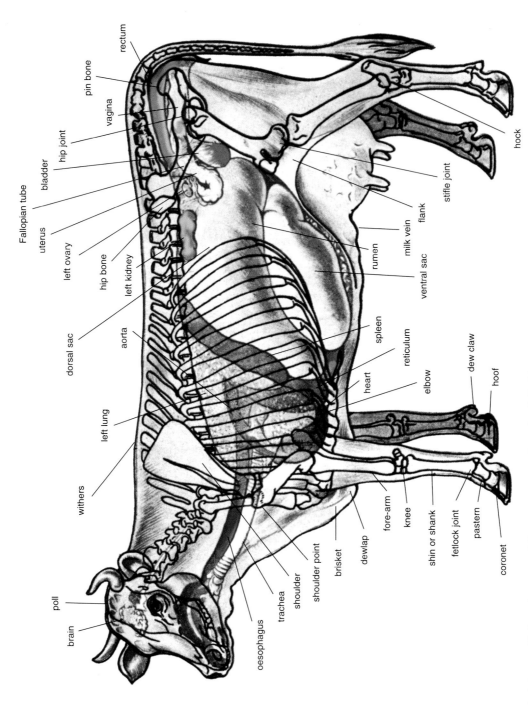

The skeleton and internal organs of the cow as seen from the left side

x

*Chapter 1*

# A CONCEPT OF DISEASE, IMMUNITY AND TREATMENT

For some diseases there is a simple relationship between the infection, the animal and the treatment needed. Examples include foul-of-the-foot, caused by a bacterial infection and treated with antibiotics, or ringworm, a mycotic infection which can be treated with antifungal drugs. However, many of the more common conditions seen on farms today are due to an interaction between the animal, its environment and a wide range of infectious organisms. Probably the best example is calf pneumonia and this will be referred to again later in the chapter. Another example of the complexity of disease is milk fever. At calving the cow's requirements for calcium may exceed her capabilities to mobilise the mineral, although she has ample reserves in her skeleton. The clinical symptoms are due to a deficiency of calcium in the blood. Milk fever is known as a metabolic disorder or a production disease.

Both the farmer and his veterinary surgeon must thoroughly understand the mechanisms of disease if we are to reduce some of the enormous losses that are incurred, and I would urge the reader to spend a short while studying this first chapter before embarking on the main text. This chapter describes the nature of disease; some of the ways in which the animal protects itself; how infection, environment and immunity interact in a clinical situation; and finally it describes an approach to the treatment of an individual sick animal.

## CAUSES OF DISEASE

Although we often think of infectious agents as the cause of disease, in fact many of the ailments we see in farm livestock are nothing to do with infection. Lameness must be the best example of this. For example, simple physical trauma to the foot has a major role in the aetiology of many hoof problems. Poisoning, or, at the other extreme, trace element deficiency, can also lead to major health problems. Overall the major causes of disease or ill health in farm livestock may be listed as follows:

- Infectious agents
- Nutritional deficiency and excess
- Metabolic disorders
- Poisoning
- Physical injury
- Congenital disorders

### Infectious Agents

There is a wide range of infectious agents which can cause disease. Some exist as normal organisms on the animal or in its environment and only cause disease when in an unusual site or when the immunity of the animal is compromised (i.e. reduced). A good example of this is the bacterium *Escherichia coli*, most commonly known as *E. coli*. It is present in the intestine of all cattle, where it usually causes no problems. However, if it gains access to the udder it can cause quite severe disease. This is especially true in the early lactation animal, whose udder defences against infection are often poor. However, for some other infections, whenever they are present disease occurs. A good example of this would be the foot-and-mouth virus.

Infectious agents may be subdivided into the following categories:

- Bacteria
- Viruses
- Protozoa
- Fungi
- Worms
- Ectoparasites

*Bacteria*

These are single-celled organisms which contain all the components needed for a separate existence. A typical bacterium is shown in Figure 1.1. It is a single cell, and consists of a thick outer polysaccharide structure, the cell wall, inside of which there is a protein membrane enclosing the cytoplasm and the nuclear material. The nuclear material contains the genetic components, the DNA (deoxyribonucleic acid), and by a complex arrangement of molecules, DNA functions as the regulator for all cell processes, determining the size and shape of the cell and the activities that take place within its cytoplasm. These 'activities' are the processes of reproduction and growth. The whole bacterium may be enclosed by a gelatinous capsule, a thick membrane which renders the bacterium more resistant to phagocytosis (i.e. being engulfed by white blood cells). Bacteria are therefore individual discrete units of life.

Given ideal conditions of warmth, nutrients and moisture most of them can also multiply outside the animal's body. Under adverse conditions some bacteria can turn themselves into a very resistant spore form, which can survive for many years. The classic example is that of anthrax, whose spores can persist in the soil for up to 40 years. Bacteria absorb nutrients for their growth from their immediate surroundings (e.g. blood, milk or body tissue) and excrete waste products. It is often these waste products which cause disease. The 'waste' is then known as a toxin and the animal is said to be suffering from a toxaemia. Typical examples of toxaemia are acute *E. coli* mastitis and severe uterine infections.

Bacteria are the major cause of mastitis, they are commonly involved in respiratory disease and they are the cause of the clostridial group of diseases such as blackleg, tetanus and anthrax. Bacteria commonly form pus and are also responsible for conditions such as navel ill, calf diphtheria and abscesses. Bacteria are killed by antibiotics, with different antibiotics being needed to kill the different species of bacteria. This is explained in more detail in the treatment section.

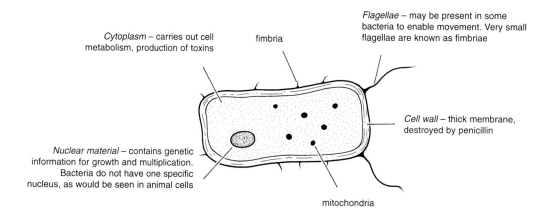

*Cytoplasm* – carries out cell metabolism, production of toxins

fimbria

*Flagellae* – may be present in some bacteria to enable movement. Very small flagellae are known as fimbriae

*Cell wall* – thick membrane, destroyed by penicillin

*Nuclear material* – contains genetic information for growth and multiplication. Bacteria do not have one specific nucleus, as would be seen in animal cells

mitochondria

Figure 1.1. A typical bacterial cell. Even the largest bacteria (e.g. anthrax) are only 0.005 mm long. They multiply by dividing into two; and under favourable conditions this may occur every 30 minutes, so that one bacterium could produce 17 million offspring in 12 hours!

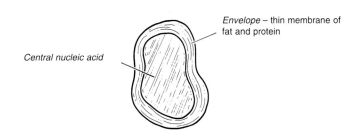

Figure 1.2. A virus particle. A virus is very much smaller than a bacterium. It uses the processes of metabolism within the animal cell for its own multiplication and growth, and as such it cannot live a separate existence away from the animal. This is very different from bacteria.

*Viruses*

Viruses are much smaller than bacteria and in fact they may even infect and cause disease in bacteria. They cannot be seen with a normal light microscope; electron microscopy is required. They consist simply of central nuclear material, which may be DNA or RNA (ribonucleic acid), and this is surrounded by a capsule of fat and protein (Figure 1.2).

Because viruses have no cytoplasm or proper nucleus, they cannot carry out their own metabolic functions of growth and reproduction and they are therefore unable to multiply outside the animal's living cells. For their survival away from the animal, and hence their transfer from one animal to another, viruses must be protected, for example in sputum (pneumonia viruses), milk (foot-and-mouth virus) or blood (EBL virus).

Once inside the animal, viruses inject their own RNA or DNA into the animal cell and then use the metabolic processes within the cytoplasm of that cell for their own purposes of multiplication and growth. When a cell is packed full of viruses, it bursts and virus particles are released to penetrate and infect adjacent animal cells. It is the bursting of these cells which generally causes the detrimental effects on the animal and hence the signs of disease, although some viruses (e.g. those causing teat warts or EBL) induce a proliferation or excessive multiplication of animal cells to produce a tumour.

Both bacteria and viruses may be very specific in the site they choose to infect. For example, certain groups will grow only in the respiratory tract – and these cause the clinical signs of a cold, influenza or pneumonia. Others can live only in the intestine and they will cause scouring. It is by this mechanism that we associate particular strains of bacteria or viruses with specific diseases. Different strains of bacteria and viruses vary considerably in shape and size, in the same way that the different species of animal or bird are so variable.

Viruses cause a wide range of disorders including foot-and-mouth and diseases of the teat skin, and they are often the primary cause of calf pneumonia. Whereas antibiotics will kill bacteria, there is no specific drug to kill viruses. This is one reason why many virus diseases are controlled by vaccination. Mycoplasma, ureaplasmas and rickettsia are organisms which have some characteristics of bacteria and some of viruses.

*Protozoa*

Protozoa are also single-celled organisms, although they are larger and more complex than bacteria and may have a free-living existence. Examples include *Babesia* and *Trypanosoma*, which live in the blood of cattle and cause redwater, and coccidia and *Cryptosporidia*, both of which live in the intestine and cause scouring. Other protozoal diseases of cattle include *Neospora*, a cause of abortion, *Theileria* which causes East Coast fever in southern Africa, and *Besnoitia* which causes skin disease and abortion.

The treatment of protozoal infections requires specific therapy. For example, there is one drug specifically used against *Babesia* (imidocarb) and another against coccidiosis (e.g. amprolium). There is no specific treatment against *Cryptosporidia*.

*Fungi (Yeasts and moulds)*

Fungi are very simple members of the plant kingdom. Yeasts are commonly found in the environment and primarily cause disease when they enter an unusual site, e.g. the udder, where they can cause a chronic mastitis. They do not respond to antibiotics and they need special therapy, e.g. iodine (see Chapter 7). In fact yeasts may grow in the oily 'carrier' used in bovine intramammary mastitis tubes. There are some specific fungal diseases of cattle, namely ringworm, and other diseases where a common environmental fungus invades an unusual site. A good example of this is abortion caused by the fungus *Aspergillus*.

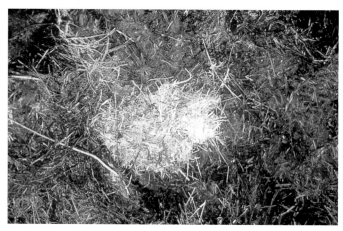

Plate 1.1. Aspergillus mould growing on silage. This led to five abortions when fed to dry cows.

*Aspergillus* may be seen as a blue-grey mould growing on silage (Plate 1.1), and if eaten by a pregnant cow it can lead to abortion.

*Worms (Helminth parasites)*

Cattle can be affected by a wide range of helminth or endoparasitic worms. In low numbers worms cause no problems, although if allowed to multiply they can cause serious disease. As with bacteria and viruses, different worms live in different parts of the body. Examples include nematodes such as the lungworm (*Dictyocaulus viviparus*), the stomach worm *Ostertagia* and the intestinal worms *Nematodirus* and *Oesophagostomum*. There is even a worm (*Thelazia*) which lives in the eye! Tapeworms (cestodes) can also occur and are found in the intestine. Flukes (trematodes) are related parasites and live in the liver.

Most worms have a direct life cycle, that is eggs laid by adult worms are passed in cattle faeces, develop into mature larvae on the ground and are then ingested by grazing animals. Other helminth parasites may have an indirect life cycle, for example the liver fluke spends part of its life in the host animal and part in a snail.

An anthelmintic is the general name given to drugs which are used to treat worms (i.e. wormers). The same drug will often treat all species of lungworm and gutworm, although different products are usually required to treat liver fluke. Anthelmintics are often subdivided into white drenches and clear drenches. The white drenches are the benzimidazole group of compounds, examples of these being oxfendazole and fenbendazole. Clear drenches include levamisole and the avermectin range of products, e.g. ivermectin, doramectin and moxidectin. Each drug has a slightly different spectrum of action and length of activity, so make sure that you have read the manufacturer's instructions before use.

*Ectoparasites*

An ectoparasite is the name given to an organism which lives on the body surface of an animal (intestinal worms are known as endoparasites). The range of different ectoparasites on cattle includes lice, mange, flies, maggots and ticks. Some have a direct life cycle (lice and mange) where all stages of the life cycle can be found on the same animal. Others, such as ticks, are more complex and part of their life cycle is spent off the animal.

## Nutritional Deficiency and Excess

Deficiency disorders are the result of an inadequate supply of minerals, vitamins or trace elements. Typical examples would be copper deficiency or vitamin A deficiency. Deficiencies may be either primary, when there is a specific lack of nutrient in the diet, such as vitamin A, or secondary, when some factor interferes with the uptake of a nutrient. Examples of the latter include molybdenum, sulphur or iron interfering with copper absorption to produce an induced copper deficiency. In most cases treatment simply involves providing an adequate supply of the nutrient.

Disease can also occur as a result of ingestion of an excess of some feedingstuffs. The most common example would be overeating syndrome, where cattle gain access to a compound feed store and develop acidosis, which is an excessive fermentation of starch in the rumen.

## Metabolic Disorders

Homeostasis is the process whereby the body maintains a constant temperature, heart and respiratory rate and also ensures that the levels of various chemicals in the blood remain within a constant range. For example, when there is a sudden increase in demand for calcium (e.g. immediately after calving), the cow may not be able to draw calcium from her 'stores' (mainly bone and intestinal contents) rapidly enough to satisfy her requirements. Blood calcium levels then fall, muscle function is lost and the cow sinks to the ground with milk fever and is unable to rise.

It is not that there is insufficient calcium in the diet, or even insufficient stored in the body. It is simply that the cow is unable to cope with the sudden increase in demand for calcium sufficiently rapidly to avoid the short-term drop in blood calcium which follows. The resulting disorder is known as a metabolic disease.

## Poisoning

When we think of poisoning we usually refer to the animal eating some 'foreign' substance, for example lead (often old paint on doors) or plants such as yew trees. The clinical signs seen will depend on the poison eaten. Ingestion of lead produces nervous signs, whereas eating yew leads to sudden death due to heart failure. Poisoning can also occur from eating an excess of some substance which in small quantities is essential for growth. Copper is a good example of this, being essential for growth, but in excess causing liver failure.

Treatment of poisoning is difficult. Sometimes there are specific antidotes, but more often all that we can do is treat the symptoms (e.g. scouring) and hope that the cow can overcome and excrete the toxin herself.

## Physical Injury

Many of the cattle ailments we have to deal with are the result of physical trauma. The best example is lameness. Hoof and limb disorders are frequently associated with either trauma to the foot, for example, prolonged standing on a hard surface producing sole ulcers, or damage to the leg, for example resulting in dislocation of the joint or even fracture of a bone.

Examples of other physical injuries include:

- teat damage
- haematomas (blood blisters under the skin)
- skin cuts
- foreign bodies, e.g. barley awn or grass seed in the eye
- burns, either caused by fire or sunburn
- chemical injury, e.g. tank cleaner mistakenly used for teat dip
- abscesses (following penetration of the skin by thorns, nails, fragments of metal etc.)

## Congenital Disorders

Congenital diseases are abnormalities which are present at birth. They may be caused by genetic factors or by ingestion of teratogens during pregnancy.

*Genetic defects*

The incidence of inherited genetic defects in cattle is said to be quite high (one in 500 births), but as at least half of the calves are stillborn, they do not represent a major problem to the cattle industry. Typical examples include cleft palate (Plate 1.2), harelip (Plate 1.3), spina bifida (Plate 1.4), a very small tail or no tail at all (hypoplastic tail, Plate 1.5), contracted tendons (Plate 1.6), hydrocephalus, brachygnathia (parrot mouth, Plate 1.7) and umbilical hernias. If it is found that a particular bull is throwing a high incidence of calves with genetic defects, he should be culled. Sometimes the defect is only seen when a bull mates with a particular cow. In this case the defect is said to be caused by a recessive gene, in that the defect will only appear if both the sire and dam are carrying the gene for that defect.

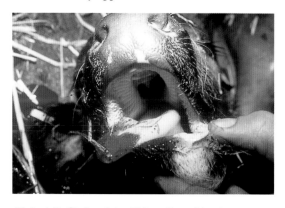

Plate 1.2. Cleft palate. This calf could not even suckle and was destroyed. Where the defect in the hard palate is smaller, the cow's teat may cover the hole during suckling and it is only when the calf starts eating solid food, or drinking from a bucket, that a severe nasal discharge indicates that something is wrong.

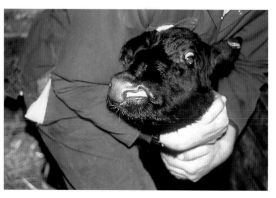

Plate 1.3. Harelip (also called cleft lip or primary cleft palate). This can also make suckling difficult, although this calf was able to drink from a bucket.

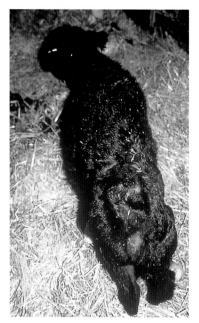

Plate 1.4. Spina bifida. The tops of two lumbar vertebrae have not closed, leaving a hole into the lumbar spine, seen here as a red area. This calf was partially paralysed in the hind legs.

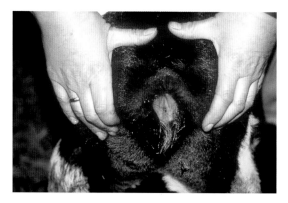

Plate 1.5. No anus and minimal tail (anal atresia and coccygeal hypoplasia). Calves with a totally blind anus rapidly develop abdominal distension, severe pain and colic. This calf was lucky and faeces were passed through the vagina. No tail or a shortened tail is commonly seen on its own without anal atresia.

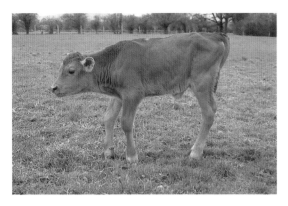

Plate 1.6. Contracted tendons at the fetlock, as in this calf, are common, particularly in larger calves. They will correct in time without treatment.

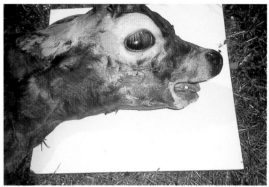

Plate 1.7. Brachygnathia (parrot mouth or overshot upper jaw) is most commonly seen in stillborn calves.

*Teratogenic defects*

Teratogenic defects result from the ingestion of toxic agents during pregnancy. The most publicised example of this must be the effect of thalidomide in man, which resulted in the birth of deformed children. In cattle, ingestion of some species of the plant *Lupinus* can produce crooked calf disease, where calves are born with malpositioned legs, either excessively flexed or excessively extended. Oral dosing of early pregnant cattle with the ringworm treatment griseofulvin should be avoided, because of the risk of producing deformed, full-term calves.

Viral and other infections can also produce congenital defects. The best examples are BVD virus and *Neospora caninum*. Infection of mid to late pregnant cows with either agent can result in defects such as cerebellar hypoplasia. In this condition the part of the brain known as the cerebellum is far too small (hypoplasia, Plate 1.9) and the affected calf is unable to stand. The calf in Plate 1.8 is a typical example. At birth it was unable to stand or suckle and when lifted it pushed its head back over its back (opisthotonos). Mid pregnancy infection with *Akabane* virus or BVD can cause arthrogryphosis (Plate 1.10), a condition in which the hind limbs become fused or deformed.

Not all congenital abnormalities are immediately apparent at birth. Strabismus is a good example. Plate 1.11 shows a Hereford heifer with bilateral convergent strabismus,

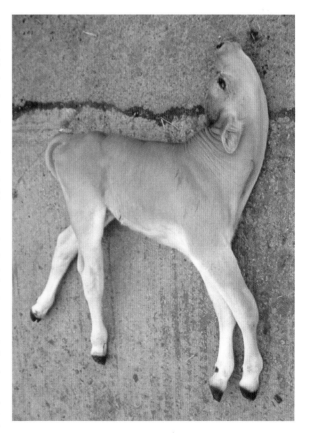

Plate 1.8. Cerebellar hypoplasia. Although this calf appeared normal and healthy at rest, as soon as it tried to feed or stand it fell over and its head went into spasm over its back (opisthotonos). BVD and Neospora are possible causes.

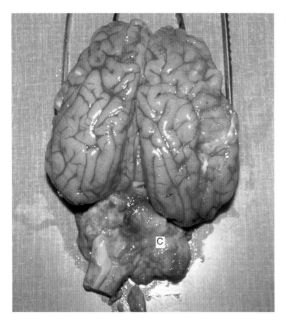

Plate 1.9. Cerebellar hypoplasia. The cerebellum (C) is the part of the brain which controls balance.

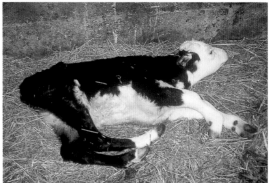

Plate 1.10. Arthrogryposis. The hind legs are fixed in this extreme flexion position and cannot be moved. Often the pelvis is also involved (when a caesarean birth is necessary). This calf also had spina bifida. Arthrogryposis can be either teratogenic in origin or inherited.

that is both eyes (bilateral) point inwards (convergent) with a squint (strabismus). This condition gets progressively worse as the calf gets older and in some instances results in almost total blindness. In one unfortunate incident I dealt with, a dairy farmer purchased a freshly calved heifer with strabismus. A few weeks after purchase she had a bad fright and ran off. Because she could not see very well she became totally disoriented and finished up by drowning in the slurry pit. Fortunately, relatively few congenital defects have such a dramatic ending!

Other congenital defects causing blindness include cataracts (Plate 1.12) and microphthalmia or anophthalmia (very small or no eyes, Plate 1.13). Cataracts are an opacity of the lens. They can be hereditary or caused by BVD infection of the dam during late pregnancy. Most cataracts are left untreated and although calves seem to manage with very limited or zero vision, treatment is possible. A very fine knife is inserted between the cornea and sclera (the clear and white parts of the eye) and one or two cuts are made across the front of the lens. The aqueous humour (the liquid in the front part of the eyeball) then slowly dissolves away the lens until sight has been restored.

See Chapter 4 for other eye disorders.

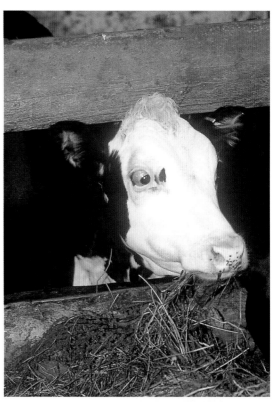

Plate 1.11. Strabismus (squint). Note how the eyeball is protruding and pointing in towards the nose. Both eyes were affected. This is a progressive condition which can eventually lead to blindness.

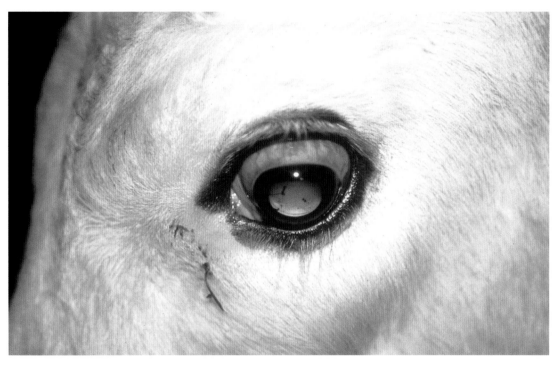

Plate 1.12. A cataract is an opacity of the lens. The centre of the eye has a blue appearance, as in this calf.

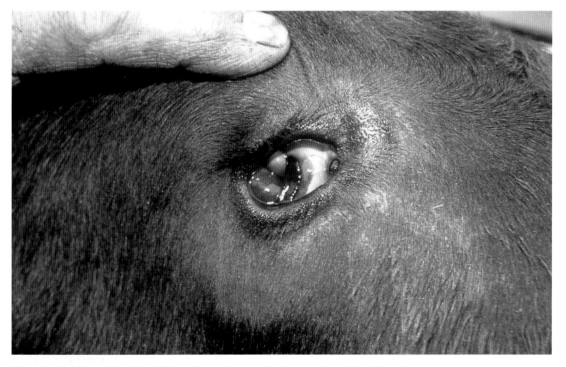

Plate 1.13. Microphthalmia. This calf was born with the eye almost totally missing.

## DEFENCES AGAINST DISEASE

Animals (and also man!) are continually exposed to a range of infectious agents and physical factors which could potentially cause disease, but fortunately disease occurs relatively rarely. This is because we all have a range of excellent defence mechanisms which afford a degree of protection against moderate challenge. These defences will be outlined briefly in the following section and can be subdivided into:

- *Physical barriers*
  - skin
  - respiratory passages
  - digestive tract
  - eye mechanisms
  - commensal bacteria

- *Chemical barriers*
  - acid in the stomach
  - alkaline in the intestine

- *Immunity*
  The body has an excellent ability to recognise materials which are 'foreign', that is materials which are not part of itself, and to control them. At the same time it has to recognise those tissues which are part of itself and leave them alone. The mechanism for dealing with 'foreign invaders' or 'non-self' materials has two components, namely:
      - cellular mechanisms: certain cells are able to recognise and engulf infectious and other foreign agents
      - humoral mechanisms: a system of 'active' proteins, most commonly known as antibodies, assist in the detection and destruction of non-self tissue

In addition, there are two categories of both cellular and humoral defence systems:

    - innate systems: these exist in all animals and do not rely on previous exposure to an infection
    - induced or acquired systems: these come into play after an animal has been exposed to an infection.

Following exposure, the precise characteristics of the invading organism are remembered and the body produces specific defences against it, using both cells and antibodies. These are then ready to attack the invader if it manages to gain entry into the body for a second time. This is the nature of vaccines. They give the unexposed animal a mild or dead form of the infection. The animal then manufactures huge quantities of specific defence materials (both antibodies and cells) and is able to repel an invasion by that infection. Different vaccines are needed for each disease.

### Physical and Chemical Defences

The skin must be the best example of a physical barrier. It consists of a thick layer of epithelial cells, with a dead and keratinised (or reinforced) surface. It is certainly a hostile environment for viral or bacterial multiplication. Should the skin get very dirty however, or if it is broken by physical damage, then bacteria may gain entry, the infection may become established and pus or abscesses may form. Bacteria retard healing and this is why wounds and cuts should always be cleaned and washed with antiseptic, thus preventing the bacteria from multiplying. Pus is an accumulation of dead white blood cells, dead cells and fluid from animal tissue and bacteria. Skin is also covered by a film of fatty acids which help to prevent bacterial multiplication. Excessive washing, especially with detergents, removes these acids and thus renders the skin more susceptible to infection. This is of particular relevance to teats, and is one reason why chapping is so common unless emollients are added to the teat dip.

The air passages (trachea, bronchi, etc.) and the intestine can be termed external surfaces because they come into contact with materials (air and food) from outside the animal's body. In the nose there are hairs which prevent large particles from being inhaled into the lungs. Their function is supported by a microscopic layer of cilia. These small, finger-like projections, which line the surface of the trachea, move in a wave motion to propel bacteria and other smaller particles back up towards the mouth, where they can be swallowed or coughed away. In addition mucus glands produce a sticky secretion to line the airways, thus trapping any bacteria or viruses which happen to land and this prevents them from reaching the susceptible tissues of the lungs. These mechanisms are described in detail in Chapter 3.

The mouth and oesophagus have a thick horny (keratinised) lining, like skin, and this helps to prevent bacterial penetration. The stomach, on the other hand, produces mucus and acid, partly to assist digestion, but also helping to prevent bacterial growth, whereas the upper small intestine is very alkaline, again inhibiting bacterial growth. These extremes of acid and alkaline conditions should perhaps be considered as chemical rather than physical defence mechanisms. Vaginal secretions are also acid.

The eye has some interesting and rather unique defences. The eyelids close rapidly when an object is approaching, and this protects the eyeball from physical damage. If a foreign body does land on the eye however, tears are produced to wash it away and rapid blinking helps to move the object to the corner of the eye where it will cause less damage. If the surface of the eye does become damaged, blood vessels grow across the cornea to supply antibodies and rebuilding materials. This is known as *pannus* formation, and is described in more detail in Chapter 4.

The final type of physical defence is provided by the bacteria which *normally* live in and on the animal as 'commensals', that is they live there without causing disease. However, they compete with disease-causing (pathogenic) infections for both nutrients and space. If these normal microbe populations are disturbed, for example by a prolonged course of antibiotics by mouth, it is possible that the more serious pathogenic infections may proliferate and cause disease. This is why it is often recommended that yoghurt or other probiotics are given at the end of a course of calf scour treatment – to recolonise the gut with 'healthy' bacteria.

## The Immune System

As stated above, the immune system can be subdivided into two parts, cellular immunity and antibodies, although within the animal the two systems will work very much in conjunction with one another to counteract disease. Although I shall be dealing with the immune response to disease-causing organisms, the reader should appreciate that an identical immune reaction is evoked against any material which the animal recognises as being foreign to its system. This is very important in the human fields of allergy and organ transplant rejection. Any material which the animal recognises as foreign is called an antigen, and antigens evoke both a cellular and an antibody response. Immunity consists of both innate and induced components.

*Innate mechanisms*
**Cellular response** The most common cells involved with innate immunity are neutrophils and macrophages. Both engulf and destroy invading infectious agents by a process known as phagocytosis. Neutrophils and macrophages are therefore sometimes collectively known as phagocytic cells, or simply as phagocytes.

The process of phagocytosis is shown diagrammatically in Figure 1.3. Neutrophils are commonly present in blood, whereas macrophages can be found in milk and other secretions. Macrophages are a type of 'bobby on the beat'. When they see something they don't like, they 'arrest it' (engulf it) and at the same time send out a signal which mobilises a 'rapid reaction force' of highly active neutrophils. The neutrophils then continue with the process of phagocytosis and destruction.

Macrophages (and cancer cells) produce matrix metalloproteinases (MMPs). These enzymes dissolve body tissue and allow the macrophages to pass between the body cells in their search for foreign invaders. MMPs also allow cancer cells to penetrate. Another important function of macrophages is that they can also hold the invading antigen in a very specific manner. They then present it to the lymphocytes (another form of white blood cell) of the induced immunity system, to ensure that the lymphocytes will recognise it in the future.

**Humoral response** The humoral part of the innate immune system consists of proteins such as complement, interferon and lysozyme. Complement coats the outside of invading agents, in a process known as opsonisation. This makes the invading organism more easily engulfed by macrophages. Interferon is best known for its effect against viruses, but it also has a role in neutralising toxins. Lysozyme is a form of 'natural antibiotic' and is highly active in killing bacteria.

*Induced mechanisms*
This also has cellular and humoral components, but each cell and each antibody is highly specific to the invading agent. The induced immune system differs from the innate immune system, in that the induced system *must* have had previous exposure to an antigen in order to be effective.

**Cellular response** The cellular response of the induced immune system is often referred to as cell mediated immunity. The major cells are lymphocytes.

There is a range of different lymphocytes. They all produce antibodies, but some may have additional functions and means of recognising and destroying invading antigens. T lymphocytes,

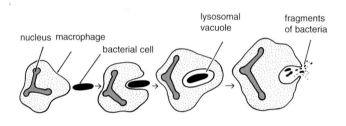

Figure 1.3. Phagocytosis, the process by which an animal cell recognises and then engulfs and destroys foreign substances such as bacteria and viruses.

The body's defences against infection are
  Physical barriers
  Chemical barriers
  The immune system
    – antibodies (humoral mechanisms) and cells
    – innate and induced systems

including killer T cells, recognise foreign cells, for example cancer cells and tissue transplants in man. Cells which are infected with virus will also be recognised and destroyed by the killer T lymphocytes. 'Helper' T lymphocytes (also known as T4 cells) hold the invading antigen so that it can be recognised by B lymphocytes. Each B lymphocyte (also known as a plasma cell) has thousands of recognition sites on its surface.

To return to our police force analogy, macrophages and T lymphocytes hold invading antigens ('suspects') and present them to B lymphocytes ('policemen'), thus enabling the suspects' fingerprints to be taken. Each lymphocyte carries up to 100,000 different fingerprints. Considering there are millions of lymphocytes, this makes the total number of combinations almost infinite. Each recognition site is different for every individual invading antigen. When a lymphocyte meets up with its specific antigen, two things happen:

- First, that single lymphocyte multiplies rapidly, producing clones of other identical lymphocytes which are immediately able to recognise that specific invader in the future.
- Secondly, these lymphocyte clones then produce antibodies, namely specific proteins to neutralise the invader.

It is interesting to note the numbers of cells which are involved. In an adult dairy cow approximately 8% of its bodyweight is blood, that is 48 litres for a 600 kilo cow. An average cow has around 7000 white blood cells per millilitre of blood, approximately 35% of which are lymphocytes, which means there are 2450 lymphocytes per millilitre of blood, or 117,600,000 lymphocytes in total! This only counts the lymphocytes in the blood. Lymphocytes are continually able to move out through the walls of the blood vessels into the extracellular fluid space, across to lymph nodes and then back into the blood again, all the time looking for 'foreign invaders'.

**Humoral response** Antibodies are large protein molecules produced by lymphocytes to combine with, and hence neutralise, the invading agents. The most interesting feature of antibodies is that they are very specific. Whereas the other defence mechanisms we have discussed so far will be effective against any bacteria, viruses or even dust, there has to be a separate and specific antibody for every type of infectious agent. Thus antibodies effective against one type of *E. coli* bacteria may not have any action against a slightly different strain of *E. coli*.

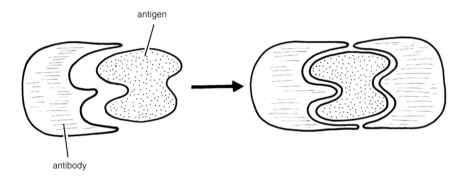

Figure 1.4. Antibodies are proteins. They work by fitting precisely into the shape of an invading antigen, thereby neutralising it.

Antibodies work by precisely fitting the shape of the invading antigen, for example, bacteria or virus. This is shown in Figure 1.4. The resultant complex neutralises the antigen, rendering it inactive and no longer capable of further invasion of body tissue. In addition, the antigen/antibody complex is more easily phagocytosed by macrophages. The 'fit' of antibody to antigen needs to be precise to be effective. Some of the less effective vaccines may produce antibodies which are not exactly the correct shape. Although they may be able to 'arrest' some of the invading infection, other 'invaders' are able to break free and still cause damage. This is shown in Figure 1.5.

Antibodies are acquired by the animal in two separate ways known as active and passive. *Active* immunisation is the process whereby the animal produces its own antibodies following exposure to an antigen.

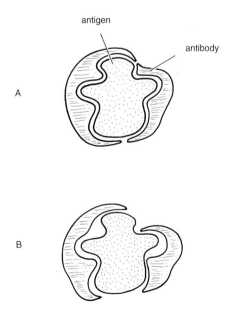

Figure 1.5. If the antibody is a poor fit (i.e. not totally specific) as in B, the antigen may break free and continue to cause damage to the host.

The cow can also produce antibodies and supply them preformed to the calf during the first few hours of its life via the thick first milk called colostrum. Because the calf has not produced these antibodies itself, they are called *passive* and they provide immediate protection against infections present in the environment.

Before an animal can produce its own active antibody against a particular infection, it must have been exposed to that infection at some time in the past, recognised it as foreign (viz as an antigen) and stored the information in a type of memory, ready to produce antibodies to overcome subsequent challenges. This initial exposure may be by vaccination, but it is much more likely to be the result of natural infection. A low dose of disease organisms which is not sufficient to cause visible symptoms will be quite adequate to stimulate antibody production and provide active immunity. This process is occurring throughout the animal's life, and re-exposure to infections helps to boost immunity levels.

Vaccines will be used when there is a risk of a heavy challenge from a specific infection, and especially if the animal has not had previous exposure to that infection. A vaccine consists of the infectious agent which has been altered in some way. When administered to the animal it stimulates the processes of recognition and antibody production, but it cannot cause disease. Vaccines may either be living, when only one dose may be required, or dead, when two doses will be needed at an interval of approximately four weeks. The presence of passive immunity, that is antibodies acquired from the mother, may prevent the calf from responding to the vaccine and this is why the instructions may state that animals under a certain age should not be vaccinated, or perhaps that if young animals are vaccinated, then an additional dose may be necessary at a later date. Passive immunity generally persists until the animal is two to three months old, depending on the amount of antibody received in the colostrum, and on the type of infection although there are exceptions to this. Vaccination of the calf should therefore be carried out at such an age that the period between passive and active protection is minimal, but not too early so that there is a risk of a poor vaccine 'take' due to persistence of passive colostral immunity.

*Antibody titres*
Antibodies are very specific: there is a group of antibodies for infection A, another group for infection B and so on. The level, or concentration, of antibody in the blood is referred to as the antibody *titre*. This may be expressed as

1:50    – blood can be diluted 50 times before the specific antibody can no longer be detected
1:100   – blood can be diluted 100 times before no antibody can be detected
1:1500  – blood can be diluted 1500 times before no antibody can be detected

Clearly the animal with a titre of 1:1500 has more antibodies to a particular disease than the animal with a titre of only 1:50.

The titre tells us nothing about the source of the antibody. It could be

● from colostrum – in which case the titre would slowly decline as the antibodies become worn out
● from a recent infection – in which case the titre would be rising, with the antibody-producing lymphocytes being in a production mode, having just been exposed to infection
● an old infection – in this case the titre would be slowly declining, unless there was a more recent exposure to the same infection, when the antibodies would start to rise again

Antibody titres are sometimes used to diagnose the cause of disease, for example calf pneumonia. If a blood sample is taken as soon as the calf is seen to be ill, then the antibody level to whatever is causing the disease is likely to be low (unless there is still some colostral antibody remaining). A second blood sample is taken two to three weeks later, by which time the amount of antibody to the infectious agent producing the high temperature should have increased considerably. The two blood samples are then tested for antibody levels to a range of possible infections, for example RSV, IBR and PI3 in the case of respiratory disease. The virus which shows a significant increase in antibody titre between initial infection and three weeks later is likely to be the cause of disease.

It is because of antibodies and other defence mechanisms that an animal can have bacteria living in it without succumbing to disease. The situation can rapidly change however if we mix groups of animals, for example calves from different sources. Calves from one farm may be carrying infection A and have antibodies to A. Calves from a second farm have infection B and the corresponding B antibodies. When the two groups are mixed, calves from A farm are exposed to infection B, but they only have antibodies to A. If the dose of B infection is large enough (for example if the groups were mixed and crowded into a poorly ventilated building), then B disease may occur in A calves before they are able to build up sufficient antibodies against B for protection. This is shown diagrammatically in Figure 1.6.

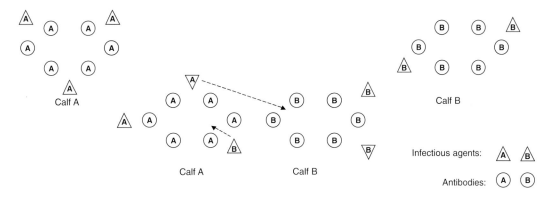

Figure 1.6. Specificity of antibodies. Calf A can exist in the presence of infection A because it has antibodies to A. Similarly calf B can exist with infection B. Problems occur when the calves are mixed. Calf A may be totally overwhelmed by infection B before it has had time to develop antibodies to it.

## Stress and the Immune System

Environmental stress in cattle (and all farm animals) is a major problem, because it *decreases* the functional capacity of the immune system. Put another way, we have discussed the many remarkable ways in which an animal is able to counteract invasion by disease agents. However, if an animal is stressed, then these defence mechanisms simply do not work as effectively. Stress leads to the release of hormones such as adrenalin and cortisone, adrenalin preparing the animal to run away, cortisone specifically reducing the activity of its immune mechanisms. So what is stress? Examples of stress leading to a reduced immune response include:

● poor nutrition, including specific deficiencies of vitamins and minerals
● overcrowding, for example the lack of a loafing area. Animals are unable to move away from one another to find any 'personal space'
● fear, for example young heifers introduced into a large dairy herd
● uncomfortable accommodation. Perhaps heifers which are not cubicle-trained lie outside on hard, wet concrete. Poorly ventilated cubicle buildings, with condensation dripping onto the cows' backs, are also a stress
● rough and unsympathetic handling: driving cattle hard, using dogs or tractors, all produce fear
● excessive noise (this would be important for sows in farrowing houses)
● transport. Transport stress is interesting. Experimentally it has been shown to cause an increase in antibodies but a decrease in cytotoxic T cells, ie the lymphocytes which destroy virus-infected cells. This is probably one reason why animals succumb to virus infections after transport

- severe competition for food or water
- concurrent diseases, e.g. chronic lameness or rumen acidosis
- weather. Temperatures above 25°C have been shown to decrease the white blood cell count and therefore compromise the immune response
- calving. Both the cow and calf have a poor immune response for the first week after calving and should therefore be housed and managed to minimise further stress. Stress in heifers is also discussed in Chapter 9

Not only will the above environmental influences reduce the animal's resistance to disease but perhaps equally as important, they can reduce the effectiveness of vaccines. In other words, a stressed animal will not respond as well to vaccination.

## Inflammation and Hypersensitivity

We have seen that when a foreign virus or bacterium invades the body, there is a response in terms of cells and antibodies. To increase the effectiveness of this response the body assists as follows:

- blood vessels in the area are dilated, thus allowing more cells to get to the invader
- small holes appear in the walls of the blood vessels, allowing cells and plasma (the fluid part of blood) to leak out into the area
- plasma contains fibrin which can coagulate to form a sponge effect. This is important to prevent blood loss if the animal has been injured, but it is also important in that bacteria and viruses stick to the 'sponge'

Externally these changes are seen as heat (increased blood flow) and swelling (plasma leaking into the tissue) and are called the changes of inflammation. Although they may be beneficial in counteracting disease, they cause discomfort to the animal. For example, inflammation in a leg due to entry of infection would lead to lameness.

Sometimes the inflammatory response can be so marked that it can be detrimental to the animal, or even be the cause of death. Probably the best example of this is in the lungs. Infection entering the lungs may produce such a marked inflammatory response, especially in terms of release of plasma, that the animal 'drowns' in the excess fluid and suffocates. In this instance we would need to give specific drugs (anti-inflammatory agents) to slow down the inflammatory response and to promote recovery.

On other occasions an animal over-reacts to the presence of a foreign invader, for example to a drug or vaccine injection. The immune system throughout the body may start to react and the animal will be seen shivering and shaking, perhaps frothing at the mouth, and eventually collapsing and possibly dying. This is known as an *allergic* or *anaphylactic* reaction and we say that the animal has a *hypersensitivity* to that particular invading antigen.

## THE BALANCE OF DISEASE

As we have described the types of infectious agents and the physical and immune defence mechanisms of the animal, their interaction can now be examined and related to the production of disease. Take a case of human typhoid. The disease itself does not matter and the figures used are not accurate, but it serves to illustrate the point very well. Putting one typhoid bacterium on the tongue of a healthy person would probably have no effect on him at all. Give him a hundred bacteria and he may feel rather off-colour and would probably get diarrhoea. Using a dose of a thousand bacteria, our 'guinea-pig' would develop a severe illness, with sickness, diarrhoea and generalised symptoms.

Now if this particular man had been drinking heavily, had lost his way home and had spent 24 hours in the cold without food and was suffering from exposure, in this case we would expect different results. Possibly one bacterium would cause mild diarrhoea, a hundred would cause a severe illness and a dose of a thousand would be fatal.

This simple example serves to illustrate two extremely important points, namely that the severity of a disease is dependent upon:

● the dose of infection received
● the state of health of the infected animal

This is extremely common in animal disease, where there is often a multiplicity of factors affecting the severity and spread of a condition. It is more easily understood by saying that health and disease are on each side of a balance, with the animal acting as the pivot of that balance. One of the best diseases to illustrate this point is enzootic pneumonia (sometimes called virus pneumonia) of calves, although *E. coli* and the other causes of environmental mastitis would serve as an equally good example. This is illustrated in Figure 1.7. Along each arm of the balance can be 'hung' various items which will either boost health or exacerbate disease. Provided the animal can be maintained with the balance in the level position, it can cope quite happily with infection, living with it but suffering relatively few adverse effects. This is the basis of preventive medicine. There is a risk of certain diseases occurring on every farm, and so it is necessary to take various husbandry and other preventive measures to minimise those risks.

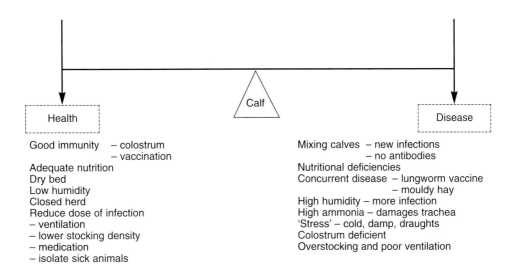

Figure 1.7. The balance of disease, using calf pneumonia as an example.

## PRINCIPLES OF TREATMENT

Treatments needed for each condition are given throughout the book. Only outlines of treatment are described, because drug availability changes very quickly and it is likely that the text will be out of date in this respect, before it is even published!

This section describes a general approach which could be applied to the treatment of any animal. Treatment may be divided into:

● specific drug treatment
● supportive therapy
● nursing

## 1. Specific Drug Treatment

If the disease under consideration is caused by an infectious agent, then it is likely that a drug is available to kill, or at least neutralise, that agent. For example:

- bacteria – use antibiotics
- viruses – no specific drug therapy is available
- protozoa – use specific antiprotozoal drugs
- fungi (yeasts and moulds) – use specific anti-fungal drugs
- worms – use anthelmintics
- ectoparasites – organo-phosphorus or pyrethroid products are often used

*Antibiotics*
Antibiotics are chemicals which destroy bacteria but have little or no adverse effect on the animal. Some act by actively killing the bacteria (e.g. penicillin, which damages their outer membrane) and these are called *bacteriocidal* antibiotics. Others simply prevent bacterial growth and multiplication (e.g. chloramphenicol interferes with their protein synthesis) and the bacteria then either die at a normal rate or are killed by the animal's defence mechanisms. These are known as *bacteriostatic* antibiotics. It is important to appreciate this difference.

Bacteriocidal and bacteriostatic antibiotics should not be used simultaneously in an animal, since one counteracts the effects of the other. This is because the bacteriocidals work best against rapidly growing and dividing bacteria, whereas bacteriostatics actually inhibit bacterial growth and multiplication. In addition, if the animal's immune defence mechanisms are likely to be severely impaired and unable to destroy bacteria, for example after calving or as a result of toxaemia, then it is probably best to use a bacteriocidal rather than a bacteriostatic drug. Bacteriocidal antibiotics are also used in the treatment of endocarditis. However, the distinction is not that precise, in that some antibiotics are bacteriostatic when used at low doses, but are bacteriocidal when given in large amounts.

Different antibiotics are effective against different types of bacteria. Some, for example the tetracyclines and chloramphenicol, are known as broad-spectrum antibiotics and are effective against most organisms. Others, such as penicillin, are only effective against staphylococci, streptococci and a few other groups. Even then, certain strains of staphylococci produce *penicillinase* which destroys penicillin and thus prevents its action. These strains of staphylococci are called penicillin resistant. (This is discussed in more detail in Chapter 7.) Even when the correct antibiotic has been chosen to counteract the cause of the disease, consideration must still be given to the tissues within the body which are harbouring the infection. Following administration to the animal, some antibiotics (e.g. tylosin and tilmicosin) are found in particularly high concentrations in the lungs and would therefore be effective as a pneumonia treatment. Others (e.g. ampicillin) achieve high levels in the urine and could be used to treat kidney and bladder infections. In both cases this assumes that the bacteria concerned are sensitive to tilmicosin or ampicillin.

If antibiotics are used indiscriminately, and especially for prolonged periods, there is a danger of bacteria mutating into forms which are resistant to the particular antibiotic. Sometimes this resistance is 'infectious' and can spread extremely rapidly in the form of genetic material to other strains of bacteria which have not been exposed to the antibiotic. The particular genetic material is unusual in that it is not part of the nucleus of the cell. Chloramphenicol is currently one of the drugs of choice in the treatment of human typhoid and certain other enteric infections and, to maintain its effectiveness, it has been requested that its use in the veterinary field is restricted to only essential cases, thus decreasing the risk of bacterial resistance developing.

There are many other factors which must be taken into account when using antibiotics and these few examples were given merely as an illustration of the complexity of the subject. It was for reasons like these that antibiotics became prescription-only medicines (POM), that is they may be used only under veterinary guidance and supervision.

There are usually milk- and meat-withholding periods following the administration of antibiotics and these need to be carefully observed. Some of the newer antibiotics, for example ceftiofur, are interesting.

They are so effective against bacteria that they can be used at extremely low concentrations, so low that they have no adverse effect on man but are still high enough to kill the bacteria. This means that they have no milk withholding period and only a short meat withdrawal period prior to slaughter.

*Antiprotozoals*
There is a range of drugs specifically aimed at protozoal infections. These include monensin, sulphonamides and amprolium, which are used against coccidiosis, and imidocarb, which is effective against the blood parasites *Babesia* and *Anaplasma*.

*Antifungals*
Antifungal drugs include griseofulvin, which is given by mouth, and nystatin, which is applied to the skin.

*Anthelmintics*
These are drugs which destroy helminths, that is intestinal worms, lungworms or liver fluke. As with antibiotics, each drug has its own spectrum of activity, some (thiabendazole) being effective against adults only, others (levamisole) being effective against adults and mature larvae, while the avermectin group (ivermectin, doramectin and moxidectin) can be used against adults and larvae. Specific products (e.g. rafoxanide or nitroxynil) are needed for liver fluke. The avermectin group persists in the animal to provide protection against reinfection for three to six weeks, depending on the type of worm and the type of product in use. This is discussed in greater detail in Chapter 4.

*Insecticides for ectoparasites*
Once again, there is a wide selection of products available.

The avermectin group of chemicals (ivermectin, doramectin and moxidectin) have good activity against warbles, mange and sucking lice, but are less effective against biting lice. They also give an extended period of cover.

Pyrethroids are used as fly repellents and for lice treatment only. They produce a rapid action by a 'knock-down' effect, and are sometimes supplied as a combination with piperonyl butoxide.

Organo-phosphorus compounds produce death by an excessive stimulation of the insect's nervous system. In high doses they can be toxic to animals. They are often available as pour-on preparations, having been combined with a chemical which carries the drug through the skin of the animal and throughout its body via the blood. They are a common treatment for lice, mange and warbles, and are particularly effective because they give whole-body cover. Phosmet is a commonly used example.

## 2. Supportive Therapy

This is aimed at treating the *effects* of the disease rather than its basic cause. The best example is undoubtedly the administration of electrolyte solutions to the scouring calf. Electrolytes positively promote the uptake of water and so prevent dehydration. They are often of greater benefit to the calf than the use of antibiotics to eliminate infectious agents.

Other examples of supportive therapy include B vitamins to assist in detoxification processes, cortisone to reduce the adverse effects of the inflammatory reaction, antipyretics (e.g. aspirin) to reduce the temperature in the fevered animal and analgesics (painkillers) to encourage the animal to move and eat. Analgesics can be particularly important after surgery. One commonly used drug is the chemical flunixin. It is known as a non-steroidal anti-inflammatory derivative (NSAID). It is able to reduce the adverse effects of inflammation without compromising the immune defence mechanisms. It is commonly used in the treatment of toxic *E. coli* mastitis and is also a very effective analgesic.

All of these treatments are designed to assist the animal in overcoming the damage caused by the disease, to improve its feeling of well-being, to restore its appetite and thus return it to health.

## 3. Nursing

A sick animal is less able to compete with the remainder of the group for food, water and even shelter, and there are many instances when it is best moved into a loose-box or a small pen of its own for a few days to convalesce. This allows more attention to be given to the animal and also makes it much easier to monitor the animal's progress. Is it eating and drinking? Are its faeces normal? Special succulent food may be offered to tempt it to eat, and for the animal with a high temperature, a warm, well-bedded dry environment is essential.

Any necessary medicines can be given much more easily if the animal is on its own, and if medication is easily administered it is more likely to be given at the correct dose and at the correct frequency. The other advantage of separating a diseased animal is that it reduces the risk of that animal spreading its infection to the remainder of the group; that is, its removal effectively reduces the challenge dose of infection to the others.

*Chapter 2*

# THE YOUNG CALF

This chapter deals with the health of the calf from birth to weaning, that is until approximately six weeks old. Current UK figures give a national calf mortality of approximately 5% of live births, and it is disappointing that this has remained unchanged for the past 20 years. In North America, the mortality rate from birth to weaning is even higher, at 8.5%, with scour accounting for over 50% of the total losses. Taking the 1998 UK value of a calf at £150, this means a loss of £750 per annum to the average 100 cow dairy herd. If there are four million calves born each year, it represents a national annual loss of £30 million.

There are many reasons why the young calf is particularly susceptible to disease. Its defence mechanisms are not fully developed, it will be going through the transition from passive to active immunity, it may have several changes of diet, and on top of all this it has an additional route by which infection may enter the body, that is through the navel. As many of the diseases of young calves are the result of failures of proper housing, feeding and colostrum intake, these factors will be discussed in some detail before specific health problems are dealt with.

## HOUSING

Undoubtedly the healthiest calves are those born outdoors, but this is impractical in the winter and presents its own problems of management (e.g. when assistance is required) in summer. Individual calving boxes are ideal, as it is then easier to ensure that the calf is not mismothered, that is, that it suckles its own mother first and therefore receives adequate colostrum. The majority of calves from dairy herds are moved into rearing quarters after a few days and the most important criteria for their housing are:

- a warm dry bed
- shelter from direct draughts and extremes of weather
- cleanliness
- preferably separation from other calves

One of the most common faults I see is wet beds. As you step in, the pen fails the *squelch test*: water can be heard squelching under your foot when you stand on the bedding. Not only does this lead to chilling (and therefore poor antibody production, see Chapter 1), but it also increases the ammonia in the atmosphere and predisposes to pneumonia. One of the best ways of bedding individual calf pens is to cover the floor of the pen with 10–15 cm thick wads of compressed straw taken straight out of the bale. The large 300 kg square bales are ideal for this. A conventional layer of loose straw is then scattered on the top. Yes, it uses more straw, but the improvement in calf performance is well worth the extra cost.

Although sub-zero conditions are best avoided, provided that the calf has a dry bed with ample straw, it is doubtful if house temperature is too important. However, ventilation as a pneumonia preventive is vital.

Individual penning is a great advantage in that feed intakes for each calf can be monitored and the slower drinker will not be penalised. Any sick calves are much more readily apparent and there is a reduced risk of the spread of disease, especially scouring. Pen size and construction will vary with the manufacturer but it is important to ensure that the calf has sufficient room to turn round easily. Although the majority of commercial pens have railed divisions (Plate 2.1), I prefer to see solid sides. This gives a greater freedom from draughts and a reduced risk of the spread of disease, and at the same time the calves have some contact with each other during feeding times. The pens shown in Plate 2.2 were constructed of 2.4 m by 1.2 m sheets of 95 mm marine ply and the fronts were home made. The whole assembly can be dismantled for cleaning out. Calf hutches (Plate 2.3), widely used in North America, are gaining popularity in the UK for a variety of reasons. Their main advantages are:

- individual attention
- reduced spread of disease. However, to achieve this the hutches must be sufficiently far apart so that calves cannot have any contact with one another. Licking and sucking can transmit both scour and pneumonia
- open air space and good ventilation. Hutches need to be well ventilated and in summer the backs should open to allow an adequate airflow; otherwise they become too stuffy and uncomfortable. Remember that a stressful environment reduces a calf's ability to produce antibodies
- some say that calves tethered and reared in hutches are quieter and more easy to handle as heifers

I do not like the severe conditions provided by calf crates, as in Plate 2.4. While faeces and urine may drain rapidly away, the calf has no protection from draughts and cannot adjust its own environment. The wet floor will provide high humidity. It is not surprising that the farm had a bad *E. coli* scour problem.

Where fixing is required it is important to use bolts, screws or wire. String is best avoided. It will be sucked by the calves and even the most secure knots can come undone. Calves then chew and eat the string and may develop indigestion, or even a fatal obstruction from string in the gut.

Whatever the construction, it should be possible to dismantle the pens, take them outside for cleaning, then thoroughly clean out, wash, disinfect and rest the calf house. If calves are purchased, they should be reared in groups preferably of the same age and size. When the first group is weaned, empty the whole house and clean it, then rest it for at least a week before introducing the next batch. This is known as the 'all in, all out' system and it is a most important factor in preventing the spread of disease between groups of calves.

On dairy farms where calves may be born throughout the year, at least two different buildings

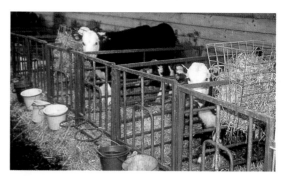
Plate 2.1. Calf pen with rail division.

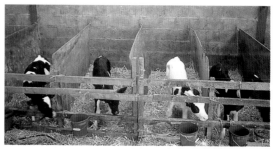
Plate 2.2. Calf pen with solid side divisions.

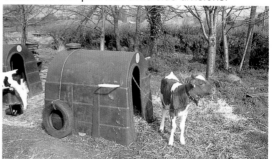
Plate 2.3. Calf hutch.

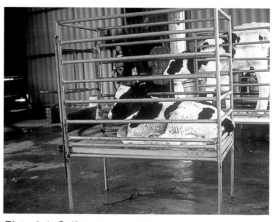
Plate 2.4. Calf crates provide a harsh environment.

should be used for calf rearing. As soon as the calves have been moved from the first building, dismantle the pens, remove all dung and bedding and give the pens and fittings a good soaking with water. Then thoroughly clean them using a detergent to remove the layer of fat which would otherwise remain as a thin film and obstruct the penetration of the disinfectant. Disinfect the pens and leave the building empty for at least a week, and preferably longer. Cleaning and disinfection must be carried out *before* the rest period to maximise its benefits. This routine should be followed even when healthy calves have been reared, although it is of course more important if disease has been present. It is good preventive medicine. It is aimed primarily at reducing scouring and pneumonia but it will also improve growth rates generally.

## THE IMPORTANCE OF COLOSTRUM

Colostrum, the thick first milk produced by the cow immediately after calving (and sometimes called beastings), is the calf's 'passport to life'. Without an adequate intake of colostrum, life will be an uphill journey and a proportion of such calves will never survive. It cannot be emphasised too strongly how extra effort after calving, leading to improved colostrum intake, will be beneficial to the calf for at least the first two to four months of its life. For example, colostral antibodies for both pneumonia and BVD may persist and protect the calf for up to four months.

The main characteristics of colostrum are:

- It contains antibodies which protect the calf from the wide range of diseases that its mother has been exposed to during her recent life.
- It is highly nutritious. The high food value of colostrum is an important factor in getting the calf warmed up and moving around soon after birth. Colostrum-deficient calves are often dull, listless and hypothermic.
- Its increased fat content acts as a laxative and assists in the passage of meconium, the foetal dung.
- The presence of colostrum (or milk) in the abomasum stimulates the production of acid and digestive enzymes. At birth the abomasal pH is quite high, falling to pH 3–4 at two to three days old, when acid is produced. This acid kills many ingested bacteria and is therefore a very important defence mechanism.

The difference in composition between colostrum and milk is shown in Table 2.1. Colostrum is twice as concentrated as milk (25% vs. 12.6% solids) and contains a higher percentage of protein and the fat-soluble vitamins A, D and E. At birth the calf may have very little of these vitamins stored in its liver. That is why many farmers inject calves with multivitamins at birth, particularly when they suspect low-quality colostrum, for example because of poor dry cow feeding during the winter.

The production of antibodies was explained in Chapter 1. In late pregnancy the cow concentrates antibodies in her colostrum, so that the calf can receive immediate preformed immunity to many of the diseases to which it will be exposed. The final concentration of antibodies in colostrum is much higher than that originally present in blood, and is the reason why the protein content of colostrum is so high. The immunity given to the calf is of course only related to the infections which the cow herself has contacted (see Figure 1.6). If a cow is purchased and moved into a new herd only a few days before calving, then clearly there is a risk that the calf will be challenged by infections for which it has no colostral protection.

Table 2.1. Some of the differences between milk and colostrum, expressed on a fresh weight basis.

|                                        | Colostrum | Milk |
|----------------------------------------|-----------|------|
| Total solids %                         | 25        | 12.6 |
| Fat %[1]                               | 5.1       | 3.8  |
| SNF %[1]                               | 19.6      | 8.8  |
| Protein %[1]                           | 16.4      | 3.2  |
| Lactose %[1]                           | 2.2       | 4.7  |
| Immunoglobulins (antibodies) g/kg[2]   | 60        | 0.9  |
| Vitamin A mg/g fat[2]                  | 45        | 8    |
| Vitamin D mg/g fat[2]                  | 23–45     | 15   |
| Vitamin E mg/g fat[2]                  | 100–150   | 20   |

[1] From Godsell, personal communication; [2] from J.B.H. Roy, *The Calf*.

# 24 A VETERINARY BOOK FOR DAIRY FARMERS

## Absorption of Antibodies

Antibodies are proteins and as such they would normally be digested (viz broken down) in the calf's intestine. However, during the first few hours of life the intestine has a special ability to absorb whole proteins into the bloodstream, rather than digest them. This ability of the calf to prevent digestion of a certain fraction of its first feed of colostrum is extremely useful and is assisted by:

- specialised cells lining the intestine which are capable of pinocytosis, that is the absorption of whole molecules. These specialist cells start to fall off within 12 hours of birth and most are gone by 24–30 hours. The calf *must* therefore receive colostrum early
- a trypsin inhibitor in the colostrum, which prevents the digestion of proteins
- the very low activity of the pancreas in the very young calf
- the quite high abomasal pH of 6–7 which prevents the pepsin (a digestive enzyme in the abomasum) from working. By 36 hours after calving the pH falls to between 3 and 4, pepsin becomes active, and ingested milk (or colostrum) then coagulates in the abomasum before undergoing digestion (see Figure 2.2). Although the lack of acid in the stomach is an advantage in terms of colostrum, it does render the calf more susceptible to infection for the first 48 hours of life, because acid would normally kill many of the bacteria ingested with the food

Absorbed antibodies pass into the bloodstream and are immediately active and available to repel invading infections. The amount of absorbed antibody can be measured in blood samples, for example by the zinc sulphate turbidity test (ZST). The sodium sulphite test and electronic methods are now more commonly used. On some farms all purchased calves are blood sampled on arrival, to ensure that the farm of origin has been taking enough care in giving their calves colostrum.

## Inadequate Colostrum Intakes

The absorption of colostral antibodies is of vital importance to the calf, not only for the first few days of life, but continuing for weeks and even months. Calves which have not received adequate colostrum have been shown to:

- have a higher overall death rate, especially from septicaemia and joint-ill
- be more likely to develop scouring (one trial reduced scouring from 12% to 2% by improving the supervision of colostrum intake)
- be more likely to develop pneumonia, even at two to three months old

Table 2.2 shows the colostrum status and subsequent performance of 1050 calves reared at the National Agricultural Centre, Stoneleigh. On the basis of the ZST test, 50% of calves were shown to have inadequate colostrum status, which was defined as less than 20 ZST units, and this significantly influenced the incidence of scouring and pneumonia in these calves, even up to five months of age.

Colostrum therefore has a profound effect on subsequent calf performance and as such it is vitally important to have some idea of the factors involved in its absorption. Whole antibodies are most efficiently absorbed during the first few hours of the calf's life, although the

Table 2.2. Of 1050 calves reared at the NAC, half had inadequate colostrum status and this led to an increase in mortality, general illnesses (including scouring) and pneumonia.

|  | Colostrum status (ZST units) | | |
| --- | --- | --- | --- |
|  | 0–10 | 10–20 | 20+ |
|  | Low | Marginal | Good |
| % of calves | 18 | 32 | 50 |
| % of mortality | 9.8 | 4.1 | 3.2 |
| % illness | 31.6 | 23.0 | 15.1 |
| % pneumonia | 5.2 | 3.2 | 1.4 |

From Thomas L.H and Swan R.C. (1973), *Vet. Rec.* 92 454

facility may persist at a reduced level for up to 24 hours or more, provided that no other food is taken. It is the *first feed* which acts as the trigger mechanism stimulating the digestive processes and hence preventing the further absorption of whole antibodies. As such, it is vitally important that the *first feed is colostrum*. If you find a weakly calf, it is far better, if necessary, to wait for an hour or two and give it colostrum, rather than give it a feed of whole milk 'to be going on with'.

As a rule of thumb I would suggest that a calf receives colostrum

- at the rate of 6% of its bodyweight (viz 2.4 litres for a 40 kg calf)
- within six hours of birth

Half a litre of colostrum may give some protection against septicaemia, but 5 to 6 litres are needed to give good protection against scouring. It is not sufficient to leave the calf with its dam. Several studies have shown that inadequate colostral intakes may result. This could be because of a weakly calf, for example due to chilling, or following a difficult calving; a nervous heifer; an older cow with a pendulous udder and splayed teats; or simply mismothering – for example, a calf born in a crowded yard which is mothered and suckled by a cow which had calved three to four days previously and whose colostral quality would be very poor. Whenever possible, the calf should be lifted to suckle as soon as it is reasonably able to stand and suckling will need to continue for 15 to 20 minutes. Because the first feed of colostrum stimulates the production of digestive enzymes, thus reducing the

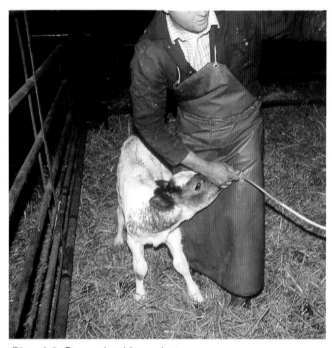

Plate 2.5. Stomach tubing colostrum.

absorption of further antibodies, this first feed needs to be as large as possible. Colostrum does *not* need to clot in the abomasum, so there is little risk of overfeeding and producing digestive upsets, even if it is given as a drench or by stomach tube (see Plate 2.5).

Some people consider that suckling is so variable that it is best to remove every calf from its dam at birth and provide colostrum by bucket and teat, or even by stomach tube. Table 2.3 shows the results of a trial which took 16 ZST units as the target of colostral intake. No difference was found in the percentage of suckled calves which achieved this target, whether assisted or not, although the range of values showed that certain individual unassisted calves achieved very poor intakes (only 3 ZST units). However, by removing the calf at birth and feeding colostrum via a teated

Table 2.3. Calves left with their dams fail to achieve adequate colostral intakes, even if assisted to suckle. A teated bucket produces the best results.

|  | Colostrum status (ZST units) | |
|  | Range | % calves above target of 16 ZST units |
| --- | --- | --- |
| Calf left with cow | 3–28 | 60 |
| Assisted suckling | 11–30 | 60 |
| Artificial suckling (teated bucket) | 21–30 | 100 |

From S. Furness, personal communication

bucket, they were able to achieve satisfactory colostrum status in all their calves. A simple teated container made from a 5 litre plastic can is shown in Plate 2.6. The handle on the top is very useful and the small filling hole prevents spillage when dealing with an excitable calf.

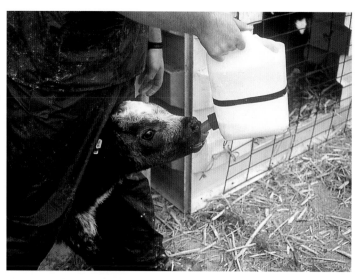

Plate 2.6. Calf drinking from a teated container, ideal for ensuring adequate colostrum intakes.

It is interesting to note that colostrum has a mainly preventive function and is of little value for treatment. In one trial, calves fed colostrum and then dosed with pathogenic strains of *E. coli* did not scour, whereas those dosed with *E. coli* and then given colostrum two to three hours later all developed diarrhoea and died. This further emphasises the need to feed colostrum soon after birth.

Mothering has an effect on the uptake of colostral antibodies and on subsequent circulating blood levels. Ideally the calf should suckle colostrum from its own dam. However, if artificial feeding is necessary (e.g. if the cow is recumbent due to milk fever, injury or mastitis, or perhaps because she has been pre milked), then antibody absorption is considered to be more effective in the presence of the cow, even when the colostrum is being given via a teat. When it is known that artificial feeding will be required, then every effort

> The main factors which can lead to poor colostral intakes include:
>
> ● weakly calves at birth – e.g. chilling, premature or difficult delivery
> ● nervous heifers: calf not allowed to suckle for long enough
> ● older cow with dropped udder, splayed or excessively large teats, making sucking difficult
> ● mismothering, e.g. a calf born into a crowded yard
> ● poor-quality colostrum, due to poor feeding of dry cows (usually winter), premature calvings or very recently purchased cows or heifers

should be made to achieve this within the first six hours of life.

Finally it has been shown that there can be a considerable variation in the antibody content of the colostrum itself. Cows which are in poor condition, affected by chronic mastitis, suffering from a debilitating disease (e.g. liver fluke) or which have been induced to calve prematurely using corticosteroids are simply unable to provide adequate protective antibodies for the offspring.

## Frozen Colostrum

Colostrum retains its nutritive and antibody potency when frozen, and the deep-freeze can be a useful emergency store *provided* that the colostrum is reheated carefully. Boiling destroys the antibodies. A microwave oven can be used, but it must be on the low or defrost setting. Colostrum 'banks' can be set up by freezing it in the quantities needed for an individual calf, viz a minimum of 2 litres. There is then always a supply available for those unexpected occasions of mastitis in all four quarters, death of the cow at calving, recumbency and other such unfortunate incidents, which would otherwise render the calf colostrum deficient.

## Stored Colostrum

Colostrum can also be stored. As in the UK milk from the first four days after calving must be discarded, many people store it, allowing it to ferment at environmental temperature and use this as milk to rear replacement heifer calves. It should be noted, however, that fermented colostrum does not have the same high levels of antibody as frozen colostrum.

To achieve the correct fermentation, the colostrum must be kept clean but exposed to air. Some advise the use of preservatives, e.g. 0.05% formaldehyde (1 ml formalin solution per litre of milk), but this is more important in hot climates and for milk discarded during treatment of a cow with antibiotics. There is, however, a body of opinion which says that antibiotic milk should not be fed to calves.

Stored colostrum is best fed fairly quickly, but it can be kept for several weeks, depending on hygiene and environmental conditions.

Some important factors to remember include:

- Plastic containers are better than metal.
- Keep the colostrum covered to prevent moulds and fungi blowing in and causing souring. A cloth covering allows the colostrum to breathe, as well as keeping it clean.
- Store in limited quantities. When one container is full, start storing colostrum in another clean container, thereby reducing contamination. Thoroughly clean the containers when they have been emptied.
- Do not add bloody milk. This has a bitter flavour and can lead to souring.
- Stored colostrum should be stirred regularly to break the crust and disperse the solid material before feeding it.
- Colostrum is much more concentrated than milk and if neat colostrum is being fed it should be diluted 1:1 with hot water.

The ideal system is to have two colostrum stores. The first is a store of colostrum from, say, the first 24 hours after calving only. This batch should be considered as a *medicine* or *vaccine* and used sparingly, for example in the control of rotavirus scour. The second batch is of milk from cows which calved two to

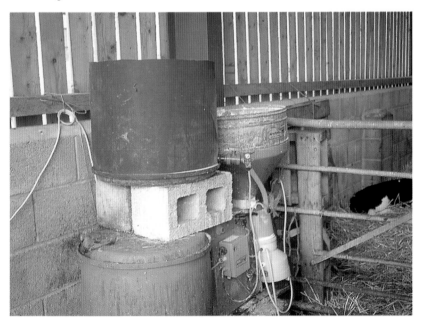

three days or more ago, plus discarded milk from cows under treatment for mastitis, or which are being given injectable antibiotics or other drugs requiring a milk withdrawal period. This batch is a *food*. It is unlikely to ferment and keep properly and thus should be used up fairly quickly.

Many milk dispensing machines (Plate 2.7) have a facility for feeding 5–10% stored colostrum with milk substitute. This provides excellent control against rotavirus and coronavirus.

Plate 2.7 Automatic calf milk feeder dispensing colostrum.

## FEEDING SYSTEMS

After the colostrum has been fed, a wide range of feeding systems is available for calf rearing. The systems vary in terms of labour input and cost, but probably largely reflect the personal preference of the calf rearer. Examples include

- twice a day bucket fed warm
- once a day bucket fed warm
- cold ad lib
- ad lib machine feeding
- computer controlled machine feeding

Twice daily bucket feeding has the highest labour input but feed costs are low and as each calf receives individual attention, management and calf performance are optimised. Ideally each calf has three buckets, one for water, one for milk and one for concentrates. The water and concentrate buckets are left in front of the calf all of the time, as in Plate 2.1. At feeding time, the concentrate bucket is removed and a bucket of milk is offered. As soon as the calf has finished drinking its milk, the milk bucket should be removed, and the concentrate bucket replaced. This encourages the calf to start eating solids. Some people leave the milk bucket in place under the concentrate bucket and never wash it out. They say that the risk of cross-contamination when washing out buckets is far too great, and provided that the calf drinks all of its milk, it is not necessary to wash the bucket and you simply put the concentrate bucket into the empty milk bucket. This system certainly saves labour and is becoming increasingly popular.

For the first five to seven days the calf will probably only drink its milk if it can suck your finger. It can then slowly be trained to drink from the bucket. An alternative system is to provide the calf with a teated bucket. If allowed to drink from this for the first two weeks, it is surprising how many calves will take directly to drinking from the bucket.

The amount of food fed will depend on the bodyweight of the calf and the growth rate required. As an approximate guide, however, calves can be left with the cow for the first one to two days, then penned and fed 1–1.5 litres of whole milk (preferably from its own dam) twice daily for the next three to four days. Milk substitute can be introduced from day five onwards, e.g. 0.75 litre of whole milk plus 0.75 litre of substitute twice daily, slowly changing and increasing to 2.0 litres of substitute twice daily from day ten onwards. If rapid growth rates are required, then feeding three times daily or increased amounts can be given. In the UK, farms over quota may use whole milk throughout rearing. The introduction of solid feed is discussed in Chapter 3.

It is commonly considered that scouring and other digestive upsets in calves are the result of an infection. Whilst this may be true in some instances, adverse management is often equally to blame. The following sections therefore describe the importance of good digestion, the significance of oesophageal groove closure, the importance of the abomasal milk clot and potential problems with feeding milk substitutes. Management deficiencies in any of these areas commonly lead to calf diarrhoea.

## DIGESTION

Figure 2.1 shows the essential anatomy of the digestive system of the calf. Food is taken into the mouth and swallowed, a process whereby the respiratory route is closed and the food is transferred into the oesophagus. Once in the oesophagus, the food is propelled downwards by *peristalsis*, which is the name given to a wave-like muscular activity which has a similar effect to the hand of a milker on a cow's teat. First the top of the teat is squeezed between the thumb and forefinger. Then, maintaining this pressure, the next finger is squeezed against the hand, then the next and so on. In this way milk is squeezed through the teat sphincter under pressure, the first few fingers preventing reverse flow back into the udder. Propulsion of food by peristalsis occurs throughout the digestive tract.

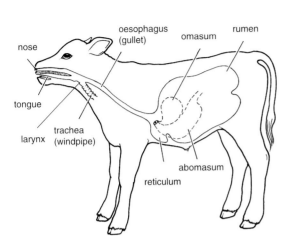

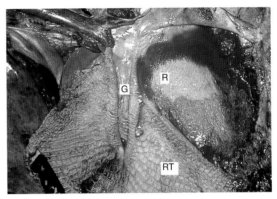

Plate 2.8. The oesophageal groove (G) in the adult cow: normal position. R = rumen RT = reticulum.

Figure 2.1. The upper digestive tract of a ruminating calf.

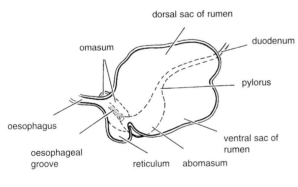

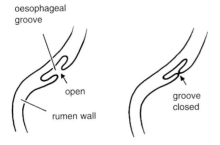

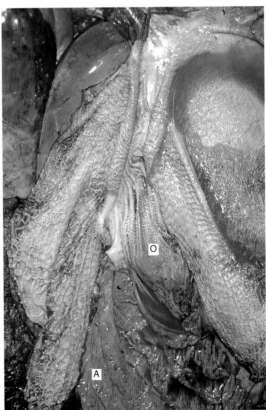

Figure 2.2. Function and position of oesophageal groove. When the groove is closed, milk flows across the rumen and into the abomasum.

Plate 2.9. The oesophageal groove in the adult cow: opened into omasum (O) and abomasum (A).

The calf is a ruminant and in common with other ruminants (e.g. sheep, goats and camels) it has four stomachs, namely the reticulum, rumen, omasum and abomasum. The very young calf uses only its fourth stomach, the abomasum, and functions essentially as a *monogastric* animal, that is an animal with a single stomach. Its rumen, reticulum and omasum would be proportionally much smaller than those in Figure 2.1.

Milk has to flow directly from the oesophagus into the abomasum, by-passing the rumen and reticulum, and this is done by a self-closing channel in the roof of the rumen, known as the *oesophageal groove*. Figure 2.2 shows the groove in transverse section, that is, as if you had cut through the wall of the rumen. When the groove is in the open position, milk passing from the oesophagus will fall into the rumen, become sour and cause a digestive upset. When the groove closes, a 'pipe' is formed which transports milk directly through to the omasum and into the abomasum. Plates 2.8 and 2.9 show the oesophageal groove (G) in an adult animal. In Plate 2.8 the groove runs across the wall of the rumen (R) to the top of the reticulum (RT). In Plate 2.9 the exit of the oesophageal groove into the reticulum has been opened to show the omasum (O) and abomasum (A). Note how close the exit of the oesophageal groove is to the abomasum.

## The Oesophageal Groove Closure Reflex

When the calf suckles there is a reflex action, activated via the bicarbonate in its saliva, which results in muscular closure of the oesophageal groove. As it gets older, simply the thought of feeding and the sight, sounds and other stimuli associated with the arrival of its milk will be sufficient to provoke closure. It is most important that closure occurs prior to feeding and hence it can be seen that the establishment of a *feeding routine* is vital. Calves should be wooed into the mood and be ready and expecting to be fed. They need to be anticipating a pleasurable experience. Only then will the oesophageal groove close securely and digestion proceed properly. Calves with wagging tails (Figure 2.3) and calves which butt the bucket (or teat or udder) are enjoying their food and the oesophageal groove is well closed. Within reason, calves on a teat need to work quite hard at the teat to get their milk – a pile of saliva beside the teat, as in Plate 2.10, is a good sign. If milk flow is too rapid, however, the calf may almost choke. This could result in milk spillage into the rumen.

I am certainly not in favour of the system seen on some farms, where a cut-off milking machine liner is fitted onto bottles and used as a teat (Plate 2.11). Milk flow is far too fast. Teats fitted onto machines

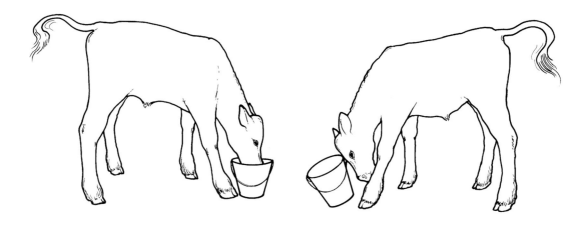

Figure 2.3. Tail wagging and 'bunting' the bucket or udder are good signs that the calf is enjoying its food and that the oesophageal groove is closed.

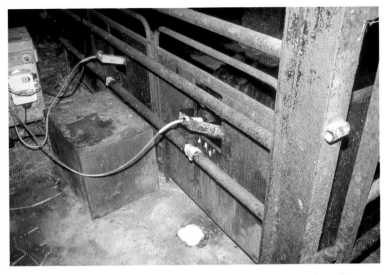

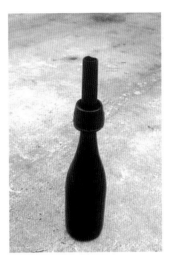

Plate 2.10. A pile of saliva beneath the teat of this automatic calf feeding machine is a good sign that oesophageal groove closure has been achieved.

Plate 2.11. A cut-off milking machine liner does not make a good teat. Milk flow is far too rapid.

and other equipment should be regularly checked to ensure that they have not become excessively worn. Plate 2.12 shows an example of a teat which produced scour, bloated rumen and abomasal dilation in a group of calves before the problem was spotted.

## Achieving Good Groove Closure

So what are some of the ways in which we can feed calves to ensure good groove closure? These include:

- Feed at the same time each day, so that the calf knows when to expect its milk.
- Keep the feed the same temperature, either always warm or always cold.
- Feed similar quantities each time.
- Let the calves know they are going to be fed. Ideally they should be able to see and hear the milk being prepared for them, so that their anticipation slowly increases (Plate 2.13). One stockperson I know says she always goes

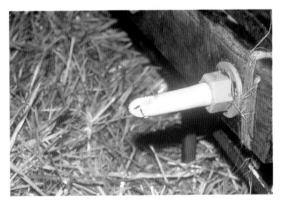

Plate 2.12. This badly damaged teat caused deaths due to scouring and abomasal bloat before the problem was noticed.

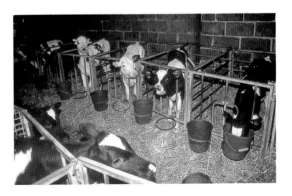

Plate 2.13. Calves waiting to be fed. Ideally they should be wooed into the mood and know they are about to undergo the pleasurable experience of feeding. This will ensure good oesophageal groove closure.

around the calves and speaks to
them before getting their milk.
Mixing milk substitute in front of
the calves works well.

- Ensure that the teat or bucket is at
the correct height. It should be
30 cm above the floor level of the
calf pen. We have all seen pens
where straw bedding has been
continually added, but the bucket
is left in the same position.
Eventually the calf has to get
down on its knees so that its head
is low enough to reach the
bucket! This was a position often
adopted by the calf in Plate 2.14.
- Do not feed calves immediately
after a stressful procedure, such
as dehorning, castration or transport (perhaps arrival from mar-

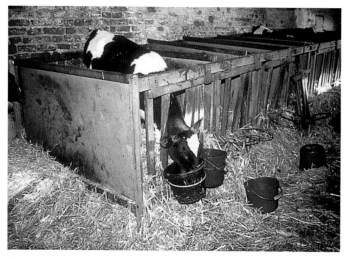

Plate 2.14. The straw in the pen has built up so high that this
calf often kneels down in order to reach the milk in its bucket.

ket). Either give them a while to settle, or for market calves, give them electrolyte solutions (page
48) for their first feed. If electrolyte spills into the rumen it will not cause problems.

*Poor drinkers and non-drinkers*

Slow drinkers present a problem. While their milk is warm, their oesophageal groove remains closed.
However, if the bucket is left in front of them and the milk cools, when they come to drink it later the
groove closure may be incomplete and some milk may spill into the rumen.

Some calves simply will not drink at all, from neither bucket nor teat, nor even from a cow. If it is a
temporary thing, stomach tubing with electrolytes for one to two days is the best option, because if you
stomach tube with milk (Plate 2.5), there is a big risk that groove closure will not occur. However, a
small proportion of calves never drink and in these stomach tubing with milk is the only option.
Although problems might occur, experienced calf feeders have said that eventually some calves get to
quite like the procedure and they can be reared to weaning by twice daily tubing!

*Consequences of poor groove closure*

Poor groove closure allows milk to fall into the rumen, rather than passing into the abomasum for proper
digestion. As there are no digestive enzymes in the rumen, once the milk enters it turns sour and this can
lead to a range of clinical signs. Poor oesophageal groove closure causes

- *bloat*, due to the gas produced by fermenting milk
- *colic*, caused by the pain associated with an inflamed and bloated rumen
- *scour*, as fermented waste products of milk pass from the rumen into the intestine and often cause
chronic diarrhoea
- *poor rumen development*, which may produce poor growth pre weaning and often bloat and scour
problems after weaning.

Plate 2.15 shows a typically affected calf. It is bloated and there is a pasty scour around its tail. With
this degree of rumen distension it is not going to want to eat solid food. Plate 2.16 shows the opened
rumen and abomasum of a calf which died as a result of poor groove closure. Fermenting milk is present
in the rumen (R). This led to such severe inflammation of the abomasum (A) that the calf died from
shock. The scissors lie in the exit from the oesophageal groove into the abomasum.

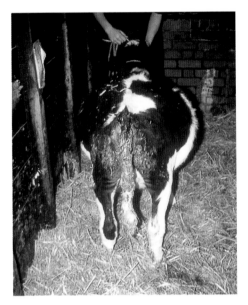

Plate 2.15. This calf has a bloated (blown) rumen and a chronic pasty scour, typical of oesophageal groove closure problems.

*Bloat treatment*

If only mild bloat is present, it is best to withhold milk for one to two days, feed electrolytes and dose the calf with oral antibiotics to try to destroy the bacteria causing the rumen fermentation. Reintroduce milk slowly, in small quantities, and preferably feed the calf four times daily, so that it gets an adequate nutrient intake without excessive risk. Badly bloated calves require deflating with a stomach tube or an operation to make a hole in the rumen. This is discussed in more detail in Chapter 3.

## The Abomasal Milk Clot

For both whole milk and the majority of milk substitutes, formation of a milk clot in the abomasum is an essential first step in the process of digestion. However, there are some milk substitute powders, especially those associated with ad libitum acidified cold milk feeding, which do not need to form an abomasal clot. Under the influence of the enzyme rennin and in an acid environment, the protein (casein) in the milk clot solidifies and then contracts, squeezing out the liquid whey fraction (containing non-casein whey proteins and sugars such as lactose)

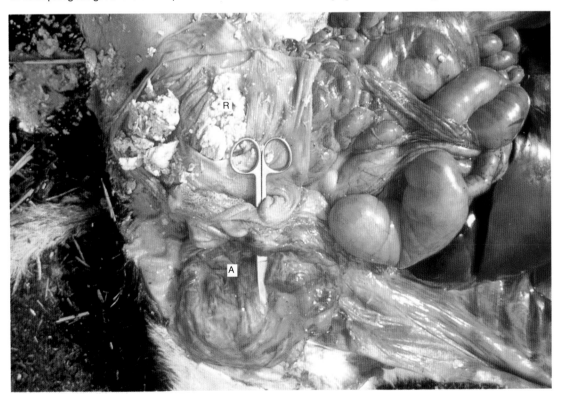

Plate 2.16. Failure of oesophageal groove closure led to souring of the milk in the rumen (R) and death due to abomasal inflammation (A).

which then passes down into the small intestine. The clot in the abomasum is slowly digested by the enzymes pepsin (digesting casein) and lipase (digesting the fat) and any remaining material forms a focus for the next milk clot. The small intestine is alkaline, digestion being carried out by enzymes produced by the villi of the intestinal wall and the pancreas. Lactose is split into glucose and galactose, two simple sugars which can be absorbed and used by the calf for energy. Protein is split into amino acids which can also be absorbed. Figure 2.4 shows diagrammatically the processes of digestion.

If abomasal milk clot formation is poor, then whole milk passes into the small intestine, where casein cannot be digested. This provides an excellent medium for bacterial fermentation, and scouring results. Some of the adverse factors associated with poor clot formation are:

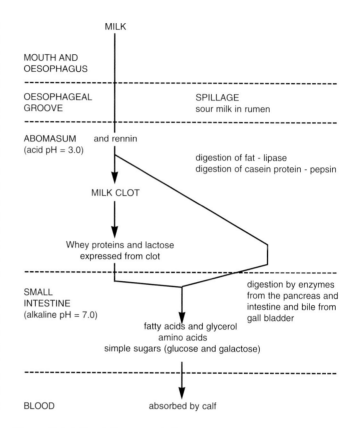

Figure 2.4 A 'flow' diagram of digestion in the calf.

- overfeeding, viz giving excessive quantities of milk at each feed. This is also important with acidified milk, although the acidification helps to prevent excessive bacterial growth
- irregular feeding times
- nervous or stressed calves
- milk fed at the wrong temperature
- milk substitute fed at the incorrect strength
- inflammation of the abomasum

*Overfeeding*
If the young calf was left with its dam it would suckle seven to ten times per day and probably take 0.5–1 litre per feed for the first one to two weeks of life. The volume of the abomasum in a young calf is 1–1.5 litres (obviously size depends on calf bodyweight) and so it is *vital* not to overfeed the calf in the initial stages. Feeding significantly too much milk will lead to undigested milk being spilled from the abomasum, which can cause scouring, or even death because of abomasal overload. You can gradually increase the amount given at each feed, and as you do so the abomasum will dilate. At the end of the first week it should be possible to feed 2 litres twice daily. If you want to grow calves very rapidly (for example to sell to market) then consider feeding them three or even four times daily.

Admittedly some people are able to achieve much higher milk intakes than this. But it's a bit like driving a car around a corner at 90 mph: you can do it if all other management factors (good tyres, good road surface, good weather, good camber etc.) are optimal. However, if one factor (perhaps poor tyres) is less than ideal, then there is a risk that the car will slide off the corner. There are many similarities with calf feeding practices.

*Consequences of poor abomasal milk clot*

As already stated, the major consequence of a poor abomasal milk clot is that some whole milk passes into the intestine, where the casein cannot be digested. This leads to scouring. Other consequences include:

- Abomasal bloat. This is seen as an acutely ill calf, with a tense abdomen and sunken eyes. Fluid can be heard splashing around in the abomasum (similar to watery mouth in lambs). Veterinary treatment is required to administer abomasal motility stimulants (e.g. metoclopramide) and perhaps a bicarbonate drip, as many of these calves have a severe acidosis (see page 40).
- Abomasal ulceration. Perforated abomasal ulcers lead to peritonitis, collapse and death. A typical example is shown in Plate 2.17. The ulcer (U) is seen as a brown hole surrounded by red inflammation of the wall of the abomasum (A) at the top of the picture. Abomasal ulcers in calves may also be the result of irregular feeding: excessive hunger may encourage the pre-ruminant calf to eat straw, which then passes direct into the abomasum and causes irritation. Many veal calves on whole milk diets have mild abomasal ulcers at slaughter, although this does not seem to affect them particularly.

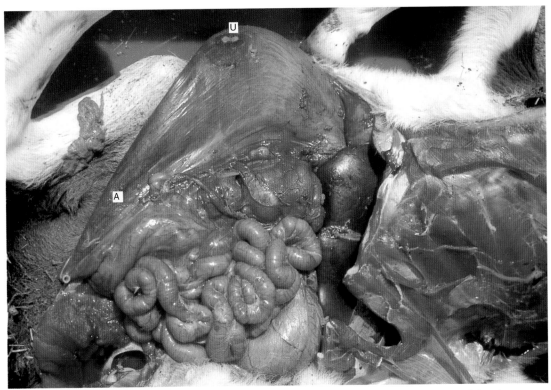

Plate 2.17. A perforated ulcer (U) of the abomasum (A). There is a peritonitis present involving the intestines.

## Problems with Milk Substitutes

There is a wide variety of milk substitutes on the market. Many are based on a high level of skim milk powder and form a clot in the abomasum, although some of the 'zero' replacers (so-called because skim milk powder is absent) do not form a clot. If milk powder is overheated during manufacture, then clot formation is poor and scouring may result. However, most of the problems associated with milk substitutes are 'on farm' in their origin.

The first rule must be to *read the manufacturer's instructions*. Many manufacturers recommend that milk powder is first mixed at a higher temperature (45–50°C) and then cooled to just above blood heat (42°C) before feeding. To do this a thermometer is needed. You *cannot* accurately judge the temperature of the milk using your hand. On a cold day you will overestimate the milk temperature and feed it too cold and vice versa on a hot day. Trials have shown that if the milk is too hot a calf simply will not drink it and no harm will be done. If milk powders are mixed and fed too cold, a variety of problems can arise:

- The fat may be poorly dispersed. It rises to the top of the milk and leaves a ring around the calf's nose, often leading to hair loss. A typical example is shown in Plate 2.18. If your calves develop bald noses, check your milk substitute mixing routine.
- Proteins and minerals may sediment to the bottom of the bucket and be wasted – and this is the expensive part of the milk substitute!

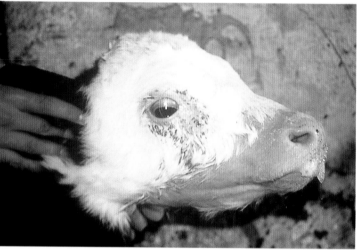

- Oesophageal groove closure is poor.
- Milk clotting time in the abomasum is retarded. A reduction of only 6°C will double the time taken for the abomasal milk clot to form. There is then an increased risk of undigested milk spilling over into the small intestine.

If a long row of calves has to be fed from a single container, the milk for the last calf in the row can be appreciably cooler – again, watch for bald noses!

Plate 2.18. Loss of hair around a calf's face is a sign of inadequate mixing of milk substitute.

Inefficient mixing is probably the biggest problem. Mixing with your hand is simply not adequate – a whisk is essential (Plate 2.19). Carelessly mixed powders leave lumps, poorly dispersed fat and a protein sediment in the bottom of the bucket. Trials have shown that *up to 60% of the oils* in the replacer may be wasted in this way, in addition to problems arising from poor abomasal clot formation and subsequent scouring. Ensure that the milk is mixed at the correct strength. This is usually 125 g per litre, but may be increased to 150 g per litre if fed once daily. Do *not* dilute milk powder, for example for a scouring calf. If fed too dilute, it will retard abomasal milk clot formation. Similarly, do not allow a calf to drink large quantities of water immediately it has finished its milk, as this will have an effect equivalent to diluting the milk. When the milk bucket is empty, it is best to put in a handful of coarse mix or calf pencils.

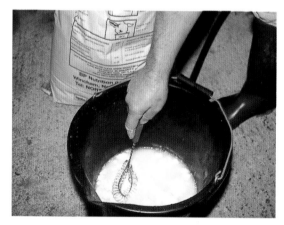

Plate 2.19. Milk substitute must be mixed at the correct temperature, using a whisk. Feeding lumpy milk is wasteful and bad husbandry.

Certain brands of electrolyte solutions can be mixed with whole milk and actually improve clotting time, but the clot formed may be less stable. In general, therefore, it is best to avoid diluting milk.

Finally, do not feed excessive quantities. Most feeding schedules are designed for a 40 kg calf and suggest starting at 1 litre per feed, increasing by 0.25 litre every second day up to 2 litres per feed. If you have a smaller calf, feed less. Overloading the abomasum can lead to spillage and scouring.

> The golden rules for feeding calves with milk substitute are:
>
> ● correct temperature
> ● correct strength
> ● properly mixed
> ● fed in the correct amount

## DISEASES OF THE CALF

Problems with young calves generally fall into two main categories. They are conditions affecting the digestive system, of which scouring is of course by far the most common, and conditions affecting the navel. Pneumonia can also occur in pre weaned calves, but as it is more common in the older animal, the condition will be fully discussed in the next chapter.

## SCOURING

Scouring is the commonest disease in young calves and it is without doubt the greatest single cause of death. It has been estimated that in the UK 140,000 calves die from it each year, which is almost 4% of the total born and 80% of all pre weaning losses. Of the calves lost, 75% were purchased through markets. In North America the same percentage applies, that is 4% of live calves die from scour, but this represents only 55% of the total pre weaning losses.

Even though mortality is high, perhaps the worst part of calf scour is the cost and frustration of treatment. One survey estimated that almost *one-third* of all calves are affected by scour. The costs of the disease can be listed as:

● death
● farm labour costs for dosing and nursing
● costs of drugs and veterinary fees
● costs of vaccines to prevent disease in adjacent calves
● costs of reduced growth and the frustration of not being able to sell the calf at the most economic time

In an analysis of 30 top herds in the DAISY recording system, Esslemont calculated that the average cost per scouring calf was £92 (at 1998 values) and that 7% of dairy herds had a serious outbreak of scouring each year. The problem is therefore both extensive and expensive.

*Fluid Balance in a Normal Calf*
In order to understand fully what goes wrong, we need to spend a few minutes discussing the normal calf. The small intestine is responsible for absorption of nutrients and water. The inner surface consists of a mat of small, finger-like projections called villi, which increase its surface area and hence its functional capacity. These are shown in detail in Figure 2.5. Each villus is covered with a lining of epithelial cells, these being produced at the base of the villus (the crypt) and passing up towards the tip. A small blood vessel (an arteriole) runs down the centre of the villus, with small branches (capillaries) radiating out towards the epithelial lining cells. The epithelial cells at the tip of the villus pump water into the central arteriole, making the blood at this point more dilute. Salts (e.g. sodium, bicarbonate or potassium) and other nutrients (e.g. glucose and amino acids) are now drawn in from the intestine by active transport and by diffusion. This flow of material is shown in Figure 2.6. There is also a flow of water from the blood into the intestine; in fact the total amount of water passing into and out of the normal intestine is

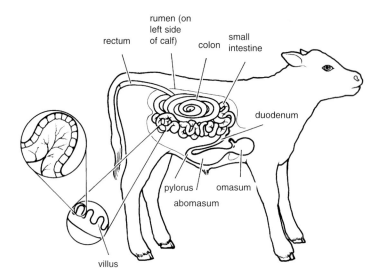

Figure 2.5. Position and function of the small intestine.

approximately 100 litres per day each way. Water therefore enters the small intestine firstly from drinking and secondly from the blood.

This flow of water into and out of the intestine is shown diagrammatically in Figure 2.7. Let us assume for this particular length of intestine that 1.1 litres/day are drunk and 4 litres/day pass into the intestine from the blood supply. In the normal calf, 5 litres/day would be reabsorbed, to produce semi-solid faeces, containing only 0.1 litre water per day, i.e.

1.1 litres *drunk* + 4.0 litres *secreted* ➜
5.0 litres *absorbed* + 0.1 litre in *faeces*

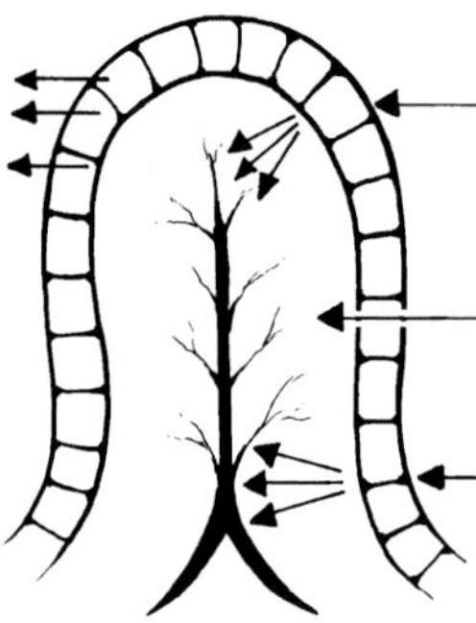

This example shows that approximately 80% of the total fluid in the intestine originates from the body itself, primarily from secretions from the salivary glands, stomach and intestines. In a normal calf around 98% of this fluid is reabsorbed, resulting in semi-solid faeces. However, a scouring calf loses much of the fluid.

Figure 2.6. Flow of water and nutrients in an intestinal villus.

*Fluid Balance in a Scouring Calf*
The main effects of scouring are loss of fluid from the body (i.e. dehydration), a loss of electrolytes, acidosis, and a reduced ability to digest food. Septicaemia may also develop.

*Dehydration*
Whatever the initial cause, the onset of scouring means that there is an increased loss of fluid in the faeces, and unless this is replaced by additional intakes by mouth, *dehydration* occurs. The blood becomes 'thicker' and more difficult for the heart to pump, poor circulation develops, body temperature drops and the calf goes into a state of shock. Inadequate blood flow through the kidneys may lead to

renal failure, with a consequent buildup of toxic waste materials further depressing an already sick calf.

The extent of dehydration in a particular calf may be difficult to assess. Ideally a blood sample could be taken to measure the proportion of fluid (serum) to cells. However, this is rarely done and clinical assessments are usually made, for example:

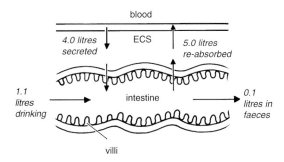

Figure 2.7. Water flow in a normal calf. (ECS = extra cellular space.)

- sunken eyes
- skin 'tent' time (Plate 2.20): with the finger and thumb pinch a fold of skin just above the calf's eyelid, and then release it. The fold should disappear almost immediately. If the skin remains 'tented' for more than five seconds, the calf is dehydrated
- loss of suck reflex. Calves which are very dehydrated (or acidotic) simply stop sucking

Bacteria have adhesive properties. They stick to the epithelial cells of the villi and produce toxins which stimulate an increased flow of fluid *into* the intestine – this is the intestine's defence to try to flush the bacteria away. The flow of fluid from the blood into the intestine increases from 4.0 litres to 6.0 litres,

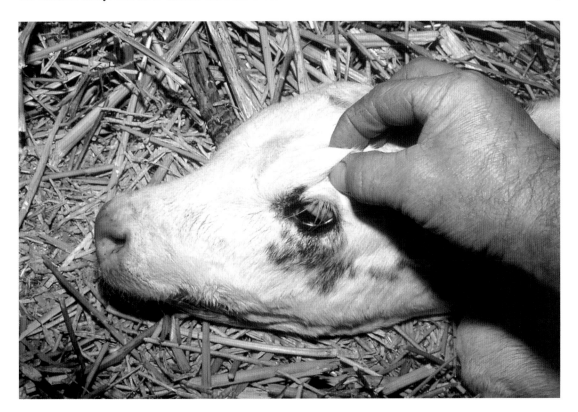

Plate 2.20. Skin 'tenting'. If the fold of the skin remains erect for longer than five seconds, the calf is dehydrated.

and so our overall fluid balance equation becomes (Figure 2.8):

1.1 litres *drunk* + 6.0 litres *secreted* →
5.0 litres *absorbed* + 2.1 litres *in faeces*

Reabsorption of fluid remains the same, so excess is voided with the faeces producing scouring.

Viruses, on the other hand, destroy the villi and reduce the rate of reabsorption of water. The rate of flow of water into the intestine remains normal (4.0 litres), but because the villi are damaged let us say that only 3.0 litres are reabsorbed. The fluid balance equation now becomes (Figure 2.9):

1.1 litres *drunk* + 4.0 litres *secreted* →
3.0 litres *absorbed* + 2.1 litres *in faeces*

Far more fluid is therefore voided in the faeces and scouring again occurs.

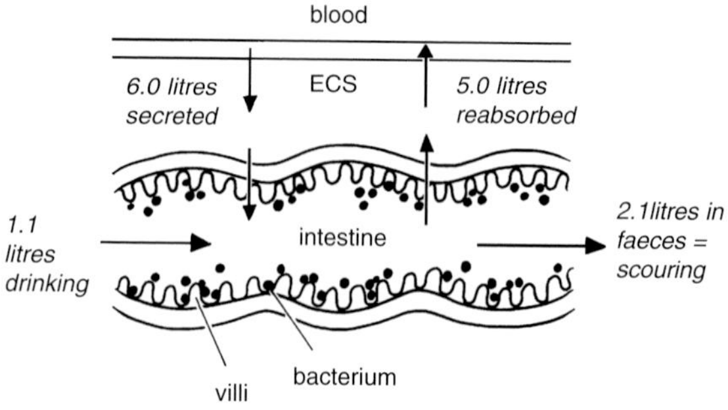

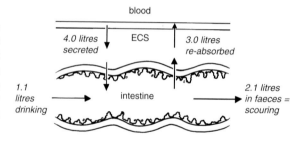

Figure 2.8. Bacteria cause scouring by sticking to the villi and causing an increased flow of fluid from the blood into the intestine. (ECS = extra cellular space.)

*Loss of electrolytes*
The excess water being voided in the calf's faeces carries with it various salts (electrolytes). As the calf's body slowly becomes depleted of salts, it loses even more of its ability to retain water in its tissues and it becomes progressively more dehydrated. The loss of body sodium is particularly significant, because the presence of sodium within the body is important for fluid retention.

*Acidosis*
The normal pH of blood is 7.4. If blood pH falls, the calf is then said to be suffering from acidosis. This is seen clinically as an increased respiratory rate, with general dullness, lethargy and a disinclination to suckle. When the blood pH falls

Figure 2.9. Viruses cause scouring by destroying the villi and preventing water absorption from the intestine. (ECS = extra cellular space.)

to 7.1 the calf will die. Next to dehydration, acidosis is the second most common cause of calves dying from scouring and this is especially so for the slightly older calf, for example seven to fourteen days old.

Acidosis in the scouring calf is caused by:

- loss of bicarbonate in the diarrhoeic faeces
- dehydration, causing poor blood circulation in the tissues and leading to a buildup of acid waste products
- fermentation of undigested milk (including lactose) in the lower gut producing acide by-products

*Reduced digestive capacity*
Damage to the intestinal villi caused by bacteria and viruses also reduces the ability of the villi to produce lactase. Lactase is the digestive enzyme which converts the milk sugar lactose into glucose and galactose:

Lactose $\xrightarrow{\text{lactase}}$ glucose + galactose

The reduced digestive capacity has two effects:

- Undigested lactose passes through the small intestine and into the large bowel, where it may undergo fermentation to produce acid and further scouring.
- As sodium and glucose are transported together, the lack of glucose means that sodium is not pumped back into the arteriole in the base of the villus as effectively (Figure 2.6). More sodium is then lost in the scour and dehydration gets worse.

*Septicaemia*

In cases of bacterial scour particularly, the wall of the intestine may become very inflamed and bacteria may 'leak' into the bloodstream to produce a generalised septicaemia (that is, bacteria growing in the blood). This can cause an even more severe illness and may lead to such secondary diseases as joint ill and meningitis.

> The main consequences of scouring are:
> - dehydration
> - loss of salts
> - acidosis
> - reduced digestive capacity
> - septicaemia

## Causes of calf scour

As dehydration and acidosis are the most important causes of illness and mortality in scouring calves, our main aim must be to control them. Perhaps surprisingly, removal of the initial infection is less important. This is because the majority of infectious causes of calf scour are self-limiting, i.e. after one wave of infection the organisms expel themselves.

The causes of calf scour may be subdivided into four categories:

- Bacterial – *E. coli* (white scour, coli bacillosis)
  – salmonella
- Viral – rotavirus
  – coronavirus
- Protozoal – cryptosporidia
  – coccidiosis (usually older calves)
- Nutritional

Nutritional causes of calf scour were discussed earlier in the chapter. Their main significance is perhaps that they make the calf more susceptible to infectious agents. For example, a healthy calf could probably cope with a low dose of rotavirus, but if it were stressed, perhaps because of gross overfeeding, then the rotavirus would cause disease. Coccidiosis and nutritional causes of scouring in the weaned calf are described in Chapter 3.

Scouring in calves may be divided into categories based on the calf's age and the prevalence of infection:

- age of the calf: Scouring at one to three days old is more likely to be bacterial (although salmonella can cause scouring at any age), whereas scouring at seven to fourteen days old is more likely to be viral or protozoal (coccidiosis can also occur in older calves, including after weaning)
- prevalence of infection: Some of the infections are present on virtually every farm all the time and it is only when the calf's defence mechanisms are compromised, or the level of that infection on the farm increases, that disease is seen. These infectious agents are known as ubiquitous or endemic. Other infectious agents are present only on some farms. These are known as exotics.

Ubiquitous infections

- rotavirus
- coronavirus
- cryptosporidia

Exotic infections

● K99 *E. coli*
● salmonella
● coccidiosis

Although it is always possible to culture *E. coli* from the faeces of calves (including normal calves), only very few strains of *E. coli* cause disease. Table 2.4 shows the results of a survey which attempted to identify the most common agents involved as primary causes of calf scour outbreaks. It clearly shows that viral causes (rotavirus and coronavirus) account for over 50% of the outbreaks of calf scour and if we add cryptosporidia, then these three agents are involved in the vast majority (79%) of cases. Bacterial infections are much less common and so when we consider treatment, antibiotic therapy, although commonly used, in many instances has only a secondary role. Before dealing with the various infections in some detail, one more general point needs to be made: it is *not possible* to diagnose the cause of calf scour from the appearance of the faeces alone. Samples need to be taken and tests carried out.

Table 2.4. This shows that rotavirus and cryptosporidia are the commonest causes of scouring in young calves. *E. coli* is a much less important cause, although it is always present in calf faeces.

| Agent | Prevalence in neonatal diarrhoea |
|---|---|
| Rotavirus | 42% |
| Coronavirus | 14% |
| Cryptosporidium | 23% |
| K99 *E. coli* | 3% |
| Verotoxin *E. coli* | 10% |
| Salmonella | 12% |
| Other viruses | 11% |

From J. H. Morgan

## Rotavirus

Rotavirus is the most common cause of scouring in calves at seven to fourteen days old. This is clearly demonstrated in Table 2.4. It is particularly frustrating for the dairy farmer who may have an excellent beef-cross calf ready for sale, only to find that it is scouring profusely as in Plate 2.21. Even if it recovers quickly, it may have hair loss over the hindquarters (Plate 2.22) which will reduce its value. Calves from both dairy and beef suckler herds can be affected.

Rotavirus is present in all herds, but only under certain conditions (usually suboptimal hygiene and/or a heavy challenge) does it cause disease. Colostrum provides a very good protection, but only while it is present in the intestine; colostrum-derived antibody absorbed into the bloodstream does *not* give any protection against rotavirus. After four to six days, when the cow is producing normal milk (Figure 2.10) or when the calf is being changed onto milk substitute, the level of colostral antibody in the intestine wanes and this is the stage when rotavirus proliferates. After an incubation period of two to five days (viz at approximately seven to ten days old) the virus destroys the epithelial cells lining the villi of the upper small intestine, thus preventing reabsorption of water, and scouring is seen (Figure 2.9). This is often a yellow or cream coloured scour as undigested milk passes through the small intestine.

In addition to scouring, the main clinical feature is dehydration – the calf is dull, its eyes are sunken and its coat feels cold. Its body temperature may be increased in the early stages, but it soon falls. Fluid therapy is vital and although antibiotics have no

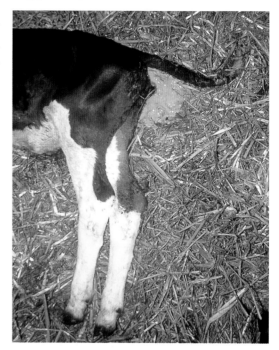

Plate 2.21. Sudden onset of scour at seven to ten days old can be due to rotavirus infection.

effect against the primary virus infection, they may be of value in preventing a secondary bacterial attack on the damaged intestinal wall. Rotavirus is not usually a 'killer'. Mortality is rarely particularly high and the main cost of the disease is the subsequent severe unthriftiness of affected calves.

Many calves will be exposed to infection and shed virus at seven to fourteen days old, but show no scouring or any other adverse effects. However, as progressively more calves pass through a house and the weight of infection increases, a greater proportion develops diarrhoea. This is one reason why scouring is more common in the later-born calves from an autumn-calving dairy herd.

*Prevention*
The prevention of diarrhoea caused by rotavirus is based on a combination of hygiene and vaccination.

*Hygiene* Rotavirus is highly contagious: only small quantities are needed to infect other calves and careful isolation and separation of affected calves is therefore essential. The virus is also very resistant: it can survive in a normal farm environment for up to six months and it is resistant to many commonly used disinfectants. However, it is susceptible to drying. If an outbreak of rotavirus diarrhoea occurs, therefore, the best preventive measure is to clean thoroughly and rest the affected shed and start rearing calves elsewhere. If convenient, pen divisions can be dismantled and affected calves left loose-housed in the same shed after weaning.

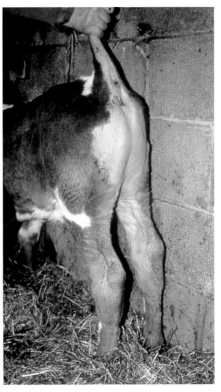

Plate 2.22. Even calves which recover from scouring may be left with hair loss over their hind legs.

*Vaccination* In the UK there is a good rotavirus vaccine commercially available, combined with one for K99 *E. coli*. One dose is given to the cow between four and twelve weeks before calving, which means that vaccination at the normal drying off time is satisfactory. This produces a high antibody level in both the colostrum and in the milk for up to one month after calving (Figure 2.10), compared with normal cows where rotavirus antibodies have fallen below protective levels by four to five days after calving. It also follows that for vaccination to provide effective protection against rotavirus, the calf must be fed on colostrum or milk from vaccinated cows during the whole period of risk.

The feeding of stored colostrum could be very useful

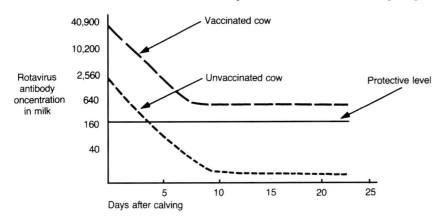

Figure 2.10. Only milk from vaccinated cows carries sufficient antibody to protect the calf from rotavirus. In a normal cow there is no protection after five days and scouring may result. (From J. H. Morgan.)

in this context. Because the concentration of antibody in the colostrum of vaccinated cows is well above that required for rotavirus protection, milk or milk substitute can be mixed with 10–15% of colostrum taken from vaccinated cows. This works out at about one cupful per feed and is a very simple and effective control measure. The machine shown in Plate 2.7 automatically dispenses this amount. This is one instance where great care should be taken to ensure that 'stored colostrum' is in fact colostrum. I have seen several breakdowns of rotavirus scour caused by excessive dilution of colostrum with mastitic and other discarded milk. Correct colostrum storage is described earlier in this chapter.

Rotavirus is a disease associated with a buildup of infection. In a batch-calving herd it may therefore be safe to allow the first cows to calve unprotected and only vaccinate later groups when the level of infection in the calf house starts to increase. Clearly if it were possible to provide several different calf-rearing houses, vaccination would probably not be necessary. This is one advantage of the calf hutches shown in Plate 2.3.

Adult cows are probably exposed to repeated attacks of rotavirus during their lives and this provides them with a good level of immunity and sufficient colostral antibody for the calf for the first three to five days. Heifers are normally reared separately from the main herd and as such they may have lower colostral antibodies and their calves may therefore be more susceptible to diarrhoea.

## Coronavirus

The pattern of infection with coronavirus is very similar to that of rotavirus. Adult cows are carriers of infection and they probably increase the excretion of virus at calving. Colostrum provides protection for the first four to six days, after which a wave of infection passes through the calf. Many calves cope without showing symptoms, but a proportion will scour at ten to twenty days old (slightly later than rotavirus). Whereas rotavirus affects only the upper small intestine and the tips of the villi, coronavirus can occur throughout the intestine and will strip the lining from the whole villus.

Outbreaks of scouring caused by coronavirus are generally more severe than those caused by rotavirus. However, the virus is more susceptible to disinfectants. There is a commercial vaccine available in the UK and control is assisted by good hygiene and colostrum feeding.

## Cryptosporidium

This is a small protozoan parasite which affects the lower small intestine (the same area as K99 *E. coli*). Affected calves may or may not develop a temperature and the clinical signs are those of scouring, dehydration, loss of appetite and, particularly, unthriftiness.

Calves with cryptosporidia may produce a very watery diarrhoea, often containing lumps of mucus, and they may strain excessively (but not as severely as with coccidiosis, see Chapter 3). Death is common. It often seems to occur in a group-feeding situation, where many calves are feeding from a single teat. Calves over three weeks old do not seem to be commonly affected. The organism is endemic in all cattle herds, i.e. it is found everywhere, and as with rotavirus and coronavirus, most calves are exposed to infection between birth and weaning, although only a proportion develop clinical signs of disease. It is highly contagious, spreading rapidly to other calves. Although it is resistant to commonly used disinfectants, it is easily killed by heat and drying.

Cryptosporidium can also cause disease in other animals and in man. Human infections are particularly important in AIDS patients, because they account for a significant proportion of their deaths.

Like coronavirus and rotavirus, there is as yet no specific licensed drug which will kill cryptosporidia. Sulphonamide injections and amprolium drenches have been tried, although success has been limited. The chemical halofuginone is currently being examined with promising results and in Australia the anti-coccidosis drug lasalocid is used at a dose of 1.0 mg per kg body weight. Alternate feeds of electrolytes and yoghurt throughout the day seem to help. Most farm houses have a warm cupboard where large quantities of yoghurt can be made (see treatment section for details). Although by no means definitely proven, prolonged feeding of colostrum could be a suitable control measure. Good hygiene is vital.

## *Escherichia coli* (*E. coli*)

It was once thought that *E. coli* was the main cause of scouring in calves. Although the organism can be isolated from the dung of all calves, whether scouring or not, it is now known that *E. coli* actually causes less than 15% of all calf scour problems (see Table 2.4).

There are more than 100 different strains of *E. coli* and those which cause scouring in calves can be subdivided into two groups, classified on their mode of action:

- Enterotoxigenic strains. These *E. coli* have small projections from their surface known as K99 antigens. The projections allow them to stick to the wall of the intestine and once in position they produce *enterotoxins*. It is these toxins which stimulate the calf to produce excessive quantities of intestinal secretions, thus leading to diarrhoea (see Figure 2.8). As it is generally the lower end of the small intestine which is affected, there are few chances of reabsorbing this fluid, so the diarrhoea can be particularly severe.
- Enteropathogenic strains. These *E. coli* usually cause scouring in older calves and are often secondary to digestive upsets or infections such as rotavirus or cryptosporidia.

A verocytoxin-producing enterotoxigenic strain of *E. coli*, known as *E. coli* 0157 and said to be carried by 2–5% of healthy cattle, can cause quite serious food poisoning in man, as in the 1996/97 outbreak in Scotland when 20 people, mainly elderly, died. In man this strain causes a haemorrhagic colitis and the toxin produced can lead to death due to renal failure. Carrier animals show no symptoms. As the incidence of human disease is quite rare in vets and farmers, carrier animals cannot be particularly infectious.

In calves the clinical signs can be very variable. In some calves the dung may not be particularly loose, but affected animals become dull and listless, and in the early stages they will have a high temperature. This is due to septicaemia, which means that some of the *E. coli* have left the intestine and are multiplying in the bloodstream and tissues. Sometimes this is called *colibacillosis*, or coli septicaemia. Typically only calves in the first week of life are affected, and the majority will have received insufficient colostrum. At this stage treatment with antibiotics by injection is necessary and careful nursing, with warmth and a dry bed, is important, in addition to the fluid replacement measures which are discussed later. In some affected calves the scour is unusually white and hence the term white scour. A white scour can also be caused by rotavirus.

A variety of measures are available for prevention and the steps most suited to your unit will depend on when the problem occurs and the feeding system in use. These include:

- Careful hygiene to prevent spread. Calving boxes are an important source of infection (because disease occurs in very young calves) and particular attention needs to be paid to the calving area. Ideally start calving cows elsewhere.
- Vaccination. There is a good K99 *E. coli* vaccine combined with rotavirus, a single dose of which is given to cows between four and twelve weeks pre calving. As *E. coli* infection is contracted soon after birth, it is vital to ensure prompt and adequate colostrum intakes for vaccination to be effective.
- Antiserum. Antiserum contains preformed antibodies to *E. coli* and can be injected into calves immediately after birth. However, as there are over 100 different strains of *E. coli*, the effectiveness of the antiserum will depend on whether the commercial product you are using contains the correct strains. Antiserum mainly protects against septicaemia.
- Oral antibiotics at birth. This may be justified in the short term as a means of reducing the bacterial challenge while management and the environment are being improved. It certainly works in the treatment of watery mouth in lambs, which is also an *E. coli* enterotoxaemia.

## Salmonellosis

Salmonella is a bacterial infection which can cause a wide range of symptoms, depending on the age of animal affected and the species of salmonella involved. There are many different species of salmonella, some of which cause severe disease, others cause mild disease and many others (the exotics) cause no problem at all. A few of the more common species (often called serotypes) are listed below:

*Salmonella typhimurium*
● can infect many different animals and birds, including man
● can cause disease in all ages of animal, with a wide range of symptoms including diarrhoea, dysentery, abortion, septicaemia and death
● has a wide range of sub-species, usually referred to as phage types

*Salmonella dublin*
● occurs only in cattle
● causes septicaemia and meningitis in weaned calves and abortion in cows

*Salmonella enteritidis*
● can cause disease in cattle and man and was implicated in the infamous 'salmonella in eggs' scare in the UK in the early 1990s

Other species of salmonella which may cause disease include *S. agama*, *S. arizona*, *S. binza* and *S. kedougou*.

Salmonella in weaned calves is discussed in Chapter 3 and salmonella in cows in Chapter 11. This section deals with the problem in young calves only.

*S. typhimurium* is the most common serotype found in young calves. Disease is seen as a profuse diarrhoea, often progressing to dysentery (dysentery means a mixture of blood, intestinal lining and faeces), with a high temperature, septicaemia and, in severe cases, death within 24–48 hours, despite treatment. More chronic forms do occur, however, in which an affected calf simply has pasty dung and is unthrifty and, at the far end of the spectrum, some calves may carry the infection without suffering any adverse effects. In some ways it is these latter animals which cause the difficulties. They probably have good levels of antibody defences against salmonella, but are *intermittent excretors*, that is sometimes they shed salmonella in their faeces and sometimes they do not. Excretion is far more likely during or after a period of stress and this has a considerable practical significance, for example:

● the stress of transport. Carrier calves are more likely to be infecting their pen-mates when they are in the market, or if they have recently been brought home from market
● the stress of a digestive upset. The primary cause of scouring in a calf unit may have been a faulty milk mixture, or some other management digestive upset but this can lead to increased salmonella excretion and then a breakdown with clinical salmonellosis
● the stress of intercurrent disease. Carrier calves may develop navel ill or calf pneumonia and this can lead to increased activity of the salmonella, either causing disease in the carrier animal itself, or spreading it to others

A most interesting survey of 589 calves purchased from markets and supplied to eleven different farms showed how common is the problem of salmonella. Calves were swabbed for salmonella three times each week. Although only four were detectable carriers when they arrived from market, by five to six weeks later *over half the calves* (51%) had been excreting infection, with a peak reached at 18–19 days. This is shown in Figure 2.11. *S. typhimurium* was the most common serotype found. On some farms antibiotics were fed prophylactically for the first few weeks but this had *no effect* on the number of calves excreting salmonella. Rather surprisingly, there was a higher proportion of calves excreting infection when penned singly than in group-housed calves. Even after cleaning out and disinfection it was still possible to isolate salmonella from the environment on six of the eleven farms, so possibly carryover from one batch to the next plays a more important part than we once thought.

These results show quite clearly that because the calf is an *intermittent excretor* of *S. typhimurium*, it is not possible to take a single faecal swab for culture and on the basis of a negative bacteriological result be sure that the animal is 'safe' to introduce into your calf unit. Swabbing daily for five days would be a better screening, but it would still not identify all carrier calves and it would also be extremely costly. Anyone purchasing calves should therefore try to reduce the risk of salmonella by taking the following measures.

1. Buy from as few different sources as possible and try to ensure adequate colostrum intake at birth.
2. Use your own transport.
3. Avoid market calves – these have been exposed to many other possibly infected calves, all of which have been subjected to the stresses of transport, cold, lack of food etc., which would increase the salmonella excretion rate from carrier animals.

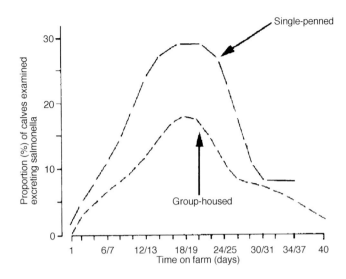

Figure 2.11. The incidence of *S. typhimurium* excretion in calves purchased from markets (from Wray, Todd & Hinton, Veterinary Record, 1987).

4. Buy only strong and healthy calves which could withstand a low level of salmonella challenge.
5. Treat calves very gently on arrival – separate penning, warm and dry bedding, feeding electrolytes only for the first 12–18 hours, then increase milk gradually.
6. Clean out and disinfect pens very thoroughly between batches. Burn bedding from isolation facilities. Store slurry for three months before spreading, and if it is spread on pasture, do not graze for two months after spreading.
7. Maintain vermin and bird control programme (mice commonly act as reservoirs of salmonella). Prevent wildlife access to cattle feeds. Provide clean, uncontaminated water.
8. Purchase feeds only from firms which operate salmonella control programmes.
9. Vaccinate. Excellent dead salmonella vaccines are available, often combined with *E. coli*. Two doses in late pregnancy will protect the cow during her highly susceptible period over calving and also the calf, via colostrum. Continued calf protection may be obtained by vaccinating at 14 and 28 days old. If the calf's immune status is unknown, serovaccines may be used, i.e. a product containing antiserum to give immediate protection, plus a vaccine to stimulate the calf to produce its own immunity. Vaccination also reduces the rate of *S. typhimurium* excretion by carrier cows and in this way decreases the overall level of contamination in the environment.

It should be pointed out that *S. typhimurium* can cause diarrhoea in man and even death in young children. Personal hygiene, especially removing overalls and washing hands, is always important after handling calves and especially scouring animals. The importance of markets and calf dealing in the spread of *S. typhimurium* was clearly demonstrated in 1977–8 when a chloramphicol resistant strain of the bacterium, called DT204C, was responsible for a severe outbreak of disease in calves in Somerset and the south-west of England. The organism travelled with calves to cause outbreaks of disease on farms in the Yorkshire area and even up to the north-east of Scotland.

Since the early 1990s a new type of *S. typhimurium*, phage type DT104, has been increasing in importance in both man and animals. In 1995 there were 2500 human cases of infection reported in the UK, this being the second most common cause of food poisoning after *S. enteriditis*. It was also by far the most common isolate from cattle, occurring at a rate of around 0.05 cases per 1000 head of cattle. It is characterised by:

- severe illness in both young and old cattle
- moderately severe illness in man, with a hospitalisation rate approaching 30%. In one survey of 200 farms having this strain of salmonella, human illness was found in 10% of them
- multiple drug resistance, in that all isolates are resistant to the antibiotics ampicillin, chloramphenicol, streptomycin, sulphonamides and tetracyclines

Other animals on the farm may be a reservoir of DT104 infection. On one farm I dealt with there was severe disease in cattle, with deaths in both adult cows and calves. Cattle deaths were controlled by vaccination, but the infection persisted on the farm, as shown by an extensive swabbing survey. The source of infection was eventually shown to be the adjacent pig unit, which was part of the farm and very close to the dairy unit. In fact slurry from the pigs was scraped across and into the cattle area. Infection was also found in mice, cats, birds, on boots and even in the foot-well of the Landrover. Vaccination of both the dairy and sow herds was carried out, using the cattle vaccine, in an attempt to reduce the excretion rate from the pigs and lower the overall challenge of infection on the farm.

## Treatment of Scour

Although it is often necessary to identify the cause of calf scour, so as to prevent and control further cases, the treatment of an individual calf is very similar whatever the cause. Treatment is discussed under the following headings:

- withholding of milk
- correction of dehydration and salt loss
- correction of acidosis
- intensive intravenous therapy
- use of antibiotics
- supportive therapy

Of these, the first three are by far the most important.

*Withholding of milk*
Opinions vary regarding whether milk should be withheld from scouring calves. Because the intestinal villi are damaged and no longer able to digest milk (and especially lactose), most people consider that milk should be withheld for at least 24 hours; otherwise undigested milk passing into the lower intestine could cause further scouring. However, do not withhold milk for too long. It is the presence of milk in the intestine which *stimulates* the growth of the specialised cells which produce lactase, the enzyme required to digest milk. Therefore if you withhold milk for four to five days and then give the calf a full feed, you may cause it to scour because at this stage the intestine is unable to digest any more than a small quantity of milk. Milk should therefore be reintroduced in small feeds by the third day, even if the calf is still scouring.

*Correction of dehydration and salt loss*
The scouring calf is suffering a massive loss of fluid and salts and this must be replaced. In addition to replacing salts, electrolyte solutions *actively promote* the uptake of water. For example, if a scouring calf with a damaged gut is given 1.5 litres of water to drink, it will probably only absorb 0.75 litre. However, if the same calf is given a drink of 1.5 litres of an electrolyte solution, it will probably absorb 1.25 litres of fluid. This is because electrolyte solutions contain glucose, sodium and other substances which are *actively transported* across the wall of the villus. This then increases the concentration of substances within the villus and water is drawn across into the blood by osmosis (see Figure 2.6).

If dehydration is marked (e.g. the calf's skin is tight and its eyes are sinking), electrolytes should be given frequently throughout the day, for example 1 litre per feed every two to three hours. Do not mix electrolytes with milk. Although there is some evidence that certain products increase the rate of milk clotting in the abomasum, it is likely that the milk clot formed will be less stable. There is then a risk of only partially digested milk passing into the intestine to cause further scour. When reintroducing milk, give a feed of electrolytes followed one to two hours later by a *small* (for example 0.75–1.0 litre) feed of milk *at full strength*. Diluting milk may reduce the rate of clotting and digestion in the abomasum and is best not done.

Electrolyte solutions are palatable and are generally drunk voluntarily. However, for calves which will not drink, a plastic dispensing bag combined with a stomach tube may be purchased (Plate 2.23). The tube is gently inserted so that its tip runs along the roof of the calf's mouth. This then ensures that it enters the oesophagus, which is situated *above* the trachea (see Figure 2.1). The tube needs to be inserted to almost the full length of the stiffest part (Plate 2.24). Fluid will thus be administered into the lower oesophagus, or perhaps even the oesophageal groove, and can be run in under gravity.

Do not be too alarmed if scouring appears to increase in the short term. When fluids are first given, although they will be correcting the dehydration, they also allow the faeces to become more liquid, thereby increasing the volume passed. It is interesting that in the short term at least, it does not matter how much the calf scours, provided that you can maintain an adequate circulating blood volume by giving ample fluids. This might entail giving as much as 6–8 litres daily, preferably in four or more feeds.

Scouring primarily produces low blood sodium and high potassium levels and so fluids should contain high sodium and low potassium. They should also be as close as possible to the same concentration as in blood. If too concentrated they may draw fluid from the body and into the intestine and make the dehydration worse! If too weak, they may not contain enough sodium and bicarbonate to correct electrolyte imbalance and acidosis respectively. If the calf has only a mild scour, then the use of a simple home-made mixture of salt and glucose might be adequate, for example 120 g glucose plus 1 teaspoonful of salt in 5 litres of boiling water, cooled to blood heat before feeding. However, if the calf is looking sick, then much more intensive therapy is needed, with three or four daily feeds using a quality product.

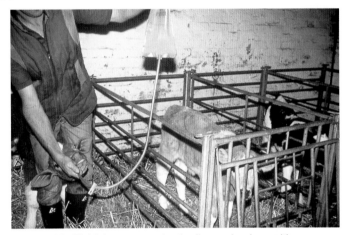

Plate 2.23. Fluid therapy: a plastic dispensing bag with a stomach tube for the calf that will not drink.

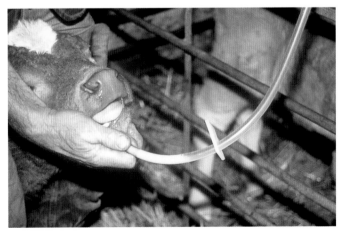

Plate 2.24. The stomach tube needs to be inserted to almost the full length of its stiffest part.

*Correction of acidosis*

Most of the better (and unfortunately more expensive!) electrolyte solutions now contain bicarbonate or bicarbonate precursors, such as citrate, which assist in the correction of acidosis. This is vitally important in ensuring a speedy recovery, especially in the older calf of seven to fourteen days old in which acidosis is likely to develop.

There is an increasingly wide range of products on the market and when selecting one for use consider:

● Does it contain adequate sodium? Sodium is needed to hold fluid in body tissues, and should be present at 100–120 mmol/litre.
● Does it contain adequate bicarbonate? Bicarbonate (or bicarbonate precursors) is needed to correct acidosis, and should be present at 70–80 mmol/litre.

*Intensive intravenous therapy*

Calves which are dull but will still suckle will almost certainly respond to oral electrolytes. Calves which are standing and able to move can be given electrolytes by feeder bag. However, calves which are collapsed, with sunken eyes and severe dehydration, are unlikely to respond unless they are given intravenous fluids. This is because they are so badly dehydrated and their circulation is so poor that they are unable to absorb sufficient electrolyte solution from the intestine. The skin 'tent' test is a good way of measuring dehydration (see Plate 2.20).

Ideally, intravenous fluid therapy needs to be given in a veterinary hospital, where the calf can be constantly monitored and blood tests carried out to ensure that the correct levels of bicarbonate are being given to correct acidosis. The calf in Plate 2.25 is receiving intravenous fluids in a veterinary hospital. Recovery can be remarkably rapid (12 hours or less) although intravenous therapy may need to be continued for two to three days if the intestine is badly damaged. If fluids are discontinued too quickly, relapses occur, with disappointing results.

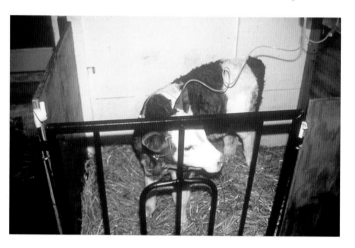

Plate 2.25. A calf being given intravenous fluid therapy. This is needed for badly affected calves.

*Use of antibiotics*

Although commonly used, antibiotics are perhaps over-rated in the treatment of calf scour. This is because:

● The majority of causes are not bacterial. Of the causes cited in Table 2.4, only *E. coli* and salmonella would be killed by antibiotics.
● Even bacterial causes are self-limiting, because the bacteria may die off quite quickly, leaving just a damaged intestinal lining (and a badly scouring calf!).

Others would say that if the gut wall is inflamed, or the calf has a raised temperature, then the use of antibiotics is justified to kill any bacteria which might leak into the bloodstream. And if bacteria are known to be the cause of scouring on your farm, then antibiotics are *definitely* indicated.

There is a wide range of antibiotics available. The one used needs to be:

● active against *E. coli* and salmonella (e.g. penicillin would not be effective)
● active in the gut (e.g. neomycin or apramycin, which stay in the gut and are not absorbed)

New drugs are constantly being developed and your veterinary surgeon will advise you on the best choice for your circumstances.

*Supportive therapy*
In addition to the above treatments, there is a wide range of measures which may help in the recovery of the calf. Some are discussed in Chapter 1. Supportive therapy includes:

● Nursing. Move the calf to its own pen, possibly with a heat lamp, so that it no longer has to compete with others in the group. This also reduces the spread of infection.
● Anti-inflammatory drugs such as flunixin may decrease shock if bacterial toxins are involved.
● Vitamins may assist in recovery, especially when the intestinal lining is badly damaged.
● Physical adsorbent agents such as attapulgite, activated charcoal and kaolin may be used. Bacterial toxins and other agents stick (adsorb) onto their surface and this will decrease the intensity of scouring.
● Eggs are sometimes used. A very traditional remedy for calf scour is to push an egg into the calf's mouth and break it as it reaches the back of the tongue. The calf then swallows both egg and shell. There are many farmers who use eggs, with or without the shell, and report good results.
● Probiotics. Probiotics could be used at the end of a course of scour treatment, before or at the same time as reintroduction of milk. They are said to colonise the gut with 'healthy' lactobilli and other bacteria and in so doing prevent pathogenic (disease-causing) bacteria and viruses from becoming re-established.

The commonest, and probably the best, probiotic is yoghurt, which can easily be made at home. Heat a small bucket of milk to boiling point (to destroy existing bacteria), cool to blood heat, stir in a carton of natural yoghurt and stand in a warm place (e.g. by the fire or in an airing cupboard) for four to five hours. Most calves will drink yoghurt. It contains millions of lactobacilli and these are normal inhabitants of the calf's intestine. Yoghurt can be a very useful treatment in cases of recurrent scouring. It has, of course, been traditionally used in certain unresponsive human conditions, e.g. vaginal thrush, a fungal infection in women. Probiotics are also commercially available in powder or liquid form and can be used for prevention as well as treatment. The majority contain lactobacilli, but may be mixed with other organisms such as *Streptococcus faecalum* to give an overall concentration of up to *one billion* bacteria per gram. Probiotics may also work by producing their own antibiotics in the intestine. For example, *Lactobacillus acidophilus* from yoghurt produces the three antibiotics acidophilin, acidolin and lactolin.

## Prevention and Control of Scour

When the stockman first sees a scouring calf it is unlikely that he will immediately know the cause. He has to treat the calf using the measures discussed above. At the same time he needs to take steps to *prevent* the spread of infection and *control* or limit the number of new cases which might occur. This is particularly so if several calves have already been affected. While the veterinary surgeon is determining the precise cause from samples taken, the following measures will help to prevent further cases.

● Separate scouring calves from the remainder of the group, thus reducing the challenge dose of infection to otherwise healthy calves.
● Pay strict attention to cleaning buckets after each feed, or ensure that each calf has its own individual bucket. Salmonella, for example, can be spread via the saliva.
● Ensure that the milk substitute is fed at the correct strength and temperature and that feeding times

are regular each day. This promotes both oesophageal groove closure and subsequent abomasal clot formation and digestion.

- If it is necessary to enter calf pens, consider providing a disinfectant foot dip to prevent infection being carried from one pen to another.
- As soon as possible, depopulate the calf house for cleaning as described earlier in this chapter. Start introducing new calves into a different building with clean pens and make sure that these calves are fed and attended each day before the scouring group.
- Ensure beds are dry and warm and that calves are not exposed to draughts. Sick animals may have a fever or a subnormal temperature from dehydration and shock. In both cases a heat lamp will be beneficial.
- Pay extra attention to achieving adequate colostrum intakes for any future calves.
- Vaccinate. Once the cause of the scouring has been established, then vaccination becomes a possible option.

In addition to these control measures, there are specific measures for each disease listed in the preceding sections.

## NAVEL PROBLEMS

### Navel Structure

During pregnancy the navel is the calf's lifeline, supplying it with nutrients from the placenta and removing its waste products. The navel is a complex structure, as shown in Figure 2.12. Plate 2.26 is the post-mortem appearance of a calf which died as a result of navel ill. Fresh blood (which carries food and oxygen) enters from the placenta via the two umbilical arteries (A) which feed into the calf's aorta, the main blood vessel running along its back under its spine. The blood then passes around the body and eventually reaches the liver. 'Used' blood (low in oxygen and carrying waste products) exits from the calf's liver and back out into the placenta via a single umbilical vein (V). The calf produces urine and this is passed back to the placenta via a single tube, the urachus, which exits from the tip of the bladder. The whole structure (two umbilical arteries, one vein and the urachus) is covered by a layer of peritoneum

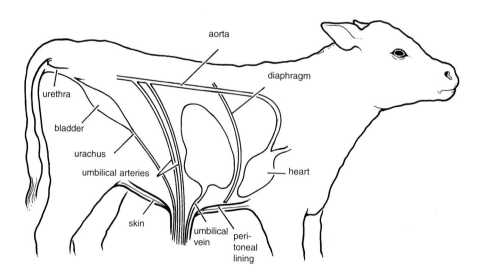

Figure 2.12. The structure of the navel

which becomes continuous with the placenta. There is a hole in the muscle and skin of the body wall (the umbilical ring) to allow unrestricted passage of the navel cord.

At birth the navel cord is the only external part of the animal not covered by a protective layer of skin. It is therefore very susceptible to infection, especially when damp, since bacteria much prefer moist conditions.

## Navel Ill

Navel ill is generally seen in calves in their first week of life and, despite very simple control measures that are effective, it is still an extremely common condition. In the early stages the calf may show no generalised signs of illness, but the navel cord feels enlarged and painful and the tip is generally moist and has a purulent smell.

Plate 2.27 shows a typical example. The calf's temperature will be raised. More advanced cases will be dull, reluctant to move and the pain makes them stand with an arched back. In most cases the infection is localised at the tip of the cord and generally responds well to treatment. However, pus may track up any of the internal structures shown in Figure 2.12 and particularly along the umbilical vein. This is because the arteries have strong muscular walls which contract and expel any remaining blood, whereas residual blood may be left pooling in the vein. Internal abscesses are therefore more common in the umbilical vein and they may even track up into the liver. The calf in Plate 2.28 was four weeks old when it was found dead one morning, having been off-colour for only two days. Note the large abscess in the navel cord tracking up towards the liver. Infection may also track up along the urachus and into the bladder, where it causes cystitis.

**Treatment** Daily antibiotic injections should be given for several days, depending on the severity of the condition, and it is useful to keep the moist end of the cord bathed in warm dilute antiseptic to encourage pus to drain. Sometimes a persistent navel discharge continues. In these cases there is probably a deeper internal abscess which needs to be flushed out. Introduce a catheter through the discharging sinus (as in Plate 2.29) and *gently* syringe in 5–10 ml of dilute antiseptic solution. This will either run back out again on its own or it may have to be sucked out with the syringe.

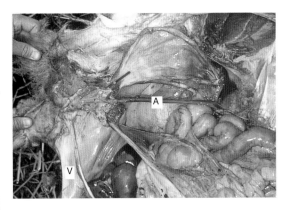

Plate 2.26. Navel ill at post-mortem, showing the umbilical artery (A) and vein (V). A matchstick has been placed at the exit of the bladder into the urachus.

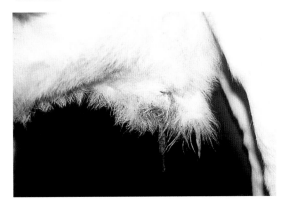

Plate 2.27. A typical case of navel ill. Note the enlarged fleshy navel with a wet tip, which will be painful and have a purulent smell.

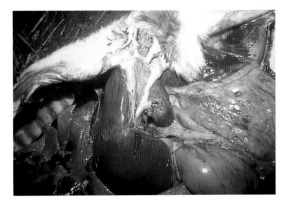

Plate 2.28. Navel abscess extending into the liver from a four-week-old calf which died from navel ill.

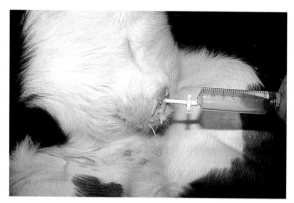

Plate 2.29. Deeper navel infections can be treated by flushing out the internal abscess with a mild antiseptic solution.

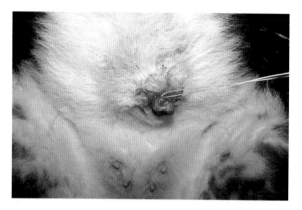

Plate 2.30. A fleshy lump of granulation tissue (proud flesh) protruding from the navel. This needs to be ligated.

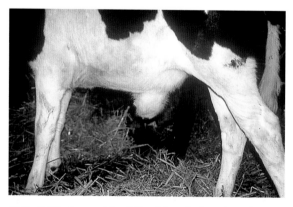

Plate 2.31. A navel (umbilical) hernia is soft and fluctuating and can be gently pushed back into the abdomen.

Repeat daily for four to six days. Do *not* attempt this procedure when you first see a case of navel ill. Wait four to five days until the internal abscess has been reasonably well walled off. Pumping in fluid too aggressively or too early can lead to internal rupture of the abscess, resulting in peritonitis and death.

Sometimes a red fleshy lump is left protruding from the end of the navel as in Plate 2.30. This should be tied off flush with the skin, using a piece of nylon. Tighten the nylon every three to four days and the lump will fall off, usually in seven to ten days.

**Prevention** Ensure that cows calve down in a clean environment and immediately after birth thoroughly spray the fleshy navel cord with an antibiotic aerosol, or dip it into iodine. This has two functions. Firstly it dries the cord, making it less attractive to bacteria, and secondly it destroys any bacteria which may have already become established.

It is probably the drying of the cord which is the most important part in the control of navel ill and hence alternative navel dressings, for example copper sulphate crystals, which produce a drying effect, may be beneficial.

Calves with large fleshy navels (more common in beef breeds) are particularly susceptible to navel ill.

## Umbilical Hernia (Navel Rupture)

The blood vessels from the placenta pass through a small hole in the skin and muscle of the calf's abdomen, and this should close at birth. Sometimes the hole in the muscle is larger than necessary however, and, after birth, this allows a length of small intestine to prolapse through and lie between the skin and the muscle, producing a swelling in the navel region (Plate 2.31). The condition is correctly termed a hernia and should be differentiated from a rupture:

- hernia: a prolapse of intestine or some other body organ through a natural opening in the body wall, e.g. a scrotal hernia or umbilical hernia
- rupture: a split in the body wall at an unnatural site, due to injury or excessive strain, and the prolapse of intestine or some other organ through this artificial opening.

An umbilical hernia may not be noticed until the calf is two months old or more, often after weaning, when the abdomen becomes full of solid food.

In the younger calf hernias have to be distinguished from navel ill. The main differences between a hernia and navel ill are:

- A hernia is soft, fluctuating and painless. In a calf with navel ill the swelling is hard and the tip is likely to be damp and foul-smelling.
- A hernia can normally be pushed back into the abdomen manually, or it will disappear when the calf sits upright on its tail.
- With a hernia the calf has no temperature and is not ill.

If a hernia is small it will eventually resolve, since the hole in the body wall remains the same size, but the intestine enlarges with age until it is eventually too big to pass through the opening in the body wall. Other cases require surgery. On smaller hernias some veterinary surgeons apply a metal or plastic clamp (Plate 2.32) to the loose fold of skin covering the hernia. The calf must first be anaesthetised, then rolled on to its back so that its belly is facing upwards. The intestine then falls back into the abdomen and the clamp is applied, making sure that all the loose skin is pulled through. The screws can be tightened every two to three days and the clamp eventually falls off in one to two weeks, during which time the skin has healed at the base. Continuous antibiotic cover should be given to prevent infection. The procedure does not seem to be particularly stressful for the calf, presumably because by the time it has recovered from the anaesthetic the segment of skin protruding through the clamp has lost its nerve supply.

*Strangulated hernia*

This is a rare phenomenon, but is one good reason why large hernias should be treated. Sometimes a segment of

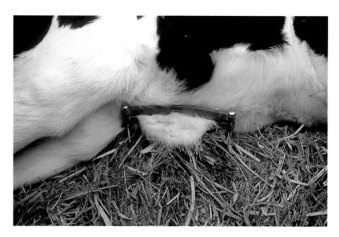

Plate 2.32. A metal hernia clamp.

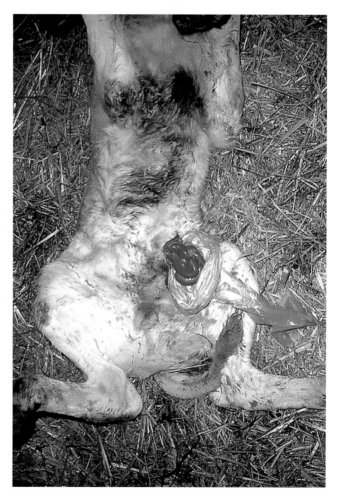

Plate 2.33. Intestines prolapsed through the navel of a newly born calf.

intestine in the hernia sac twists over on itself, leading to a blockage. The blocked intestine dilates, producing enormous pressure and pain inside the hernia, until it eventually ruptures. Death is due to peritonitis.

*Intestinal prolapse*

On occasions, large quantities of intestine prolapse through the fleshy navel cord immediately after birth and lie exposed on the ground. Plate 2.33 shows a good example. This is a serious condition, but if the calf is operated on promptly it can be saved. Keep the calf warm and still, the intestines clean and covered, and call for veterinary assistance. Sometimes it can be very difficult to decide if a large sac hanging from the navel contains intestines or simply fluid.

## Joint Ill

We have already said that infection entering the navel at birth can pass along the cord to the liver and then spread around the body via the blood stream, and this is especially so in colostrum-deficient animals. The bacteria often localise in the joints, and this produces *joint ill* (Plate 2.34). Joint ill is seen at a later stage than navel ill, probably at two to four weeks old, and although the infection may have originally entered at the navel, calves with joint ill do not necessarily have an associated navel ill.

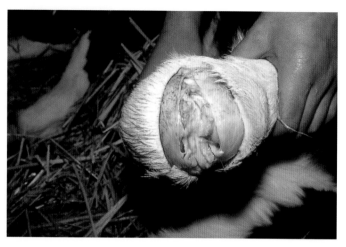

Plate 2.34. Joint ill. When pus has filled the joint, as in this calf, treatment is very difficult.

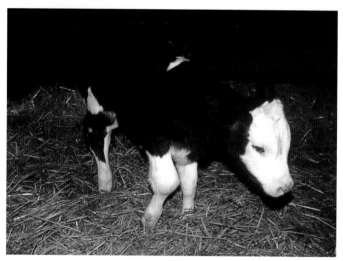

Plate 2.35. Joint ill. Note the very swollen knee. The calf is not taking weight on this leg.

Some calves which recover from a severe bout of scouring may also develop joint ill. This is caused by bacteria which have leaked into the circulation from a damaged and inflamed intestine. A range of different bacteria may therefore be involved.

The first sign of joint ill is likely to be lameness. The calf in Plate 2.35 has an obviously swollen right knee and is not taking its full weight on that leg. If more than one joint is involved, the calf may be seen as generally lethargic and reluctant to move. It will have a high temperature. Later, heat and a fluid swelling appear in one or more joints, and it is the hocks and knees in particular which are commonly affected. Because there is no blood flow into the joints, the condition is difficult to treat. If a case is caught in the early stages, then a prolonged course of antibiotic, for example up to three weeks, may produce a cure.

If a fluid swelling can be palpated around the joint, then an improved response may be obtained by getting your veterinarian to drain pus from the joint and inject antibiotic into the joint space. However, great care with hygiene is needed; otherwise more infection may be introduced, making matters worse.

Once a calf has become totally recumbent from joint ill it is not worth treating. Probably half of the calves developing serious joint ill die. Early treatment is essential. Prevention simply consists of dressing the navel at birth, as described for navel ill, and ensuring adequate colostrum intake.

## OTHER CALF DISEASES

### Meningitis

The meninges are the fibrous layers which surround the brain and separate it from the skull. Meningitis simply means inflammation of the meninges and may be caused by a range of bacteria including streptococci, salmonella species and *E. coli*.

The initial source of infection is often the navel, although meningitis can also be secondary to scouring and enteritis. Colostrum-deficient calves are much more susceptible. The clinical signs depend on the nature of the infection invading the meninges and on the part of the brain affected. The calf may or may not be blind, but often the pupils are dilated and the eyes move from side to side in a jerking movement known as *nystagmus*.

The calf in Plate 2.36 was a typical case. It walked around the pen with its head on one side, continually pushing against the wall. Some calves appear to have an intense headache, in that they stand apart from the others with their head down, possibly pushing it against a feeding trough or into a corner. In this respect the symptoms resemble lead poisoning. More severe cases tremble and eventually fall to the ground with fits and spasms. There is usually a raised temperature and some calves develop a white cloudy debris inside the eye (Plate 2.37). This is panophthalmitis and shows that the whole eye is affected. It is not commonly associated with meningitis.

For treatment your veterinarian will prescribe an antibiotic which can pass across the blood–brain barrier. This is a physiological barrier which normally protects the brain from large molecules and which certainly prevents many drugs from entering. Anti-

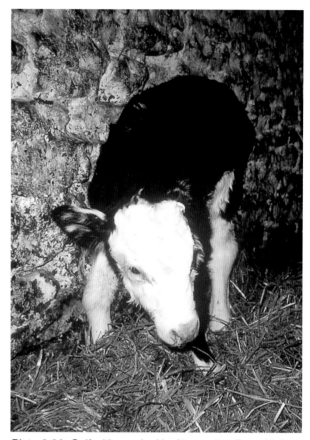

Plate 2.36. Calf with meningitis. It was standing with its head on one side, continually walking around the pen, pushing its head against the wall. There may also be a middle ear infection present.

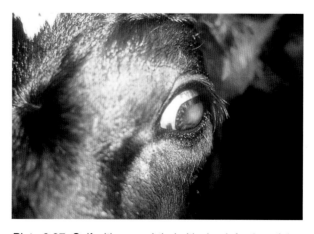

Plate 2.37. Calf with panophthalmitis, i.e. infection of the whole eye resulting from meningitis.

inflammatory drugs and painkillers will also help. Nursing is very important. The affected calf should be penned on its own and if it has stopped eating, it should be given milk to drink to maintain its strength and/or drenched with electrolytes to prevent dehydration.

## Middle Ear Disease

This can be confused with meningitis but it is a much less severe condition. Affected calves hang their head to one side (because they have earache), but otherwise they continue to feed, eat and grow normally. In some animals the ear-drum eventually bursts and a moist purulent discharge oozes from the ear canal. This assists recovery.

Injectable antibiotic for four to six days is needed to overcome the infection.

## Calf Diphtheria

This occurs mainly in the mouth and may be seen in calves both before and after weaning and occasionally even in yearlings. Although the name is identical to the condition in man, the disease has a different cause and is far less serious. The bacterium concerned, *Fusobacterium necrophorum*, gains entry to the soft tissues after the thick epithelial lining of the mouth has been damaged. Once established, the infection forms an ulcer covered by a layer of thick pus and this can be seen inside the calf's mouth.

The common sites affected are the inside of the cheek and at the back of the tongue. The cheek form is probably caused by the calf accidentally biting the inside of its mouth and it is seen as a swelling of the skin between the upper and lower teeth (Plate 2.38). This often causes little adverse effect on the calf, whereas the tongue form leads to difficulty in swallowing and affected calves drool and often froth at the

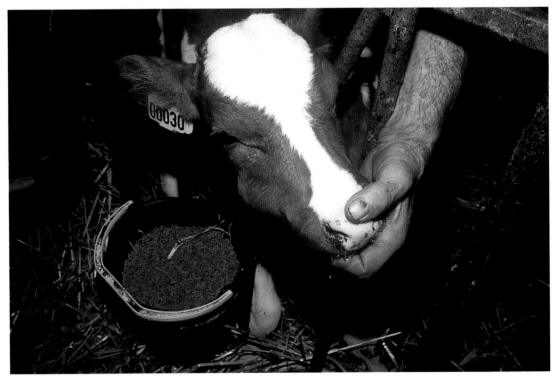

Plate 2.38. Calf diphtheria: the cheek is swollen. This usually responds well to a few days of injectable antibiotic.

mouth. When examined, they may have a mass of partially chewed food at the front of the tongue and this needs to be removed in order to see the pus and blood associated with the diphtheria ulcer. These calves will also have a high temperature and often a foul-smelling breath. If left untreated, infection can pass down into the lungs and cause a fatal pneumonia, or into the rumen to produce digestive upsets.

*Laryngeal diphtheria*
Occasionally the larynx (voice box, Figure 2.1) is the primary site of infection. Affected calves breathe extremely noisily, a 'roaring' or 'snoring' breathing, but they are not particularly ill and their respiration rate may be normal. This syndrome should not be confused with calf pneumonia, where breathing will be quieter but faster, and the calf will be very sick.

Antibiotic therapy by injection is needed and your vet will prescribe a suitable drug. If the calf is badly affected, it needs to be fed liquids, preferably three or four times daily, and removed from the rest of the group, since it could act as a source of infection to the others. Laryngeal diphtheria is slow to respond, and may need continual antibiotic treatment for three to four weeks.

The calf in Plate 2.39 had already been given a long course of antibiotic, but the infection on its larynx was so severe that its breathing was almost totally obstructed. A tube was inserted into the trachea (an operation known as a tracheostomy) and the calf breathed through the tube until the larynx healed.

For prevention of diphtheria, avoid dirty feeding troughs and hay containing thistles or other sharp material which might damage the lining of the mouth. If there is an infected calf, make sure that it has its own bucket and does not suckle from the same teat as the other calves in the group.

## Heart Defects

Figure 2.13 shows the normal circulation of blood in the body. The heart is divided into four compartments, two atria and two ventricles. In the adult animal the left ventricle (LV) pumps blood around the body and back into the right atrium (RA). The right atrium drains into the right ventricle (RV) which then pumps blood through the lungs. From the lungs the blood returns into the left atrium (LA) and then into the left ventricle, where the whole circulation starts again.

The developing calf in the uterus has two modifications to this, shown as dotted lines in Figure 2.13:

● From its body there is a direct flow through its navel to the placenta of its mother and back again.
● Because the placenta supplies the calf with oxygen its lungs are not needed and so there is a bypass or 'shunt' mechanism whereby blood can flow directly from the right to

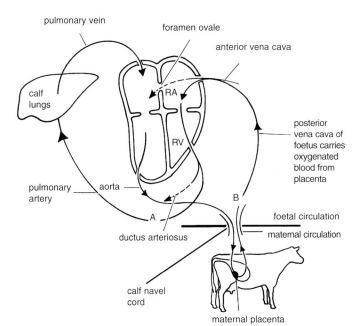

Figure 2.13. Blood circulation in the cow, showing the attachments of the placenta. Pathways indicated by the broken line apply to the developing calf only, although sometimes the foramen ovale (RA to LA) fails to close at birth.

the left atrium (RA to LA). This is called the foramen ovale.

At the point of birth the foramen ovale should close so that as soon as the calf draws its first breath, all of its blood can be pumped through its lungs to collect oxygen. Unfortunately in some calves the foramen fails to close. Insufficient blood is pumped to their lungs and they are, in effect, short of oxygen. Such calves will appear to be short of breath and they will pant and have a racing pulse after relatively mild exercise. They will also be much more susceptible to pneumonia. There is no specific treatment, although heart stimulants and antibiotics to prevent or treat the pneumonia will help. In some calves

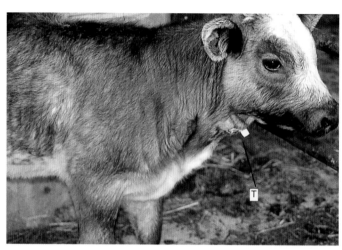

Plate 2.39. Laryngeal diphtheria. This calf had such badly obstructed breathing that a tube (T) had to be inserted into the trachea to allow airflow while the treatment was taking effect. The tube was removed two weeks later.

the foramen slowly closes and by three to six weeks old they will have fully recovered. Others remain permanently affected and become so stunted that they have to be put down.

Similar syndromes are caused by other heart defects; for instance occasionally there is an interseptal ventricular defect (a connection from LV to RV) or a patent ductus arteriosus (a blood vessel connecting the aorta (A) to the pulmonary artery (B).

*Chapter 3*

# THE WEANED CALF

Traditionally calves were weaned at almost eight weeks old, although in recent years this has been reduced to six or even five weeks old. Calves may be weaned as soon as they are eating significant quantities of concentrate, for example 1–1.5 kg per day for three consecutive days. The concentrate being offered needs to be highly palatable to achieve these intakes. Some calves are abruptly weaned, but it is more common to reduce to once-daily feeding for a few days before totally withdrawing milk. Fresh water and palatable forage (hay or straw) should be freely available throughout. The change from a liquid to a solid diet is a critical time for the calf, and to be successful it is important that pre weaning feeding has allowed the rumen to develop to its full size and that it is functioning correctly. Inadequate ruminal development before weaning can lead to many post weaning digestive problems, with bloat and scouring being the most common.

After weaning the calf needs to be given a highly nutritious diet to compensate for the loss of milk. It has probably been moved from individual pens to group housing, where it must compete with others for trough space. If the stress of this is combined with an overall reduction in nutritional status, then the calf is rendered more susceptible to disease, and this is at a time when its passive antibody levels are declining. As with the young calf, many health problems are exacerbated by poor management, and one of the most important preventive measures for all the diseases of the weaned calf is to provide adequate space, good housing and a well-balanced diet.

The following diseases of the weaned calf will be considered on the basis of their main symptoms:

**Digestive problems**
- pot-bellies
- chronic diarrhoea
- rumen bloat
- colic
- coccidiosis
- salmonellosis
- necrotic enteritis

**Respiratory problems**
- calf pneumonia

**Deficiency diseases**
- nutritional deficiencies
- muscular dystrophy

**Urolithiasis**

**Nervous diseases**
- hypomagnesaemia
- meningitis
- tetanus
- lead poisoning
- cerebrocortical necrosis (CCN)

## DIGESTIVE PROBLEMS

The rumen is very small at birth and digestion of milk takes place in the abomasum. The calf quickly learns to eat solid food and by two weeks old ruminal movements and cudding should have started. Continued development and expansion of rumen size are stimulated by propionic and butyric acids, the rumen fermentation products of the concentrate fraction of the diet. These substances also stimulate the development of papillae, small finger-like projections which increase the absorptive surface of the rumen. Rumen *movements* are stimulated by the presence of long fibre which physically 'pricks' the rumen wall. Straw is ideal for this, which is why so many farmers now rear calves on a straw and concentrate diet. The type of concentrate is important. The rumen is not fully developed until ten to twelve weeks old and so prior to this the calf is best fed fairly high levels of concentrate (2–3 kg/day) with ample high-quality protein (e.g. 20% CP). It is cost-effective to do so, because food conversion is much more efficient at the younger age, as shown in Table 3.1.

The rumen of the young calf is also much more acid than in the adult, partly due to low saliva production by the calf. This high acidity, if not checked, can depress food intake. High-quality concentrates, containing a high level of digestible fibre, are therefore needed at this stage. Only after calves are 12 weeks old, when the rumen is fully developed, can concentrate quality be reduced and greater reliance placed on forages. Feeding straw stimulates rumen contractions and promotes cudding. This in turn increases saliva flow which decreases rumen acidity. High-starch concentrates without adequate balanced fibre should be avoided as they ferment rapidly, produce acidosis and retard rumen development.

Table 3.1. Food conversion ratio (FCR) is most efficient in the young calf and deteriorates with age.

| Bodyweight | FCR |
|---|---|
| 50 kg | 2:1 |
| 100 kg | 3:1 |
| 300 kg | 5.5:1 |
| 500 kg | 8.5:1 |

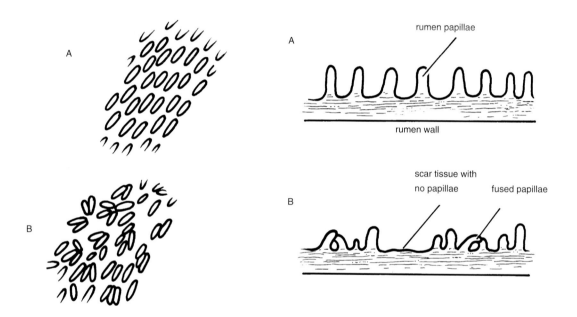

Figure 3.1. The development of the rumen wall is strongly influenced by diet:
A – normal, high fibre diet     B – high starch and no fibre

Figure 3.1. is a diagrammatic representation of the rumen wall of calves fed two different diets. Diet A was well balanced and produced good rumen papillae. Diet B was high in starch concentrates, leading to shorter papillae, some fusion of papillae and some areas so badly scarred by acidosis that they were totally devoid of papillae.

The physical form of the concentrate can also have an effect. Finely ground products (e.g. ground barley or maize) are bad because they ferment rapidly in the rumen and could cause acidosis. At the other extreme, a coarse mix is a big advantage because

- Calves eat coarse mix more slowly.
- They chew it more and in so doing produce more saliva.
- They often start eating it earlier than pellets.

Many farms feed pellets or pencils without any problems and I am certainly not recommending that everyone should change. However, if you are experiencing digestive problems like bloat or scour with your calves around weaning, I would certainly recommend changing to a coarse mix ration. This should be offered from one to two weeks of age and fed until at least one to two weeks after weaning.

One of the problems of ad lib feeding of milk, either cold or warm, is that although calf growth is very good, concentrate intake, and hence rumen development, is depressed and there is often a greater check at weaning. This is particularly the case if calves are abruptly weaned. Gradually reducing milk over the two weeks prior to weaning helps to stimulate dry food intakes and ruminal development. This can be done by putting the milk bucket much lower than the teat, by placing a constricting clip on the pipe, or simply withholding access to milk a few hours each day. All three systems encourage concentrate intakes.

## Pot-bellies

At one stage it was thought that plenty of good hay was needed to stimulate rumen development. In fact this is not true and if concentrate is restricted (for example, either in the amount given or by inadequate feeding space) and the calves have free access to unlimited supplies of palatable hay, then the rumen becomes overstretched and a pot-bellied calf may result. This is because concentrates are needed to act as 'food' for the rumen micro-organisms which digest the hay. Absence of this 'food' leads to an accumulation of very slowly digesting hay in the rumen, eaten because the calf was hungry. In fact any rumen upset or poor rumen development could result in pot-bellied calves.

## Chronic Diarrhoea

It is not uncommon to see a dark, pasty grey chronic scour in calves either just before or just after weaning. The scour often has a 'cakey' appearance, looking as though it is associated with overfeeding of concentrates. In the majority of calves it simply causes stunting and poor growth. A typical example is shown in Plate 3.1. Probably the whole group will be affected to a greater or lesser extent and although the stunting is severe, deaths are rare.

I find it a particularly difficult condition to deal with and I suspect that we do not know the true cause.

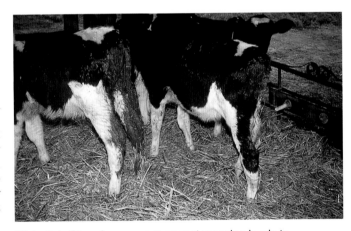

Plate 3.1. Chronic scour pre or post weaning leads to unthriftiness and, if not corrected, can even cause death.

Although digestive upsets are suspected, the rate at which the scour can pass through several groups of calves would suggest that infectious agents are also involved. One suggestion is a protozoal infection of the large bowel, precipitated by dietary upsets, very similar to colitis in pigs. However, this has yet to be proven. Group-housed calves and calves which consume large quantities of concentrates are more likely to be affected. The condition is rare in individually penned calves or calves reared in hutches.

*Treatment*
There does not seem to be an effective treatment and sometimes I wonder if it is better to let things run their course! However, I would suggest the following:

● Get your vet to test for coccidiosis, cryptosporidia and salmonella. Results are likely to be negative, but if positive, then specific treatment can be given.

- Try injecting with sulphonamides, which sometimes help.
- Badly affected calves must be taken off concentrates and put onto a generous and good-quality whole milk ration for two or three weeks; otherwise they will die. This suggests that the problem is in the rumen or large bowel and that the abomasum (where *milk* is digested) is unaffected.
- Try feeding yoghurt, for its probiotic effect (see Chapter 2). Badly affected calves seem to respond well to it.
- Change from ground concentrates to coarse mix and ensure that future batches of calves are reared on coarse mix.
- Check general feeding and husbandry procedures, especially in relation to oesophageal groove closure (see Chapter 2) and the type of concentrate and fibre being fed. The feeding of adult dairy cake to young calves is particularly dangerous, as part of the protein is likely to be indigestible for young calves.

## Rumen Bloat

The mechanics of rumen function are described in Chapter 13 and the reader should refer to that section before reading the following. Rumen bloat can be caused in three ways:

- lack of rumen movements
- oesophageal obstruction, i.e. choke
- gas produced in the rumen forming a stable foam, known as *frothy bloat*, which cannot be released

In young calves the bloat is almost always due to lack of rumen movements, technically known as rumen *atony*, although I have occasionally treated calves which have had an apple stuck in their oesophagus. Rumen atony is most commonly the result of a digestive upset and/or poor rumen development.

Some of the more common causes of bloat are:

- Oesophageal groove failure, where milk falls into the rumen, rather than passing into the abomasum. The milk sours and ferments, producing gas which cannot be released because the immature rumen does not contract. A typically affected calf is shown in Plate 2.15. This is seen mainly in young calves.
- Poor rumen development. Calves may develop bloat one to two hours after a feed of concentrates. Some may be normal again by the next feed, whereas in others the rumen stays dilated. The discomfort associated with this prevents the calf chewing the cud, or eating straw or other long fibre, and this makes the problem worse.

If there is a high incidence of bloat in your calves, check that:
- Their concentrate is not too finely ground.
- It does not contain excessive levels of starch and inadequate digestible fibre.
- Good-quality palatable straw is available at all times. This may simply mean that the calves are freshly and liberally bedded with clean straw every day, as in Plate 2.2.

*Treatment*
The treatment given must depend largely on the severity of the bloat. If it is only mild and disappears two to three hours after feeding, then putting the calf onto reduced quantities of a coarse mix may be adequate. More severely affected calves, or calves which repeatedly blow up, will need additional treatment. This could be one or more of the following, again depending on the severity of the bloat:

- Return to a whole milk diet.
- Deflate the calf with a stomach tube, trocar or needle.
- Surgically prepare a permanent rumen fistula.

**Return to a whole milk diet** Sometimes the removal of all concentrates, dosing with an oral antibiotic for three to four days (to suppress rumen fermentation) and returning the calf to a whole milk diet for two to three weeks will work. Then slowly reintroduce concentrates. This is laborious, but works well in many calves. However, a proportion continue to get blown.

**Deflate the rumen** Although many people use a needle or a trocar and cannula and mechanically puncture the calf's skin, I think that a stomach tube is the best option. It is less traumatic for the calf and carries less risk. A length of flexible 15 mm garden hosepipe will suffice, provided it does not have sharp ends. If you reverse the calf into a corner, stand beside it and hold its mouth upwards (as shown in Plate 3.2) the stomach tube can be used quite easily.

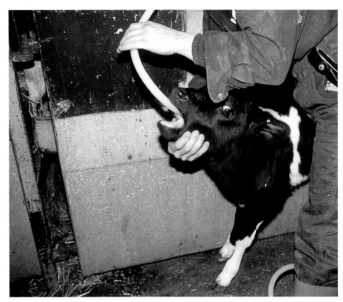

Plate 3.2. Passing a stomach tube is an easy and effective way of relieving rumen bloat.

From Figure 2.1 it can be seen that when the tube is inserted into the calf's mouth it must pass over the top of the larynx and trachea before it can be swallowed and fed down into the oesophagus. If you are in any doubt about whether the tube is in the oesophagus or the trachea, simply place your ear over the end of the tube and see if you can feel or hear air moving in and out in parallel with the breathing. If the answer is yes, the tube is in the trachea and it needs to be withdrawn and reinserted.

If a large-bore needle or trocar and cannula is to be used, it should be inserted on the *left side* of the calf, at a point mid-way between the last rib and the edge of the spine. The correct position is shown in Figure 3.2 and more details are given in Chapter 13. The needle or trocar should be pushed downwards and forwards, towards the calf's elbow on the opposite (right) side. Hold the needle or trocar in position, pushed firmly into the rumen, while the gas escapes and, if possible, at the same time squeeze the rumen by lifting it upwards with your knee to expel all the gas. Injectable antibiotic cover should be given for several days afterwards, to avoid the risk of peritonitis.

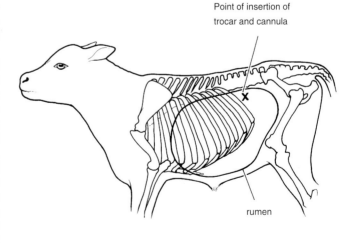

Point of insertion of trocar and cannula

rumen

Figure 3.2. The correct position for inserting a needle or a trocar and cannula is on the LEFT side, at a point in a triangle mid-way between the last rib and the spine.

**Permanent rumen fistula** For calves which repeatedly develop ruminal bloat, construction of a permanent hole, opening the rumen onto the skin wall on the left side is by far the best option. It is one of the most common operations I perform and the improvement in the calf in terms of growth and food intake is dramatic. It is a simple (and therefore inexpensive) procedure, with an almost 100% success rate.

Plate 3.3 shows a calf after the operation. Although rumen contents may spill down over the side of the calf, it usually worries the calf less than the owner! Sometimes the hole slowly closes on its own, but more often it is necessary to have it closed

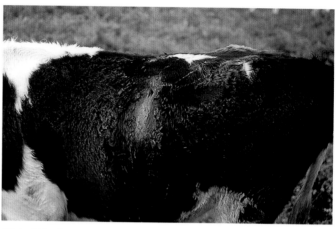

Plate 3.3. Construction of a permanent rumen fistula (a hole directly into the rumen) is the safest way to deal with a chronically bloated calf.

with sutures when the calf is 12 months old or more. Beef animals may be sold for slaughter with the hole still discharging.

## Colic

The word 'colic' simply means severe abdominal pain; it does not give any indication as to what is causing the pain. It may be due to a twisted gut or an intussusception or one of the other serious conditions discussed in Chapter 13. On occasions calves may be seen kicking at their stomachs or even rolling on the ground and bellowing with pain, due simply to a spasm, that is an excessive contraction, of the intestine. They can make a rapid recovery, less than one to two hours following the administration of drugs to relax the intestine. A similar syndrome may be seen in calves still on liquid diets.

## Coccidiosis

This is caused by small protozoan parasites, *Eimeria zurnii* and *E. bovis*, which burrow into the wall of the lower gut. Typically, affected calves pass semi-solid or very loose faeces, usually containing variable quantities of chocolate-brown blood. Scouring is a feature and the calf's tail becomes soiled, but the faeces are not as liquid as in some cases of diarrhoea in younger calves. If the faeces are examined carefully, small lumps of a fawn-coloured gelatinous material may be seen. This is the mucosa, or lining, of the intestine.

Probably the most characteristic clinical sign of coccidiosis is strain-

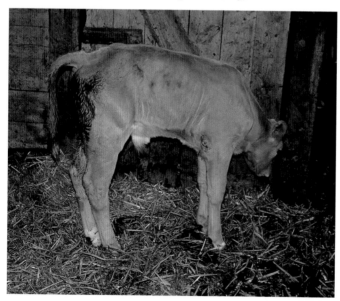

Plate 3.4. Calf continually straining due to coccidiosis. Note the raised tail, protruding rectal mucosa and bloody scour.

ing, technically known as tenesmus: the calf stands with its tail raised and appears to be continually trying to force out small quantities of blood, mucus and faeces. A typical example is shown in Plate 3.4.
After a few days the calf is dull, and it runs a moderate temperature and loses weight rapidly. Death can
occur in untreated cases. You will need your vet to confirm the diagnosis so that specific anticoccidiosis
therapy (e.g. sulphonamides, to toltrazuril or amprolium) can be given. Affected calves should be dosed
at treatment level and any in-contact animals at preventive level, because it is likely that all calves are
exposed to the same source of infection and the condition can rapidly spread. The drugs monensin and
lasalocid can be used for prevention.

*The coccidian life cycle*
This is shown in Figure 3.3. The
coccidiosis eggs or oocysts are taken
in by mouth, pass through the acid
barrier of the abomasum and hatch
out in the large intestine (the colon,
caecum and rectum), where they
invade the cells lining the gut wall.
Once inside the cell the oocyst
repeatedly divides, to produce thousands of vegetative forms, the mero-
zoites. These rupture the cell and are
liberated into the intestine to infect
and destroy adjacent healthy cells.
Resistant forms, the oocysts, are produced sexually at a later stage and are
passed out in the faeces. The oocyst
has a very thick wall and as such it
can survive in the environment for
many months, waiting to be eaten by
another calf so that its life cycle can
start again.

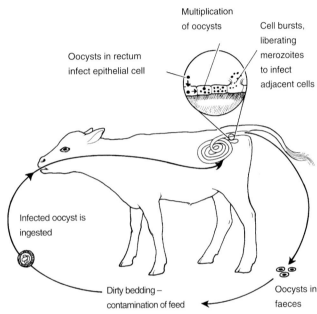

Figure 3.3. The life cycle of *Eimeria zurnii* and *E. bovis*, the
coccidiosis parasites.

The initial source of infection is
most probably the cow, since many
adult animals carry the infection at low levels without showing any symptoms. Affected calves excrete large
numbers of oocysts which can pass to their pen-mates, however. This occurs especially where hygiene is
poor and there is an increased risk of faecal contamination of the feed, for example when water and food
troughs are dirty, or inadequate bedding is used. The oocyst is an extremely resistant form and is not
affected by many of the standard disinfectants. Dirty pens should be thoroughly cleaned, washed and then
soaked with an ammonia-based product or a specific proprietary anticoccidial disinfectant, before a new
group of calves is introduced. Hygiene is important in control although the ideal way of stimulating immunity is for calves to ingest oocysts during the first few days of life when they are still receiving colostrum.

## Salmonellosis

The disease in young calves, usually involving *S. typhimurium*, has been described in Chapter 2, and the
overall problem of salmonellosis is dealt with in Chapter 11, where the wide range of other species of salmonella, called serotypes, is described. A less common type in weaned calves is *S. dublin*. Infection is
contracted from symptomless carriers (see Chapter 2), either the dam or from other calves when groups
are mixed at weaning. One of the peculiar and often frustrating aspects of *S. dublin* is that infection may
exist within the herd for several years without ever being seen as disease. When disease appears, and no
stock have been purchased, it is difficult to explain why the outbreak has occurred. In the carrier animal,
infection persists in the mesenteric lymph glands, the small 'drainage' organs associated with the intestine.

Excretion of infection, i.e. the passing of salmonella in the faeces of carrier calves, is likely to be very intermittent and may not occur at all for quite long periods. This means that it is difficult to identify carrier animals simply by taking faecal swabs and trying to isolate *S. dublin* in the laboratory. A positive result shows that infection is present and action can be taken. However, a negative result can either mean that the calf is not a carrier, or it may simply mean that the calf was not shedding infection when the swab was taken. Serial swabbing of a group of calves, e.g. at weekly intervals, would give a better chance of identifying carriers, but even then a negative result would not be conclusive proof of absence of infection.

## Clinical signs

*S. dublin* can cause scouring, and in this respect it resembles *S. typhimurium*, but it can also cause other clinical signs such as septicaemia, pneumonia, joint ill or meningitis, and these may occur without any obvious change in the faeces. The affected calf will run a high temperature in the early stages and scouring may occur, but it may not be particularly severe. Sometimes scouring is profuse, however, and lumps of intestine wall, blood and mucus are passed, viz the calf has dysentery. The calf will be dull, its coat bristling rather than smooth, its appetite reduced and there may be some coughing. On occasions a group of

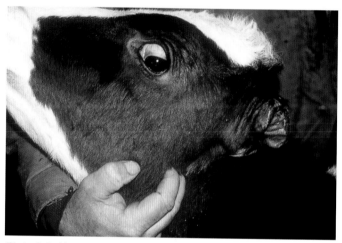

Plate 3.5. Necrosis and loss of the ear tips can follow a *Salmonella dublin* infection.

calves may simply appear unthrifty and sudden deaths occur, but following post-mortem examination and bacterial culture, salmonella can be isolated from throughout the carcase.

Some calves recovering from septicaemia develop necrosis of the extremities. The calf in Plate 3.5 had shown an unidentified illness two months previously; then its ear tips were found to be falling off. *S. dublin* was isolated from the faeces of several other calves in the group, even though many had apparently recovered fully. Two others were not so lucky. Although their ears were not affected, their feet developed necrosis and started to fall off. Obviously these calves had to be culled.

Salmonella in weaned calves is often an extension of the disease which has been present earlier in life. The acute phase is over and the calves remain unthrifty with pneumonia and/or arthritis.

*S. typhimurium* and other salmonella serotypes can also cause scour, dysentery, pneumonia and death in weaned calves.

## Treatment and control

Diagnosis is difficult and your vet will need to examine the calves and take faecal samples to the laboratory for culture. Once the presence of *S. dublin* has been confirmed, antibiotic therapy may be administered to affected calves and, whenever possible, the calves should be isolated, to reduce the weight of challenge of infection to the remainder of the group. A good dead vaccine is available, and other calves can be vaccinated to give them protection before entering the infected area.

Although antibiotics need to be given to avoid fatalities, there is now some evidence that they in fact *prolong* the period of excretion of the organism, and in so doing they reduce the chances of self-cure and increase the risk of an animal becoming a carrier. Treatment needs to be considered very carefully, therefore, since many animals will throw off the infection themselves and achieve a full cure.

*S. dublin* can infect adult cows (see Chapter 11), so careful hygiene is needed to prevent the spread of infection. When the infected group has left the building, clean out and rest as described in Chapter 2.

Ideally, soiled bedding needs to be stacked and heated to avoid pasture contamination, since it has been shown that faeces may remain infectious for up to three months even when spread onto pasture.

**Necrotic Enteritis**

This condition primarily affects home-bred single-sucked beef calves around six to eighteen weeks old. Affected calves often have bloody diarrhoea, due to the presence of ulcers throughout the intestinal tract. Ulcers may also be seen in the mouth, and necrotic enteritis can therefore be confused with BVD/mucosal disease. Most affected calves die, although fortunately the incidence in any one herd is likely to be fairly low. The cause remains unknown.

# CALF PNEUMONIA

Calf pneumonia (virus pneumonia or enzootic pneumonia) must be the most common of all the diseases of the weaned calf and it undoubtedly causes the highest losses in this age group in terms of both mortality and reduced growth rates. Pre weaned calves can also be affected, but generally they are protected by antibodies obtained from the colostrum. Passive colostral antibody levels drop significantly by two to four months old, however, and it is at this age that pneumonia starts to be seen, although it may occur in housed animals of any age, including adult dairy cows.

*Clinical signs*
Probably the first indication of the presence of pneumonia will be that a few calves have a slightly red eye and there is a clear discharge, making a wet mark over the calf's face (Plate 3.6). This should not be confused with New Forest disease or a foreign body in the eye. Both of the latter conditions produce a discharge, but they are also painful and the calf keeps its eye tightly closed. With calf pneumonia, the eye remains open.

Soon after, or maybe at the same time, coughing will be heard and the cough is generally a deep 'chesty' type, almost as if the calf is trying to bring up phlegm. Some calves may then develop a noticeably faster breathing rate, while more severely affected animals will be standing with their heads down, backs arched and breathing very heavily, finding it difficult to get enough air. The hair on their backs often stands up with a 'spiky' ungroomed appearance as in Plate 3.7, the result of sweating from a high temperature. These calves will not be eating and are likely to be standing apart from the rest of the group. Even in the early stages, affected calves may be off their food and running a high temperature (40.5–42.0°C), and sometimes acute outbreaks may occur, with fatalities, before any significant coughing has been heard.

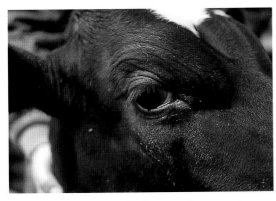

Plate 3.6. A clear eye discharge, often seen in conjunction with a reddening of the eye, may be the only indication that a respiratory infection is present.

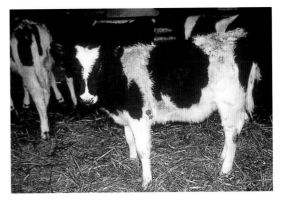

Plate 3.7. Typical 'sweating backs' of calves with pneumonia. Very rapidly growing calves may show similar dampness along their backs.

*Causes*

Calf pneumonia is known as a multiple aetiology syndrome, that is it is caused by one or more of a whole range of organisms, including bacteria, viruses and mycoplasmas. Environmental factors are also extremely important.

Some of the more commonly found infectious agents involved in pneumonia are:

**Viruses**
- respiratory syncytial virus (RSV)
- para-influenza type 3 (PI3)
- infectious bovine rhinotracheitis (IBR)
- bovine viral diarrhoea (BVD)
- coronaviruses

**Bacteria**
- *Pasteurella multocida* and *P. haemolytica*
- *Haemophilus somnus*
- *Actinomyces (Corynebacterium) pyogenes*

**Mycoplasmas**
- *Mycoplasma dispar, M. bovis*, ureaplasmas
- *Acholeplasma laidlawii*

It is almost impossible to diagnose the different causes of calf pneumonia on clinical signs alone. Swabs, blood tests or post-mortem tissues are needed for a full diagnosis. However, a few of the infectious agents have some specific properties which are worth noting. For example:

- RSV can be involved in acute outbreaks of pneumonia, leading to sudden death. The calf in Plate 3.8 was one of a group of eight calves which surprisingly developed pneumonia while outdoors. Despite treatment the calf died within 24 hours. A post-mortem examination showed the typical swollen emphysematous 'burst lung' appearance of RSV (Plate 3.9) and the virus was demonstrated in the tissues. Emphysema can sometimes be detected with a stethoscope as crackling and squeaking sounds in the chest.
- IBR can cause very red eyes (as in Plate 4.7) and a severe infection of the trachea (Plate 4.6). The disease is described in detail in Chapter 4.
- *Pasteurella haemolytica* (-especially serotypes A1 and A2) is often present in the noses of healthy cattle, and it is only

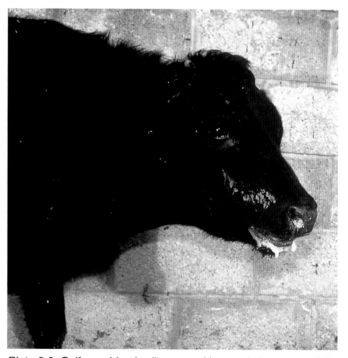

Plate 3.8. Calf coughing badly, caused by respiratory syncytial virus (RSV) infection.

when animals are stressed that it invades the lungs to cause pneumonia. Stresses include sudden temperature or other environmental changes, concurrent infection or even calving. Shipping fever is the name given to acute pasteurella pneumonia seen in cattle after a long journey. Typical signs are a high temperature, panting and appearing very sick, with minimal coughing.

However, pasteurella most commonly invades after viral infections. For example, it has been shown that the lungs are particularly susceptible to pasteurella infections for up to 30 days after an RSV infection. This is one reason why repeat treatments are commonly needed in outbreaks of calf pneumonia. It is not that the antibiotic is ineffective; it is simply because the damaged lung tissue is highly susceptible to reinfection by pasteurella living in the nasal passages. Recently pasteurella has become an increasingly common cause of acute toxic pneumonia, producing severe lung damage and even death in adult dairy cows. Toxins produced by *Pasteurella haemolytica* damage the phagocytic cells in the lungs, allowing some strains of the organism to multiply almost unchecked. It is highly probable that pasteurella would be isolated from the dark purple consolidated areas (A) of lung seen in Plate 3.10. The small remaining area of pink lung (B) is normal tissue.

- *Haemophilus somnus* may cause a 'sleepy' pneumonia.
- *Actinomyces pyogenes* produces chronic abscesses in the lung tissue, which may persist for the whole of the animal's life. Typical examples are shown in Plate 3.11.

All calves, on every farm, will be carrying some of these infectious agents, but disease occurs only when natural defences are low or when there is an excessively high load of infection in the environment. The latter is known as the atmospheric load. These two aspects will be discussed separately. Some of the points were covered in Chapter 1 in discussion of the 'balance' of disease.

*Natural defences*
The defence mechanisms of the respiratory tract are shown diagrammatically in Figure 3.4. They

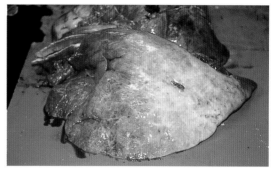

Plate 3.9. Burst lungs, typical of RSV infection. Note how the lung tissue is grossly swollen, with free air producing grey areas just under the lung surface. These are technically known as emphysematous bullae.

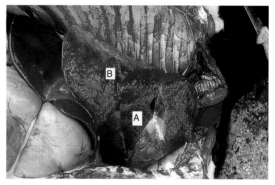

Plate 3.10. Typical lung seen in calf pneumonia. The dark consolidated areas (A) could be infected with Pasteurella, and it is unlikely that any air is flowing through this part of the lung. The pink area (B) is normal lung.

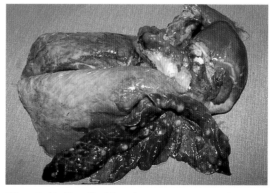

Plate 3.11. Small white abscesses scattered throughout the lung are a common consequence of inadequately treated pneumonia. They may remain with the animal for the rest of its life.

consist of

- hairs in the nose, which prevent entry of large particles
- nasal turbinate bones with a covering of mucus. The bones warm the in-coming air and the mucus traps air-borne particles
- mucus glands lining the trachea. These secrete a sticky mucus which traps particles as they swirl past in the air
- cilia, which moving in a wave-like motion, propel the mucus and any entrapped particles back up the trachea and into the mouth, from where it is either swallowed or coughed back into the environment
- alveolar macrophage cells line the terminal air sacs (respiratory alveoli) and continually patrol the area. They engulf any particles which succeed in penetrating to this depth.
- antibodies

It is only when infection has penetrated all of these defences that respiratory disease, e.g. pneumonia, occurs.

Antibodies to pneumonia organisms are obtained via the colostrum, and calves receiving inadequate colostral intakes are therefore more susceptible.

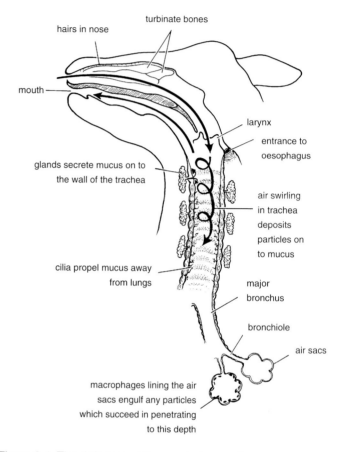

Figure 3.4. The defences of the respiratory system.

However, very high levels of infection and an unsuitable environment can overcome even good levels of immunity.

The activity of the cilia can be damaged by high levels of ammonia and other gases (e.g. from wet bedding and poor ventilation), by dust, by certain viruses and by chilling. Once lung damage has occurred, it is easier for infection to gain entry and cause pneumonia. In this state we say that the defence mechanisms have been compromised and the calf is more susceptible to disease.

*Atmospheric load*

This is the term given to the combined amount of infection and particulate matter carried in the air. Probably 99% of the different bacteria, viruses, dust and fungi present in the air could not cause disease on their own, but if present in sufficiently high numbers they overload, and therefore compromise, the calf's defences. The lung macrophages and other defence systems do not distinguish between dust, 'normal' bacteria and pathogenic bacteria and viruses. They attempt to remove all of them. Hence if the defence systems are over-loaded dealing with dust, this may allow the few disease-forming agents to cause problems. A good example of this is RSV. It is difficult to produce RSV pneumonia experimentally by infecting calves with RSV, but if the same calves are first exposed to a high level of dust, then pneumonia develops.

Outdoors there are probably only 150 particles (dust, bacteria, fungi and viruses) per cubic metre in the air, whereas in a typical enclosed calf house this can rise to 400,000 per cubic metre! Where do all these particles come from? There are several sources:

● the bedding, especially if the straw is mouldy from poor harvesting or storage
● the calf's skin
● breathed out from the calf's lungs. The mucus and cilia are a very efficient filtering system, however, and probably some 95% of all inhaled particles are retained. Infection breathed out in expired air is, therefore, not as important as we once thought

Surprisingly, the disease-causing organisms which the calf does breathe out do not live very long. For example, RSV survives for only 40–60 seconds in the air! This very short survival time for disease-causing organisms has two important consequences:

● Calves have to be in very close contact in order to pass pneumonia from one to another. This is one reason why stocking density is so important and why calves licking one another is thought to be an important way of spreading infection.
● Once a building has been depopulated, it is highly unlikely that it will retain pneumonia infections for very long.

The size of the atmospheric load at any one time (i.e. the number of particles present in the atmosphere) will depend on:

● the amount being given off by calves and bedding
● the amount being removed by
  – death of the organisms
  – sedimentation (falling to the ground)
  – inhalation by calves (and therefore filtration by mucus and cilia)
  – ventilation (carried out of the building)

Humidity is a vitally important factor for both processes. If a house is humid and the bedding is wet, far more infection will be given off from the straw. Secondly, humid air can support considerably more micro-organisms than dry air, because their death rate is lower. Increasing humidity from 60% to 90% is said to lead to a ten-fold increase in the atmospheric load. Thirdly, the high ammonia often associated with humid buildings reduces the action of cilia, leads to chilling and generally lowers the calf's defences. This is why we see far more pneumonia in damp, humid and foggy weather. In fact in one trial a sudden change from cold and dry to warm, humid conditions was the only environmental factor which precipitated disease when calves were experimentally exposed to infection.

*Prevention*
From the above, it can be seen that the quality of the calf's environment is vitally important in the prevention of pneumonia, the main factors being:

● The calf should have a warm, dry bed.
● Calf pen floors should have a slope of 1:20 to facilitate drainage.
● All surface water should be swept or drained into channels and taken out of the building
● Stocking density *must be kept low*. For example, a decrease in stocking density by 50% is equal to increasing the ventilation rate by 20 times!

The approximate target stocking densities for calves up to ten weeks old are 1.5–2 square metres per calf of floor area and 8–9 cubic metres air space. If your house only allows 1–4 cubic metres per calf, then pneumonia is almost a certainty. In the face of a pneumonia outbreak it is worth considering a reduction of the number of calves in a house. This is especially so for intensively reared calves on high concentrate diets, which breathe faster and need more air space anyway. Pneumonia sometimes occurs in outdoor calves, especially in large groups during hot weather. This is thought to be because the calves lie quite close to one another in a group and this allows the rapid spread of infection from one calf to the next. If faced with an outbreak of pneumonia in a large group of calves, whether housed or outdoors, it is a good idea to subdivide them into smaller groups, ideally in separate air spaces, to reduce both the severity and the rate of spread of infection.

- Provide adequate ventilation but freedom from draughts. The lying area for calves should have a wind-speed barely detectable on your face (this is approximately 0.2 metre per second). Provided that calves have a dry bed and are free from draughts, temperature is not too important, particularly for weaned calves. Given the option, many calves will lie outside even on quite cold days, which is why I think that open-fronted, naturally ventilated, mono-pitch buildings are ideal housing.

> **Some important factors in the prevention of calf pneumonia**
>
> - minimise dust (including moulds)
> - ensure adequate ventilation, which
>   - removes dust and noxious gases
>   - removes respiratory pathogens
>   - reduces humidity
> - ensure a dry bed, which
>   - reduces chilling
>   - reduces noxious gases
>   - improves humidity
> - avoid mixing
>   - differing age groups
>   - animals from different sources
> - minimise
>   - group size and stocking density
>   - stress and intercurrent disease
> - maximise immunity
>   - colostrum
>   - vaccination
> - medicate with antibiotics
>   - inject whole group when 20% are affected
>   - put into milk for pre weaned calves

- Regularly clean out the shed, for example, every four to six weeks, depending on the number of calves present. If the straw bedding is allowed to build up and compost, this will have several effects:
  - it may significantly decrease the air space in the building.
  - it produces ammonia and other noxious gasses which reduce the effectiveness of the calf's respiratory defence mechanisms.
  - it generates warmth and humidity, both of which favour the survival of bacteria and viruses in the air and both of which make calves uncomfortable.
- Avoid mixing calves from different sources, since they may well be carrying different infections and have differing levels of antibody protection (see Figure 1.6).
- Avoid mixing different age groups, as they will have different antibody levels. In this context mixing means sharing the same air space.
- Straw used for food or bedding should be free of moulds and stored under cover.

*Treatment*

The first factor one should consider when faced with a group of coughing calves is whether any treatment is necessary. If coughing and eye discharge are the only symptoms, all the calves are eating and none have a significantly elevated temperature, I would not treat. The infection should spread and the calves should develop their own active immunity without any disease. On the other hand, if a proportion are panting, off their food and have elevated temperatures, I would treat the whole group.

- Isolate individually sick calves. Not only is this good nursing which aids recovery, but it also reduces the challenge dose for other calves.
- Give medication. Although mainly used for treatment, antibiotic medication of a whole group of calves will reduce the spread of bacterial causes of pneumonia and decrease the effects of viral agents. Antibiotics may be given:

– as long-acting injections for older calves
– in the milk of pre weaned calves, because milk passes directly into the abomasum

It is best not to give oral antibiotics to weaned animals as they may interfere with rumen function, although there are some exceptions to this.

Antibiotics only provide protection during their period of activity. They do not give the longer term protection given by vaccines. Some of the newer antibiotics reach high concentrations in the lungs and are particularly effective against pneumonia. Tilmicosin is especially interesting. It reaches high concentrations in lung tissue, it is effective against bacteria and mycoplasmas, it decreases toxin production and a single injection gives five days of 'bacterial killing' in lung fluid, followed by two to three weeks of antibiotic persistence in the lung macrophages, the bacterial killing cells (see Chapter 1 and Figure 3.4). As lung damage from RSV will render the lungs susceptible to infection for the next 30 days (see previous section), this degree of persistence is ideal.

New products are being developed all the time and your vet will advise you on the most suitable drug for your circumstances. Remember also that antibiotics do not have any effect against viruses. Treating the whole group may help to lower the overall level of bacteria and mycoplasmas in the environment to the extent that the calf's own defences will then be able to cope with the reduced challenge and develop an immunity.

Severely ill animals will need respiratory stimulants, anti-inflammatory drugs and other supportive therapy, and veterinary attention should be sought for these. Others may develop chronic lung infections, leading to poor growth and intermittent bouts of pneumonia for weeks after the initial outbreak. I have found prolonged antibiotic cover to be well worthwhile in such cases; for example giving daily antibiotic or a long-acting penicillin or tetracycline injection twice weekly for three weeks or more. It eventually worked on the Charolais heifer in Plate 3.12.

*Vaccination*
This is a complex area and definitely needs veterinary advice. The type of infection involved in a particular pneumonia outbreak can be assessed by:

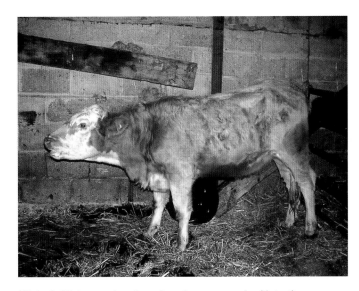

- nasal swabs
- tissue from calves which have died
- blood samples taken when the calf is first affected and again two to three weeks later, looking for a rising antibody titre (see Chapter 1). Unfortunately in calves less than four months old, the presence of colostral antibodies may interfere with the interpretation of results.

Good live intranasal vaccines are available against IBR and PI3 and a live intramuscular vaccine for RSV. These are the three most common causes of pneumonia. IBR and PI3 vaccines are temperature attenuated strains, i.e. the virus can multiply in the lower temperatures of the nose (and this stimulates the calf to develop an immunity), but the normal

Plate 3.12. Long-standing chronic pneumonia. Note the open mouth breathing as this Charolais heifer fights for breath. A three-week course of antibiotic by injection eventually produced a cure.

body temperature of the calf's lungs inhibits growth of the vaccine and so disease cannot develop. With a special applicator, 2 ml of the vaccine is sprayed into the animal's nose (Plate 3.13). There is also evidence that these vaccines stimulate the production of interferon and as such can be used during an outbreak of pneumonia to give protection against a whole range of viruses.

## DEFICIENCY DISEASES

Because growing animals generally have a higher requirement than adults for minerals, vitamins and trace elements, it is in this age group that nutritional deficiencies are most likely to be seen. Weaned calves are

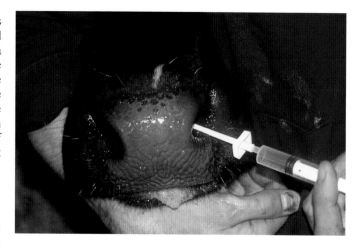

Plate 3.13. Administering an intranasal vaccine, for example against IBR or PI3 viruses. The applicator on the syringe produces a spraying effect.

normally reared indoors on a forage and concentrate diet, and problems may occur towards the end of the winter, especially when feeding and management are poor. The mineral and vitamin requirements of the animal and the effects of the various deficiencies are given in detail in Chapter 12, and in this section I shall be dealing with only one of the slightly unusual deficiencies, that is muscular dystrophy or white muscle disease. CCN, which is an induced deficiency, is listed under nervous diseases later in this chapter. Deficiencies of copper and vitamin A are common in calves and dealt with in Chapter 12.

### Muscular Dystrophy (White Muscle Disease)

The name muscular dystrophy means 'abnormal development and function of the muscles' and it is a muscular abnormality which causes the clinical signs and the white areas seen in the muscles at post-mortem. Disease generally occurs at turnout in the spring and can be precipitated by the stress of bad weather. Calves which have been fed rations containing inadequate levels of vitamin E and/or

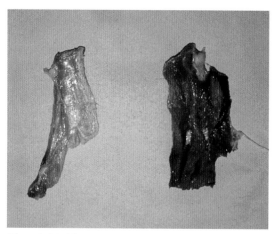

Plate 3.14. Muscular dystrophy caused by a deficiency of vitamin E and/or selenium. The dark-coloured muscle on the right is normal.

selenium during the winter develop muscles which are weak and have areas of degeneration. Often no clinical signs are seen indoors, where the calves are relatively inactive. A few days after turnout, however, when they have been running around, a stiffness of gait may be noticed, with the legs unusually rigid. Some animals may be so badly affected that they become recumbent, while others may be found dead from heart failure, the heart muscle having degenerated. Muscle degeneration leads to release of the pigment myoglobin and this is occasionally seen as a red discolouration in the urine. If the chest muscles are involved there will be difficulty in breathing and affected calves may appear to have pneumonia.

Plate 3.14 shows a piece of pale, white muscle (left) taken from a calf which died from muscular dystrophy, compared with a normal coloured piece of muscle on the right. In addition to being very pale, the affected muscle has a 'gritty' appearance, due to precipitation of calcium. Only very limited areas of the carcase will be affected and so it is essential that a thorough post-mortem is carried out. Blood samples from live, affected calves can be tested for selenium, vitamin E or muscle degeneration to assist in the diagnosis. Occasional animals exhibit what is known as the 'flying scapula' effect. The muscle attachment between the shoulder blades and the chest degenerates, the spine drops and the shoulder blades start to protrude above the backbone, as shown in Figure 3.5.

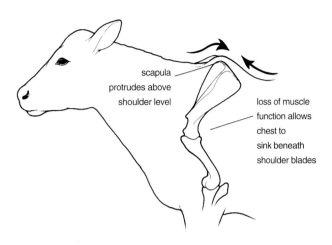

Figure 3.5. 'Flying scapula'. Degeneration of the muscle attachment between the shoulder blades and chest leads to the shoulder blades protruding over the spine.

*Occurrence*

With improvements in testing procedures for selenium and vitamin E, surveys have shown that deficiency is very common. Deficiency does not always seem to be associated with disease, however, and the cost benefits of treatment must be carefully evaluated before embarking on any control programme. Traditionally disease occurred in beef suckler herds which had been over-wintered on a diet of straw and turnips. Many pastures have now been found to be deficient, however. Table 3.2 gives an idea of the feedingstuffs which are good or bad sources of vitamin E.

Table 3.2. Some dietary sources of vitamin E.

| *Good* | *Average* | *Poor* |
|---|---|---|
| Grass and dried grass | Cereal grains | Poor hay |
| | Maize silage | Straw |
| Grass silage | Good hay | Root crops |
| Kale | Brewer's grains | |

Total dietary selenium requirement = 0.1 ppm in dry matter.

*Vitamin E and selenium*

Although they are two totally unrelated chemicals, they act on similar mechanisms (involved with the metabolism of unsaturated fatty acids) within the animal. In intensively fed animals, an increase in the oil content of the concentrate, and particularly in the proportion of unsaturated fatty acids in the oil, leads to an increase in the vitamin E requirement. Animals with a marginal selenium status can be precipitated into disease by vitamin E deficiency and vice versa. Selenium deficiency is closely related to soil type and hence all crops grown in certain areas may be deficient. On the other hand, vitamin E levels are more related to the type of plant, its stage of growth and the method of conservation. For example, vitamin E levels are very low in hay which has been badly weathered in its making and in grain which has been stored using propionic acid as a preservative.

*Treatment and control*

This is an area where you will undoubtedly need veterinary advice, since an excess of selenium is extremely toxic. There is a wide range of possible courses of action, however. For example:

● Inject a selenium/vitamin E preparation. This is essential in the treatment of affected animals to achieve a rapid effect. A long-acting product is also available as a control measure.

- Selenium bullets. These are given by mouth and slowly dissolve in the reticulum. A variety of products are available, some containing selenium only and others combined with additional trace elements such as copper and cobalt. Consult the manufacturer's instructions for dosage rates.
- Add sodium selenite to the ration to produce a final dietary concentration of 0.1 ppm. This is an extremely low level however, only one-tenth of a gram in one ton of mix, and it is impossible to achieve an even distribution of selenium unless specialist mixing facilities are available.
- Water-soluble preparations are available, which can be placed in the drinking water and slowly dissolve at a specified rate to provide the animal's selenium requirement. One such system is known as Aquatrace. The pellets are formulated so that when the selenium concentration in the water reaches a level which will satisfy the animal's requirements, no further selenium will dissolve. If some of the water is drunk, fresh water flows into the tank, the selenium concentration falls and this then permits more pellets to dissolve.

## Tendon Rupture

Not all calves which go lame immediately after turnout have white muscle disease. Plate 3.15 is a good example. This nervous Limousin heifer ran wildly around the field for three to four hours when first turned out, eventually stopping because of exhaustion. The next day her lower limbs were badly swollen and her fetlocks drooped towards the ground – in fact the fetlocks were almost resting on the ground. Although a blood sample would show severe muscle damage, her vitamin E and selenium status was normal. She was simply suffering from tendon rupture associated with gross over-exercise. She was returned to the farm and kept in a loose-box with plenty of feed, but took three to four months to recover.

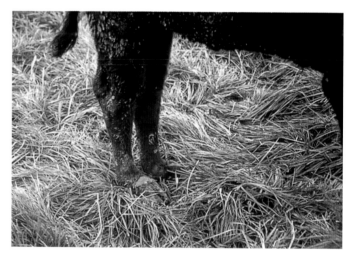

Plate 3.15. Tendon rupture, caused by excessive exercise at turnout, led to the fetlock collapsing onto the ground.

I have seen the same syndrome several times. On another occasion a group of calves were repeatedly chased around a field by a donkey when they were turned out!

## NERVOUS DISEASES

There are several diseases which can produce nervous signs in calves and these include lead poisoning, cerebrocortical necrosis (CCN), meningitis, tetanus and hypomagnesaemia.

Hypomagnesaemia can occur in milk-fed or suckler calves of three to six months old where little or no supplementary concentrates are being fed, and it may produce sudden death or nervous signs. Milk is a poor source of magnesium and any reserves in the skeleton are quite quickly depleted. Hypomagnesaemia in calves occasionally results from scouring or from excessive drenching with liquid paraffin, both of which prevent the absorption of magnesium from the gut. Further details of hypomagnesaemia are given in Chapter 6.

Meningitis is caused by a wide range of different infectious agents, but as it is most commonly seen in the young calf it is discussed in Chapter 2.

Tetanus is the least likely of the disorders. Of the few cases I have seen, one was the result of a rubber castration band being applied to an excessively large calf. Tetanus then developed in the necrotic stump.

The clinical signs and methods of control are similar to those for adult animals and are dealt with in Chapter 4.

## Lead Poisoning

Lead is still the most common cause of poisoning in farm animals and it is usually young calves or heifers which are affected, probably because of their inquisitive nature and tendency to lick and chew at unusual objects. There are several possible sources of lead, the most common being paint. Old doors are still used in the construction of calf pens. This is extremely dangerous, since old paint invariably contains large quantities of lead and calves tend to chew at woodwork. The door shown in Plate 3.16 was the cause of lead poisoning in a Gloucester suckler calf. Although the condition was diagnosed and treatment given, the calf did not recover.

Other possible sources of lead include:

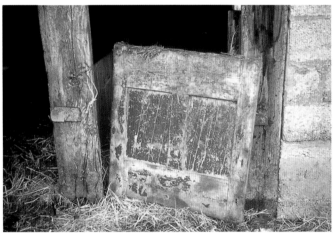

Plate 3.16. The paint from this old door was the source of lead for a Gloucester calf, which eventually died from lead poisoning.

- putty and traditional 'liniment' or 'white lotion'
- golf balls and lead shot
- lead plates from batteries (Plate 3.17)
- pasture contamination, e.g. beside motorways (from petrol), near lead mines and from certain types of industrial workings. The latter are now very carefully controlled.
- contaminated food. In 1989 a batch of lead-contaminated rice bran became incorporated into compound animal feed and was quite widely sold to farms in the south-west of England. There was an outbreak of animals showing signs of lead poisoning, but perhaps economically more significant was the fact that Food Safety legislation was brought into operation. This prohibited the sale of milk or beef from those herds which had consumed the food until blood levels of lead in the affected animals had fallen to below acceptable values. Some herds were unable to sell stock for several months. Not surprisingly, the compensation claims were enormous!

*Clinical signs*
The signs of the disease vary, depending on whether there has been a high intake of lead over a short period (acute poisoning), or a lower intake over a more prolonged period

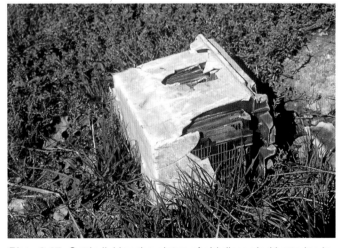

Plate 3.17. Cattle licking the plates of old discarded batteries is another common cause of lead poisoning.

(chronic poisoning). Acute poisoning is more common and calves may show symptoms a few days after eating the lead. The affected animal is blind and experiences periods of extreme excitement, bellowing, frothing from the mouth and trying to run up the wall. Quiet periods may follow, when the calf stands almost motionless, often pushing its head into a corner or against the feeding trough. It stops eating, it will probably be constipated and it may run a temperature. Death may occur in as little as one to three hours after the onset of symptoms, with the calf finally lying on its side, kicking with its legs and bellowing, as if it has severe abdominal pain.

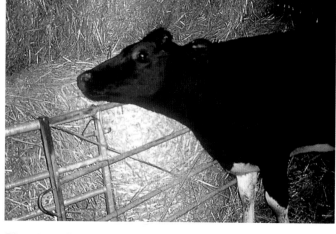

Plate 3.18. Chronic lead poisoning. Some animals are dull and simply push their head against a wall, as in this case. Acute poisoning produces more violent nervous signs.

Chronic lead poisoning produces a dull animal, which may be reluctant to move or simply stands pushing its head against a wall or bales of straw, as in Plate 3.18. This is probably a sign of a severe headache.

*Treatment*

Lead poisoning is a serious condition and you should consult your veterinary surgeon if you suspect it. He will most probably take blood and dung samples to confirm the diagnosis and then administer calcium disodium versenate by intravenous injection. This chemical combines with the lead in the animal's blood, producing an inert form which is readily excreted from the body. The affected calf, and the others in the group, should be given 100 g of magnesium sulphate (Epsom salts) by mouth. This has the double action of producing insoluble lead sulphate in the gut, thus reducing the rate of lead absorption and also acting as a purgative to quickly carry ingested lead out of the intestine. All possible sources of lead should be carefully considered and removed.

## Cerebrocortical Necrosis (CCN) or Polioencephalomalacia (PEM)

The name means degeneration of the grey matter of the brain. Disease can occur in any age of calf, although it is most commonly seen at three to nine months old and especially in housed calves on a fairly high concentrate diet. The cause is an infection by two bacteria, *Bacillus thiaminolyticus* and *Clostridium sporogenes*, both of which live in the rumen and produce a substance, thiaminase, which destroys thiamine (vitamin B1). Although there is plenty of thiamine in the rumen initially (partly from the diet and partly from thiamine-producing bacteria), with CCN large quantities are destroyed before it can be absorbed and thiamine deficiency results.

Thiamine is needed for the manufacture of glucose, and as glucose is essential for brain function, lack of thiamine leads indirectly to degeneration of the grey matter in the brain. CCN is most commonly seen on low fibre/high concentrate diets. Not only do these diets produce an acid rumen, which favours the growth of *B. thiaminolyticus* and *Cl. sporogenes*, but they also increase the requirement for thiamine in ruminal metabolism.

There are other syndromes in calves which produce almost identical polioencephalomalacia changes in the brain and similar nervous signs. These include:

● bracken poisoning. Bracken contains thiaminase
● molasses toxicity, due to decreased propionate levels in the rumen and consequently low glucose

- water deprivation, especially if it is combined with high sodium and/or sulphate intakes, e.g. brackish water.
- lead poisoning
- sulphate toxicity. Ammonium sulphate has been incorporated into animal feedingstuffs at 0.5% to prevent urolithiasis. If high levels are fed, toxicity, seen as a form of CCN, has been reported. Ammonium chloride is now more commonly used and is safer, although it is more expensive

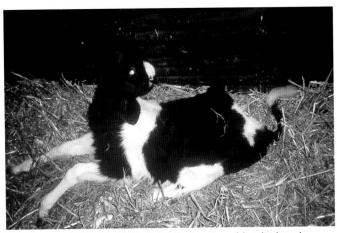

Plate 3.19. Calf with CCN. It is blind and pushing its head backwards.

*Clinical signs*

Blindness is a common clinical sign and the affected calf tends to wander around the pen with its head held up and nose forward, often walking into things. Its temperature will probably be normal, although it may stop eating and soon develop a very hollow appearance. If the disease is allowed to progress, the calf becomes recumbent, often with its head pushed over its back, as in Plate 3.19. This is known as opisthotonos. Eventually the animal rolls onto its side and may die following bouts of kicking and struggling.

*Treatment and prevention*

Treatment consists of giving large doses of thiamine and it is surprising how quickly quite severely affected calves recover. The first dose will most probably be administered by your veterinary surgeon as an intravenous injection, to obtain rapid action. He may use a multivitamin complex or a simple thiamine solution. If several cases have occurred in a group of calves, it may be worth supplementing their ration with thiamine-rich sources, e.g. 60 g of brewer's yeast per calf per day, or 20–30 mg of synthetic thiamine per kilogram of concentrate, although it has been suggested that feeding additional thiamine simply encourages the proliferation of *B. thiaminolyticus* and *Cl. sporogenes* and makes the situation worse. Sometimes CCN is preceded by, or associated with, a bout of scouring. As diets leading to an acid rumen may be involved, sodium bicarbonate added to the concentrate at 1.5–2% or the addition of chopped straw to the concentrate may be useful preventive measures.

## UROLITHIASIS (BLADDER STONES)

Calculi are small stones of calcium or magnesium ammonium phosphate which form in the urine in the bladder. They cause few problems in the bladder, but when they pass out of the bladder into the urethra they may cause a blockage.

Because of the longer length and smaller internal diameter of their urethra, it is usually only males which are affected and castrates more commonly than entire males. The most common point of blockage is at the sigmoid flexure of the penis, just above the scrotum (Figure 3.6). Initially the calf will stand apart from the others, not eating and disinclined to move. With a grossly distended bladder, the symptoms are not too surprising! At this stage the condition is difficult to diagnose. Later the penile urethra may rupture at the point of impaction of the calculi and the urine flows out and collects under the skin to form a large swelling, as in Plate 3.20. Note the dry crystals on the hairs of his prepuce, which are effectively 'external' calculi.

*Treatment*

The only treatment option is surgical. A new opening for the penis is created above the scrotum. Unfortunately the skin covering the urine swelling often drops off and recovery is then very slow.

Sometimes the bladder ruptures before the urethra. The calf then dies.

*Prevention*
Various dietary measures are available and these will reduce the likelihood of calculi forming. These include:

- Ensure the correct dietary ratio of calcium to phosphorus, especially avoiding excessive phosphorus intakes.
- Avoid excess dietary magnesium. No more than 200ppm should be added to the diet. (Magnesium is added to prevent hypomagnesaemia in milk-fed calves.)
- Add urinary acidifiers, e.g. ammonium chloride or ammonium sulphate to the ration (but note that excess ammonium sulphate can cause CCN).
- Ensure there is adequate and *easy* access to a plentiful supply of fresh, *clean* water. Some people suggest adding salt to the ration to encourage even further water consumption, thereby diluting the urine and decreasing the risk of urinary calculi.

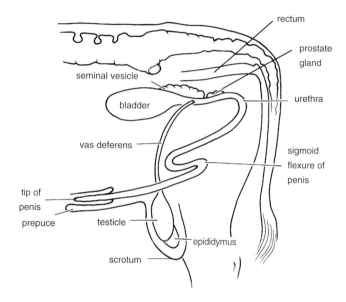

Figure 3.6. The diagram shows the urinary and genital organs of a bull. Calculi can cause a blockage of the penis at the sigmoid flexure, just above the scrotum.

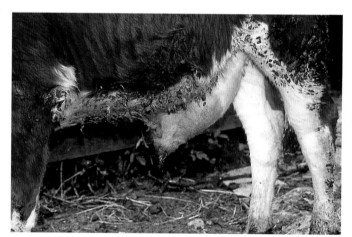

Plate 3.20. Urolithiasis. Note the swelling caused by rupture of the penis and accumulation of fluid under the skin. There are dry crystals on the hairs of the prepuce.

# Chapter 4

# REARING DAIRY HEIFERS

For profitable heifer rearing, the age of calving needs to be decided well in advance. It is now common practice to calve heifers in batches and if at all possible growth rates should be adjusted to ensure that the animals in a batch are all approximately the same weight at calving. Generally the faster-growing animal is more efficient, because a smaller proportion of its food is used for maintenance and a greater proportion for growth. It is for this reason that the two-year-old calving heifer is now very common. The age of puberty is also affected by growth rate, with well-fed animals showing their first oestrus as early as nine to twelve months old. Approximate targets for growth are given in Table 4.1.

These targets are for standard crossbred Holstein–Friesian heifers. Clearly the larger, pure-bred Holstein will be heavier. As an approximate guide, the growth rate should be the mature bodyweight in grams per day, so a Holstein cow with a mature bodyweight of 700 kg needs to grow at 700 g per day to achieve two-year calving.

To achieve high growth rates such as these, a high protein diet is essential throughout the rearing period. Calves should be weaned off milk, eating 1–1.5 kg of a 20–22% crude protein concentrate, reducing to an 18–20% rearing ration, depending on the forage on offer. Even if grass silage quality is high, protein intakes need to be maintained at 17–18%, perhaps increasing to 18–20% immediately pre calving, once again to avoid excessive deposits of fat. If protein intakes are maintained at 18–20% in the total diet, then high liveweight gains can be achieved without the risk of heifers getting overfat.

Table 4.1. Growth targets for Holstein–Friesian cross heifers calving at two years old.

| Age | Target wt (kg) | Daily gain (g/day) | Height at withers (cm) |
|---|---|---|---|
| Birth | 45 | 550 | |
| Weaning (6w) | 65 | 550 | |
| 4 months | 115 | 750 | 100 |
| Puberty (11 m) | 280 | 750 | |
| Service (15 m) | 375 | 820[1] | 130 |
| Pre calving (24 m) | 580 | 720[2] | 142 |
| Mature cow | 660 | | |

[1]Higher growth rates are sometimes recommended for the period 6 weeks before to 6 weeks after service.
[2]Growth rates may have to be reduced to around 600 g/day for the final 3–4 weeks before calving to avoid overfat heifers.

Probably the worst approach is to stunt growth during the early rearing period by inadequate feeding, poor housing, poor disease control or poor pasture management, then overfeeding in later pregnancy to try to compensate. This will produce overfat heifers with an increased risk of calving problems and early lactation metabolic disorders. An increasing number of people now rear their heifers entirely indoors on a straw and concentrate regime. This certainly gives good control of growth and enables targets to be achieved. However, it does mean that the heifers have no immunity to lungworms and intestinal worms when they first join the grazing dairy herd and this can cause complications.

Another good growth target is height at the withers (Table 4.1). A well-grown Holstein–Friesian heifer will be around 130 cm withers height at the time of service, with the Friesian animals slightly less.

There are many different types of management and feeding systems for rearing. The most important factor is to decide on a policy and then adhere to it. As general guidelines, the following points are important:

- Excessive growth rates in the early rearing period, particularly prior to puberty, can be detrimental. Overfeeding of energy may limit protein intakes and this can depress secretion of growth hormones.

Excess fat is then deposited in the udder and this in turn suppresses development of the milk-producing secretory portion of the mammary gland. Concentrate intakes should be restricted after three months of age to avoid this. Reduced concentrate intakes also encourage increased forage consumption and this may make the heifer a more efficient eater and converter of roughage.

● For optimum conception rates, heifers need to be above a certain minimum size (Table 4.1) and *gaining weight* at around 0.8 kg/day at the time of service. To achieve this, supplementary feeding with 2.0 kg concentrates will probably be necessary, particularly if conserved forage is being fed. Further details of service regimes and the advantages of batch calving heifers are given in Chapter 5.

● Underfeeding during pregnancy, leading to low maternal bodyweight at calving, will depress yields. In a survey of Holstein– Friesian heifers calving at two years old, Drew (1988) showed that heavier heifers at calving gave significantly higher yields:

| Weight of heifer at calving | 1st lactation, 305 day milk yield |
|---|---|
| <480 kg | 4278 litres |
| 480–520 kg | 4578 litres |
| >520 kg | 4770 litres |

However, although the three-year-old calver may produce more milk in her first lactation, numerous trials have shown that the two-year calver is more efficient and will produce 20% more milk per day of her lifetime (see Table 8.5). Three-year calvers tend to be fatter and experience more calving problems. On the other hand, heifers calving at less than 23 months old are not sufficiently mature, may be bullied, and will give reduced yields irrespective of their bodyweight and condition.

● Weight gains in the last two to three months of pregnancy should be moderate only. Since the majority of the bodyweight of the calf is laid down in late pregnancy, some increase in feeding will be required. A high-protein, moderate energy ration, with ample access to good-quality forage, should be given to avoid laying down excess fat. Excessive fat deposited around the inside of the pelvis can lead to serious calving problems (see Chapter 5).

● When a heifer has calved at two years old she is then both a growing and a lactating animal, and feeding levels should be adjusted accordingly. If she does not reach her full mature size, total lifetime production will suffer and many of the advantages of calving at two years old will be lost.

The achievement of reasonable growth rates depends on adequate feeding, full utilisation of the feed and minimising the effects of disease. Disease contracted during rearing can have great carryover effects on longevity and total lifetime production. Problems of the young calf and the post weaning animal have been described in Chapters 2 and 3. Now we can turn our attention to the diseases which are encountered in the first grazing season, the second winter indoors and miscellaneous conditions of the second grazing season leading up to calving.

Many of the diseases affecting the growing heifer cause few symptoms apart from reduced growth rates and failure to thrive, and this means that it is even more important to be aware of the weight targets for specific ages of animal. The growing heifer is often a grazing animal, and if she receives little or no concentrate supplements she will be particularly susceptible to deficiency diseases. This is especially true during her second grazing season when she will have the requirements of pregnancy added to her needs for growth. Some of the more common causes of failure to thrive are listed below.

Some of these conditions have already been dealt with, and others (for example liver fluke and deficiency diseases) are included in later sections. In this chapter I shall be discussing ostertagia and lungworm, a number of viral conditions, eye problems and the clostridial diseases.

## Common Causes of Failure to Thrive

**Parasites**
- *Ostertagia* = stomach worm
- *Dictyocaulus* = lungworm
- *Fasciola hepatica* = liver fluke
- ticks and tick-borne disease
(redwater and tick fever)

**Trace element deficiencies**
- copper
- cobalt
- selenium/vitamin E

**Inadequate feed levels and poor housing**
A very common cause of poor growth
but not discussed in this section.

There will, of course, be many other diseases affecting heifers where failure to thrive is not the main symptom. Examples include:

**Virus infections**
- IBR, infectious bovine rhinotracheitis
- BVD, bovine viral diarrhoea
- MCF, malignant catarrhal fever

**Clostridial diseases**
- tetanus
- blackleg
- black disease and botulism

**Udder problems**
- summer mastitis
- teat warts

**Eye problems**
- New Forest eye
- other causes of damage

**Conditions of the mouth**
- tooth abscesses
- lumpy jaw
- wooden tongue

**Skin conditions**
- ringworm
- mange
- lice
- photosensitisation

# STOMACH AND INTESTINAL WORMS

Although there are some 18 species of stomach and intestinal worms in Great Britain, relatively few cause disease and those which do follow a similar life cycle. By far the most important worm is *Ostertagia ostertagi* and this is discussed in detail. *Nematodirus* can be a problem in lambs and occasionally causes disease in early spring and late autumn grazing calves. *Cooperia oncophora* may cause disease on its own, especially later in the grazing season, and also in second season grazing cattle. This suggests that development of immunity to this worm may be poor. Depressed weight gains of up to 50% have been reported for heavy infestations, so if grazing calves appear unthrifty in the autumn, consider dosing. Probably the main effect of *Cooperia* is that moderate infections may exacerbate the adverse effects of *Ostertagia*. Significant worm infestations, that is enough to retard growth, are a problem of grazing cattle only. Calves which are housed, even if they are fed grazing or conserved forage, will not be affected.

## Ostertagia

The adult worm lives in the abomasum and lays eggs which pass out in the faeces (see Figure 4.1). The eggs have small larvae developing inside them and after a period of time they hatch, releasing the third-stage larvae, $L_3$. Under suitable conditions the $L_3$ swim up blades of grass in a film of moisture and remain there ready to be eaten by grazing animals. This migration from the dung pat to grass occurs best in warm, wet conditions. Once eaten, the $L_3$ burrows into one of the gastric glands lining the wall of the abomasum and here it feeds and grows (Figure 4.2) and develops into an adult. As an adult it emerges into the abomasum and begins to lay eggs. The period between eating the $L_3$ on pasture, and eggs appearing again in the faeces, is three weeks.

## Clinical signs

Disease is the result of the damage caused by the developing worms in the gastric glands of the abomasum. The gastric glands produce hydrochloric acid and the enzyme pepsinogen, both of which are essential for protein digestion. Following ostertagia infestation there is less acid produced, the pH of the abomasum rises, protein digestion is impaired and this is seen clinically as scouring. Mildly affected calves may have only semi-solid dung and this may be difficult to detect in animals on lush grazing. As the condition progresses, however, the scouring becomes profuse, watery and bright green, and calves lose weight rapidly. Severely affected animals may show a fluid swelling under the chin ('bottle jaw'), which is in fact oedema (dropsy) caused by the protein lost in the scour. Death is not common, the main symptoms being weight loss due to impaired digestion and subsequent growth retardation.

In the northern hemisphere, disease from type I ostertagia (the development of recently ingested larvae) is seen from July until October. Type II disease (the sudden development of arrested larvae) is much more acute, and it occurs in February/March the following year.

To understand why this occurs and how to control outbreaks we must look carefully at the life cycle.

## Type I ostertagiasis

Start with calves turned out in mid April onto a pasture which is contaminated with $L_3$ (see Figures 4.1 and 4.3). The infective $L_3$ are eaten with the grass, they develop into adults in the abomasum and begin to lay eggs some three weeks later, that is in early May. The rate of development and

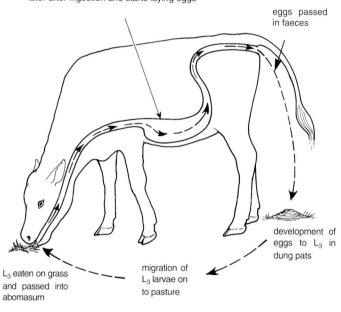

L₃ enters gastric glands in abomasal wall and develops to L₄, L₅ and then on to an adult. It emerges 3 weeks later after ingestion and starts laying eggs

eggs passed in faeces

development of eggs to $L_3$ in dung pats

migration of $L_3$ larvae on to pasture

$L_3$ eaten on grass and passed into abomasum

Figure 4.1. Life cycle of a stomach worm, *Ostertagia ostertagi.*

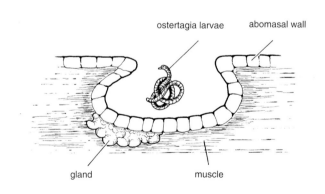

ostertagia larvae          abomasal wall

gland                muscle

Figure 4.2. Ostertagia larvae developing $L_3$ to $L_4$ in gastric gland in the abomasum.

hatching of these eggs depends on temperature, so that eggs deposited on the pasture in April and May take several weeks to develop, while those passed in the warmer midsummer months complete the transition to infective $L_3$ in only two weeks. Consequently all the eggs passed in the dung from May onwards develop at approximately the same time, namely mid July, and this can produce a massive increase in the level of herbage $L_3$ infestation. The calves are now eating the $L_3$ which developed from the eggs which

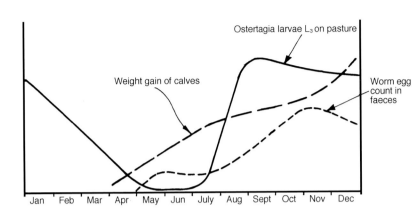

Figure 4.3. The pattern of summer ostertagia infection. Overwintered $L_3$ are the primary source of infection, and these are present on pasture until mid June. Disease is caused by the secondary wave of $L_3$ produced in July.

they themselves passed earlier in the summer, and this massive increase in the challenge dose may be sufficient to produce disease. Even where clinical symptoms are not seen, the worm burden may be sufficient to reduce weight gains (see Figure 4.3).

Towards the end of the grazing season an immunity develops. This has the effect of restricting the life of the adult worm to approximately one month and hence only moderate worm burdens are then likely to be carried. This feature has two important consequences. Firstly if calves are moved to and maintained on pastures free of infestation in September, their worm burdens will quite quickly decrease, because the adult worms die in four weeks. Secondly, anthelmintic treatment without moving onto a clean pasture will give only a very temporary relief, because the worms killed by the anthelmintic would soon have died anyway and new infections are rapidly established from fresh larval intakes.

Even if no further worm eggs are passed from July onwards, herbage larval infestations (that is the number of $L_3$ present on the grass) will persist at a high level over the winter and will only start to decline during the spring of the following year. If there are no calves grazing this pasture, i.e. no way in which the larvae can be multiplied, then the pasture should be virtually free of worms by mid June of the following year. These points are illustrated graphically in Figure 4.3. If calves are left until late June before being turned out and they are then put onto pasture which has not been grazed that year, larval intakes will be very low and hence the risk of disease will be minimal.

The incidence and severity of disease will therefore be affected by a variety of factors, namely:

- the level of pasture larval infestation produced during the previous grazing season
- the time of year chosen for turnout
- stocking density. Heavily stocked fields lead to tighter grazing, greater larval intakes and more extensive faecal contamination of pasture. All these factors could lead to a high larval challenge in mid/late July
- rainfall. Heavy rain physically scatters dung pats and hence spreads larvae over the pasture. In addition, high moisture levels make it easier for $L_3$ to swim up blades of grass, whereas larvae are killed by direct sunlight and very dry weather
- intercurrent diseases, especially debilitating conditions such as copper, selenium or cobalt deficiency. These reduce the calf's ability to develop an immune response and hence increase the severity of the ostertagiasis

*Control of ostertagia*
There are a variety of control measures available and each farmer must choose the system best suited to his own farm. The following are the most common:

**Three-weekly anthelmintic dosing** Dose calves with anthelmintic at intervals of three weeks after turnout. The length of time from ingestion of larvae to their development into egg-laying adult females is

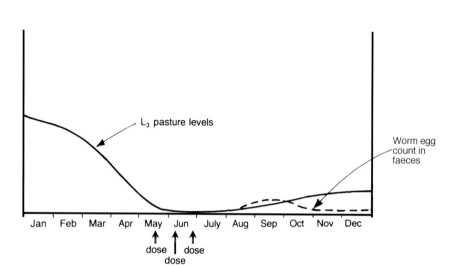

Figure 4.4. Dosing calves at three-week intervals after turnout in late April reduces the level of ostertagia larval infection on the pasture.

three weeks. Hence anthelmintic dosing of the calves at regular three-weekly intervals from turnout kills the females just before they reach the egg-laying stage. The pasture does not become heavily contaminated with worm eggs and there is no massive increase in pasture larvae from mid July onwards. This situation is shown in Figure 4.4, which should be compared with the undosed calves in Figure 4.3. Calves turned out in late March/early April should be dosed four times at three-weekly intervals, while for those turned out in late April, three dosings may be sufficient. The calves can then be left on this pasture for the remainder of the year.

An inexpensive levamisole drug can be used, either by drench, injection or pour-on, whichever is most convenient. Levamisole only gives an 82–88% kill of adult worms, however, and it is not very good at killing larvae, so when using it you are still relying on the calf to build up a degree of its own immunity. One of the benzimidazoles, e.g. fenbendazole or oxfendazole, would give better protection.

| Anthelmintic | Days of Protection Against Re-infection | | |
|---|---|---|---|
| | ostertagia (stomach worm) | dictyocaulus (lungworm) | chorioptes (mange) |
| ivermectin | 21 | 21 | 14 |
| doramectin | 28 | 35 (pour-on) 28 (injection) | 21 |
| moxidectin | 35 | 42 | 28 |

**Prolonged activity anthelmintics** Use prolonged activity anthelmintics. The avermectin/milbemycin group of anthelmintics, namely ivermectin, doramectin, abamectin and moxidectin, all have the unusual property of persisting within the animal to give protection against reinfestation by intestinal worms (as well as lungworms, lice and mange) for several weeks. The quoted period of prolonged activity depends on the anthelmintic, the worm, and the test used. Approximate figures are:

ivermectin – two weeks for ostertagia and four weeks for lungworm
doramectin – five weeks for ostertagia and five weeks for lungworm
moxidectin – five weeks for ostertagia and six weeks for lungworm

When using strategic dosing with ivermectin, therefore, an additional two weeks can be allowed, and the equivalent three-weekly dosing strategy becomes:

- first three-weekly dose at three weeks after turn-out gives cover to five weeks
- second three-weekly dose at five weeks + three weeks for larvae to mature = eight weeks + two weeks anthelmintic persistence, gives cover to ten weeks
- third three-weekly dose at ten weeks + three weeks = thirteen weeks + two weeks, gives cover to fifteen weeks

Instead of worming every three weeks until June, therefore, ivermectin can be used at three, eight and thirteen weeks after turnout and this gives protection against ostertagia for fifteen weeks and against lungworm for sixteen weeks.

When using doramectin, only two doses are required for a full season's cover and so one dose can be given at turnout and the next eight weeks later:

- dose at turnout gives five weeks protection, plus a further three weeks before ingested larvae start to lay eggs: five weeks + three weeks = eight weeks
- second dose at eight weeks gives five weeks protection, plus another three weeks before ingested larvae lay eggs: eight weeks + five weeks + three weeks = sixteen weeks protection

An alternative regime would be to give the first dose of doramectin three weeks after turnout. This would then give cover for nineteen weeks and would have the added advantage of early exposure to larvae, allowing the development of immunity. Moxidectin can be used in a similar regime to doramectin.

It is likely that developments in anthelmintics will produce further new products in the future and you will therefore need to consult your veterinary surgeon before selecting a particular system.

**Pulse release boluses** Pulse release boluses (sometimes called 'multiwormers') can be used, which will automatically deliver a dose of anthelmintic every three weeks. One such bolus is shown in Figure 4.5 and Plate 4.1. It consists of five separate doses of 750 mg oxfendazole, each separated by a plastic ring

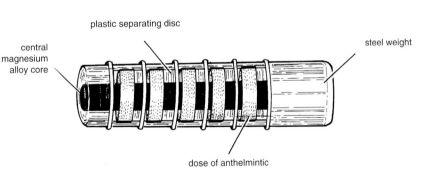

Figure 4.5. The structure of an oxfendazole pulse release worming bolus.

plastic separating disc

central magnesium alloy core

steel weight

dose of anthelmintic

and all enclosed in a PVC case. A core of a special magnesium alloy runs through the centre and is attached to a heavy weight at one end. This end weight has two functions:

- It retains the bolus in the reticulum of the calf.
- It acts with the magnesium core to produce a galvanic current and, in so doing, the core is corroded away.

The rate of core corrosion is constant (11 mm per three weeks) and this allows one plastic collar to fall off, releasing its dose of oxfendazole every three weeks. Calves are given the bolus at turnout, so with five doses at three-weekly intervals it will provide protection for fifteen weeks, well past the end of June, by which time all the overwintered larvae should have died. Despite its cost, this bolus has proved very popular and has produced excellent weight gains in treated calves. It can also be used in an outbreak of clinical ostertagiasis, where the calves cannot be moved onto clean pastures.

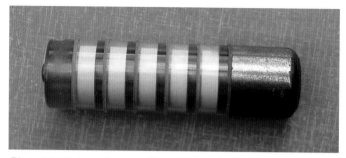

Plate 4.1. Pulse release bolus, which delivers a dose of anthelmintic every three weeks.

**Slow release boluses** Use a continued slow release bolus. These are also given at turnout, but instead of producing a pulse of anthelmintic every three weeks, they continually release small quantities, thus preventing the development of any worms. The danger with this product is that total inhibition of larval development may also inhibit any development of immunity in the calf. Hence when the effects of the bolus have worn off, the calf can still be susceptible to worm challenge. The anthelmintic morantel causes few problems because it kills the worm at such a late stage of its development that immunity is produced. However, there has been considerable concern over the use of ivermectin, which is so effective that very little immunity develops. In fact ivermectin released in the faeces also kills dung beetles and in so doing prevents the degradation of dung pats.

**Dose and move** Figure 4.3 shows that the secondary wave of larvae on the pasture reaches a peak from mid July onwards. If calves are given a dose of anthelmintic just before this date it will eliminate their burden of egg-laying adults. They can then be moved onto larvae-free pasture, for example silage aftermaths which have not been grazed by calves earlier that year. The disadvantages of this system are:

- Any delay in the 'dose and move' may allow an outbreak of clinical disease.
- The pasture that the calves grazed during the early summer will remain highly infested until June of the following year, and should not be used for calf grazing during the remainder of the season.

**Delay turnout** Ensure that calves are turned out onto pastures which have a very low level of larval herbage infestation; for example those which were used only for conservation and/or sheep in the previous year, or on which new seeds were planted after an arable crop. Alternatively, delay turnout until after early June. However, research has shown that larvae may pass down into the soil and maintain pasture infestation for up to three years after the last grazing, so no pasture can be considered completely 'safe'.

**Rotational grazing** Rotational grazing of cattle and calves, or sheep and calves is a possibility. Two-year grazing plans can be devised whereby calves are turned out onto pastures with low larval herbage infestations and moved again before any significant worm burdens are established. Such procedures require careful planning and I would recommend that anyone considering such systems seek veterinary advice well in advance. They tend to be cumbersome to administer and not very popular.

It is important to realise that anthelmintic treatment of clinically affected calves *without* moving them to a clean pasture will give relatively little relief, because new infestations are rapidly established. Some people treat cattle at turnout. This is *never* necessary for calves which have not previously been grazing, and it could only be justified in second-season cattle if they had been inadequately treated the previous year. The exception to this is when dosing at turnout is part of a doramectin control system (see heading on the use of prolonged activity anthelmintics above).

**Housing and other dosing strategies** The patterns of infection and control measures described above relate to the most common sequence of events for ostertagiasis, but, as so often happens in nature, there are numerous variations. Sometimes the peak of pasture larval infestation occurs in August, or even early September, in which case it would not be properly controlled by three-week worming up to the end of June. Sometimes there is a second rise in pasture larval numbers in November, especially if there has been a warm, wet autumn. This is why a dose of wormer is always required at housing, whatever system has been used during the summer or if cooperia is present.

The best housing treatment is undoubtedly an avermectin derivative. Not only does it control very effectively the adult and larval stages of almost all intestinal

Options for ostertagia control include

- three-weekly anthelmintic dosing
- prolonged activity anthelmintics
- pulse release boluses
- slow release boluses
- dosing and moving in early July
- delaying turnout until July
- rotational grazing

worms (the exception is *Nematodirus*, which is not important at this time of the year), but it also gives very good control over lungworm, warbles, mange and lice. The only other treatment which may be necessary is against liver fluke, although fluke treatment is generally best carried out six to eight weeks after housing. Avermectins also control winter ostertagiasis.

Some think that benzimidazoles should be used at housing, because they have the added property of killing worm eggs in the intestine. However, as worm eggs last only a short while in slurry and straw bedding, particularly if it heats up, this is unlikely to be important.

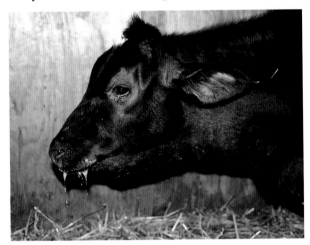

Plate 4.2. Bolus gun injury. A few days before this photograph was taken, this calf had been given a wormer bolus which penetrated the pharynx and became lodged in the adjoining tissues.

*Dosing gun injuries*
Whether giving oral drenches or administering boluses, take great care not to penetrate the back of the calf's throat with the dosing gun. Read the manufacturer's instructions carefully before use. Penetration of the throat can lead to infection and abscesses which are very difficult to heal. Occasionally a dosing gun may penetrate the pharynx (throat) and deposit a pulse release bolus into the surrounding tissues, as with the calf in Plate 4.2. This is a serious condition. The bolus is very difficult to remove and few affected calves recover.

The correct angle for holding the gun is shown in Plate 4.3, which is a photograph of the same calf as in Plate 4.2. (Note the hole A in the pharynx wall, through which food passed and accumulated, causing the neck swelling seen in Plate 4.2.) When the bolus is discharged the gun should be positioned no further back than the back of the tongue; otherwise the bolus may penetrate the pharynx. Note the angle of the dosing gun as it enters the mouth.

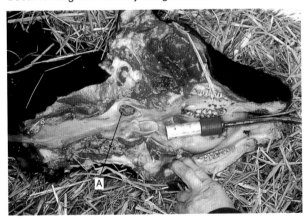

Plate 4.3. Bolus gun injury. The bolus penetrated the pharynx at A and thereafter food passed through the same hole each time the calf swallowed. The bolus gun is now in the correct position for delivery.

*Winter ostertagiasis (type II)*
Earlier in this section we discussed the way in which ingested $L_3$ larvae completed their development in the gastric glands of the abomasum (Figure 4.2) before emerging as adults. From September onwards, however, many of the ingested $L_3$ undergo *arrested development*. Known as hypobiotic larvae, they remain dormant as $L_4$ in the abomasal gastric glands. This is the fate of a large proportion of the larvae eaten in the autumn and, by the time of housing, a calf may have a burden of some 80,000 ostertagia, 40,000 of which are adults in the abomasum and 40,000 are $L_4$ larvae in the gastric glands. The latter may remain as dormant $L_4$ until February or even up until April of the following year, when their sudden development into adults and emergence from the gastric glands can produce an outbreak of profuse, watery diarrhoea. The 'calves' will be 12–18 months old at this stage and may be housed or out-wintered. Diarrhoea is the most prominent clinical sign, although bottle jaw, rapid weight loss and anaemia are also seen. Calves may die if treatment is not given quickly, which is in contrast to the summer (type I) disease, when deaths are relatively rare.

Prevention of winter (type II) ostertagiasis is achieved simply by dosing with a suitable anthelmintic at housing (or in December for stock which are to be out-wintered); 'suitable' means an anthelmintic which is effective against inhibited $L_4$ larvae. For summer treatments, almost any anthelmintic can be used, but at housing the choice is restricted to the benzimidazole derivatives (e.g. fenbendazole, oxfendazole) or the avermectins. If you are in any doubt you should seek veterinary advice before dosing.

*Worms in older stock*
After the first year, cattle develop an immunity to ostertagia, although it may take a complete grazing season for this immunity to fully develop and worm burdens may still be high (e.g. 80,000) in the first October following turnout. Heifers in their second grazing season will carry much lower burdens however (perhaps 5000 worms) and at least half of these may be present as arrested $L_4$ larvae. Not only does immunity act by restricting the number of worms present, but it also reduces their egg-laying capacity. Using a faecal worm egg count to check the presence of worms in second-season cattle and cows may therefore give a false impression.

Adult cows will be carrying even fewer worms than heifers and although the risk of clinical disease in cows is virtually zero, you may still see improvements in growth rates and milk yields following treatment. For example, one large trial involving 9000 dairy cows in the UK showed a 42 litre improvement in the milk yield of treated cows compared with untreated controls in the same herds and this would more than cover the cost of treatment. As one might expect, the response varied enormously from herd to herd, with some herds showing a dramatic improvement and others no effect at all. As any animal under stress is more susceptible to disease, it would seem sensible to at least give two-year-old heifers a pre calving treatment even if you do not treat all the milking herd. In lactating animals there may be a milk withholding period after treatment. I would also recommend dosing beef cattle at housing after their second grazing season, in both cases ensuring that the anthelmintic used is effective against arrested $L_4$ larvae.

If infection with *Cooperia* is a possibility, then the dosing of second-season cattle becomes even more relevant, because immunity against *Cooperia* may be poor.

## Lungworm (Husk)

Lungworm, husk, hoose, or parasitic bronchitis is caused by the small worm *Dictyocaulus viviparus*, whose life cycle is depicted in Figure 4.6. The

---

The circumstances when worm treatment of older cattle *may* be beneficial

- if calves were turned out late (or not at all) in their first season and had a reduced chance of exposure
- if there is a very heavy pasture larval challenge
- in first lactation heifers under stress
- if *Cooperia* is present
- in adult cows showing signs of lungworm

adult lungworms live in the trachea and bronchi (the air passages to the lungs), laying eggs which rapidly hatch into first stage larvae, $L_1$. These larvae cause irritation and are coughed up into the throat. They are then swallowed, passing through the intestine and out onto the pasture in the faeces. Maturation of the larvae from $L_1$ to $L_3$ (i.e. the growth from the first to the third stage) is dependent on temperature, but takes a minimum of seven days even under ideal conditions of warmth and humidity. When mature, the $L_3$ move up the blades of grass in a film of moisture, are eaten by the calf and pass into the intestine. They then burrow through the intestinal wall and travel via the bloodstream to the lungs. Up to this stage no clinical signs will have been observable. However, as the larvae penetrate the air sacs of the lungs (Figure 4.7), clinical signs of panting will be seen. Coughing does not occur until $L_3$ have matured into adult worms in the bronchi.

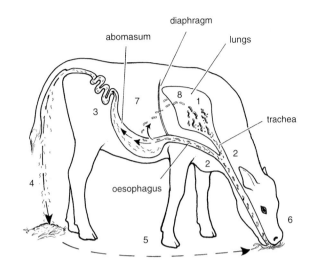

1 Adult worms inhabit bronchial tree and lay embryonated eggs.
2. Eggs and hatched larvae are coughed up and swallowed.
3. Eggs hatch during pasage through alimentary tract.
4. First stage larvae passed in faeces.
5. Development, from first, through second stage, to third (infective) stage larvae upon pasture.
6. Infective larvae consumed with herbage.
7. Infective larvae penetrate intestinal muscosa and migrate via lymphatic and blood circulaton to lungs
8. Development to fifth stage, and maturation to adulthood, in lungs

Figure 4.6. Life cycle of the lungworm dictyocaulus viviparus.

*Clinical signs*
Usually disease is seen in calves at their first season at grass, although second-year heifers or even adult cows can be affected following a heavy larval challenge. Outbreaks occur from late July until September and are most common in the milder and wetter parts of the country. No symptoms are seen immediately following the ingestion of large numbers of larvae, but ten to fifteen days later, as the larvae penetrate the lungs, rapid breathing and grunting may be noticed, especially when the calves are moved. Heavily infested animals

Figure 4.7. Lungworm larvae begin to penetrate the air sacs of the lungs ten to fifteen days after being eaten. Symptoms are first seen at this stage.

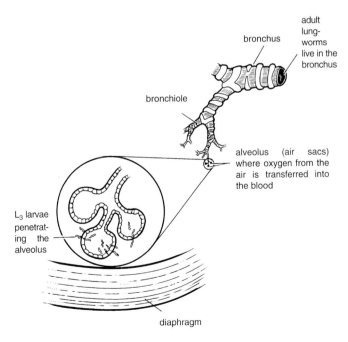

will have an increased temperature, they may be reluctant to move, they stand with their backs arched and their mouths open, and they are often fighting to obtain enough air. A typical case is shown in Plate 4.4. Because they are not eating there will be a rapid weight loss. Deaths may occur in as little as 15–20 days after exposure to heavily infected pasture.

As the worms move up the airways to become adults and begin egg laying, coughing becomes more pronounced, a deep abdominal cough, as the calf is trying to clear the worms from its trachea and throat. Plate 4.5 gives an idea of how many worms may be present in the trachea. By this stage (25–50 days after infection), larvae will be present in the faeces and your veterinary surgeon can take a dung sample to confirm the diagnosis.

A word of caution, however. Severe panting and even deaths may occur at 15–20 days after infestation, when the larvae are penetrating the lungs. At this stage there may be no larvae in the faeces and no coughing, because there are no adult lungworms in the trachea or bronchii. This is known as *prepatent husk* and can be difficult to diagnose.

A similar condition occurs in adult dairy cows exposed to a heavy challenge. In this case the cows may cough badly, making milking difficult, but no larvae develop in the faeces because the cow's immunity

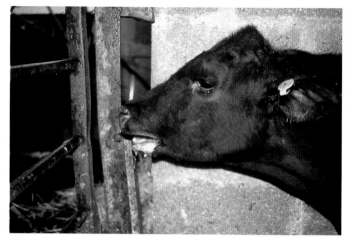

Plate 4.4. Calf with open-mouthed, laboured breathing, typical of severe lungworm infestation. Coughing may not occur until a later stage.

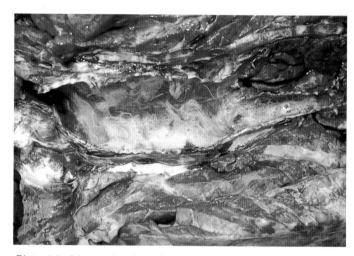

Plate 4.5. A heavy burden of adult lungworms in the trachea caused the death of this young Charolais bull.

prevents reproduction in the worm. This is known as *superinfection husk*. Blood testing is the best method of diagnosis in such cases and the test differentiates between vaccine and field infection. Alternatively try test therapy, i.e. dose the cattle and see if they improve. This would be a quicker approach.

*Treatment*

Remove the calves from the infested pasture, possibly by bringing them indoors, and dose with a suitable anthelmintic. Injectable preparations (e.g. levamisole or avermectins) probably provide a more rapid effect. Unfortunately anthelmintic treatment causes death or paralysis of the lungworms and this allows many of them to fall back into the air sacs, so the treatment itself may lead to a fatal pneumonia in some calves. A severe outbreak of husk can be a crippling condition and many of the calves which do survive may be so badly affected that they never reach mature bodyweight. Antibiotics and general supportive therapy may be prescribed by your vet for animals which develop a secondary bacterial pneumonia.

*Reservoirs of infection*
Contaminated pasture, leading to a clinical outbreak of husk, may arise from a variety of sources, for example:

- Overwintered $L_3$ larvae, passed by calves infected in the previous summer, are the most likely source of infection. These larvae will certainly persist on pastures until April or May. Lungworm larvae have also been found deeper in the soil, even in earthworms, and both may remain potential sources of infection for a year or more.
- Carrier animals. Six to eight weeks after exposure to infection an immunity develops which has the effect of restricting the number of adult lungworms living in the air passages at any one time. Even after treatment there will be a few worms remaining, however, and this produces carrier animals which can infect pastures the following spring. Young calves should not be turned out with second-season cattle therefore, or to areas where they have been grazing. It has been estimated that around 4% of adult cows are excreting lungworm larvae, albeit at very low levels. Therefore grazing young calves behind adult cattle is unsafe.
- A somewhat more unusual method of spreading infection is provided by a fungus called *Pilobulus*. This grows on bovine dung pats and produces a seed head which explodes when it is ripe (Figure 4.8). Lungworm larvae climb onto the seed head and they are then carried up to 3 m away from the dung pat with the explosion. This takes them beyond the foul area around the dung, which cattle are normally reluctant to graze, and is a very effective way of increasing the larvae's chance of finding a new calf to infect.
- Other methods of transmission of infection from one field to another, or even from farm to farm, include infected dung on boots and tractor wheels, the spreading of slurry, and even earthworms. Lungworm larvae are surprisingly resistant and mechanical transmission of infection in this way is often overlooked.

Figure 4.8. Lungworm larvae are dispersed by the explosion of the spore of the *Pilobulus* fungus. There may be as many as fifty larvae on one seed head, and they are thrown well clear of the foul grazing area around the dung pat by the explosion.

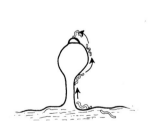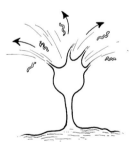

*Occurrence of disease*
Young calves turned out in the spring may be exposed to only low levels of $L_3$ infection. However, these rapidly multiply. For example, each $L_3$ eaten and established as an egg-laying female can be producing over 3000 new larvae per day in the faeces. This means that in one month a single female can shed approximately 100,000 larvae onto the pasture and, should weather conditions become favourable for their simultaneous development, calves can be exposed to a very high challenge of infection. With ostertagia it is possible to predict when outbreaks of disease are likely to appear. High intakes of lungworm larvae occur far more randomly, however, and hence control of husk by strategic anthelmintic treatment during the summer is *not reliable*.

The buildup of infection can be so rapid that, in the face of a very high challenge, disease occasionally occurs even between the pulses of a multi-worm bolus, and there has certainly been some evidence of lungworm infestation after the end of the dosing period.

Unless there is repeated exposure, immunity to lungworms lasts on average 12–18 months. Hence disease may be seen in adult milking cows if they have not been exposed to infection for several years. Persistent coughing can be a problem and can cause a significant milk drop.

*Lungworm in adult dairy cows*
Recent years have seen a marked increase in the incidence of lungworm in adult dairy cows in the UK. The effects vary from a nuisance effect of the milking units falling off because cows are coughing excessively, to severe weight loss and stunting and even deaths in badly affected cows. There is likely to be a milk drop. Suggestions for the increased incidence in cows include

> Clinical signs of lungworm
> – panting and weight loss
> – coughing (a later sign)
>
> Sources of infection
> – overwintered larvae in soil
> – carrier animals
> – *Pilobulus* fungus
> – faeces (via boots, tractors, etc.)
>
> Control
> – vaccination (the only reliable method)
> – anthelmintics

- there has been a reduced use of lungworm vaccine
- the use of highly efficient wormers has led to reduced natural exposure to lungworm larvae and hence reduced development of immunity
- worming of second season cattle further reduces natural exposure
- larger dairy herds produce larger heifer groups, and therefore an increased number of susceptible animals in a group at any one time

The balance between exposure which is adequate to develop immunity, but at the same time does not provide an excess challenge which might produce disease, is quite difficult to achieve. 'Pulse release' anthelmintic boluses are generally preferable to 'slow release' ones because the former allow a 'window' without anthelmintic cover which can give some natural exposure.

*Prevention*
The only reliable way of preventing lungworm is by vaccination. Strategic anthelmintic dosing (as for ostertagia) provides protection during treatment, but does not give any lasting effect.

**Vaccination** The vaccine consists of larvae which are alive but have been rendered harmless by irradiation. In the UK it is a 'prescription only' medicine available from your vet. Each dose is in an individual bottle to be administered as a drench. It must be stored in the fridge and used within a few weeks of arrival, so carefully check the expiry date given by the manufacturers. Two doses, each of a thousand larvae, are given at six weeks and two weeks before turnout, and calves should ideally be eight weeks old before receiving their first dose. Other dosage regimes are possible, however, and if you have a late-born group of calves or have simply forgotten to order the vaccine, reasonable levels of immunity are produced by dosing at intervals of less than four weeks. There is also no reason why calves should not be given vaccine after turnout, except of course that they will not have adequate protection until two weeks after the second dose, and that no anthelmintics can be given over this period. This could interfere with ostertagia control programmes. Once turned out, calves will hopefully be exposed to low levels of natural infection and this boosts their immunity.

Vaccinated calves can still become carriers and can infect pastures the following year, however, so vaccination cannot be discontinued after a few years simply because no outbreaks of disease have been seen. It takes only a very small number of larvae, under favourable conditions, to build up to significant disease levels if susceptible calves are available. A morantel slow release bolus can be used two weeks after the second vaccine dose has been given since by this stage the vaccine will have stimulated an immunity in the calf. Morantel is not absorbed from the intestine and hence is not effective against adult lungworm. It also allows a low number of larvae to develop into adults, thus maintaining a good level of immunity.

**Strategic anthelmintic** Ivermectin at three, eight and thirteen weeks after turnout or doramectin at turnout and eight weeks gives protection for sixteen to eighteen weeks. Calves turned out in April would therefore be covered until August, but have no protection thereafter.

One of the concerns over the use of ivermectin slow release boluses is that they are so effective that they totally inhibit the development of lungworm larvae and therefore leave the calf with no immunity. This renders the calf susceptible to the next exposure of lungworm, which may occur in the second grazing season, or in the September or October of the first year, when a rise of pasture lungworm larvae may occur, especially if these two months are warm and wet.

Similar considerations apply to the pulse release bolus which provides almost the same period of cover (15 weeks), although with the bolus the development of immunity from natural exposure is much better than with the ivermectin slow release bolus.

A heavy lungworm infestation is a severely debilitating disease. Some calves can be so badly stunted that they eventually represent a greater economic loss alive than dead. Prevention is always better than treatment therefore, which is another reason why vaccination is to be preferred. One survey of 36 farms, none of which had vaccinated against lungworm, showed that two-thirds had been exposed to lungworm (on the basis of blood tests) and yet only one farm had seen any adverse clinical signs. One can only speculate on the growth-retarding effects of lungworm on the farms subclinically infected.

## THE VIRAL DISEASES

Husk is likely to be the most common condition affecting the respiratory system of grazing cattle, although as herd sizes have increased and cattle have tended to be kept in progressively larger groups, there are three viral conditions which have increased in prevalence:

- IBR (infectious bovine rhinotracheitis)
- BVD (bovine viral diarrhoea and mucosal disease)
- MCF (malignant catarrhal fever)

All these conditions affect organs other than the respiratory system, and all may also cause problems in adult dairy cows. Although they occur in grazing cattle, they are perhaps a greater problem in housed animals, when nutrition is generally poorer and where crowding increases the risk of animal-to-animal transmission. All three diseases may also play a part in the enzootic pneumonia complex of calves described in Chapter 3, when they would not necessarily be recognisable as a single clinical condition.

A fourth viral disease, BPS (bovine papular stomatitis), will also be described. It chiefly affects younger cattle and rarely causes significant illness. Its main importance is in being differentiated from foot-and-mouth disease.

### IBR (Infectious Bovine Rhinotracheitis)

This is a virus disease of cattle and, as its name indicates, it affects primarily the nose (rhino-) and windpipe (-tracheitis), although there are other manifestations. First reported in Scotland in 1968, the condition is now widespread throughout Great Britain. Disease is seen in a variety of forms, depending on the age of the animal and on its previous level of immunity. All ages of animals can be affected, from the young calf to the adult cow. The five main groups of clinical signs caused by IBR are:

- acute respiratory disease
- conjunctivitis

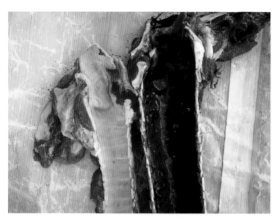

Plate 4.6. IBR. The normal trachea (left) should be compared with the acutely inflamed trachea from an animal which died from the acute respiratory form of IBR.

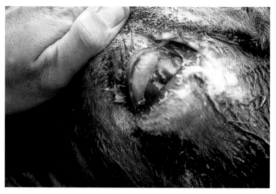

Plate 4.7. Conjunctivitis associated with IBR. Note the swollen brick-red conjunctiva. Small errosions may also be seen and these can produce a purulent discharge.

- abortion
- genital infections
- nervous signs

**Acute respiratory disease** This is the classic type of the disease. Affected animals run a very high temperature, are off their food and a discharge is seen from the nose and sometimes from the eyes. Panting and coughing do occur, but may be fairly late clinical signs. Roaring breathing may develop, with a strong purulent smell on the breath due to secondary bacterial infection of the lining of the trachea, as in Plate 4.6. The smell can be quite obvious and it is worth making a special check when examining the animal. If detected, antibiotic treatment is needed urgently. In severe outbreaks deaths can start within a few days of clinical signs first being noticed. At the other extreme the disease may be quite mild, for example simply as an additional agent in the calf pneumonia complex, while other animals may contract the infection and develop immunity, but never even produce symptoms.

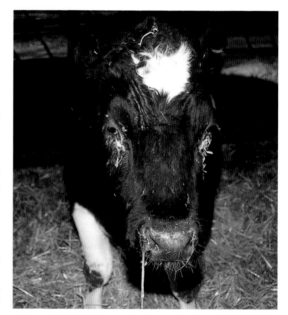

Plate 4.8. IBR. Several other animals in the group also had a high temperature, a slight cough, an eye discharge and were off their food. Immediate intranasal vaccination was indicated.

**Conjunctivitis** Conjunctivitis may be seen on its own or in association with respiratory symptoms. The conjunctiva lining the eye becomes very red and swollen and, if examined carefully, small erosions can be seen, which are caused by the IBR virus (Plate 4.7). A white, purulent discharge may appear and may be so severe that the eyelids totally close. Although it looks unpleasant, it does not seem to be particularly painful. The beef heifer in Plate 4.8 is a typical example. She had a high temperature, was off her food and had a slight cough. As there were several animals similarly affected the farmer decided to vaccinate the whole group immediately, using the intranasal route (Plate 3.13) to get a rapid response.

**Abortion or foetal death** This can occur at any stage of pregnancy and may be quite difficult to diagnose. It is thought that the virus multiplies in the placenta and this may well occur without any other clinical signs of generalised illness being seen in the cow. Abortion occurs some weeks or months after the initial infection, by which time the virus has disappeared from the placenta. Diagnosis is usually based on blood sampling the cows to look for high antibody titres and on presumptive evidence, for example eye lesions having occurred in these or other cows in the herd a few weeks or months before the abortions.

**Genital infections** In addition to the conjunctiva, cattle may also develop erosions on the penis and vagina, leading to inflammation and irritation. In the vagina the condition is known as IPV (infectious pustular vulvovaginitis). Badly affected cows have a purulent vaginal discharge, which can interfere with fertility.

**Nervous signs** These can occur with IBR, but are rare. They are usually seen in calves infected at or immediately before birth.

*Treatment*
With the disease showing such a variety of symptoms, treatment depends on the type of IBR present. For the acute disease, your veterinary surgeon will prescribe a suitable antibiotic to prevent secondary bacterial pneumonia, but there is no specific treatment against the virus. Non-steroidal anti-inflammatory drugs to reduce the temperature and aid recovery may also be used. If there is a purulent eye discharge, then topical antibiotic ointment or a subconjunctival 'depot' injection (described later in this chapter) is indicated. There is no treatment for the abortions.

*Prevention*
The best method of control is by vaccination. The vaccine is a live, *temperature-attenuated* strain of IBR, which means that it can only live at the lower temperatures found in the nose. It would be killed by the normal body temperature in the lungs. The vaccine can be administered in two ways:

- intranasal spray. With a special applicator (Plate 3.13), the vaccine is squirted into the nose as an aerosol. The production of interferon gives almost immediate protection and is used to protect animals if an outbreak has already started
- intramuscular injection. This is obviously much easier and gives equally good immunity, but it takes seven to ten days to achieve full protection

Vaccination by injection is used for routine prevention, and annual boosters are necessary to maintain full immunity. This could be required if herd replacements are purchased from the open market, although even then vaccination of incoming animals may be sufficient without resorting to whole herd vaccination. As herd sizes increase, heifers are often reared totally separate from the main dairy animals, and when they first enter the herd they may have lost their immunity to IBR. In such circumstances the vaccination of late pregnant heifers is advisable, especially as the freshly calved heifer has a reduced immune response, making her more susceptible to a whole range of diseases.

As IBR is quite widespread in the national herd, one of the problems is deciding whether or not vaccination is necessary. This is especially so if animals from different sources have been mixed and only one animal in the group is showing symptoms of IBR. In such a case it is impossible to know how many of the group have been previously exposed and are therefore already solidly immune. For these immune animals vaccination would clearly be a waste of money. To be safe, however, you should always vaccinate the whole group as soon as a single case has been confirmed. On occasions I have done this and when no more cases have occurred I have felt that perhaps vaccination had not been necessary. On the other hand I have also delayed vaccination on a 'wait and see' basis and this has led to a serious outbreak of disease!

## BVD (Bovine Viral Diarrhoea and Mucosal Disease)

At one time it was thought that there were two separate diseases, mucosal disease in the young animal and bovine viral diarrhoea in the adult. They are now known to be caused by the same virus, namely BVD, which is closely related to Border disease in sheep and swine fever in pigs. There are two strains of BVD virus, known as cytopathic (BVDVc) and non-cytopathic (BVDVnc) because of their effects on tissue culture preparations (BVDVnc has no effect on tissue cultures). It is BVDVnc which initially affects an animal. This infection may have relatively little effect until the virus mutates into BVDVc (some authorities consider that there is secondary infection by BVDVc rather than mutation), when quite severe mucosal disease may develop.

To understand the nature of this complex disease, it is best to start with a non-immune cow infected in early pregnancy. In early foetal development – less than 100 days old – the calf's lymphocytes are unable to recognise foreign substances, that is they are *antigenically incompetent*. BVD virus is very small and BVDVnc can pass across the placenta and into the foetus. This may cause embryo death or early abortion but if it does not, the foetus, having been exposed at a very early age, will then consider that BVDVnc is part of itself and the virus stays within the calf. The calf will then never produce antibodies against the virus and it will remain *permanently infected* with BVDVnc. Such animals are said to be persistently infected (PI) and they will excrete high levels of virus for the remainder of their lives.

Infection of the dam just after 100 days may occasionally lead to a PI viraemic calf, but because the immune system is starting to develop, there may also be a low level of circulating antibodies. However, this is not a common occurrence. For most cows, infection after 120 days leads to one of the following:

- abortion (often with mummified calves)
- birth of normal calves but with circulating antibody (because the virus passed the placenta)
- birth of deformed calves, for example having cataracts (Plate 1.12) or brain damage such as cerebellar hypoplasia (Plate 1.8) or skeletal defects such as arthrogryposis (Plate 1.10)

The effects of BVD infection on the pregnant animal can be summarised as follows:

| Stage of pregnancy | Effects of BVD infection | If calf survives, presence of: | |
|---|---|---|---|
| | | virus | antibody |
| 0 to 100 days (foetus immunologically incompetent) | Foetal death with irregular return to service or mummified calf *or* | | |
| | Foetal infection leading to persistently infected live calf | + | – |
| after 100 to 200 days (foetus able to produce antibodies) | Abortion/mummified calf *or* | | |
| | Congenitally deformed calf *or* | – | + |
| | Normal calf | – | + |
| after 200 days | Normal calf | – | + |

*Primary BVD in Adult Cattle*

Whatever the stage of pregnancy and whether pregnant or not, most adult cows will only be mildly affected. They may have a raised temperature and be mildly off-colour for one to two days, but most cases pass unnoticed. However, in a few herds (and this syndrome is becoming more common) primary

BVD infection in adult cows with a 'group two' virus which destroys thrombocytes can produce a haemorrhagic diarrhoea and can cause quite severe illness, including milk drop, scouring and even occasional deaths. This seems to be more common when BVD enters a herd for the first time, e.g. by a hire bull, and is probably exacerbated by stresses such as mixing cattle, cold weather and digestive upsets, all of which can reduce the immune response of the cow. A severe outbreak of BVD in adult cattle is unlikely, because 70% of adult animals in the UK have antibody, the majority of cows having been exposed to infection. However, BVD should always be considered as a cause of acute scour in cows. I have known several occasions when BVD caused a wave of scouring to pass through a dairy herd, resulting in the birth of persistently infected calves five to seven months later.

*BVD in calves*
Primary BVD in young calves can produce a severe bloody scour, with haemorrhages throughout the body due to destruction of blood platelets.

*BVD and infertility*
As well as causing abortions, a primary BVD infection in cows or heifers at service can lead to poor fertility. A recent UK trial in dairy herds showed that vaccination against BVD improved conception rates from 51% to 68%. Infected bulls can shed BVD virus in semen for several months, rendering them infertile. Even six day old embryos flushed out by embryo transfer can carry the virus.

*BVD and immunosuppression*
An animal of any age infected with BVD for the first time suffers a temporary suppression of its immune system, that is it is more susceptible to other diseases. Hence calves infected with the pneumonia viruses RSV, IBR and PI3 are much worse affected if BVD is also present. A similar syndrome of immunosuppression is seen with Border disease in sheep, gumboro disease in chickens and, of course, AIDS in man.

*Fate of persistently infected BVD calves*
It is estimated that up to 10% of all calves born in the UK are persistently infected (PI) and it is the fate of these calves which is the major economic loss associated with BVD. Many die at or soon after birth and are not recognised as BVD-PI. As mentioned above, there are two strains of BVD virus, known as cytopathic and non-cytopathic, because of their effects on tissue culture preparations. It is the non-cytopathic strain (BVDVnc) which infects the PI calf. If the calf is then exposed to the more virulent cytopathic virus later in life (or possibly there is a mutation from non-cytopathic to cytopathic), then the very severe syndrome of mucosal disease develops. This is usually fatal.

Not all PI calves develop mucosal disease, however; some may reach maturity and as cows they can give birth to further PI calves. On the other hand, I have dealt with a case where infection passed through a herd (probably brought in with a purchased cow): it initially caused an increase in abortions and retained placenta in the late pregnant cows, and then eight to ten months later, fourteen out of sixteen calves being reared for beef developed mucosal disease and died over a period of two months.

Before calves develop full-blown mucosal disease, BVD can be a cause of poor growth and stunted development, possibly because they have lower thyroid hormone levels than normal calves. The two animals shown in Plate 4.9 were born on the same day, on the same farm, from heifers which were sisters! The calf on the left was generally a 'poor doer', with occasional attacks of mild scouring and pneumonia, a raised temperature, but no definite symptoms. It was eventually shown to be persistently infected with BVD virus.

*Clinical signs of mucosal disease*
When the persistently infected calf eventually becomes superinfected with the cytopathic strain of BVD, i.e. BVDVc, the syndrome of mucosal disease then develops. This is almost always fatal.

The virus attacks all the mucosal surfaces in the body, causing inflammation and ulceration, and it is the results of this which cause the symptoms seen. As with IBR, the clinical signs can vary enormously from one animal to another, depending on which of the mucosal surfaces is the worse affected, and on the severity of the attack. The mucosal surfaces which may be affected are:

- the mouth, oesophagus and sometimes the abomasum: these may be ulcerated. A typically affected calf is shown in Plate 4.10. Note the pus on its hard palate. It was reluctant to eat and drooled from its mouth and nose
- the nose and trachea: small ulcers may be seen around the muzzle. Ulcers in the nose undergo secondary bacterial infection and this causes a thick white nasal discharge. If the lungs are also affected, the animal will take very short, shallow breaths because of the pain of breathing
- the abomasum and intestines: scouring is then the most prominent feature, sometimes a black scour, the dark colour being blood from bleeding intestinal ulcers. Very often whole lumps of intestinal lining are shed and these are seen as gelatinous tissue mixed with the dung. The other characteristic feature is the severity of the scour. The dung may be almost 100% water, with so little solid material that the tail is not soiled and you are not even aware that the animal is scouring

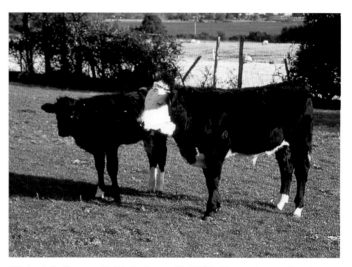

Plate 4.9. Congenital infection with BVD. These two animals are the same age but the one on the left is persistently infected with BVDVnc, leading to stunted growth. It died from mucosal disease soon after this photograph was taken.

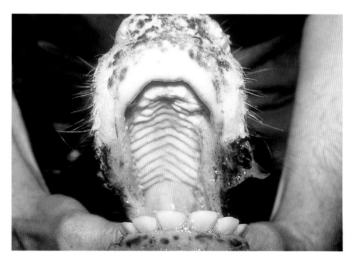

Plate 4.10. Early mucosal disease, caused by congenital BVD infection. Note the pus and ulcers on the roof of the mouth. This calf will not recover.

*Treatment*

The treatment of cases of mucosal disease is hopeless and once the diagnosis has been confirmed the animal should be culled. Whilst waiting for the test results there are a few symptomatic measures which would be worth trying – and anyway, the results may be negative!

Treatment is based on alleviating the symptoms and providing antibiotic cover to prevent secondary bacterial infection. Affected animals run a moderate temperature, they are off their food and they usually stop cudding, so appetite stimulants may be indicated. Vitamins, especially A and D, will help in the repair of the mucosal membranes, and B vitamins will act as a general tonic. Animals with very sore mouths may have to be given liquid gruel and those which are scouring should be given kaolin or kaolin and chlorodyne. I find 250 g kaolin twice daily to be a useful symptomatic treatment for scouring cows and your veterinary surgeon may prescribe a suitable antibacterial to mix with this. Copper sulphate is another useful astringent drench.

*Prevention*

The vaccine available in the UK since 1998 acts by preventing the BVD virus from crossing the placenta and in so doing prevents the development of persistently infected calves. Two doses are given, at four weeks and one week before service, and an annual booster is needed. The effect of the vaccine on early foetal death, abortion and enteritis in adult stock has not yet been determined, but it is highly probable that it will give protection. Some vaccines do not protect the dam against placental transfer and other vaccines may precipitate a breakdown with mucosal disease in persistently infected cattle. However, vaccines are continually changing, so check with your vet which is the best product for your cattle.

In the absence of vaccination, there are other possible BVD control measures. For example:

● blood sample all incoming stock (for example, purchased cattle and hire bulls), prior to arrival, to ensure that they are not persistently infected (PI) with BVDVnc
● once a persistently infected animal has been identified, it *must* be moved away from pregnant cattle
● some farms leave known PI calves with non-pregnant calves and maiden heifers in the hope that they will become infected. Once heifers have been infected they remain immune for life and even if they then contract BVD for a second time when they are pregnant, they will not be affected, nor will their calf. However, the spread of BVD from a PI animal can be quite slow, as virus is only excreted in oral, occular and nasal discharges and not in faeces. The other major disadvantage is that the farm remains infected with virus.
● eradication of BVD from the farm by blood sampling all calves over four months old (when colostral antibodies have gone) and removing persistently infected animals. The improvement in health in BVD-free herds is said to be dramatic.

The BVD status of a dairy herd can be monitored by measuring antibody and virus levels in bulk milk.

# MCF (Malignant Catarrhal Fever)

This is the third in the group of virus infections which cause respiratory disease.

It is much less common than either IBR or BVD, although infection results in a more severe illness, almost always fatal, but luckily affecting only one or, at most, two animals in a group. The clinical signs are similar to those of the acute respiratory forms of IBR.

In the acute disease, affected animals run a very high temperature and are extremely ill in themselves, standing motionless with a dejected appearance. Severe depression and dullness are prominent features.

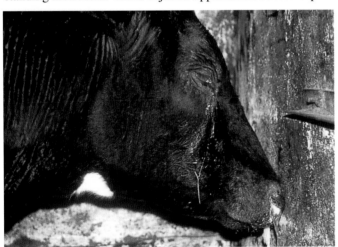

There is a purulent discharge from the eyes, nose and mouth (see Plate 4.11) and the animal stops eating. Diarrhoea is often present, arising from ulcers which may occur throughout the intestinal tract, and this can sometimes develop into a bloody dysentery. There may be skin changes in other parts of the body and some animals show nervous signs, although many have died before reaching this stage.

One feature which is almost diagnostic but unfortunately does not necessarily develop in every animal is an accumulation of a white flocculent material in the anterior chamber of the eye, and at the same time the cornea may become blue/grey in colour and

Plate 4.11. Malignant catarrhal fever. The animal is very depressed, drooling and has a cloudy white eye.

opaque. This obscures the colour of the iris and leads to blindness as in Plate 4.11. It is often associated with the development of nervous signs.

MCF is an interesting condition because, although it is thought to be caused by a virus, the virus itself has still not been isolated. The most widely held theory is that the causal virus, which originates from sheep (especially at lambing), wildebeest and possibly deer, becomes incorporated into the genetic material of one of the strains of the animal's lymphocytes. (A similar situation exists with EBL.)

The class of lymphocyte affected is called the 'large granular lymphocyte'. This cell line has two functions. Firstly it regulates the growth and activity of T lymphocytes (see Chapter 1), and secondly it destroys animal cells which have become infected with virus. When MCF virus becomes incorporated into the large granular lymphocyte, it loses its ability to control the growth of T lymphocytes, and so these cells continue to multiply. This is seen in the clinical disease as enlargement of the lymph nodes. At the same time the large granular lymphocytes themselves get out of control and begin to destroy normal healthy tissue cells, rather than just those infected with virus. This produces ulcers in the nose, mouth and intestine, and in so doing leads to the drooling and scouring seen in clinical MCF.

*Treatment*
Symptomatic only, as for IBR and BVD. However, once the diagnosis of MCF has been made, most animals are culled, as the condition is invariably fatal. No vaccine is available. There is one report of recovery following prolonged antibiotic and cortisone dosing.

## Bovine Papular Stomatitis (BPS)

Although disease can be seen in any age of animal, young calves are most commonly affected. The virus, which also causes pseudocowpox on cows' teats (see Chapter 7), produces a circular area of erosion, usually on the gums, hard palate or inside the nose. The outside of the ring is reddened (again like pseudocowpox) and there may be pus in the centre. Affected calves may drool slightly and have a mild temperature, but they are rarely seriously ill. Very occasionally vesicles may be seen on the feet. Probably the main importance of BPS is in being differentiated from other conditions such as mucosal disease and foot-and-mouth.

# EYE DISORDERS

Because growing heifers are affected by a range of eye conditions, I have used this section as a general review of all eye disorders in cattle. Congenital defects such as strabismus (Plate 1.11), cataracts (Plate 1.12) and microphthalmia (Plate 1.13) are described in Chapter 1. New Forest is undoubtedly the most common eye disease and will be considered first. To enable the reader to follow the description of eye disorders, the first section will outline the anatomy and function of a normal eye.

## The Normal Eye

The eye is spherical in shape and covered by a thick, fibrous membrane (the sclera) but with a transparent front section (the cornea) which allows light to enter. These structures are shown in Figure 4.9. The lens focuses light onto the retina, which is a sensitive membrane at the rear of the eye. Focusing is achieved by the muscles in the ciliary body, which allow the lens to expand and contract for far and near vision respectively.

The amount of light entering the eye is controlled by the iris, a circular membrane with a central hole known as the pupil. The iris is equivalent to the shutter in a camera. In bright light the iris moves across the lens and this leads to constriction of the pupil. It is the iris which is the coloured portion of the human eye. The iris is an extension of the choroid, a vascular and coloured structure lying between the retina and sclera, which helps to absorb light falling onto the retina. When the retina has been activated by light, electrical impulses pass along the optic nerve and the brain interprets this into a picture.

If a foreign object is approaching at speed, or if the eye is damaged, sore or inflamed, the eyelid passes over the cornea. The inside of the eyelid, the part in contact with the cornea, is lined with the conjunctival membrane and it is this structure which is inflamed when an animal has conjunctivitis.

## New Forest Eye

Sometimes known as pink eye and, scientifically, as infectious bovine keratoconjunctivitis (IBK), this is an extremely painful condition affecting all ages of stock, and particularly calves of up to one year old during their first summer grazing. Winter infections are becoming much more common, however, especially in tightly housed calves, and sometimes

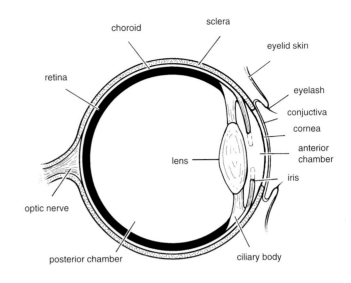

Figure 4.9. Diagram of a normal eye.

in groups of calves purchased from a range of sources. This is possibly because animals are being kept in larger groups and there is therefore a much greater risk of transmitting infection from one animal to another.

Disease is caused by the bacterium *Moraxella bovis*. When it lands on the cornea, *Moraxella* starts to burrow inwards, forming a pit or ulcer and this is seen as a small white spot or a white ring on the surface of the eye as in Plate 4.12. The reaction of the eye to the infection is a fascinating series of events. Firstly, with only mild infections, tears are produced. This has the effect of washing away the bacteria, and the tears also carry antibodies to counteract the infection. At a slightly later stage the

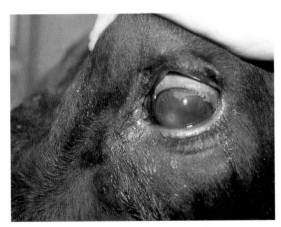

Plate 4.12. New Forest eye at the early stage. There is a small white circle and an early ulcer on the centre of the cornea.

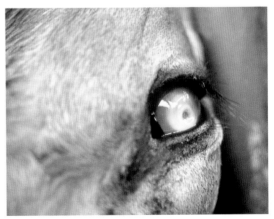

Plate 4.13. New Forest. A deep ulcer is present, and pressure changes within the eye have resulted in the cornea becoming opaque.

eyelids may close to reduce pain and protect the eyeball. This is especially true in bright sunlight, which acts as an irritant. In fact ultra-violet light itself can damage the corneal surface of the eye and this reduces healing.

As the ulcer becomes deeper (Plate 4.13 shows a particularly deep one), an alarm signal is sent out. Blood vessels start to grow rapidly across the front of the eye, carrying antibacterial cells and antibodies to kill the infection, as well as 'building materials' to repair the ulcer. The blood vessels appear as a red ring progressing inwards from the rim of the cornea and this is known as pannus formation, as in Plate 4.14. The eye may become totally red and sight may be temporarily lost but there is still a chance of recovery. The creamy appearance of the centre of the eye (Plate 4.14) is due to a change in pressure within the eyeball, leading to corneal opacity, plus pus in the anterior chamber (Figure 4.9). The latter is known as hypopyon.

When the bacteria burrow completely through the cornea and the ulcer perforates, the fluid (the aqueous humour) in the anterior chamber of the eye starts to leak out. The iris is then sucked forward from behind to block the hole. This stage, known as a staphyloma, is shown in Plate 4.15. This maintains the remaining fluid pressure in the eye, but vision has been lost. Provided that the cornea has not ruptured in this way, once the pannus blood vessels have finished their repair work they eventually withdraw and sight is restored, with the only blemish being a small white dot in the centre of the eye. However, sometimes other bacteria get into the eyeball, producing pus, so that the eye becomes totally white and sight is permanently lost. The bull in Plate 4.16 had lost his sight one to two years before the photograph was taken. The rough edges of the perforated corneal ulcer plugged by the staphyloma can still be seen.

*Treatment*
Antibacterial ointment applied to the surface of the eye is very effective in killing the infection and your vet will recommend a suitable preparation. Most need to be applied for at least four days, although there are now longer-acting topical preparations which should persist for 72 hours. Antibiotic powders may be easier to apply, but tears very quickly wash away the antibiotic and the powder itself may be an irritant.

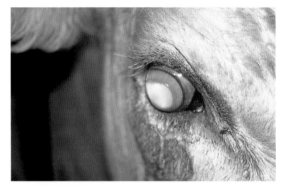

Plate 4.14. New Forest, late stage. The reddening of the cornea is due to a ring of blood vessels – known as pannus – growing across to repair the ulcer. This calf also has hypopyon (pus in the anterior chamber of the eye).

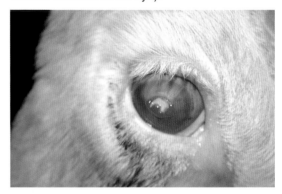

Plate 4.15. New Forest, late stage. Protrusion of the iris through a perforated corneal ulcer is called a staphyloma.

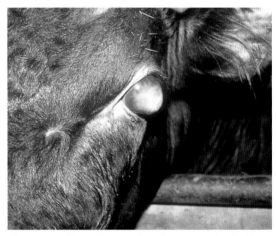

Plate 4.16. New Forest, chronic stage. The bull's eye is no longer painful, but it is unlikely to heal any further.

First hold the animal's head and tilt it to one side and then the other, to see if you can find the typical white spot of the New Forest Disease ulcer (Plate 4.12). Next turn the eyelids back to make sure that no barley awns or other foreign bodies are present (see next section). Finally, very carefully apply a line of ointment across the front of the eyeball, holding the tube at an oblique angle to the eye as shown in Plate 4.17, and moving the tube from the inside to the outside of the eye so that the tip does not penetrate the eye.

An alternative is to inject a deposit of antibiotic behind the conjunctiva, that is the membrane lining the eye. This is released slowly over seven to ten days and provides continual antibiotic cover against the bacteria. There are several techniques for giving the injection. One method is shown in Plate 4.18. In all cases the animal must be held very still; otherwise severe eye damage could result.

Sulphonamide injections given into the muscle are excreted in quite high concentrations in the tears and this is another useful treatment for severe cases.

Whatever is used, treatment *must* be applied *early*, before the eye is severely damaged. The speed of healing is almost entirely dependent upon the severity of the initial eye damage which in turn depends on the dose of bacteria received and the length of time before treatment is applied. Prompt treatment also reduces the risk of spreading the infection to other animals. Ideally, infected calves should be removed from the remainder of the group and placed in a dark box for their own comfort.

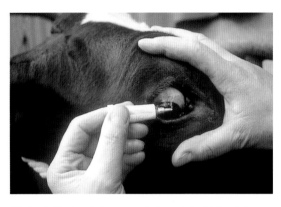

Plate 4.17. Applying eye ointment: hold the tube almost parallel to the eye and move it carefully backwards across the surface of the eye, to avoid damaging the cornea.

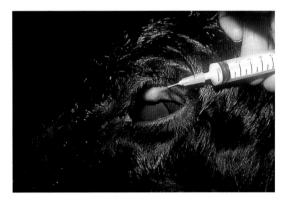

Plate 4.18. A subconjunctival depot injection provides a more prolonged period of cover.

*Prevention and control*

New Forest infection is thought to be spread by flies and hence fly control, by pour-on, spraying or ear-tagging, should be helpful in reducing the condition. (Fly control is dealt with in more detail in Chapter 7.) If several animals in a group are affected, and especially if disease is spreading rapidly, it is well worth while asking your vet to inject both eyes of every animal in the group with antibiotic. This sharply reduces the reservoir of infection and it therefore decreases the challenge dose to other animals. Often no further cases are seen. Anything leading to irritation of the eye, such as dust, grass seeds, ringworm and overhead feeding racks, will be important in the spread of disease.

Inadequate trough space and overcrowding will increase the likelihood of contact spread and if calves are grazing areas with a heavy fly burden (e.g. near water or trees), they are likely to group together in a bunch and this in itself increases the risk of disease. There is also a small nematode worm called *Thelazia* which lives in the eyes and tear ducts of cattle and this may be a further contributory factor.

Some immunity develops after recovery from infection, although the other eye could still develop disease. So far no effective vaccines have been produced, possibly because there are many different strains of *Moraxella*.

## Foreign Bodies

Grass seeds and barley awns often become wedged in the corner of the eye and may cause damage to the cornea, leading to white opaque areas, as shown in Plate 4.19. However, the white corneal opacity is usually at the side of the cornea (thus differing from New Forest where it is invariably towards the centre), and there may be more haemorrhage present, with blood vessels growing in from one side of the eye only. Before treating for New Forest, the eye should be carefully checked for foreign bodies, which can be easily missed if they have penetrated deep into the conjunctival sac at the corner of the eye. Forceps are needed to remove them. Sometimes the foreign body penetrates the cornea itself, as in Plate 4.20. These can be particularly difficult. The eye will need to be anaesthetised and a scalpel used to remove the object. Overhead racks (Plate 4.21) are a great danger because grass seeds and other debris can fall into the calves' eyes when they are pulling food from the rack. Hay and straw should always be fed from ground level.

## IBR (Infectious Bovine Rhinotracheitis)

This was discussed earlier in the chapter. Although it leads to a red and painful eye (Plate 4.7), often with the eyelids closed, the discharge is more of a white, creamy pus rather than clear tears, and it is the conjunctiva which is inflamed. The cornea is normal, and there is no white ulcer present.

## Irritation Caused by Flies or Ultra-violet Sunlight

This can lead to calves rubbing their faces which in turn produces runny eyes during the summer, particularly in white-faced animals. Even if the eyes are examined very carefully it is sometimes difficult to tell whether New Forest disease is present or not. New Forest infection *may* cause nothing more than a mild eye discharge, when no ulcer is visible. This would be impossible to differentiate from fly or ultra-violet irritation. Therefore if there are a large number of calves with New Forest and others with running eyes, it is advisable to treat them all.

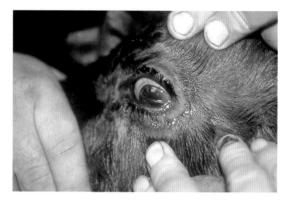

Plate 4.19. Foreign body in eye. The corneal opacity is now at one side of the eye, rather than central as with New Forest. A small piece of plant material can be seen running across the surface of the cornea.

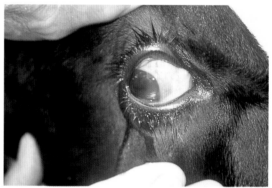

Plate 4.20. This foreign body (a grass seed) has become totally embedded in the eye and can be quite difficult to remove.

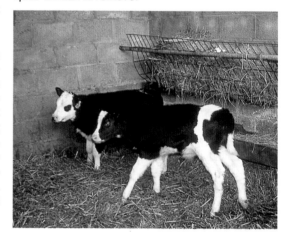

Plate 4.21. Overhead hay racks such as this increase the risk of debris falling into the eye.

## Tumour of the Third Eyelid

This is seen as a red, fleshy lump protruding from the inner (medial) corner of the eye. A typical example is shown in Plate 4.22. Early cases can be easily removed by your vet who will anaesthetise the eye, pull the third eyelid out and, using scissors, cut across below the tumour. Suturing is not required, but it is essential to remove all of the tumour; otherwise it will regrow. Occasionally tumours grow onto the cornea itself. These are much more difficult. If neglected, the tumour will invade the whole eye, or even occasionally pass into the lungs. Treatment is then hopeless. Tumours generally occur in older cows and not heifers.

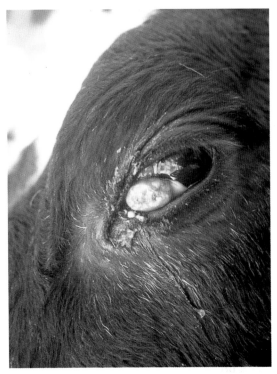

Plate 4.22. A squamous cell carcinoma (tumour) of the third eyelid.

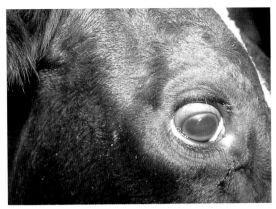

Plate 4.23. Blood in the anterior chamber of the eye (hyphaema) caused by trauma to the head.

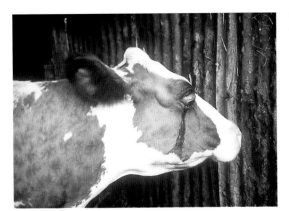

Plate 4.24. Prolapsed eyeball. This is a rare condition but easily treated.

## Physical Injury and Hyphaema

Scratching or other physical damage to the surface of the eye can produce a corneal ulcer which may be difficult to distinguish from New Forest. A bang on the head may lead to bleeding into the anterior chamber of the eye. This is known as hyphaema and is shown in Plate 4.23. This cow came in for morning milking one day almost totally blind, but the blood slowly dispersed on its own and within two weeks she was normal again, without treatment. Very occasionally the eyeball will even prolapse from its socket, as shown in Plate 4.24. Although this looks dramatic, it was quite easy to sedate the cow, push the eye back in and leave the eyelids sutured together for a week. The cow recovered without any problems.

## Bovine Iritis

This disease, first reported in 1988, has now been seen in most parts of the UK. It occurs primarily in dairy cows although beef cattle and occasionally growing calves may be affected. A cursory glance might suggest that the cow has New Forest, but closer inspection shows that there is no corneal ulcer present. The earliest changes consist of a thickening and wrinkling of the iris (the coloured part of the eye, Figure 4.9).

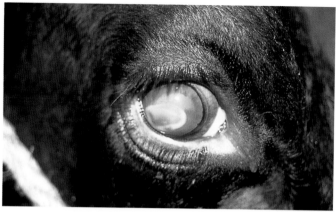

Plate 4.25. Bovine iritis is generally associated with the feeding of big bale silage, especially in windy conditions. The cause is unknown, but may be associated with Listeria.

Increased pressure within the eye (glaucoma) leads to corneal opacity (i.e. the outer covering of the eye turns cloudy) and plaques of white material develop on Descemet's membrane, which is the inner surface of the cornea. In severe cases, extensive plaques produce white lumps on the outer corneal surface, a red rim of pannus develops from the periphery, and sight is totally lost. A typical example is shown in Plate 4.25. This is normally only temporary, however, since subconjunctival injections (see Plate 4.18) of antibiotic and cortisone produce good recovery.

Outbreaks with up to 50% of the herd affected have been associated with feeding big bale silage. Its higher pH allows the proliferation of the bacterium *Listeria monocytogenes*, which is the proposed but as yet unconfirmed cause of bovine iritis, and the long fibre length of big bales means that cows are more likely to drop irritant and possibly infected particles into their eyes when they are feeding.

Iritis seems to be more common in cattle feeding from round feeders, perhaps because they shake silage into the faces of adjacent cattle. Outbreaks often follow windy weather, when silage has been blown into their eyes. An increased incidence may be seen when the ends of silage bales are frozen or mouldy, presumably because the cattle then burrow their heads into the centre of the bale to reach more palatable silage. Stage of maturity of the crop may also be important: there is evidence that if the bale silage is made from less mature grass with fewer seed heads it causes less iritis.

## THE CLOSTRIDIAL DISEASES

There is a group of infections in cattle all caused by one family of bacteria, the *Clostridia*. The clostridia are also responsible for some of the major diseases of sheep, that is pulpy kidney, lamb dysentery, entero-toxaemia, braxy etc., and they are the cause of gas gangrene in man. In cattle there are five major syndromes, namely:

|  | causal agent |
|---|---|
| tetanus | *Clostridium tetani* |
| blackleg | *Cl. chauvoei* |
| black disease | *Cl. novyi (oedematiens)* |
| botulism | *Cl. botulinum* |
| malignant oedema | *Cl. septicum* |

All five diseases are similar in that infection can persist in the soil in a very resistant spore form and the bacteria grow best in the absence of air, that is, they are anaerobic.

Malignant oedema (necrotic cellulitis) is a skin disorder described in Chapter 10. Anthrax, caused by *Bacillus anthracis*, is a very closely related organism. It is dealt with in Chapter 11.

# Tetanus

Tetanus can occur in cattle of any age and should always be considered as a possibility if an animal is showing nervous symptoms. It is generally associated with a deep and dirty wound, although in cattle the original wound may no longer be detectable by the time the symptoms of tetanus have developed. Wounds caused by an object originally coated with soil, for example penetration by a muddy nail, are especially dangerous because they take infection deep into the tissues and away from air, and anaerobic conditions such as this are exactly what the clostridia prefer. Improper application of castration rings to calves which are too old can also lead to a festering wound and tetanus. Traditionally wounds were flushed out with a solution of hydrogen peroxide. This not only kills the tetanus bacteria, but it also supplies a large quantity of oxygen to prevent their growth by destroying their anaerobic environment. Modern antiseptics have a similar effect but it is important that wounds are always cleaned first to remove dirt and soil contamination. The use of an antibiotic aerosol after cleaning is also beneficial.

## Clinical signs
When infection has gained entry to the body the bacteria start to multiply and produce neurotoxins. The neurotoxins pass via the bloodstream to affect the nerve cells in the brain, and this causes either spasms or loss of function of the muscles. It is this effect which produces the clinical signs of tetanus. Initially the affected animal is dull, shows a small trembling of the muscles and is disinclined to move. A slight bloat may be noticed on the left flank because the rumen muscles have stopped working and the paralysed third eyelid passes part way across the front of the eye.

Problems with swallowing may lead to drooling and later it becomes very difficult to open the animal's mouth, the classic lockjaw syndrome. This can be very helpful in making a specific diagnosis. As the disease progresses, stiffness becomes more apparent, then waves of muscle tremors occur, especially if the animal is excited, and its whole body may shiver uncontrollably. Eventually it is unable to stand and death follows periods of more severe muscle spasm, when all four legs and the neck become completely rigid. It is a most distressing condition to witness and as in the final stages treatment is hopeless, such animals should be humanely slaughtered.

## Treatment
Your veterinary surgeon will undoubtedly be advising you on this, since treatment is extremely complex. The clostridial bacteria are easily killed by penicillin and this should prevent any further toxin from being produced, but only time and the natural defences of the animal can remove the toxins which are already present. Antiserum, containing specific antibodies to tetanus toxin, may be used and muscle relaxants and sedatives will help to overcome the muscle spasms. Animals which are not drinking should be *carefully* drenched (the swallowing reflex may not be functioning correctly either) and in severe cases fluids may be given intravenously. Provided the condition is diagnosed and treated in the very early stages, it is surprising how many cattle will recover from tetanus.

## Prevention
There are two important aspects in the prevention of tetanus. The first is to ensure that all deep wounds are thoroughly cleaned and dressed, especially if soil contamination is a possibility.

Secondly, vaccination is highly effective and comparatively inexpensive. If animals are to be grazing areas of known tetanus risk, then they should be given two doses of vaccine at ten weeks and four weeks prior to turnout, plus an annual booster where there is a high risk. On occasions, hard swellings may develop in the skin at the site of vaccination. These will slowly disappear without treatment. Sometimes large numbers of animals from a single group develop tetanus over a short period of time and no cause is found. This is known as *idiopathic* tetanus. If a single animal is affected it is therefore a wise precaution to immediately vaccinate the remainder of the group to prevent further cases.

## Blackleg

Blackleg most commonly affects cattle approximately six to eighteen months old and it is almost always a disease of grazing animals or of housed animals which have previously grazed infected pastures. It is caused by the bacterium *Clostridium chauvoei*, which is present in the soil and is eaten during grazing. The factors which lead to the development of blackleg in an animal carrying spores in its muscles are unknown. It is possible to dose calves with *Cl. chauvoei* spores and produce no effect. Muscle bruising, e.g. trauma or 'bulling' activity, may be important, as bruising can produce anaerobic conditions in muscles which just happen to be carrying blackleg spores. However, soil or pasture must be implicated because disease seems to be more prevalent on certain fields and especially fields which flood.

*Clinical signs*

It is unlikely that you will see anything but a dead animal, because the disease is so acute. However, on occasions you may witness an animal which is very dull, standing apart from the others and perhaps panting. Characteristically there will be a swelling somewhere in the muscles where the bacteria are growing, and this is seen in both the live and the dead animal as an enlargement under the skin, often along the back or in the hind legs. If squeezed, a cracking sound is heard, due to the massive accumulation of gas produced by the bacteria. After death the affected muscles have a butyric or rancid smell and are much darker in colour – hence the name blackleg.

Plate 4.26 shows a typical example. Note the very dark muscle in the right leg compared with normal muscle in the left. This animal was in a field bordered by the River Severn. For many years the farmer had vaccinated his cattle prior to turnout, but that year he simply forgot. The animal was seen alive, but acutely lame with a huge swelling in the muscles of the right hind leg. Although massive doses of penicillin were given, it died within a few hours. In some animals only the heart is affected. This could be missed at post-mortem.

*Treatment and control*

Treatment is rarely possible, although if a live affected animal is seen, massive doses of penicillin may be

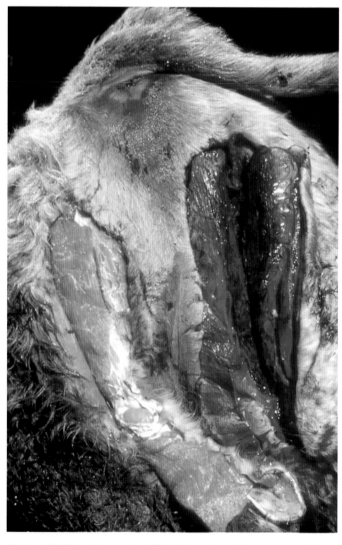

Plate 4.26. Blackleg, a clostridial infection of the muscles. The right hind is swollen and the muscle is very dark compared with the normal left leg.

effective. Vaccination is the only means of prevention and a combined blackleg and tetanus vaccine is commonly used.

## Black Disease (Infectious Necrotic Hepatitis)

This is certainly not a common disorder, but may occasionally be seen in grazing calves. The organism *Cl. novyi (oedematiens)* is ingested with soil-contaminated food and multiplies in the liver, where it causes a type of 'gas gangrene' similar to blackleg, and, again, very rapid death. If a live affected animal is seen, then penicillin would be the drug of choice for treatment.

Control is by vaccination and this is highly effective. Liver fluke larvae migrating across the liver are thought to cause damage which encourages the growth of *Cl. novyi*, so fluke control (Chapter 13) is also important in prevention. Combined tetanus, blackleg and black disease vaccines are available and cost little more than the tetanus vaccine alone. Vaccination would be advisable in fluke areas.

## Botulism

This is a rare disease of cattle in the British Isles, although it occurs more commonly overseas. Botulism is an intoxication, not an infection. The bacteria, *Cl. botulinum*, may be present in the gut of normal healthy animals and cause no problems. After death, however, the bacteria may multiply rapidly and produce a toxin. If other cattle then consume (probably inadvertently via contaminated feed or water) part of the dead carcase containing the toxin, they will develop a progressive paralysis, eventually causing death from loss of function of the respiratory muscles. The toxin of *Cl. botulinum* is one of the most deadly substances known to man, with minute quantities being fatal. Outbreaks in the UK are usually associated with cattle grazing pasture which has been fertilised with chicken manure containing dead chickens.

## Ryegrass Staggers

Ryegrass staggers is not a clostridial infection, but it is included here because it is seen in grazing animals and it produces nervous signs and peculiarities of gait which could be confused with the early stages of tetanus or botulism. Affected animals are normal when resting, but when moved they may tremble slightly, drag one or both hind legs behind them, or collapse if their front legs give way. Sheep are more commonly affected than cattle. The condition is seen after a very dry summer, when cattle or sheep are grazing perennial ryegrass pastures tight to the ground. It is caused by ingestion of the toxin Lolitrem B, produced by the fungus *Accremonium lolii*. If cattle are removed from the perennial ryegrass pasture they recover within a few days without treatment.

# Chapter 5

# THE COW AT CALVING

## GESTATION LENGTH AND DYSTOCIA

The average gestation period for a Friesian cow is approximately nine months, usually quoted as 281 days, although male calves tend to be carried for one day longer and Holsteins one day more than Friesians. There is considerable variation between the other breeds. For example Table 5.1 shows the effect of varying breeds of bull on subsequent gestation length when used to serve Friesian cows.

It is interesting to note that although the Limousin bull gives the longest gestation length when used on Friesian cows, its calves are not the heaviest at birth. There is a certain amount of compensatory growth however, and the Limousin cross steer reaches a final slaughter weight approaching (but not equal to) the Charolais cross. The heaviest calves are sired by the Chianina and Charolais, and these are the two breeds which lead to the highest number of births requiring assistance. This is known as the incidence of *dystocia*, and is usually expressed as a percentage.

The Belgian Blue is a breed which is heavily muscled over the hind quarters and which some say always requires caesarean birth when pure-bred. Cross-bred on a Holstein–Friesian cow, it produces far fewer problems, however. The first 1106 calvings recorded from three Milk Marketing Board bulls showed a reasonable incidence of dystocia, at 4.3% seriously difficult calvings, resulting in 5.4% calf mortality at birth. This calf mortality is only slightly higher than the Charolais and less than the South Devon (see Table 5.1). It is the shape of the inside of the pelvis of the pure-bred Belgian Blue which produces the extreme calving difficulty. Figure 5.1 shows diagrammatically how the pelvic shape differs in the Friesian, Continental and Belgian Blue breeds. The Friesian provides much more room for the calf to pass through.

Table 5.1. The influence of the breed of the bull used on Friesian cows and its effect on gestation length, calf birth weight, calving problems (in cows and heifers) and calf mortality.

| Breed of sire | Gestation length Friesians (days) | Calf birth wt. rating | % Dystocia | | | Heifers | Calf Mortality % |
| | | | Cows | | | | |
| | | | Male calf | Female calf | Mean - | | |
| --- | --- | --- | --- | --- | --- | --- | --- |
| Aberdeen Angus | 278.8* | - | - | - | - | 1.4 | 5.3* |
| British Friesian | 281.0 | 1 | - | - | 2.7 | 5.7 | 2.4 |
| Hereford | 282.1 | 2 | 1.3 | 0.4 | 1.2 | 2.7 | 2.3 |
| Charolais | 284.2 | 7 | 7.9 | 2.2 | 3.4 | 6.7 | 4.7 |
| Simmental | 284.3 | 6 | - | - | 1.0 | 8.8 | 3.8 |
| South Devon | 284.9 | 4 | 3.3 | 1.4 | 2.7 | - | 5.6 |
| Chianina | 286.1 | 8 | 9.6 | 2.2. | 6.1 | - | 6.5 |
| Blonde d'Aquitaine | 287.3 | 5 | - | - | 2.0 | - | 3.6 |
| Limousin | 287.4 | 3 | 3.0 | 1.7 | 2.4 | 3.2 | 3.3 |

* Aberdeen Angus bull on Friesian maiden heifers, not cows.
From J.W. Stables, *Bovine Practitioner* (1980) 15 26

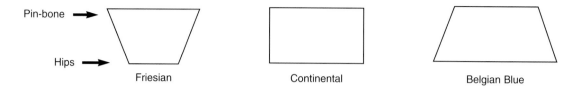

Figure 5.1. It is the internal pelvic shape of the Belgian Blue dam which produces calving difficulty in the pure-bred animal. Cross-bred to a Holstein–Friesian there will be few problems.

As one might expect there is a higher dystocia rate in heifers than in cows (Table 5.1) even if the same bull is used. The number of calving problems also increases when a male calf rather than a female is born, and in the data used to construct Table 5.1 the highest incidence of dystocia was given by the Chianina bull producing male calves, although the figures would undoubtedly have been worse had the bull been used on heifers and not cows. Calf mortality, possibly better called the full-term stillbirth rate, is the percentage of calves born dead, and this increases with the relative birth weight of the calf, with the Charolais and Chianina giving the heaviest calves and two of the highest mortality figures. In addition to the interbreed variations, individual bulls *within* a breed will also vary in gestation length and in the ease of calving of their offspring. Provided that heifers are not overfed for the six weeks prior to calving, there is no reason why an 'easy-calving' Holstein bull should not be selected to give an additional crop of Holstein–Friesian heifer calves. (This is considered in more detail in Table 8.4.) One potential disadvantage of an easy-calving short gestation length bull is that he may well produce offspring which develop to a low mature bodyweight and height, which is usually not a desirable characteristic.

Although the average incidence of dystocia using a Friesian bull on Friesian heifers is given as 5.7%, this could be reduced by careful bull selection. For example, an extensive UK survey by Dr Drew involving 6609 Friesian heifers from 321 farms and served by 223 different Friesian AI bulls showed a wide variation in calving difficulty, depending on the bull used and the gestation length he produced. Although the average number of seriously difficult calvings was 4.5%, and the overall calf mortality 11%, careful selection of bulls with a short gestation length could have produced fewer assisted calvings and a much lower calf mortality. However, the bull used was not the only important factor. For a single bull there was still a wide variation in gestation length and the longer gestation length gave a much greater proportion of difficult calvings. So be warned: if your heifer is overdue, expect problems!

The same survey showed a higher incidence of calving problems with heifers served below a certain weight (260 kg), with heifers overfat at calving (above condition score 3) and with older heifers. Even the month of calving has an effect, with gestation length and the incidence of calving problems increasing from August to November/January. The reason for this is unknown, although possible factors include changes in day length and nutritional status.

The factor which had the greatest influence on the incidence of dystocia was the farm on which the heifers were reared, served and calved, showing the vital importance of good management and stockmanship. It is this final category of management and stockmanship which is so difficult to define and yet has a big effect.

I definitely believe that stress at calving has an effect. When a cow at

In addition to abnormal positions of the calf, the factors which can lead to an increased incidence of difficult births include

- breed of bull
- an individual bull within a breed producing large calves
- heifers have more problems than cows
- male calves are larger than female calves
- heifers underweight at service
- heifers overfat at calving
- older heifers
- time of year
- management and stockmanship

pasture is close to calving she stops ruminating and wanders off on her own to a more secluded part of the field (often near a deep ditch!). During the early stages the outer allantoic sac of the placenta (the waterbag) bursts and the fluid falls to the ground. Its smell then marks the spot where she would prefer to give birth. If you try to bring her into the yard she will often attempt to run back to this spot.

Now imagine a heifer in a crowded calving yard. She would find it almost impossible to find a secluded spot. Even when she has 'marked' her preferred calving area with placental fluids, she may well be moved on again by another higher ranking cow or heifer. This is undoubtedly a cause of stress and can lead to poor vaginal dilation and consequently slow calving and an increased percentage of stillborn calves. There is a muscle encircling the vagina which must dilate to allow the calf to pass through. If the heifer is unsettled, the muscle will not relax.

One interesting trial compared heifers which were left in a field and watched intermittently with heifers which were housed and exposed to regular disturbance and supervision. When someone was present all the time there was a much higher percentage of vaginal constriction, difficult calvings and stillbirths than when heifers were left quiet and allowed to calve on their own. I am certainly not advocating a total lack of intervention. If the calf has a leg back or some other postural problem, then assistance is obviously necessary. However, I am sure that sometimes we intervene too quickly and in so doing can actually cause problems.

## The Birth Process

It is the developing calf which determines exactly when birth will occur. Increased activity of its adrenal gland immediately prior to calving leads to a marked rise in foetal cortisone. This triggers off a reaction in the cow to produce a rise in her oestrogen levels and a fall in progesterone, which in turn leads to the sequence of events which induces birth.

To understand the mechanisms of the birth process, it is necessary to appreciate the basic anatomy of the reproductive tract and the structure of the calf in the uterus. Figure 5.2 and Plate 5.1 show the reproductive organs viewed as if you were standing above the cow and looking directly down onto her back. The opening to the outside is known as the *vulva* and the fleshy folds of skin surrounding it are the *vulval lips*. The passage leading forwards from the vulva into the cow is known as the vagina and this goes as far as the *cervix*, a thick fibrous structure which seals off the inner tract, thus preventing the entry of infection and protecting the calf during pregnancy. The *uterus* is the womb, the part of the tract which enlarges during pregnancy to accommodate the calf. It consists of a main *body* which divides into two horns. From the tip of each horn a very narrow and convoluted tube, the *oviduct* or *fallopian tube*, runs forward to the *ovary*, the organ which produces the eggs to initiate pregnancy. These structures will be referred to later in the chapter on fertility control and for the moment we will return to the cow at calving.

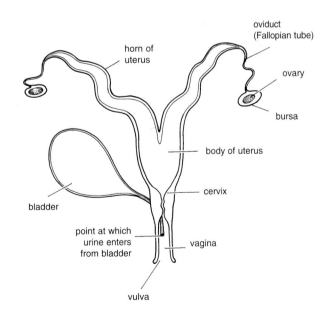

Figure 5.2. The reproductive tract of a cow (as shown in Plate 5.1).

## Structure of the Placenta

Figure 5.3 shows the position of the calf in the cow's uterus towards the end of pregnancy. The calf is floating in fluid which acts as a 'shock absorber', protecting it from the cow's movements. This fluid is contained in a thick membrane called the placenta. The placenta is expelled from the uterus after the calf has been born and for this reason it is often referred to as the afterbirth. It is also known as the cleansing. The placenta is a highly complex structure with two distinct layers. These are shown in Figure 5.4 and are:

- the allantoic sac, which is the outer layer and contains straw-coloured allantoic fluid. This is the 'waterbag'
- the amniotic sac, the inner layer containing the more gelatinous amniotic fluid which lubricates the passage of the calf during the final stages of delivery

The placenta is attached to the wall of the uterus only at certain specific areas, known as cotyledons. A placenta with placental cotyledons exposed appears in Plate 5.2 and their structure within the uterus is shown in Figure 5.4. The uterine or maternal cotyledons to which the placental cotyledons attach can be seen protruding from the exposed inner surface of the prolapsed uterus in Plate 5.44. A combined maternal and placental cotyledon is known as a *caruncle*. These are sometimes amputated from inside the uterus to assist in the diagnosis of causes of abortion.

The cow and the calf each have completely separate blood supplies;

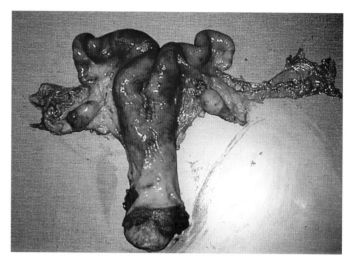

Plate 5.1. The reproductive tract of the cow showing the vagina opened to the cervix, the two uterine horns and the two ovaries. The ovary on the left has a red corpus luteum protruding from its surface. The convoluted fallopian tube running from the ovary to the uterus is clearly visible.

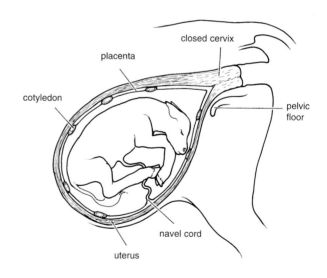

Figure 5.3. Position of the calf in the uterus towards the end of pregnancy but before the first stage of labour.

there is no direct flow of blood from one to the other. Instead, their blood vessels grow very closely together at the cotyledon so that food and oxygen can diffuse from the cow's blood supply into the placenta, while urea and other waste materials flow from the calf to the placenta and back into the cow. All the nutrients which have passed from the cow into the placenta at the cotyledons are collected together by a series of blood vessels and eventually these join as one and enter the calf via the *umbilical* or navel cord. The blood vessels running from the placenta towards the calf's navel cord can be seen on the right of Plate 5.2.

The structure of the navel cord was shown in detail in Figure 2.12. To summarise, the navel cord consists of:

- two arteries
- one vein
- the urachus, carrying urine from the foetal bladder
- a membranous outer covering

The point of interchange at the cotyledon also acts as a filter, allowing only small molecules of nutrients and waste products to pass. Bacteria, moulds, large viruses and certain drugs are unable to gain access into the normal calf, and if bacteria cause abortion they do so by destroying the placenta and 'starving' the developing foetus. Although the placental filter is a useful protective mechanism, it means that the calf is not exposed to the majority of the infectious organisms and other antigens in the cow's environment, and so it cannot produce its own antibodies before birth. In addition, antibodies from the cow are such large molecules that they cannot pass the placenta either. The newborn calf is almost totally devoid of immunity therefore, and this is why the antibodies it receives in its colostrum are of such vital importance to its survival. There are a few very small viruses, for example BVD (Chapter 4), which can cross the placenta. These may result in either the loss of the developing calf, the phenomenon of immune tolerance, or, if the calf is old enough, antibody production.

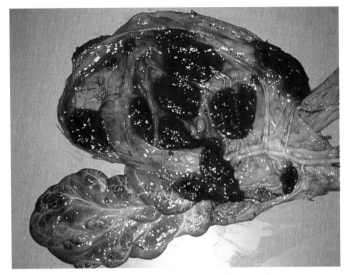

Plate 5.2. The placenta. The dark red circles are the cotyledons, the fleshy structures which attach to the wall of the uterus. Blood vessels running to and from the navel cord can be seen on the right.

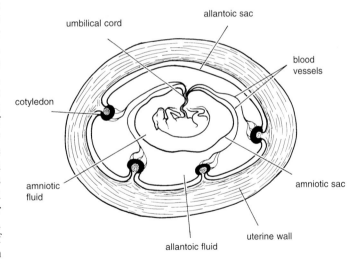

Figure 5.4. Structure of the placenta.

## Freemartin Calves

The twinning rate for Holstein–Friesians varies from approximately 3.5% in heifers to 5% in older cows. Unless they are identical twins, the sexes of the calves will be randomly distributed, that is 25% of the twins will be male–male, 25% female–female and 50% male–female. In the latter combination, over 90% of the female calves are infertile due to incomplete development of their reproductive tract, and they are known as *freemartins*.

The cause of this occurs in very early pregnancy. In all but a small proportion of twin calves, the placentae fuse together and have a common blood supply. Because male hormones are produced at an earlier stage than those of the female, the heifer calf starts its development as a male. Later, its own female hormones take over, so the calf is born with almost normal external reproductive organs (the vulva etc.), but parts or all of the cervix, uterus and ovaries are missing. Often the freemartin vagina ends just in front of the point where the urethra enters from the bladder which would be the equivalent position of the hymen (see Figure 5.2). By measuring the vaginal length of your female twin calf and comparing it to a normal calf, your vet may be

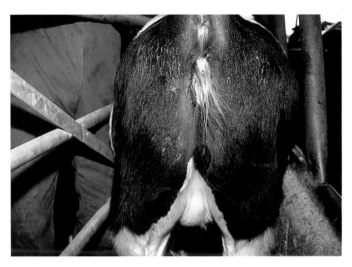

Plate 5.3. The external genitalia of a freemartin calf. Note the enlarged clitoris and thick tuft of protruding hair. This calf was unusual in that testicles were also present: the enlarged left scrotum can be seen in this picture.

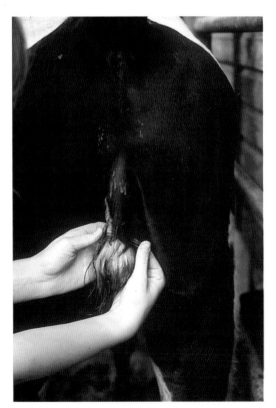

Plate 5.4. A freemartin with extensive abnormalities. Note how the rudimentary penis/vulva opens well below the anus.

able to decide whether your heifer, born twin to a bull, has an abnormally short vagina and is therefore one of the unfortunate 90% which will be unable to breed. Another useful sign of a freemartin is the presence of an enlarged clitoris and a tuft of hair between the lower lips of the vulva, as shown in Plate 5.3. This was an unusual case in that there were also testicles present. A more advanced case, with a rudimentary penis, is seen in Plate 5.4.

However, the only accurate tests are either to take a blood sample from the calf and perform a chromosome analysis, or wait until the young heifer is mature when your vet will be able to carry out a rectal examination. A chromosome analysis consists of culturing certain blood cells (the lymphocytes) and then examining the chromosomes (that is the genes) in their nucleus. True female calves will have only XX chromosomes, true males XY, whilst the freemartin will have a mixture of XX and XY because of the interchange of blood in the early stages of pregnancy.

There is one final point of interest. A very small proportion of *single* heifer calves are also freemartins. This is because they were originally twin to a bull, but the male calf died early in pregnancy. However, the *hippomane*, the small irregular-shaped rubbery mass approximately 3 cm in width and often seen in the foetal fluids at calving, is not the remains of an original twin. It is simply an accumulation of fibrin and placental cells.

## Calving Facilities

Calving is the most critical time of a cow's life. A smooth calving will help to ensure a successful and profitable lactation, and so it is important to provide adequate facilities. Ideally there should be sufficient loose-boxes to allow each cow to calve on its own, and the boxes ought to be positioned within easy access of the dry cow yard so that the herdsman doing his late evening rounds can easily separate an individual cow for the night.

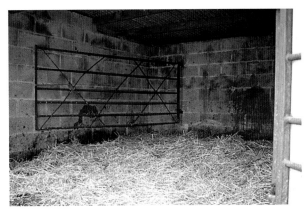

Plate 5.5. A gate hinged to the front wall can be used as an excellent handling facility. Note there is a large door on the right allowing good access to the box.

Ideally, I would like to see a cow moved into her own calving box *well before* the waterbag ruptures to release the placental fluids. She then has time to settle and if the placenta ruptures while she is in the box she is more likely to accept the box as her 'chosen spot' and this should help towards a more successful delivery. The other advantage of a separate calving box is that the calf is less likely to be mismothered and so colostrum intakes will be better. However there is a proportion of cows and heifers who get very upset when put into a box on their own and this will probably make calving slower.

Calving boxes should be large enough for several attendants to enter should assistance be required, and I strongly favour an internal handling gate, as shown in the box in Plate 5.5. If it is easy for one person to restrain and examine a cow, there is far less risk of problem cases being overlooked or neglected. The cow should remain with her calf for the first 24 hours when every effort must be made to ensure an adequate colostrum intake. This period of isolation also allows a regular check for milk fever mastitis and the other post calving complications described at the end of this chapter.

There must be facilities for food and water and there must also be good lighting. Boxes ought to be regularly cleaned to decrease the risk of mastitis and uterine infections, although this means there will then never be more than a shallow bed of straw present, and this may not be sufficient to provide an adequate grip for cows with nerve damage. A thin layer of sand spread over a concrete floor before the straw is added is an enormous improvement. The door should therefore be large enough to carry a cow through on a gate, and also to remove the unfortunate fatalities that are bound to occur.

## Signs of Calving

During late pregnancy the cow's abdomen enlarges, especially the lower part, and her udder progressively fills. There is no set time scale for these changes to occur, and they seem to vary with the individual animal. The secretion in the udder changes from a tacky, clear, honey-coloured fluid in the dry cow, to a much cloudier, off-white thick liquid, the start of the colostrum.

At 48 hours or so before calving, the ligaments of the pelvis relax to

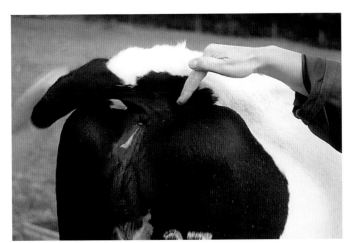

Plate 5.6. 'Dropping in' immediately prior to calving is caused by relaxation of the pelvic ligaments. The vulva is also swollen.

allow additional room for the calf to pass through and this can be seen as a depression in the skin on each side of the tail at its base, that is where it joins the main body. This point is shown in Plates 5.6 and 5.7 and the cow is said to be dropping in. The junction between the coccyx (held in the operator's hand in Plate 5.7) and the pelvis loosens and this allows the tip of the coccyx to move upwards, making more room for delivery. There is also enlargement of the lips of the vulva and the cow shows increasing discomfort. Given the opportunity she will wander off to a secluded area, rumination frequency decreases and she stops eating.

## Stages of Labour

Traditionally, the process of giving birth has been divided into three parts, known as the three stages of labour.

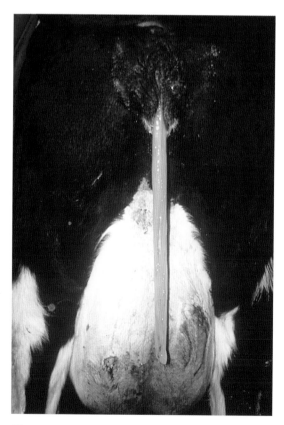

Plate 5.8. A thick mucus 'plug' is often passed just before calving starts.

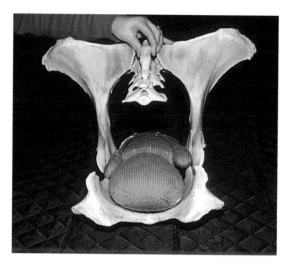

Plate 5.7. The pelvis of this cow has the coccyx (the fused tail vertebrae) in the lower pre calving position, and the woollen toy indicates the position of the calf. Immediately prior to birth, relaxation of the pelvic ligaments allows the two wings of the pelvis to move apart slightly, at the point of the assistant's fingers, and the coccyx lifts upwards.

*First stage labour*
This is the opening of the cervix. Waves of contraction pass through the muscles of the wall of the uterus leading to discomfort but the cow is not seen straining. A thick, cloudy, slimy discharge may occur as in Plate 5.8 and this is the plug which was originally blocking the cervix. The calf alters from the position shown in Figure 5.3, bringing its front feet up, so that they are extended forward ready to lead the way through the cervix, and its nose also comes upwards.

*Second stage labour*
This is the actual delivery of the calf. Externally it is seen as the start of the contractions of the abdominal muscles, that is the cow begins to strain. The contraction of the muscles of the uterus forces the calf and the fluid-filled placenta through the cervix and into the vagina and it is the presence of these large objects, dilating the vagina, which stimulates the cow to contract her abdominal muscles, thus giving further help to the expulsion of the calf. The hormone *oxytocin* is involved in these reflex actions.

After a period of forceful straining, the outer placenta ruptures and liberates a large quantity of straw-coloured allantoic fluid. This is known as the bursting of the *waterbag* or allantoic sac. The calf is still enclosed in an inner placental bag, however, and this inner bag (the amniotic sac) contains the thicker and more lubricant amniotic fluid which will assist the birth process. As the contractions increase in strength and frequency, the feet of the calf may be seen appearing at the vulva, usually covered by the inner placental membrane. See Plate 5.9 and Figures 5.5 and 5.7. When the calf's head reaches the vagina, the cow often lies flat on her side as her abdominal muscles contract to push the calf's head through the vulva. After this stage has been passed, the cow may rest for a few minutes before making the final effort to expel the calf's chest and then its hips.

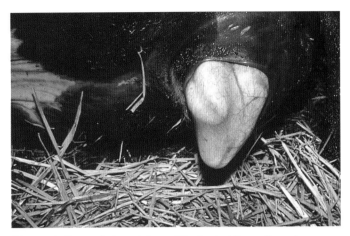

Plate 5.9. Second stage labour. The feet of the calf can be seen at the vulva, still covered by the inner placental membrane (the amnion).

If the inner placenta has not broken during birth, the calf's own movements should be sufficient to clear it from its face and nose, thus allowing breathing to start. If you happen to be present at the time of birth, however, it is always worth checking that the airways are clear and that the calf cannot suffocate. The navel cord breaks very quickly, either when the calf moves or by the cow standing up, and the blood vessels, which have elastic walls, spring back into the calf's umbilicus to prevent bleeding.

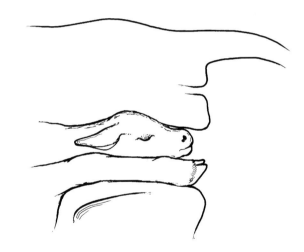

### Third stage labour

During birth there has been a slow separation of the placenta from the uterine cotyledons (see Plate 5.2) and

Figure 5.5. Calf at the second stage of labour. (Usually the nose and feet are still covered by placenta.)

the third stage of labour is the expulsion of the placenta. Under normal circumstances this should occur within one to six hours after the birth of the calf and the cow will eat its afterbirth if given the opportunity. In the natural state there is some evidence to suggest that the placenta even supplies hormones required for mothering and early lactation. However, others have associated eating the placenta with digestive problems and there have also been a few cases of sudden death in cows following inhalation of the placenta and subsequent choking. On balance therefore I would recommend removal of the placenta from the calving yard. This would also be good practice in reducing the spread of uterine infections.

Usually the calf is standing and suckling some 30 minutes after birth and the suckling itself leads to the release of oxytocin, which in turn stimulates uterine contractions and helps with the expulsion of the placenta.

The stages of labour

● First – opening of cervix
● Second – delivery of calf
● Third – expulsion of placenta

*Time sequence*

One of the great questions with regard to calving is 'How long should I wait?' Unfortunately no specific time sequence can be given. Heifers, especially, can show discomfort some two or three days before calving and this may be due entirely to distension and tightness in the udder. The first stage of labour, leading to the opening of the cervix, involves only uterine contractions: the cow is not seen to be straining. Straining is the second stage of labour and a vaginal examination at this time should show that the cervix is open. If the calf is still covered in the inner placental membrane, as shown in Plate 5.9, there is usually no hurry. As a very rough guide I would suggest the following:

> *First stage:* allow nine hours
> *Second stage:* allow three hours

This assumes that the birth is proceeding normally. If any abnormality is suspected, the cow should be examined so that any necessary help can be given. Heifers may need considerably longer than the times quoted.

## Manual Examination

You can learn a great deal from examining the cow yourself and it is unlikely that any harm will occur, provided that you follow these simple instructions.

1.  Restrain the cow, preferably by standing her behind a gate, rather than using a halter which may cause her stress. I think all calving boxes should be fitted with gate hinges slightly offset from one corner, so that a gate can be brought in and the cow easily and calmly restrained by one person, as in Plate 5.5.
2.  Ask an assistant to hold the tail to one side, and wash the vulva with warm soapy water, possibly containing a mild antiseptic.
3.  Thoroughly wash your hand and arm, then, with your sleeve rolled well back and using ample lubrication, insert your hand through the vulva and into the vagina. At the time of insertion your fingers and thumb should be together and pointing forwards, with the thumb uppermost. This will cause least discomfort to the cow.
4.  Once your hand is in the vagina, push it slowly forward towards the cervix. If the vagina ends in a hard protruding button, and in the centre of that button there is a hole into which only one finger can be inserted, then the cervix is fully closed and the cow should be left (Figure 5.6) as calving has not started.
5.  If the cervix is open, you will be able to push your hand into the uterus. Now it should be possible to feel the calf's head and two front legs, although they will most probably be covered by a placental membrane, probably the amnion. Do not break this membrane. Withdraw your hand into the cervix. If the rim of the cervix can easily be felt as a ring or a thick fibrous band running around the inside of the vagina (Figure 5.7), then the cervix is not fully dilated and the cow should be left for a little longer. Sometimes you need to wait until the

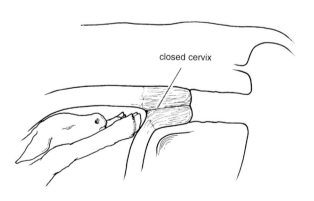

closed cervix

Figure 5.6. The cervix is still tightly closed: you may be able to insert one finger but no more.

cow is straining and forcing the calf into the vagina to be able to feel this incompletely dilated cervical ring.

## Births Needing Assistance

The majority of cows calve quite easily without assistance and one of the great features of stockmanship is knowing precisely when additional help is necessary. If the calf's feet and nose are appearing at the vulva, then clearly the cervix must be opening and at this stage I would not leave the cow for more than an hour or so, especially if she is lying down and straining regularly. If the nose is present and the tongue swollen, as in Plate 5.10, then assistance is definitely needed and delivery should be attempted.

The next step is to confirm that you have two front legs and a head in the vagina and that they all belong to the same calf. The latter point is easily checked by sliding your hand along each leg until you can confirm that both join the same body and that the head in the vagina also comes from that body. If there is any doubt, check that you have two front legs and not two back legs. This is done by bending the legs: starting from the foot, if the first two joints bend the same way it is a front leg. If the first joint moves the foot up and the second joint moves the leg down, then you are dealing with a hind leg. These differences are shown in more detail in Figure 5.8. It is most important to check for these features when the calf's head cannot be felt. The commonest cause of two feet with soles uppermost in the vagina is a calf coming backwards, although the possibility of it being a forwards delivery, but with the head back and the calf upside down, must not be overlooked, and this can also be checked by bending the leg.

Having satisfied yourself that the

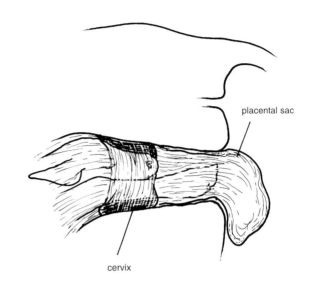

Figure 5.7. Although the calf's feet covered by placenta may be appearing at the vulva, careful examination would reveal that the cervix was detectable as a thick ring running around the vaginal wall. The cow is still not ready to calve.

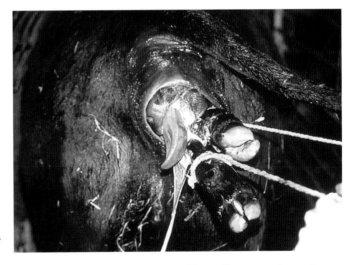

Plate 5.10. Second stage labour. The calf's tongue is swollen and protruding and hence delivery should proceed. Note the tightness of the vulval ring around the face of the calf. This is a typical heifer problem. The ring should first be dilated manually, and then the calf is pulled through after additional lubrication has been applied to its head.

calf is positioned correctly, next attach the ropes. I would strongly recommend that you purchase a special set of calving ropes, that these are used *only* for calvings and that they are washed and stored in the same place after each occasion. Calvings seem to occur at the most inconvenient times and there is nothing worse than not having the equipment to hand when it is needed. The rope should be looped *above* the calf's fetlock as shown in Figure 5.9B and Plate 5.10 and you must make sure that there is no placenta between the rope and the calf's skin; otherwise there is a risk of it slipping off when you start to pull. The rope could also slip if it is attached just above the hoof and below the fetlock (Figure 5.9A).

Next tie short bars to the ropes (sawn-off axe handles are ideal), ready for the pull. A steady but continual pressure can be applied with one man on each rope, but as the cow strains the pull should be increased, so that the increased forces of man and cow coincide. In the early stages of the pull it is

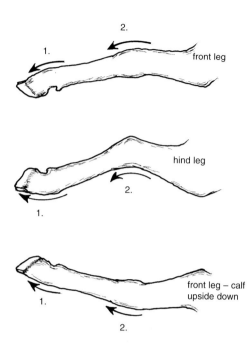

Figure 5.8. Distinguishing the presentations of the calf in the uterus by examining its leg.

vital that two factors are checked. First, check that the head is coming with the feet. If not, a third rope may have to be attached to the head as shown in Figure 5.10 and Plate 5.16. Second, check that there is enough room for the calf's head to enter the bony pelvis of the cow. If not, then you are dealing with an impossible case and a caesarean section will be necessary.

With a pull, the feet should pass through the vulva fairly easily. However, as the head approaches there may be some difficulty, especially in heifers, and an additional operator can provide very useful assistance by standing beside the animal and manually stretching the vulva with both hands. The vulva in Plates 5.10 and 5.16 is quite tight and would definitely benefit from being dilated and lubricated prior to delivery. Even well before this stage and when the vagina is quite tight, with time and patience it is remarkable how much dilation can be achieved. With your hands and arms well lubricated, and your hands together (with fingers closed), insert them into the vagina and then start to move them apart. As the vagina dilates, more space will be available and both arms can be inserted. I have also heard of people inserting the inner tube of a car tyre and

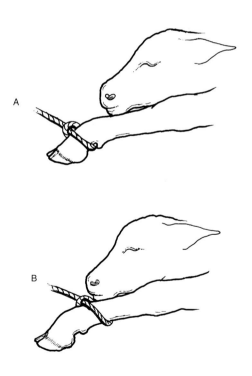

Figure 5.9. Rope should be attached above the fetlock (as in B), not below the fetlock (as in A).

gently inflating it to dilate the vagina. It is much better to dilate a tight vulva with your hands rather than pulling the calf, since excessive pulling will reduce the calf's chances of survival, and there is also a risk of tearing the vaginal wall.

Sometimes it is simply not possible to stretch the vagina and vulva enough to allow the calf to pass, and in this case your vet could cut through the constriction, cutting back to a point beside the operator's first finger in Plate 5.6. This is known as an *episiotomy*. The incision has to be sutured afterwards, but a controlled cut through soft tissues is far better than a tear which might rupture blood vessels and lead to fatal haemorrhage.

Adequate lubrication is vital at all stages of the birth, but especially when the head is stretching the vulva. If there is any dryness, the friction between the skin of the calf and the wall of the vagina can easily lead to tearing and even severe bleeding. Proprietary lubricants are available. Personally I find that soapflakes are the easiest to use, while others recommend lard. Choose a moment when the cow is not straining, allow the ropes to slacken and, taking a handful of dry soapflakes, briefly immerse your hand in a bucket of water and then push the now pasty soap into the vagina. The top of the calf's head is especially important, but put soap all around the head and shoulders if you are at all doubtful. Failure to provide adequate lubrication is a commonly made mistake.

When the head is passing through the vulva, the calf's ribs will be passing through its mother's pelvis and if the birth is tight the umbilical cord may be constricted. Time is now more important. Continue to pull, co-ordinated with the cow's straining, ensuring that the calf's legs are pulled obliquely down towards the cow's feet as shown in Plate 5.11, rather than straight backwards. This enables the calf to pass in an arc through the mother's pelvis and facilitates the passage of the calf's hips. Additional pressure may be required to get the calf's hips through and a slight rotation of the calf may also help, so that the calf's hips pass obliquely through the mother's pelvis. This is shown diagrammatically in Figure 5.11. In a more difficult birth it may be necessary to pull the head of the calf under its front legs and over

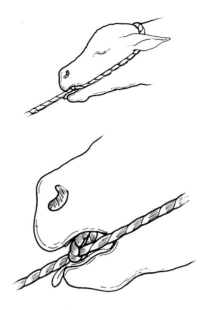

Figure 5.10. The head rope must go behind both ears of the calf, and passing it through its mouth will help to lift the nose when traction is applied.

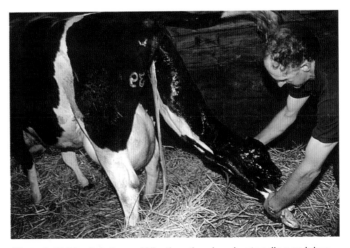

Plate 5.11 Final delivery. Whether the dam is standing or lying, at the final delivery the calf should be pulled in an arc towards the hind feet of the cow. The calf is then gently brought to the ground.

Diagrammatic representation of the hips or pelvis of the calf, in this case too large to pass through the mother's pelvis.

Pelvis of cow in cross-section

Rotating the calf provides slightly more room and may facilitate delivery.

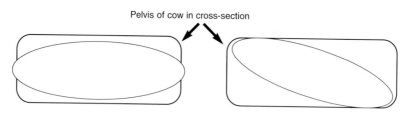

Figure 5.11. Rotating the calf facilitates delivery of its hips and pelvis.

its body to achieve a more forceful rotation while traction is being applied.

If the cow pushes well, then delivery of the calf with the cow remaining standing may be acceptable. Some cows do not strain well however (they are said to have *uterine inertia*), and if the calf has to be drawn with relatively little help from the cow, she is best cast. Figure 5.12 attempts to demonstrate this in diagrammatic form. Provided that the cow contracts her uterus, then the floor of the uterus lifts the calf up towards the horizontal canal and delivery is relatively easy, even pulling downwards in the direction shown (Figure 5.12A). However, with a difficult birth or uterine inertia, it would be much easier with the cow lying on her side (Figure 5.12B) The calf then falls towards the birth canal by gravity and the pull can initially be done in less of an arc, thus drawing the calf into the birth canal.

As a veterinarian I am usually only involved in the more difficult births, but I frequently cast the cow with a single rope (see Figure 14.7) and am amazed at how much easier the delivery then becomes. Once the cow has

When assisting at births remember to

- check that the head and legs belong to the same calf
- attach ropes above the fetlock
- pull when the cow strains
- use ample lubrication, especially when the head is being delivered
- lay the cow onto her side if delivery is difficult

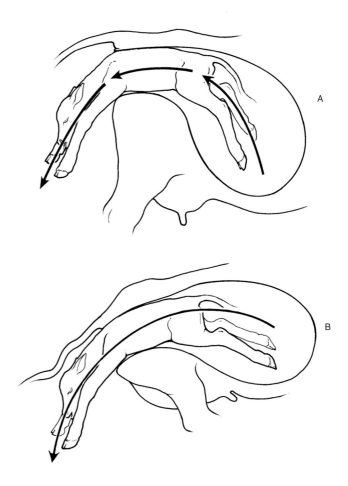

Figure 5.12. Provided the floor of the uterus lifts the calf up towards the birth canal, delivery in the standing position should be possible. The lying position is preferable for difficult births and uterine inertia.

been cast, the rope must be released to allow her to strain. The majority of cows remain lying down, without attempting to rise.

## Calf Resuscitation

Whether the mother is standing or lying, when the calf reaches the ground, immediately clear any placenta from its nose and mucus from its mouth. Although a large quantity of placental fluid may run from the mouth, most of this comes from the calf's stomach. The calf should only be lifted for a short while. Although calves were once commonly left hanging upside down, it is now considered that this impedes breathing (because of the weight of the liver and stomach pressing on the diaphragm), and the calf should be moved to a more suitable breathing position as soon as possible.

At birth the lungs *should* contain fluid. When in the uterus the calf is compressed by fluid, in a similar way to our bodies being compressed by water when we dive into a swimming pool. At birth, the pressure on the calf's chest is decreased and at the same time a lack of oxygen and a buildup of acid in the calf's blood encourage it to inhale. It is interesting that the *first* breathing movement of the calf must be to breathe in. Provided the airway is free, breathing should then continue normally.

Some of the main points to consider in regard to breathing are as follows:

- Remove any placenta from the nose and clear all mucus from the nose and mouth, either manually or by using a small suction device. Ideally this should to be done before the calf takes its first breath, to prevent fluid being inhaled into the lungs.
- Remove straw bedding from around the calf's nose and keep its neck reasonably extended. This is so that the airways are not obstructed by a tightly bent neck. Some say that the best position for a calf is sitting on its chest, not left lying on its side. This is because both lungs can then get expanded with air and also because it is the upper part of the lungs, adjacent to the spine, which is the larger and more important part. The lungs are quite thin towards the sternum.
- Encourage breathing by
  – tickling the calf's nose with straw (Plate 5.12). This may make it sneeze, that is breathe out, which is ideal to clear any obstruction.
  – putting cold water into its ear.

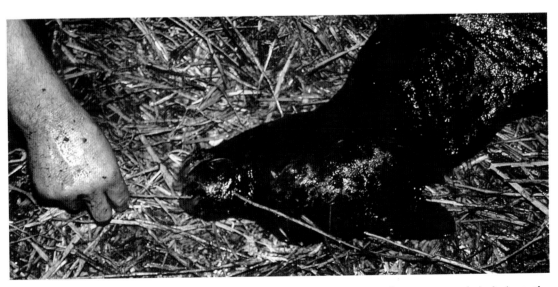

Plate 5.12. Calf resuscitation. Note how the neck is extended to ensure a free passage of air. A piece of straw placed in the nose may make it sneeze, thereby stimulating respiration.

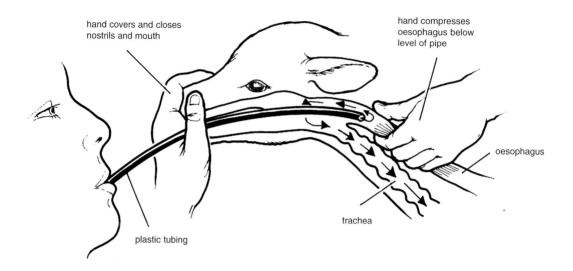

hand covers and closes
nostrils and mouth

hand compresses
oesophagus below
level of pipe

oesophagus

trachea

plastic tubing

Figure 5.13. Artificial respiration.

– mothering, i.e. getting the cow to lick her calf. Unfortunately heifers sometimes do not start mothering the calf until it begins to move and of course it is the 'non-moving' calf that needs the stimulation. Rubbing the calf's body with a towel may help. Not only does this dry (and therefore warm) the calf, but it may also mimic licking by the cow and stimulate breathing.

- Artificial respiration may be given. Simply blowing into the mouth or nose is of only limited value, as much of the air passes down into the stomach. It is not particularly easy to get a tube into the trachea. One way around this is to pass a short tube into

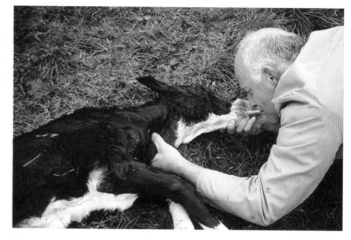

Plate 5.13. Calf resuscitation. The tube is in the oesophagus. The operator pinches off the oesophagus just below the tube, to ensure that any air blown in passes back into the pharynx and then down to the lungs.

the calf's oesophagus and pinch off the oesophagus just below the tube with finger and thumb, as shown in Figure 5.13 and Plate 5.13. Then cover the calf's nose and mouth with your other hand and blow into the tube. This increases the pressure in the calf's mouth and consequently air is forced into the lungs.

- A variety of drugs are available, some of which stimulate breathing while others improve heart function. These can be used and many people claim benefits. Your veterinary surgeon will advise you on the best product. However, it is interesting that artificial respiration is used in human obstetrics in preference to stimulatory drugs.
- Try heart massage. If the heart is not beating, then things are bad. With the calf lying on its side,

compress the area of chest wall under the front legs with your hands approximately 60 times per minute. This will produce some heart function and blood flow. However, you must allow some time for the calf to breathe and if you are on your own it will be difficult to do heart massage at the same time as artificial respiration!

- Some calves, so-called 'dopey calves', seem incredibly dull and lethargic after birth, even if they have already had their colostrum. These calves could be suffering from acidosis (see Chapter 2). A degree of acidosis is normal at birth and this encourages the calf to breathe. However, if the acidosis persists producing a calf which is dull, with a low temperature and disinclined to suckle, then treatment with high bicarbonate electrolytes to correct the condition may be beneficial.

---

Calf resuscitation

- remove placenta and mucus from nose and mouth
- keep neck straight
- encourage natural breathing by
  – tickling nose
  – putting cold water into ear
  – rubbing/mothering
  – drugs
- try artificial respiration and heart massage
- treat acidosis

---

## Calves Born Dead

It is disappointing for both the cow and the owner when a calf is born dead. Examine the calf's eye: if the cornea has lost its turgidity and turned a blue, opaque colour, then the calf has probably been dead for at least six to eight hours. Examine its hindquarters for the presence of foetal dung (meconium). If the calf is badly soiled, this demonstrates that death occurred *during* the birth process, with the calf struggling to breathe. Finally, leave the dead calf with the cow and allow her to lick it dry. I believe that this enables the cow to complete her part of the birth process and causes far less stress to her than removing the dead calf immediately. An average herd will have 5% of calves born dead.

## The Post Calving Check

With the cow still restrained, wash your arm and then reinsert it into the uterus to check for a second calf. If you remove the second, check for a third! Check all four quarters of the udder for mastitis and check for vaginal tears and excessive bleeding. The technique for this is described in detail later in this chapter. Then release the cow, putting the calf in front of her head to encourage her to lick it dry (Plate 5.14). This stimulates the calf's breathing and prevents it from getting too cold. As soon as the licking has stopped, spray the wet umbilical cord with an antibiotic aerosol to prevent navel ill, and when the calf can stand, guide it to the teat for a good feed of colostrum. If it does not stand within six hours, it is very important that it is kept warm and that colostrum is given by bottle or stomach tube.

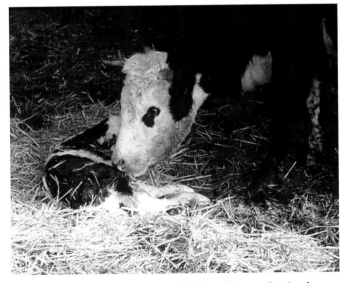

Plate 5.14. Allowing the cow to lick the calf immediately after birth cleans and dries it, thereby keeping it warm and stimulating its breathing.

## Calving Aids

The most common calving aid is the calving jack (Plates 5.15 and 5.16). It can exert considerable additional force when pulling a calf and so it is vital that you are *absolutely* sure that the calf is positioned correctly for delivery before operating it. Restrain the cow, check the posture of the calf and apply the calving ropes as described previously. Next slide the ratchet down to the bottom of the jack, attach the ropes to the hooks and place the transverse buffer bar of the jack (the black crosspiece) on to the thick muscle of the cow's hind legs. You are now in a position to start pulling. Slowly work the ratchet handle and start to draw the calf. As the cow strains, extra pressure can be applied by pushing the free end of the calving jack downwards in a lever action; when the contraction ceases, ease the handle back up to the horizontal position and take up any additional slack rope using the ratchet. In this way the calf can be slowly delivered.

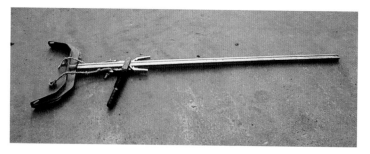

Plate 5.15. A calving jack. Some have a bar which fits across the back end of the cow, just below the vulva.

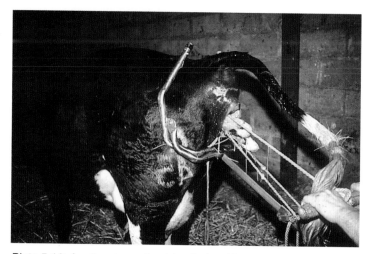

Plate 5.16. Another type of calving jack, with a frame which fits over the cow's pelvis.

An alternative form of calving jack is shown in Plate 5.16. This has a large frame which fits over the sides of the cow to hold it in place. It has the advantage of staying in place much better when the cow moves, although it is slightly more difficult to fit on when a cow is lying down. In Plate 5.16 the ratchet handle is obscured by the cow's tail. A rope attached to the calf's head is being pulled by hand. Great care is needed at this stage: a slow, gentle pull and ample lubrication over the calf's head will reduce the risk of tearing.

The calving jack is particularly useful for the single-handed stockman, and for assisting calvings in a field. However, in inexperienced hands or if handled incorrectly, it can be very dangerous. The main danger is that it is used in the wrong circumstances, for example before the cervix or vagina has fully opened, or before the calf has been correctly positioned for delivery, or simply when the calf is too large and veterinary assistance should have been sought. Another misuse is that the calf is drawn far too quickly. If the tissues of the vulva and vagina are not allowed to dilate naturally as the calf's head is being delivered (this critical stage is shown in Plates 5.10 and 5.16), tearing of the vagina may occur. This in turn can lead to severe infections or even fatal blood loss.

A disadvantage of the jack is that it is not easy to rotate a calf stuck at the hips to facilitate its passage through the maternal pelvis (Figure 5.11). Rotation may be a critical part of delivery at this stage. Great care therefore needs to be taken with its use. If in doubt, call for veterinary assistance. The possibility of losing a cow from vaginal infection, blood loss or nerve damage following an excessively tight delivery is never worth the risk. Once the calf becomes locked in the birth canal, it may be too late for the vet to carry out an embryotomy, episiotomy or caesarean section to effect a safe delivery.*

*Embryotomy* – cutting up the calf inside the cow and delivering it piecemeal.
*Episiostomy* – cutting through the vulva and posterior vagina to increase the space available for the calf.
*Caesarian* – cutting through the flank and into the uterus so that the calf does not have to be drawn through the pelvis.

## Abnormalities Requiring Correction

There are some abnormalities which can be easily corrected and others which need to be recognised so that veterinary assistance can be sought. The following gives a few ideas on when a manual vaginal examination should be carried out:

1.  Any cow due to calve which has been in discomfort for more than 24 hours without any positive signs of the birth process starting should be examined.
2.  If a piece of placenta is hanging from the vulva, and especially if deep red/purple cotyledons are visible on it, this indicates that placental separation is already occurring and intervention is needed.
3.  Towards the end of pregnancy the calf straightens its nose and forelegs so that these are the first parts to enter the birth canal (the name given to the opened cervix and vagina leading through the pelvis). If head and both forelegs do not appear at the vulva, assistance may be needed.

Some of the common abnormalities which require attention are described in the following sections.

*Uterine torsion*
The shape of a normal closed cervix has been described as a protruding button (Figure 5.6). If this bulging structure cannot be felt, but it is still not possible to pass your hand through the cervix, you may be dealing with a twist, or *torsion of the uterus*. This would feel similar to the effect of trying to push your hand along the sleeve of a jacket which has been rotated through 180° or 360° at the elbow. This is shown diagrammatically in Figure 5.14. If uterine torsion is suspected, veterinary attention should be sought. The condition is thought to be caused by the calf making excessively violent movements within the uterus at the start of calving and in almost every case there is a large calf involved. Although it is possible to untwist the uterus or roll the cow and correct the torsion, in some cases the cervix then fails to dilate adequately and delivery by caesarean section may be necessary.

*Uterine inertia*
Sometimes even though the vagina and cervix are fully dilated and the calf is lying normally, the cow simply refuses to push to effect its delivery. This is the condition of *uterine inertia*. The calf will now have to be delivered by traction, and it is preferable to have the cow lying on her side before starting (Figure 5.12B). It is also worth giving her a bottle of calcium in case milk fever is a predisposing factor.

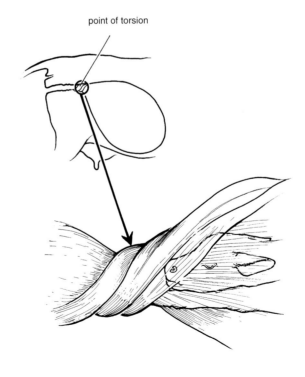

point of torsion

Figure 5.14. Uterine torsion.

*Leg back*

The bend may be at the calf's knee (Figure 5.15), when the point of the knee will be felt by pushing your hand along the calf's neck, through the bony canal formed by the cow's pelvis and into the uterus. It may be possible to cup the calf's hoof in the palm of your hand and draw it forwards (Figure 5.16). This is especially so if the abnormality has been detected at an early stage and the head and normal leg of the calf are not already tightly locked in the pelvis.

At the other extreme you may need to ask for veterinary help to inject an epidural anaesthetic into the spine of the cow to stop her straining, so that the calf can be pushed back into the uterus and the leg brought forwards.

On occasions the whole leg may be turned backwards from the shoulder (Figure 5.17) and your first impression when examining the cow is that you are about to witness the birth of a three-legged calf! With a good long reach, however, it should be possible to pull the leg forwards into the 'knee flexed' position (Figure 5.15), either pulling it with your hand or by attaching a rope. It is very rare that it is not possible to push a rope around the leg, even if it is fully extended backwards.

The cases which pose problems are those in which the head and one leg have passed through the vulva, as shown in Plate 5.17. The cow was found like this early one morning and the calf's head had become dry and swollen. Note the protruding and swollen tongue. The calf is clearly dead. After an epidural injection was given (to stop the cow straining), the calf's head was thoroughly cleaned, lubricated and then pushed back into the uterus so that the second leg could be pulled forwards.

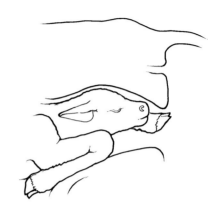

Figure 5.15. Abnormalities of posture: leg flexed at knee.

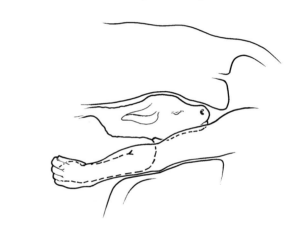

Figure 5.16. Correction of simple leg flexed (leg back) presentation. Cup the calf's foot in your hand and draw it forwards.

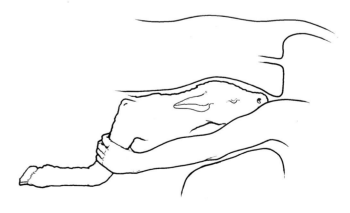

Figure 5.17. Full leg flexion from the shoulder, showing an attempt to draw the leg forwards to the simple knee flexion position.

*Head back*

In this posture two legs will be presented in the birth canal and it is vital that you confirm that they are front and not back legs, using the method described in Figure 5.8. Once you are sure that they are front legs, try to locate the top of the calf's neck and follow the direction of its curve. This will tell you if the head is on the right or the left. If possible, gently cup the calf's nose in the palm of your hand (Figure 5.18) and draw it forwards so that it will enter the vagina. Sometimes it may be necessary to apply a rope as shown in Figure 5.10. If the posture cannot be corrected easily, for example as in Plate 5.18, call for veterinary assistance. Pulling the head round with excessive force can rupture the wall of the uterus and there will be occasions when correction is not possible and delivery will have to be by embryotomy or by caesarean section.

*Hiplock*

It can be particularly frustrating if you have managed to draw a large live calf into the pelvis, only to then find that it gets stuck at the hips. Options available to deal with hiplock calves include

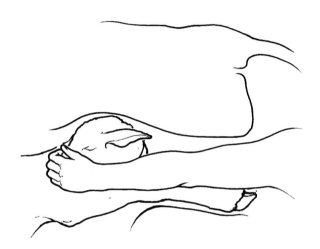

- Stop pulling, lubricate the calf's hips well and then re-apply traction.
- Twist the calf at the same time as you are applying traction. This can be done by one person pushing the calf's head to one side while one or two others continue to apply traction to the legs. Alternatively, if there are two of you pulling one leg each, simply exchange ropes. If the person on the left pulls the rope attached to

Figure 5.18. It may be possible to correct a 'head back' simply by drawing the nose around with your hand. On other occasions a rope is needed.

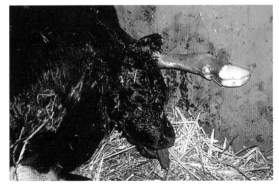

Plate 5.17. Head and one leg out. Note how the tongue is protruding and swollen. The calf is dead. The head will have to be pushed back into the uterus to bring the second leg forwards.

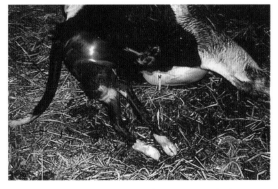

Plate 5.18. Head back, but front legs and chest presented. This is an unusual presentation and could only occur with a small calf. The heifer was given an epidural to stop her straining, the calf carefully pushed back into the uterus and the head brought forwards. The calf was obviously dead.

the right leg and vice versa, this will rotate the calf at the same time as pulling it.

- Lay the cow down. It is surprising how often this effects a delivery.
- If the calf will not come through the pelvis with reasonable traction, and especially if the calf is now dead, then it is best to call for veterinary attention rather than risk damaging the mother. The vet will probably cut the calf in half across its chest, then feed an embryotomy wire between its hind legs so that the two halves of the pelvis can be delivered separately.

*Backwards delivery*

A proportion of calves are born hind legs first without any trouble. There are a few additional complicating factors, however. Firstly the presence of only the feet in the vagina (that is without the head) does not dilate the vagina to the same degree, so there is thus a reduced release of the hormone oxytocin and reduced abdominal contractions. Secondly, because the vagina has not dilated properly, extra care needs to be taken to avoid tearing the vagina as the hips are drawn through the vulva (Plate 5.19). Thirdly, when the hips eventually pass through the vulva, the chest is entering the cow's pelvis and so the umbilical cord is constricted well before the calf is able to breathe. The danger of it inhaling uterine fluids is therefore much greater and calves born backwards should be delivered quite quickly after this stage.

The situation is sometimes exacerbated by the fact that the umbilical cord may be passing back between the hind legs of the calf and over its hock, as shown in Figure 5.19. In this instance the cord would rupture as soon as delivery commenced, and the chances of obtaining a live calf are even more seriously impaired. If you detect this abnormality of the cord I suggest you call for immediate veterinary assistance to reposition it before delivery commences.

The final danger with backward deliveries is that the tail may be pushed towards the calf's head (Figure 5.20). If this is not corrected it can cause serious damage to the roof of the vagina.

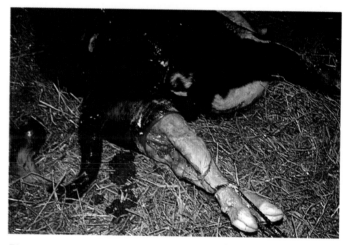

Plate 5.19. Calf backwards. Generous lubrication and a slow, steady pull are needed at this stage to avoid tearing the vagina.

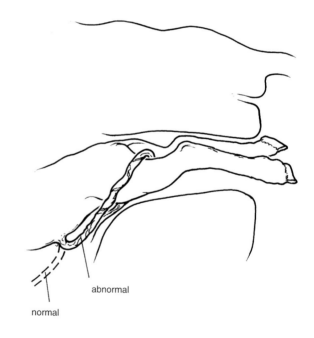

Figure 5.19. Backwards presentation showing normal and abnormal positions of the umbilical cord. With the latter, veterinary assistance is needed.

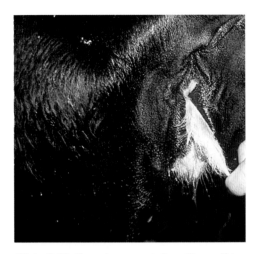

Plate 5.20. Breech presentation. The calf is coming backwards, but both hind legs are forwards, so only the tail is presented. Often the cow is not seen straining and a dead calf results.

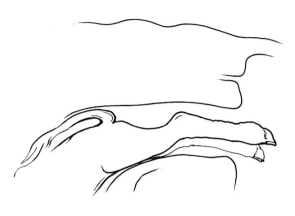

Figure 5.20. Backwards presentation: always check that the tail is not being forced into the roof of the vagina as it is in this diagram. It should be lying between the hind legs during the birth.

## Breech presentation

This is probably the most difficult of all the abnormalities to correct and I would suggest that you call for veterinary assistance. In this posture the calf is coming backwards, but with both of its hind legs pointing forwards (Figure 5.21), so that only the tail enters the birth canal. The absence of any object dilating the vagina means that the cow does not strain, nor is any part of the calf or placenta seen at the vulva, except perhaps the tail, as in Plate 5.20. As a consequence, cows with breech births tend to be left too long and in the majority of cases the calf is already dead before assistance is thought necessary. Decomposition may have set in, and the calf may even have to be delivered piecemeal by embryotomy. Correction involves pulling the calf's foot backwards at the same time as its hock is pushed upwards and forwards. The rope needs to be looped above the fetlock and then run down between the claws, so that pulling bends the hoof backwards. There is then less danger of rupturing the wall of the uterus with the calf's foot, but great care needs to be taken with the position of the hock.

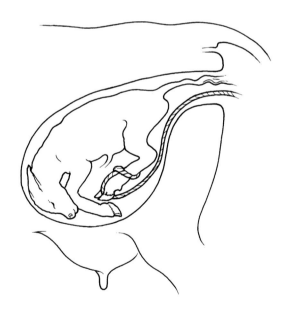

Figure 5.21. Breech presentation: the calf is coming backwards but with both legs forwards so that only the tail is felt in the vagina. Because there is nothing dilating the vagina the cow often does not strain, and consequently many breech births may go unnoticed for several hours and produce a dead calf. Attaching the rope like this folds the foot back as the leg is lifted.

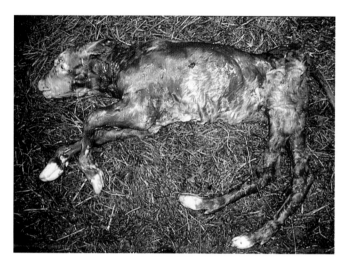

Plate 5.21. Arthrogryposis. Both hind legs are longer than normal and fused at the joints so that they will not bend.

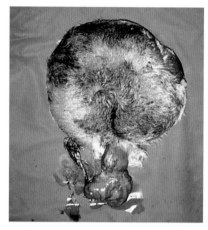

Plate 5.22. Amorphous globosus, a hairy ball of tissue but with its own heart and circulation. Most are born twin to a normal calf.

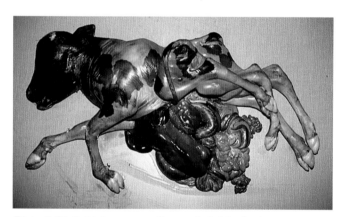

Plate 5.23. Schistosomus reflexus. A cleft in the lower abdomen allows all the contents to float free in the uterus. This calf had the additional abnormality of four hind legs!

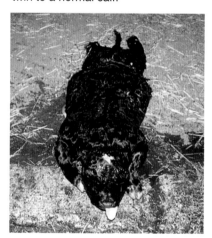

Plate 5.24. Bulldog calf. Note the very large head.

*Monster calves*

These are relative rarities and are only mentioned for the sake of completeness. Some have massively enlarged heads, some have two heads and some may have the hind legs totally fused with the pelvis so that they cannot bend. This fusion of joints is known as ankylosis and the calf is said to be affected by *arthrogryposis*. A typical example is shown in Plate 5.21. This was a dead, cross-bred Charolais calf coming backwards and I had enormous difficulty in getting both legs lined up in the pelvis to effect delivery. Occasionally just a ball of hairy skin is delivered, as in Plate 5.22. These are known as *amorphous globosus* and are nearly always twin to a normal full-term calf. Internally this calf even had a heart and circulation!

   Probably the most bizarre abnormality, although one of the most common, is the condition of *schistosomus reflexus*. A cleft in the lower abdomen allows the prolapse of all the foetal abdominal contents. Plate 5.23 shows a schistosome calf which also had leg abnormalities. It was aborted with a normal twin at approximately seven months of gestation. Achondroplastic calves (dwarfs or bulldogs) also occur, although the majority are born dead. The calf in Plate 5.24 was coming backwards. Its hind legs were so short that it was very difficult to attach ropes to pull and the very large head made delivery difficult. Foetal monsters can be due to exposure of the pregnant dam to toxins or they may be genetic (Chapter 1). They should therefore be reported to the breeder or AI centre, thus allowing selective culling if indicated.

Any foetal abnormality can lead to difficulties at calving, with a risk to the dam which can be avoided only by caesarean section. I would therefore recommend that you request veterinary assistance as soon as a problem has been detected.

> Births requiring attention include
>
> - oversized calves
> - uterine torsion
> - uterine inertia
> - leg back
> - head back
> - hiplock
> - backwards delivery
> - breech presentation
> - monster calves

## THE 'DOWNER' COW

### Causes of the 'Downer' Cow

Cows which do not get up after calving, or, after standing for a few hours, sit down and will not rise are sometimes known as 'down' or 'downer' cows, although some authorities reserve this term for cows that fail to respond to milk fever treatments. The expression simply describes the symptoms of the animal, that is its inability or disinclination to rise, and the cow is said to be recumbent. There is a whole range of possible causes, and considering that the life of both the cow and calf may be in danger, I would strongly recommend that veterinary advice is requested.

Some of the possible causes of the downer cow are as follows:

*Blood loss*

After the birth of the calf there will always be a certain amount of free blood released, due to the breaking of the umbilical cord. If large quantities of bright red blood continue to run from the vulva following a difficult birth as in Plate 5.25, this is an *extreme emergency*, as it most probably indicates rupture of a major blood vessel in the vaginal wall. First ask someone to telephone for immediate veterinary help.

Next insert your hand into the vagina as far as wrist depth, and then hold your fingers against any tears which may be present. The blood vessels in a normal cow can be felt as pulsating tubes, approximately the size of a pencil, covered by a relatively thin membrane which is the

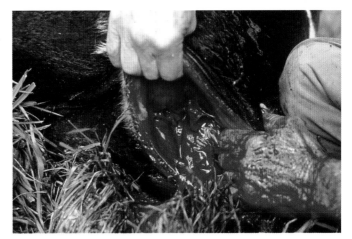

Plate 5.25. Profuse haemorrhage after calving. If one of the blood vessels in the vaginal wall has ruptured, immediate assistance should be sought.

wall of the vagina. You should get used to feeling these in a normal cow. A rupture is felt as a tear in the membrane and almost always occurs at the four or eight position of a clock face, that is, just below halfway down the vaginal wall on either side, and a broken blood vessel will be felt as a pulsating jet of fluid on the fingertips. If possible, catch hold of this blood vessel and pinch it between your finger and thumb to stop the bleeding until veterinary assistance arrives.

If this cannot be done, push a small towel into the wound with as much pressure as possible, to try to stop the bleeding. If this approach is used, however, it may make it much more difficult for the veterinarian to identify the actual bleeding point when he arrives. I have known heifers bleed to death in less than an hour, so anything which can be done must be an advantage.

Just one word of warning. Sometimes the umbilical cord bleeds profusely for one to two minutes after the calf is born (as in Plate 5.26), so do check that there is not a simple reason for the blood loss before you panic!

Post calving haemorrhage is especially common in very fat heifers. Fat laid down in the space between the wall of the vagina and the cow's pelvis tends to reduce the overall size of the birth canal and it also reduces the strength of the attachments of the vaginal wall to the bony pelvis. If force now has to be applied to draw the calf, and especially if there is inadequate lubrication, the wall of the vagina tends to fold over on itself and tearing can occur. Small globular lumps of off-white fat as in Plate 5.27, which have been passed with the calf, are indicative of vaginal damage. If these are seen in conjunction with profuse bleeding, you know that time may be limited. Even in the absence of bleeding, it may be worth seeking veterinary assistance to suture the vaginal wall to prevent severe and possibly fatal infections or peritonitis a few days after calving. Correct pre calving feeding of heifers will help to prevent vaginal tearing.

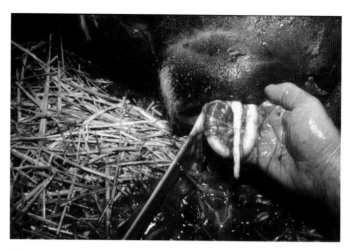

Plate 5.26. Blood loss from placental vessels may continue for 1–2 minutes after calving and must not be confused with rupture of a vaginal artery.

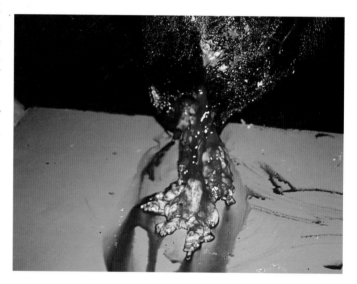

Plate 5.27. Prolapse of fat such as this indicates that the vaginal wall has been ruptured. Even though there may be no blood loss, the cow would benefit from suturing and/or antibiotic cover.

### Milk fever
This is the commonest cause of down cows and is dealt with in Chapter 6. Low blood magnesium or phosphorus may also be involved.

### Nerve, muscle and bone damage
The cow may have been injured during calving, especially if excessive force was applied to an oversized calf. Injuries can also be the result of the cow falling on slippery concrete, either accidentally or because she is unsteady on her feet from milk fever, or the nerve damage may be simply the result of the cow having had milk fever and having been left in an incorrect posture on a hard surface for too long. Whatever the cause of its recumbency, the cow should always be positioned so that she is sitting correctly, that is with the upper hind leg flexed in front of its udder and sitting on the lower leg with it

also in a flexed position (Plate 5.28). It should not be possible to see any more of the lower leg than the foot to the fetlock in front of the udder. If you can see the lower leg up to its hock or beyond (as in Plate 5.29), then the leg is almost fully extended. Research has shown that a cow left in this position on a hard surface for as little as six hours may suffer irreversible muscle and nerve damage. In fact the heifer shown in the pictures was trying to deliver an oversized calf which got stuck at the hips. She never recovered. In such cases, and if you know that the calf is dead, it is better to carry out an embryotomy rather than risk further nerve damage. (See *hiplock* in preceding section.)

The common *injuries* which occur post calving and which can result in a downer cow are:

- obturator nerve paralysis (Plate 5.30)
- peroneal nerve paralysis, especially if both legs are affected (Plate 5.32)
- dislocation of the pelvis from the spine (Plate 5.33)
- rupture of the gastrocnemious tendon (Plate 5.34)
- severe muscle damage in the hind legs (Plate 5.35)
- fractured femur and dislocation of the hip

**Obturator paralysis** This is the classic problem following a tight calving. Originating in the spine, the obturator nerve passes through the inside of the pelvis on its way to the muscles of the hind leg. It can therefore be easily damaged by an oversized calf being pulled through the pelvis. The nerve supplies the muscles responsible for pulling the hind legs together, so that when it is damaged the cow literally 'does the splits'. She may attempt to stand, but one or both legs start to slide outwards. If obturator paralysis is suspected, the cow should immediately be moved off concrete and either onto soft pasture or into a straw yard containing a good depth of rotted straw bedding, where she can get a grip with her feet. A rope or belt can be tied just above the hocks, to prevent her legs splaying out, or a chain can be used as in Plate 5.31. If left unattended, and she 'does

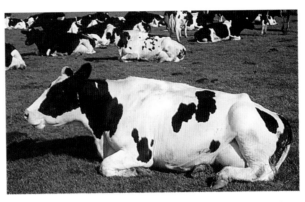

Plate 5.28. Correct position of a sitting cow: both hind legs are flexed and the foot of the underneath leg can only just be seen in front of the udder.

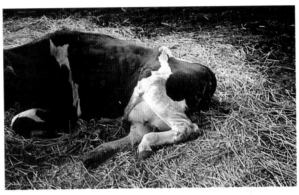

Plate 5.29. The lower leg of this cow is extended too far forwards. If left like this, nerve or muscle damage will result.

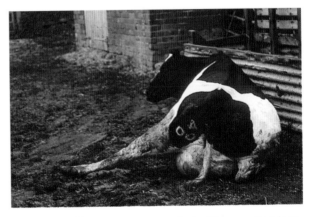

Plate 5.30. Obturator nerve paralysis. This cow has lost the ability to pull her two legs together. Her legs must be hobbled and she must be moved away from slippery concrete immediately; otherwise a broken leg will result.

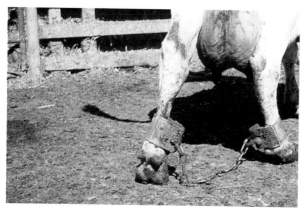

Plate 5.31. Hobbles should always be used if there is any risk of the legs splaying apart following a calving injury or milk fever.

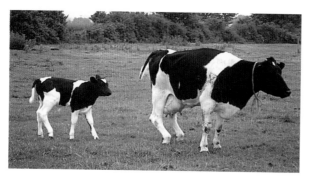

Plate 5.32. Peroneal nerve paralysis: note how both the cow's hind legs are knuckled at the fetlock. The cause of the problem (the large bull calf) is walking along behind!

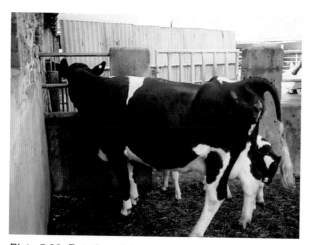

Plate 5.33. Rotation of the pelvis on the spine, a fairly common injury caused by oversized calves.

the splits' on slippery concrete, this could result in severe muscle tearing (Plate 5.35), a fracture of the top of the femur, a dislocation of the hip, or a fracture of the pelvis. All four conditions are likely to be irreversible and probably mean that the cow would have to be sent off as a casualty.

**Peroneal nerve paralysis** The other very common injury at calving is damage to the peroneal nerve, which runs from the spinal cord through the pelvis and then down over the outside of the hock towards the foot. Loss of function of the nerve results in the cow being unable to straighten the fetlock and, when she tries to walk, she knuckles forwards, as shown in Plate 5.32. In more severe cases the hock is also dropped, so that the cow walks with the stifle extended and the hock is almost on the ground (the normal position of these joints is given in Figure 9.23).

It is surprising how well cows manage to compensate for peroneal nerve injuries and provided they get up and start walking the majority of them slowly recover, although recovery may take anything from a few days to two or three months. It is doubtful if anti-inflammatory drugs (e.g. cortisone, flunixin or phenylbutazone) produce any significant benefit other than during the first few days after the injury, when they may prevent the condition from deteriorating.

**Dislocation (rotation) of the pelvis** The pelvis is attached to the spine by ligaments only (Plate 5.7). There is no bony connection. At calving the ligaments relax to allow the calf to pass and this explains why the cow 'drops in' beside her tail, as shown in Plate 5.6. However, if severe traction is applied to the calf when the pelvic ligaments are in the relaxed state, it could lead to a permanent rotation of the pelvis, as shown in Plate 5.33. This cow was able to stand again, but many are not.

**Rupture of the gastrocnemius tendon** The gastrocnemius tendon connects to the main muscle mass in the hind leg and runs down over the hock to the foot. If a severe strain is placed on the leg (or if the tendon and/or muscle is weakened by having the cow sitting or lying on it for an extended period of time), the gastrocnemious tendon may break and then the hock drops to the ground. A typical example is shown in Plate 5.34. There is no treatment and the cow is best culled.

**Severe muscle damage** The hardening and enlargement of the muscle can be seen in the left hind leg of the cow in Plate 5.35, where the left leg is swollen from the hock to the stifle. She never recovered. It is sometimes referred to as the compartmental syndrome and consists of a pressure degeneration of the muscle inside its own thick covering (the fascia). Although surgery is possible, most cases are best culled. Muscle damage results either from tearing or from excess pressure if the leg is left in the incorrect lying position.

**Fractured femur and hip dislocation** These most commonly occur when a cow, unsteady on her legs, attempts to stand and then falls over. It will be the fate of the cow in Plate 5.30 unless she is moved off concrete.

*Acute mastitis*
A high proportion of acute cases of mastitis occur around calving or soon after, and mastitis should always be suspected as a cause of the downer cow. In all the cases mentioned so far, the cow generally looks quite bright and alert (except of course in the terminal stages of blood loss). A cow with mastitis has a very dull appearance, however, often with its eyes sinking. The pathetic depressed gaze of the cow in Plate 5.36 is typical of this. It may have developed a profuse scour. In this respect it is very different from a milk fever cow which is normally constipated. Its temperature is usually raised, but not always. It may even be below normal. The pulse will be very rapid, and this is an important differential from milk fever, when the pulse is often slow. The udder of a downer cow should *always be checked* before arriving at any final conclusions, although when colostrum is present it may be very difficult to detect the early changes associated with, for example, *E. coli* mastitis. Treatment is discussed in Chapter 7.

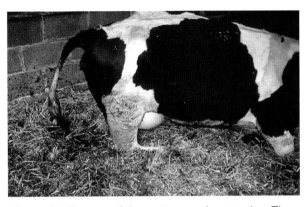

Plate 5.34. Rupture of the gastrocnemious tendon. The whole lower leg, from hock to foot, now rests on the ground. There is no treatment.

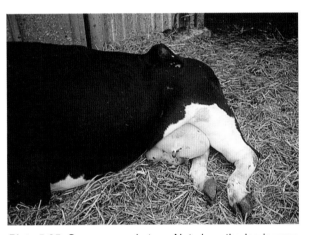

Plate 5.35. Severe muscle tear. Note how the leg is very swollen from the hock to the stifle. This cow never recovered. Often the affected muscles also become very hard.

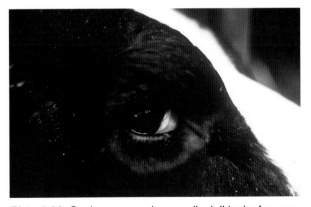

Plate 5.36. Sunken eye and generally dull look of a cow, recumbent because of toxic mastitis.

*Liver failure*

This generally occurs as a consequence of some other condition, for example an unresponsive case of milk fever, which has led to recumbency and depression of appetite for a few days. It is especially common in overfat, high-producing animals and will be dealt with in more detail in Chapter 6.

## Care of the Down Cow

The two most critical aspects of care have already been mentioned. They are moving the cow to a field or some other suitable non-slip surface, and secondly making sure that her legs are in the correct sitting position (Plates 5.28 and 5.29).

It is not difficult to move a recumbent cow onto a gate, wooden pallet or tractor with a fore-end loader. Drive the loader towards the cow and lift one front and one back leg onto the edge of the loader. Next, roll her right over so that she is lying flat on her other side. She will then be lying in the loader bucket (Plate 5.37) and can be carried away. If using a gate or pallet, attach the end of the gate nearest to her head to a tractor with a short chain. When the tractor pulls, her head will then be lifted off the ground. As she is being moved, an assistant may need to lift the lower hind leg, to avoid damaging the udder.

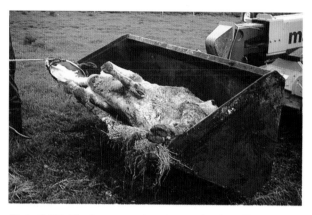

Plate 5.37. Moving a cow in a tractor bucket. If she is rolled partly onto her back she cannot fall out. The head is restrained by a halter to prevent injury if struggling occurs.

Once you have moved the cow onto a firm surface and away from slippery concrete, it is easy to roll her out of the bucket or off the gate, and with added confidence many cows will simply stand up and walk away. Those which do not, however, need to be positioned correctly, as described in the previous section, and given continual access to food and water. If she is outside in the winter, a large carpet draped over her provides excellent protection and, if it is large enough, it will not fall off when she moves. Unless recumbent cows are moving themselves, they need to be rolled from side to side at least four times each day. You will want your vet to check her periodically for illness, fractures and other irreversible injuries, and then much of her chances of recovery must depend on how long you are prepared to persist with nursing.

Some people consider cow lifting aids to be valuable. The Bagshawe hoist (Plate 5.38) fits over the wings of the cow's pelvis (the pin bones: Figure 9.23). The screw must be turned up very tight, so that the vertical part of the hoist is pressing against the edges of the bones of the lumbar spine. If the cow moves and falls from the hoist during lifting, considerable damage can occur, e.g. fracture of the pelvis. Once onto their front legs,

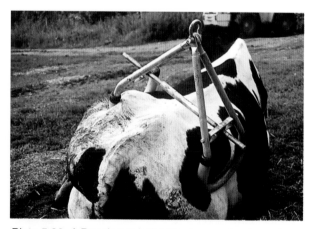

Plate 5.38. A Bagshawe hoist lifts a recumbent cow by means of clamping onto the pelvis. Although only giving support to her hindquarters, it does mean that she can get some circulation going and the big advantage is that the hoist can be used single-handed.

some cows will walk forwards, and the advantage of the hoist is that the tractor can be driven along behind her, supporting her walking. For other cows the hoist appears totally ineffective, however, because the cow simply hangs, without making any effort to stand.

An alternative device is a lifting bag, which is positioned under the cow's chest and then inflated using a small pump operated from a 12 volt battery. If the cow is then gently pushed forwards so that the bag rolls back towards her udder, the forwards lunging movement she feels is often sufficient to get her to stand on her front legs, with the bag supporting her hindquarters. When she takes her own weight, the air can be slowly released and the bag removed. Some cows try to rush forwards as soon as they are lifted and trip over the bag before it can be removed. Much larger bags are available, but I find that because they support the whole cow, like an enormous cushion, the cows make no effort to stand on their own.

Lifting nets can also be used, as in Plate 5.39. They are not easy to fit onto the cow, and it is unlikely that anyone could do it single-handed, but they give good support when the cow is hoisted. The use of a large straw bale to support some of the weight of the cow, as shown, is an excellent idea. If unsupported cows are left hanging in the net too long, the weight-bearing edges of the net can cut off the circulation to the legs, resulting in swelling and tissue damage.

At one time the use of a mobile warm water bath, to float recumbent cows into the standing position, was advocated. Great success was claimed for these, but they are not commonly used. Mobile hoists (Plate 5.40) which lift cows and then allow them to walk on their own (theoretically!) are also available.

Dealing with any recumbent cow can be a most frustrating and time-consuming experience, and when physical injuries and metabolic problems have been eliminated, it cannot be overstressed that time and careful

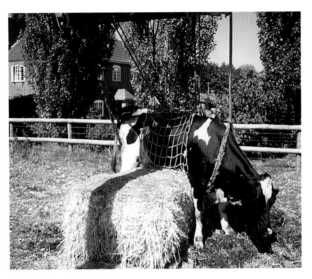

Plate 5.39. A lifting net gives much better support but is more difficult to fit. Lifting the cow onto a bale of straw also helps.

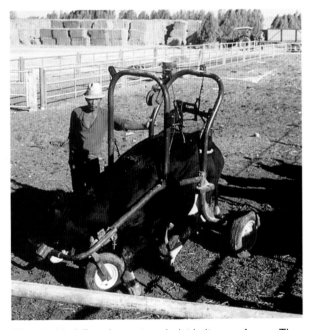

Plate 5.40. A Bagshawe-type hoist in its own frame. The idea is that once lifted by the winch, the cow can walk around on her own within the mobile frame.

nursing are the two most important factors determining recovery. Unfortunately many farms simply do not have the facilities to lift a cow and turn her several times each day, but for anyone prepared to spend the time, their efforts can be amply rewarded. I have known at least three cows get up and lead a useful productive life after being 'down' for four weeks or more.

# OTHER POST CALVING COMPLICATIONS

Blood loss and nerve damage are normally apparent immediately after calving, although occasionally cows suffer a severe haemorrhage two or three days later. Acute mastitis can also occur at any time during the first few weeks, and may be the cause of severe illness without necessarily leading to recumbency. The other important post calving conditions are retained placenta, metritis, vaginal infections, rectovaginal fistula and prolapse of the uterus, vagina or cervix. Failure of milk let-down, blocked teats and blind quarters are also evident during this period. They are discussed in Chapter 7.

## Retained Placenta

Earlier in the chapter we said that expulsion of the placenta (the afterbirth or cleansing) was the third stage of labour and should occur within approximately six hours of the birth of the calf. A proportion of cows will pass the placenta within 24 hours, but after this, uterine contractions become very weak or non-existent, and then several days will have to elapse before the attachments to the cotyledons (Figure 5.4) eventually putrefy and decompose, and the placenta is dropped.

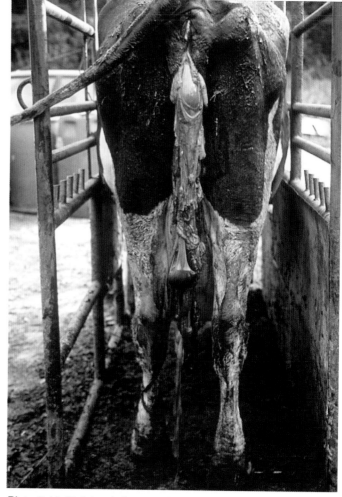

Surveys of the incidence of retained placenta have given very varying results, but if the condition exists in your herd at greater than the 10% level, it undoubtedly represents a problem. The condition is easily recognised by the fact that part of the placenta is seen hanging from the vulva as in Plate 5.41, although in a proportion of cases all of the placenta remains inside the uterus and the stockman may be unaware of its existence. The effects of a retained placenta on the overall health and well-being of the cow seem to vary enormously. Some cows are sick within two or three days, while at the other extreme a cow may pass her whole placenta ten or fourteen days later with no one knowing that retention had occurred and without any signs of ill-health. This is relatively uncommon however.

*Treatment*

This is necessary for four main reasons. First some cows may develop a bacterial infection in the uterus which can lead to illness, reduced yield and even death. Second, under the UK Dairy Regulations milk from affected cows should not be sold for human consumption. Third there could be a reduced conception rate in

Plate 5.41. Retained placenta. Most cows can be left for four to five days before any action needs to be taken.

cows which have not been adequately treated. (Retention of the placenta in itself probably does not affect subsequent fertility, whereas retention plus infection almost certainly does.) Finally, it is unpleasant milking a cow which has a putrefying placenta hanging around its udder and there must be an increased risk of mastitis.

Veterinary surgeons vary in their approach to treatment, but as a general rule cows are left for three to five days without treatment, provided that they are not sick. Illness occurs either because of bacterial infection, or simply because the cow is absorbing toxic waste products while the placenta is degenerating naturally. Even on the fourth day the attachment of the placenta at the cotyledons is sometimes so strong that separation is not possible and your vet will have to try again two to four days later, depending on how sick the cow is. It is *essential* not to tear the placenta and it is far better to get your vet to have a second attempt rather than run the risk of leaving pieces in the uterus.

Pessaries will be inserted through the cervix and into the uterus. These usually contain an antibiotic to kill the infection and possibly also drugs to help the natural uterine defence mechanisms and to stimulate its contraction. Some authorities question the wisdom of using pessaries in an otherwise healthy cow. They would say that bacterial action should be allowed to continue as it is a normal feature of placental degeneration and separation, and anyway there is a risk that any increased blood flow caused by the pessaries may increase the absorption of toxins. Whilst this may be sound theory, the change from a healthy to sick cow may be so sudden that in practice the use of pessaries would seem to be a commonsense safeguard.

Injections of oxytocin can be used, but they are only likely to have any effect in the first 24 hours after calving. Injections of oestrogens have also been suggested, but these may possibly lead to an increased incidence of cystic ovaries. If there is a large volume of stinking fluid present and the cow is very sick, your vet may attempt to wash out and drain the uterus using a length of tubing and a bucket of warm saline solution.

*Causes and control*
If the main causes of a high incidence of retained placenta can be identified, then the control and preventive measures will be obvious. Anything which interferes with the normal third stage of labour is likely to lead to placental retention. Such factors include:

- abortions and premature calvings (including those induced by prostaglandin, cortisone and other drugs). Although birth may occur normally, the processes of placental separation may not. Injections of oxytocin or oestrogen on the day of calving will certainly aid placental expulsion in artificially induced cows
- twins. Retention probably occurs because the uterus is weak after pushing out two calves, and also because a high proportion of twins are born early
- milk fever. This is a condition of lack of muscle power and in this instance the uterus simply lacks the necessary 'push' to expel the placenta
- difficult calvings. Again the uterus may be 'tired' after the calf has eventually been delivered. Sires producing large calves may increase the incidence of placental retention
- unnecessary manual interference at calving. It has been shown that inflammation and infection of the placenta at the very early stages does, in fact, *reduce* the chances of a normal placental separation and expulsion. On some farms there is definitely a tendency to provide assistance with calvings before it is really necessary. As well as the risk of a stillborn calf from excessive pulling and a torn and infected vagina, delivering a calf before the birth canal is fully opened may lead to weakness of the uterus and hence failure to expel the placenta
- dirty calving boxes. During the calving process the cow strains and the calf is partly ejected from the vagina. As she relaxes the calf falls back into the abdomen, and as it does so a volume of air is drawn into her uterus. If this air is contaminated, e.g. from dirty bedding, then there is an increased risk of retained placenta and vaginal infections
- vitamin E and/or selenium deficiency. This leads to reduced muscle power in the uterus
- any condition which leads to debility in the cow, for example liver fluke, copper deficiency or simple under-nutrition

- conversely, grossly overfat cows with fatty liver may have an increased incidence of retained placenta

If you are faced with a herd with a high incidence of retention – and on occasions this may be up to 50% of calvings – the first step towards control is a careful recording of all the calvings, with the following questions in mind: Did the cow calve on time; were there twins; was assistance or manual examination necessary; where did the cow calve; did she have milk fever; how old was she; was she overfat; was pre-calving feeding correct?

It is very easy to read through such a list and assume that the overall answer is known. Careful recording often leads to a different conclusion, however, and possibly more than one factor is involved. Your vet will probably want to take blood samples from dry cows and from cows immediately after calving, to make sure that selenium deficiency or a subclinical level of milk fever is not involved.

## Metritis

Metritis simply means inflammation of the uterus. The inflammation is most commonly associated with a bacterial infection, and we can therefore say that the majority of cows with retained placenta also have a degree of metritis. Metritis often occurs in the absence of retained placenta, however. It may be an *acute* condition, that is severe and sudden in onset and the cow is ill. A foul-smelling brown watery discharge is passing from the uterus through the vulva, the cow is running a high temperature and she is probably off her food. Treatment consists of administering pessaries into the uterus and giving antibiotic by injection, although if the cow is very sick your vet may give intravenous fluids and other anti-shock therapy.

A proportion of cases are so badly affected that they die. These are relatively rare however, and as the cow recovers the uterine discharge slowly becomes thicker, taking on a gelatinous consistency, and its colour becomes progressively lighter until you are left with white globules of pus, possibly mixed in with clear mucus as in Plate 8.20. This is now at the *chronic*, or long-standing and less severe stage, and the condition is referred to as *endometritis* (that is, affecting the inner wall, endo, of the uterus), often known as 'the whites'. The causes of endometritis are dealt with in detail in Chapter 8. Acute metritis can be caused by unnecessary or unhygienic assistance at calving; by dirty calving boxes; by difficult or rough calvings leading to uterine tearing, or by improper removal of a retained placenta that leaves small pieces of tissue attached to the uterine cotyledons.

## Vaginal Infections

These are the result of a tear in the vaginal wall at calving which was not adequately dealt with, either by suturing or by antibiotic treatment. The first signs are normally seen five to seven days after calving, and it is often heifers which are affected. They become very dull, they may have a swollen vulva (Plate 5.42) or they may simply stand with their tail raised. There may or may not be a foul-smelling uterine discharge, but they will always have a very high

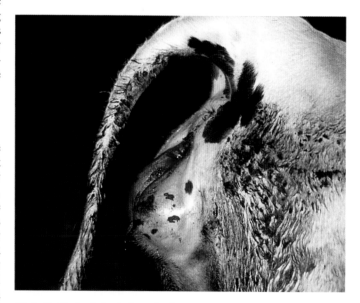

Plate 5.42. An infected vaginal tear caused at calving, leading to an enlarged vulva. This is most common in overfat animals.

temperature. At this stage it is too late to suture the vaginal wall, but immediate and high-level antibiotic treatment is necessary to prevent peritonitis. Vaginal tears are particularly common in overfat animals because the fat separates the vaginal wall from its normal close attachment to the bony pelvis.

## Rectovaginal Fistula

Sometimes the vaginal tear at calving is so severe that the roof of the vagina perforates into the rectum. This is known as a rectovaginal fistula (Plate 5.43). Unfortunately most cases are not noticed until it is too late to suture them and the cow is left with faeces falling down through the hole, i.e. from the rectum into the vagina. This produces an inflamed and infected vagina and seriously reduces the chances of the cow getting back in calf.

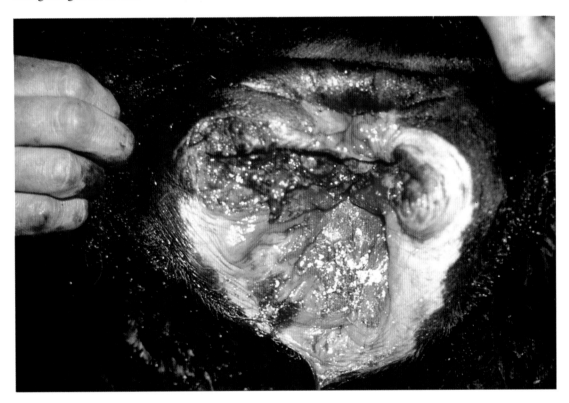

Plate 5.43. A rectovaginal fistula. A severe vaginal tear has perforated the rectum, allowing faeces to fall into the vagina.

## Prolapsed Uterus

Uterine prolapse occurs immediately after calving, sometimes as the calf is expelled, but almost always within 12 hours of parturition. It is thought to be associated with slackness of the ligaments holding the reproductive tract in position, and as such it is more common in older cows. Figure 5.22 shows that the uterus turns itself inside out and passes through the cervix and vagina. If the cow is standing, as in Plate 5.44, the prolapsed uterus will be hanging down as far as her hocks or teats, in other words it is a very large structure. The other characteristic feature is that the uterine cotyledons are clearly visible. The placenta may or may not still be attached. It is not in Plate 5.44.

The mass of exposed internal organ leads to a large heat loss for the cow, and a state of shock soon sets in. It is therefore a serious condition, and you should call for immediate veterinary attention to have it replaced. In the meantime it is important to keep the cow quiet and if possible cover the prolapse with a clean sheet. If she damages her prolapsed uterus by standing on it or catching it on a fence or similar object, the condition becomes far more serious.

I find that the best way of dealing with a prolapse is to give an epidural anaesthetic and then either suspend the cow by her hind legs from a tractor fore-loader as in Plate 5.45 or, if this is not possible, roll her hind quarters onto some bales to give extra height. Some vets put the cow into the sitting position, then pull her hind legs back out behind her. In addition to the epidural, a rope tied tightly around her abdomen, immediately in front of her udder, also helps to stop her straining, and this makes replacement easier. It is not an easy task, however. Two assistants support the uterus in a sheet, lifting it up to the vulva (Plate 5.45), and the task is to force the uterus back through the vagina and cervix. Often two people are needed to push because the uterus is so large that as you push one part of it, another part slides back out. When it is back in place, oxytocin and calcium are given to contract the cervix and uterus, and antibiotic injections and pessaries to prevent infection. There is no reason why the cow should not be served again. Most cows conceive normally and the chances of a prolapse at the next calving are only slightly increased.

Very occasionally the whole uterus, cervix and vagina prolapse, as in Plate 5.46, i.e. the prolapse is even longer than that in Plate 5.44. Although this can be replaced without too much difficulty, a proportion of such cases will die due to rupture of the uterine artery and internal haemorrhage. Unfortunately that happened to this

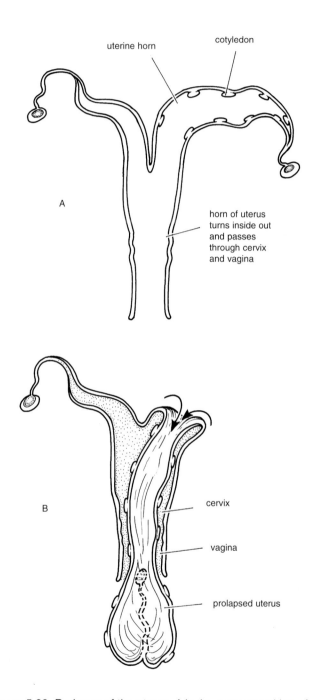

Figure 5.22. Prolapse of the uterus. A is the correct position of the uterus immediately after calving. B shows the prolapsed uterus protruding from the vulva. The cervix and vagina remain in their correct positions.

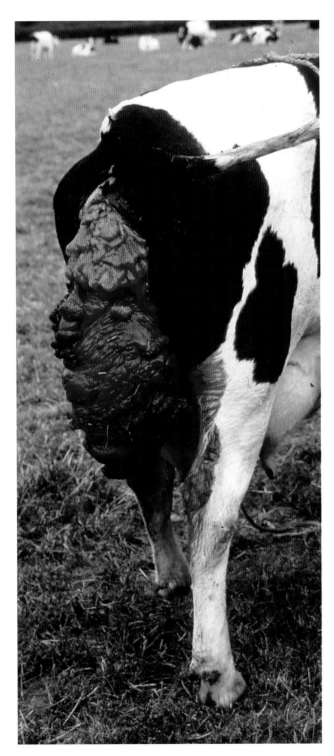

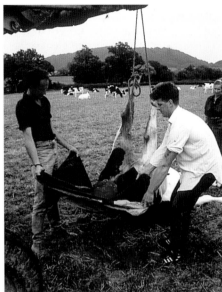

Plate 5.45. Replacing a uterine prolapse. A variety of positions are available, but I find the easiest to be the suspension of the cow's hindquarters from a tractor fore-loader.

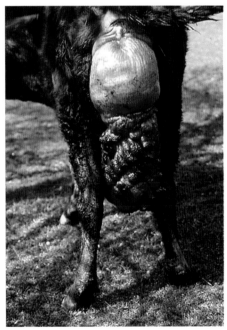

Plate 5.44. Uterine prolapse. The whole uterus has turned itself inside out and hangs down behind the cow.

Plate 5.46. Prolapse of the uterus, cervix and vagina. Although these can be replaced, there is a much greater chance of death due to internal bleeding.

cow. Uterine prolapse must be carefully distinguished from the much less serious condition of vaginal prolapse, described in the next section.

## Prolapse of the Cervix and Vagina

This is a much less serious condition than a uterine prolapse, and although it can be seen during the few days after calving, it can also occur at any stage of pregnancy. As Figure 5.23 indicates, only the cervix and vagina are everted, and the uterus remains in its normal position. You will need veterinary assistance to replace the prolapse under epidural anaesthesia and suture it into position. Make sure your vet knows that he is being called to a vaginal and not a uterine prolapse, as only the latter needs to be dealt with as a matter of urgency. A cervical and vaginal prolapse is shown in Plate 5.47 and this should be carefully compared with the uterine prolapse shown in Plate 5.44.

Occasionally a vaginal prolapse may be accompanied by a rectal prolapse, although a rectal prolapse can also occur as a separate condition. Replacement and surgical fixation are needed in both cases.

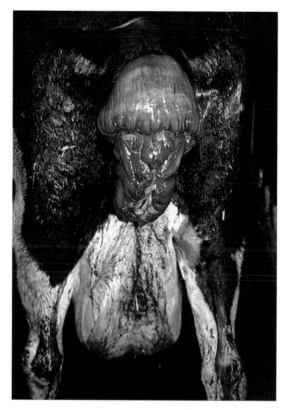

Plate 5.47. Prolapse of the cervix and vagina. This is a much less serious condition than uterine prolapse and can be easily replaced.

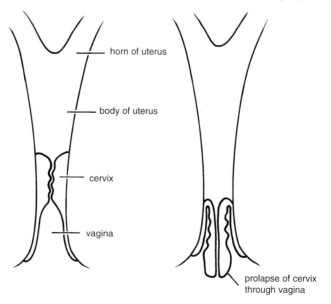

horn of uterus

body of uterus

cervix

vagina

prolapse of cervix through vagina

Figure 5.23. Prolapse of the vagina and cervix.

# Chapter 6

# METABOLIC DISORDERS

A metabolic disease, or metabolic disorder, is the name given to a group of illnesses in dairy cows which are caused by an over-exertion of their normal metabolism. These diseases are generally seen during early lactation, when milk yields are at a peak, and they are due to an imbalance between the *input* of the cow's food compared with her *output* in terms of maintenance, pregnancy and lactation. As such they are sometimes referred to as production diseases. The main metabolic disorders are:

- milk fever
- hypomagnesaemia
- acetonaemia
- fatty liver syndrome
- rumen acidosis

Rumen acidosis is slightly different from the other metabolic diseases because it is primarily a disorder of the rumen with secondary effects on the metabolism of the cow.

## The Nature of Metabolic Disease

For a better understanding of the mechanisms of a production disease, take the analogy of a cold-water header tank in the roof of a domestic house, as shown in Figure 6.1. Water enters the tank via the input pipe and when it reaches a certain level its flow is shut off by a ball-valve. There will be various uses for the water; for example, there will be one feed to the kitchen, another to the bathroom and a third to the heating plant.

When the ball-valve is open, water will enter the tank at a constant rate and the level of water in the tank will be determined by the rates of outflow; that is, to the kitchen, bathroom and heater. If the system was badly designed, it is possible that output will exceed input, in which case the tank runs dry and various problems occur (e.g. air-blocks, or the heating plant boils).

A dairy cow may be looked at in a similar way. Although she may have several feeds during the day, the rate of flow of nutrients from the rumen into her bloodstream (the *input*) is virtually constant. These nutrients, or *metabolites* as they are correctly called, are used for a variety of purposes (the *output*). Their main functions are for maintenance (for movement, warmth and tissue respiration), pregnancy (and the adult cow should spend about 75% of her life pregnant) and, most

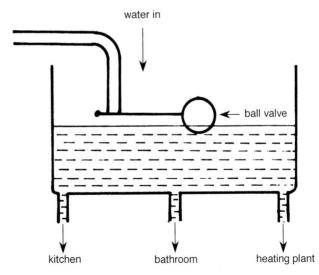

Figure 6.1. The cold-water header tank analogy – factors affecting the level of water in the tank.

important of all, milk production. For a dairy cow therefore the water tank principle can be rewritten as in Figure 6.2.

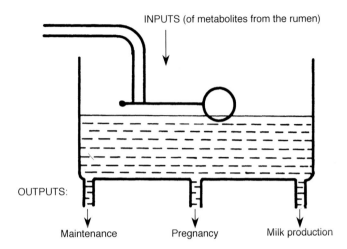

For a constant input of metabolites from the rumen, the level of 'water' in the tank (or in this analogy, the level of the metabolites circulating in the bloodstream) is governed by the over-all rate of output. If output increases without any corresponding rise in input, the level of metabolites will fall until the tank is empty and this is when *metabolic disorders* occur.

## Metabolic Profile Tests

We can take blood samples to measure the level of metabolites in the circulation and this is known as a *metabolic profile test*. The metabolic

Figure 6.2. The water tank analogy used to explain the concept of production disease and metabolic profiles.

profile is an extremely useful technique for monitoring the nutritional and health status of dairy cows in that it tries to identify problems before they are seen as overt disease. The test measures the 'balance' between input, in terms of food, and output, based on the cow's requirements of nutrients for maintenance, pregnancy and lactation. Metabolic profiles are only an *aid* in the investigation of production diseases however, and great care is needed both with the selection of cows to be blood sampled and in the interpretation of results. Even so, they can give very useful information on herd problems, such as:

● unsatisfactory milk production or milk quality
● high incidence of metabolic diseases
● assessment of dietary energy and protein status
● investigation of suboptimal fertility
● mineral and trace element deficiencies

One of the commonest mistakes made with metabolic profiles is that the wrong animals are sampled. For example take a herd where production is disappointing, the problem being that some cows fail to reach peak yield while others drop off rapidly from an early peak. Cows which have already fallen in yield have of course decreased their production to match the food intake being received, that is their output has dropped to balance input. These would be the *wrong animals to blood sample*. It can be seen in Figure 6.2 that if their milk yield has fallen to match the food intake being received, then their blood levels will have returned to normal – and the initial cause of the production failure will no longer be apparent. If you are trying to assess the nutritional status of your herd, therefore, it is essential to choose *normal* cows with average to good production; otherwise the cause of the problem may be missed. Do not choose the one 60 litre cow in your herd – we know she is being underfed!

Normally cows in the early lactation stage are sampled, for example at around four to eight weeks after calving. This is certainly the best group to examine when energy and protein balance are being checked, and there is also the advantage that cows at this stage of lactation are approaching the service period. However, there are occasions when you may wish to sample other groups of cows. When faced with a high incidence of milk fever or retained placenta, it would be best to look at the energy and mineral status of the dry cows and perhaps also a few animals immediately after calving, and analysis for magnesium, phosphorus and selenium might be particularly useful. Copper deficiency is best detected in pregnant heifers, since the requirements of copper for growth and pregnancy are greater than for milk production. Similarly, if you are investigating a possible fatty liver syndrome in your dairy herd, bloods are best taken from cows at seven to fourteen days after calving and analysed for glucose and GOT/AST (aspartate amino transferase, an indicator of liver damage).

A fuller explanation of the metabolic profile test is outside the scope of this book and those interested should discuss it in detail with their veterinary surgeon. The metabolic diseases are described individually in the following section, when the concept of the 'nutritional imbalance' should become more apparent.

## Milk Fever

This disease is best described by its technical name of parturient hypocalcaemia, which means a lowered blood calcium level around the time of calving. As Figure 6.3 shows, the cow has a massive store of calcium in her skeleton (6000 g) and plenty in the food in her intestine (100 g). She has only a small quantity (10 g) circulating in her blood however. Although this reservoir of readily available calcium is sufficient to meet the requirements of the calf in late pregnancy (8 g/day), it is not adequate to match the huge increase in the requirements of milk production in early lactation (25 g/day). There are always on-going 'obligatory' losses of calcium in the urine and faeces (12 g/day), which the cow cannot avoid, and to make matters worse, colostrum contains twice as much calcium as milk (2 g/litre versus l g/litre). There is also a tremendous loss of calcium in the birth fluids.

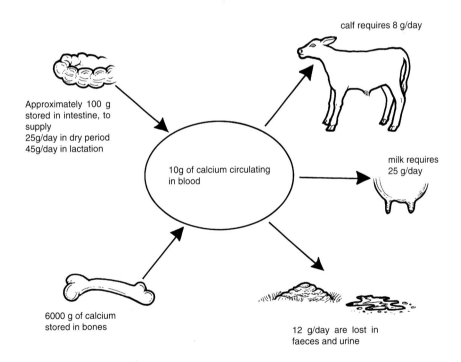

calf requires 8 g/day

Approximately 100 g stored in intestine, to supply
25g/day in dry period
45g/day in lactation

10g of calcium circulating in blood

milk requires 25 g/day

6000 g of calcium stored in bones

12 g/day are lost in faeces and urine

Figure 6.3. Calcium balance within the cow in pregnancy and lactation.

At the point of calving, therefore, there is a very heavy and sudden increase in the demand for calcium and most cows will experience a drop in blood calcium levels. This is compensated for by:

- increased activity of parathyroid hormone, leading to
- increased efficiency of calcium absorption in the intestine, from 35% pre calving to 55% immediately post calving

The effect of this is to increase the amount of intestinal calcium absorbed from 25 g/day to 45 g/day, i.e. a net increase of 20 g. Combined with the 8 g/day no longer taken by the calf, this *should* be adequate (20 + 8 = 28 g) to compensate for the 25 g/day being drawn into milk production.

Generally only a few cows will be affected by clinical milk fever, so what are the control mechanisms which maintain calcium levels? These are explained in detail in the following.

*Mechanisms controlling blood calcium levels*

The mechanisms involved are shown in Figure 6.4. The cow obtains its vitamin D either from the diet or by synthesising it in the skin under the influence of ultra-violet light. Whatever the source, $D_3$ must first go through a primary activation change to 25 hydroxy $D_3$ ($25(OH)D_3$) in the liver. Falling blood calcium levels trigger off a signal which leads to the release of parathyroid hormone. (There are two parathyroid glands on each side of the thyroid gland in the neck, Plate 12.3.) Parathyroid hormone has a *limited* ability to stimulate calcium and phosphorus release from bone, but its main action is in the kidney where it converts 25 hydroxy vitamin $D_3$ (made in the liver) into the very active form of 1,25 dihydroxy vitamin $D_3$ ($1,25(OH)_2D_3$). It is this latter hormone which is responsible for increasing the absorption of calcium from bone and particularly from the gut. The intestine is the major source of calcium around calving: the bone mobilisation mechanisms take some ten to fourteen days to come into operation. This in itself is important, because intestinal muscle is particularly susceptible to low calcium (depressing its activity) and hence milk fever is almost a self-perpetuating syndrome. Low calcium produces a decrease in ruminal movements and hence in food intake and the reduction in intestinal activity further reduces calcium absorption from the gut.

All cows show increases in both parathyroid and 1,25 dihydroxy vitamin $D_3$ at calving, and yet some are unable to mount a response which is sufficient to prevent milk fever. The activity of both hormones is

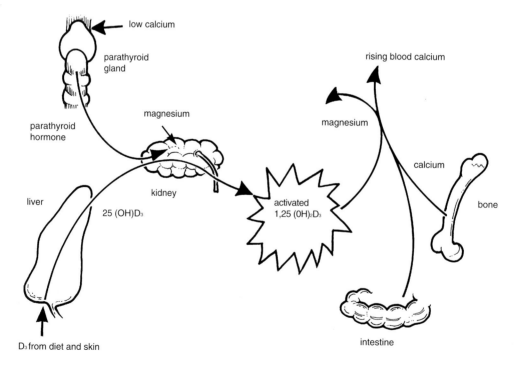

Figure 6.4. Control of blood calcium levels. Parathyroid hormone, produced in response to low calcium, activates vitamin $D_3$ in the kidney and this promotes calcium absorption from bone and gut.

stimulated by the presence of magnesium at the points shown in Figure 6.4 and this is why low magnesium intakes during the dry period can lead to an increase in the incidence of milk fever. Oestrogens inhibit calcium mobilisation mechanisms and since oestrogen levels rise at calving, this would be another reason why milk fever occurs.

An increasing number of high-yielding cows seem to be developing milk fever at six to eight weeks after calving or even in mid lactation. This is usually associated with oestrus (leading to high oestrogen levels) and/or a digestive upset (depressing calcium absorption).

Older cows are much more susceptible to milk fever because they have fewer $D_3$ receptor sites in bone and intestine and hence their calcium reserves are less available. The condition is virtually never seen in heifers and only rarely in second calvers. Cows which have had milk fever at one calving will be more susceptible at subsequent calvings.

Channel Island cattle, particularly Jerseys, are more susceptible than other breeds, and general stress on the cow, in terms of environment, can make the condition worse. Yield is important. Over the ten year period from 1960 to 1970, *yields* rose by 30% and milk fever incidence increased from 3% to 9%. In underdeveloped countries, where yields are much lower, milk fever is rare.

*Clinical signs*
In the body, calcium is needed to liberate acetylcholine, a chemical messenger from the nerve ends which activates muscles. Lack of calcium therefore results in a failure of acetylcholine release and the clinical signs of milk fever are essentially those of a lack of muscle function.

In the early stages the cow will be walking stiffly, throwing her legs out to the side in order to retain her balance. She will be slightly blown (lack of ruminal activity) and probably constipated. Later she will be found sitting and unable to rise, or possibly she is only able to half lift herself onto her hind legs and then falls back to the ground again. The list of other possible causes of an inability to stand after calving given in Chapter 5 should be read in conjunction with this section.

The milk fever cow is quiet and sits with a characteristic 'S' shape in her neck (Plate 6.1), rather than holding her head to one side in a slow bend, which is the position you would see in a normal cow (e.g. Plate 5.28). Her coat feels cold, she is likely to be cudding either irregularly or not at all, and this makes her slightly blown. Her temperature will be below normal. The rectum will be full of faeces, making the anus bulge backwards. This occurs because there is insufficient muscle power to enable the cow to defecate, and is a feature clearly seen in Plate 6.1. As blood calcium falls, intestinal movement also decreases and as a result, even less calcium is absorbed from the gut into the blood. Some cows develop a fine muscle tremor, seen as a 'shivering' especially over the neck and chest area. If left untreated, the muscle paralysis worsens and the cow eventu-

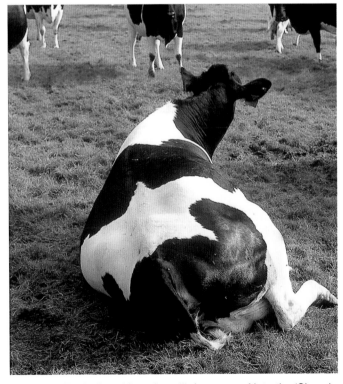

Plate 6.1. Typical position of a milk fever cow. Note the 'S' neck and the rectum bulging with faeces under her tail.

ally rolls over onto her side and lacks the power to sit up again. When she is on her side the normal rumen gases cannot escape, so she becomes bloated and death is caused by either excessive pressure on the heart or possibly by inhaling rumen contents which have been forced up into the mouth by the pressure of the gas.

These are the general clinical signs of milk fever. What is often not realised, however, is that cows which have had milk fever have a reduced resistance and are therefore much more susceptible to a whole range of subsequent conditions such as retained placenta, mastitis, metritis and fatty liver syndrome. A proportion will also develop secondary injuries to bones, nerves or muscles and will never get up. Finally, those which do recover will have poorer fertility. Table 6.1 shows that days to first service and the calving to conception intervals are both affected. At a cost of £3.50 per day (1998 values) the extra 28 days from calving to conception, that is the extra time to get a milk fever cow back in calf, will amount to £98 – and this is in addition to the cost of treatment.

Table 6.1. Cows which have had milk fever are likely to be much slower to get back in calf. There is also an increased risk of acetonaemia.

|  | Normal calvings | Cows with milk fever |
|---|---|---|
| Number of cows | 27 | 30 |
| Percentage cycling by 5 weeks | 32.5 | 12.5 |
| Days from calving to first oestrus | 54 | 71 |
| Days from calving to first service | 67 | 82 |
| Days from calving to conception | 92 | 120 |
| Number of services per conception | 1.7 | 1.9 |
| Incidence of ketosis (%) (based on ketones in urine) | 48 | 90 |

From Bouters 1986.

*Treatment*

Calcium is given by injection, usually in the form of calcium borogluconate. Various regimes are used and the important feature is to make sure that the cow receives at least 12 g of calcium in one dose. This may be given as 400 ml of a 40% solution by slow intravenous injection – if given rapidly it can cause a fatal heart failure. The technique is described in Chapter 14. Sometimes blood levels of phosphorus and/or magnesium are also low and if your vet thinks that this is a possibility, then proprietary preparations containing calcium mixed with phosphorus and magnesium should be used. There is less risk of heart failure using the 20% calcium solutions intravenously and they can also be administered subcutaneously, but two 400 ml injections of 20% would be needed. If 40% solutions are given subcutaneously there is a risk of producing a sterile abscess under the skin (Plate 10.29), and this route of administration should therefore be reserved for 20% solutions only. Calcium preparations should be warmed prior to use and subcutaneous injection sites must be massaged afterwards to promote absorption.

As soon as it is practically possible, the cow should be manoeuvred into a sitting position. If she is 'flat out', it will be better to try to get her upright while someone else goes to call for veterinary assistance and/or to collect the calcium. Although it is very difficult to do when a cow is blown, try to get her sitting upright, as even a cow with severe milk fever will live for several hours in this position. Bales of straw can be used as supports and it may be necessary to pull her head around with a halter. After the calcium has taken effect, the cow should sit upright reasonably well, although you must make sure that the hind legs are correctly positioned, as shown in Plate 5.28. This is extremely important in order to prevent permanent nerve damage. The first signs that the calcium is working are often a belch, liberating ruminal gas, and defecation, as muscle power returns to the rumen and rectum respectively. It is said that if faeces flow from the blunt end of the cow soon after calcium has been administered to the pointed end, then the diagnosis of milk fever has been confirmed! Encourage the cow to start eating as soon as possible after treatment. This will supply additional dietary calcium and also promote gut activity to facilitate absorption of that calcium. It may even be worth giving a calcium/vitamin D drench (discussed under prevention) to prevent a relapse.

Usually the cow is standing again within a few hours of being given the calcium and the only preventive measure needed then is to make sure that the calf does not suckle too much and that the cow is not 'milked out' for one or two days, as this would stimulate increased milk flow and might precipitate another attack of milk fever. In a proportion of cases treatment may improve the general appearance of the cow, but she is still not standing six hours later. This is an instance where your vet should definitely be called. A thorough examination will be given to check that none of the other factors mentioned in Chapter 5 are involved, and blood samples may be taken to see if magnesium or phosphorus levels are seriously low and possibly also to check for liver function and muscle damage. It may be that the cow simply needs a second dose of calcium, and this is often the case, with full recovery occurring one to two hours later. If she remains recumbent, however, she must be moved on to a non-slip surface and nursed as described previously.

Do not give excessive amounts of calcium at any one time. This can produce:

- temporary *hypercalcaemia* (high blood calcium), thus stimulating production of the hormone calcitonin, which in turn may produce a *hypocalcaemia* (relapse of milk fever) when the overdose of calcium has been excreted
- death from heart failure. Intravenous calcium will improve circulation in the skin, which can result in rapid absorption of previously administered subcutaneous calcium

*Prevention and control*
Spring- or autumn-calving herds grazing lush wet pasture may suffer an almost 100% incidence of milk fever. There are four probable reasons for this. Firstly, grass contains a high level of calcium. If the dry cow has been having a high dietary calcium intake, because she only needs a very small amount (8 g per day) for the calf, her calcium mobilisation mechanisms (involving vitamin D and parathyroid hormone) become 'lazy'. Then when there is a sudden increase in the calcium demand for lactation, she is unable to cope with it. If, on the other hand, instead of grass, she was fed on a low calcium diet during the dry period, her mobilisation mechanisms would be 'fit and active', because they have had to work hard to get enough calcium even for pregnancy. In this state she is more able to cope with the sudden demands of calcium for milk production.

Secondly, spring or autumn grass may contain low levels of magnesium and it has been shown that a marginal hypomagnesaemia (that is low blood magnesium levels) can precipitate milk fever. The pasture may also be low in phosphorus, so that although calcium deficiency is the prime problem, low-grade magnesium and phosphorus imbalances are acting as exacerbating factors.

Thirdly, during calving there is a period of gut stasis; that is normal gut movements cease, and this further reduces the cow's ability to absorb calcium. One of the stimuli for the resumption of normal intestinal activity after calving is the presence of bulky food in the gut and, as all dairy farmers know, lush wet autumn grass passes through the gut fairly rapidly! The incidence of milk fever can be reduced by feeding a quantity of hay, straw or silage to increase the bulk in the intestine, thus improving calcium absorption, both by decreasing the rate of passage of food and by providing a better stimulus for the resumption of gut activity after calving. Not only is intestinal activity depressed at the time of calving, but rumen motility and rumination almost cease. This is explained in more detail on page 170. If rumen movements stop, the cow will stop eating and this further reduces the flow of food (and therefore calcium) along the intestine.

Fourthly, lush grazing produces a high intestinal pH (pH 6.5–6.7) which further depresses absorption of both calcium and magnesium. This is explained in more detail in the section on DCAB that follows.

Some of the more important ways of controlling milk fever, therefore, are as follows:

1. Ensure low calcium intakes during the dry period. Rations as low as 20 g per cow per day have been suggested, but this is virtually impossible, especially if grass is part of the diet. However, it is not uncommon to put late pregnant cows onto a sparse pasture and feed straw plus a special 'down-calver' concentrate (low in calcium) as a means of control. Conventional dairy cakes are especially bad in this respect because they contain high levels of calcium. Rolled barley would be a better alternative.
2. Avoid excessive feeding or 'steaming up' pre calving, so that the risk of fatty liver is reduced and the very high early flush of milk production does not occur.

3. Ensure adequate dietary magnesium and phosphorus intakes.
4. Supplement with hay, straw or silage and provide a highly palatable diet to maintain appetite immediately prior to and after parturition, and at this stage supplement with high calcium products.
5. Try the dietary cation–anion balance (DCAB) approach, pioneered by Bede in North America. It is
   almost the reverse of trying to achieve low pre calving calcium intakes. The system is based on feeding
   anions to acidify the diet for the three to five weeks prior to calving. This then allows increased
   calcium absorption from the intestine.

   • Anions are negatively charged salts such as sulphur and chloride (which are electrically
     attracted to the anode).
   • Cations are positively charged salts such as sodium and potassium (attracted to the cathode).

   The calculation is quite complex, but it involves analysing the ration for these salts (something
   which is not normally done) and then calculating the dietary cation–anion balance (DCAB) as:

   $$DCAB = (Na^+ + K^+) - (Cl^- + S^-) \text{ mEq/kg DM}$$

   (Na = sodium K = potassium, Cl = chloride S = sulphur, mEq/kgDM = milliequivalents per kilogram
   dry matter)

   The actual equation is

   $$DCAB = (43.5 \text{ Na} + 25.6 \text{ K}) - (28.6 \text{ Cl} + 62.5 \text{ S}) \text{ mEq/kg DM}$$

   where the mineral contents are expressed in g/kg DM (see Chamberlain & Wilkinson, page ix).

   By having a high $(Cl^- + S^-)$ relative to $(Na^+ + K^+)$ the cow develops a mild metabolic acidosis, with
   acid urine, and this in turn increases the responsiveness of bone and intestine to parathyroid hormone. In other words, calcium mobilisation is increased. Measuring the urinary pH with a dip stick
   gives an indication of the DCAB: on most diets cows have alkaline urine due to high potassium
   excretion, whereas this system is trying to achieve acid urine. Because grazing has such high levels
   of the cation potassium it would be impossible to achieve an adequate DCAB on lush grazing –
   which is perhaps another reason why we see such high levels of milk fever in cows grazing lush
   autumn pastures.
   Suggested targets for DCAB vary from –20 to –150 mEq/kg DM. This can often only be achieved by
   careful selection of forages and by supplementing the diet with ammonium chloride, ammonium
   sulphate and magnesium sulphate. The drawback is that these supplements can make the diet unpalat-
   able (as much as 0.75 kg per cow/day may be needed) with a risk of depressed dry matter intakes.
   Caustic wheat (soda grain) and caustic treated straw can have the opposite effect: by increasing the
   sodium content of the diet, they make the urine very alkaline and the DCAB may rise to
   +1000 mEq/kg DM. If such diets are fed to dry cows, the incidence of milk fever can increase dramatically.
   The DCAB system is said to make it possible to feed high calcium and magnesium diets pre calving
   (for example, 120 g and 30 g/day respectively) and to feed high concentrates at the same time without any risk of milk fever, fatty liver, displaced abomasum etc. Yields are also said to increase.

Other control measures which can be used are:

6. Give vitamin $D_3$ derivatives by injection. The best of these has the enormous name of 1-alphahy-
   droxycholecalciferol (1-HCC) and in the UK is marketed under the trade name of Vetalpha. 1-HCC
   is converted in the liver into the very active form 1,25 $(OH)_2D_3$ and hence it avoids the kidney pathway
   which relies on falling blood calcium and parathyroid hormone for activation (see Figure 6.4). Even

so, it still takes 18–24 hours for 1-HCC to become activated and its effect starts to wane after 96 hours, although some increase in blood calcium is maintained for up to seven days after injection. Although the product is highly effective, it is still difficult to predict exactly when calving will occur, and this is one of the main problems with this treatment. However, it is widely used.

Very high doses of vitamin $D_3$ (10 million units, 30–50 times the normal dose) can also be given, but these take four to five days to work and have to be activated via the liver and kidneys and are therefore less effective. There is also the risk of calcium being laid down in the arteries, a process known as metastatic calcification.

---

Control of milk fever is based on

- Diet
  - ensure low Ca and adequate Mg in the dry period
  - increase Ca and Mg immediately before and after calving
  - optimise dietary cation–anion balance (DCAB) to acidify the gut and promote Ca absorption

- Management
  - avoid flush feeding prepartum
  - feed long forage to stimulate rumen and intestine motility
  - avoid lush grazing

- Preventive treatments
  - give oral or subcutaneous Ca at calving
  - inject vitamin $D_3$ or $1,25(OH)_2D_3$ analogues

---

7. Give vitamin D mixed with 100–150 g calcium chloride, either in the feed or as a drench, for four or five days before calving. Calcium is absorbed better from acid gut conditions and this can be produced by adding ammonium and magnesium salts to the ration, or even drenching with 100 ml of 10% hydrochloric acid. Commercial oral preparations containing calcium, magnesium and phosphorus are available, although they are not used routinely, perhaps because of the difficulty in treating cows which are very close to calving as a separate group. They are a useful adjunct to therapy, especially for the recurrent case of milk fever. Adding a bottle of 40% calcium injection to a bucket of warm water and giving it to the cow to drink immediately after calving will also help.

8. If faced with an outbreak, or if certain cows are known to have had milk fever in previous lactations, it is worthwhile giving 400 ml of a 20% calcium solution (preferably with a low level of magnesium and phosphorus) subcutaneously, immediately after calving. This will help the cow over her first four to six critical hours and possibly prevent the occurrence of full-blown milk fever.

9. There is some Dutch evidence that supplementing pasture with sodium helps to control milk fever, because sodium and calcium uptakes from the intestine are linked. This would be contrary to the DCAB principle discussed above.

## Hypomagnesaemia (Grass Staggers)

As its name implies, hypomagnesaemia is caused by a deficiency of magnesium in the blood. The disease occurs in beef cows on very bare pastures and in single-suckled calves (Chapter 3), but here we will be confining our attention to the condition seen in milking cows. The balance of magnesium for a dairy cow is shown diagrammatically in Figure 6.5. Although there is some 200 g of magnesium present in the body (much less than calcium), most of this is unavailable and to fill any short-term deficit the cow has an 'available' store of only 4–6 g. Consequently she must receive a regular dietary intake to prevent blood levels falling. The absorption of magnesium is not very efficient: only 17% of ingested magnesium is absorbed from the gut, the remainder being excreted in the faeces. The cow also does not have the luxury of increasing her efficacy of absorption in periods of deficit, as she does with calcium.

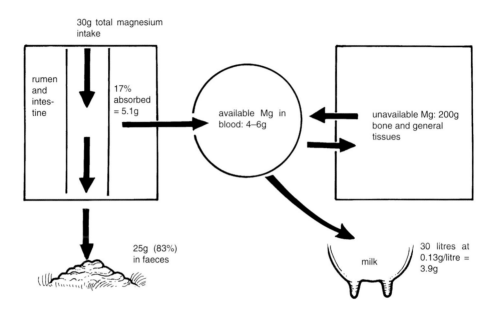

Figure 6.5. Magnesium balance in the cow.

*Intake and requirements*

Milk contains 0.13 g of magnesium per litre, so a 30 litre cow would have a daily magnesium requirement of 30 x 0.13 = 3.9 g per day (Figure 6.5). Lush grazing could contain as little as 0.1% magnesium in the dry matter, so a cow eating 18 kg DM daily would be receiving only 18 g of magnesium, of which only 17% (3.1 g) is available – not enough to satisfy her requirements. Hypomagnesaemia could develop within a few days. However, this is a very low pasture magnesium value.

The level of magnesium obtained from the forage is depressed by factors such as:

● heavy nitrogen fertiliser
● modern rapidly growing swards. The inclusion of clover helps in correction
● high potassium in the soil: the use of potassium fertilisers should be avoided
● lush low fibre and high nitrogen result in a rapid passage through the gut and an increased ruminal pH, both of which further decrease magnesium absorption (most of the magnesium is absorbed in the rumen)
● low dietary sodium. The absorption of magnesium (and calcium) from the intestine is partly dependent on sodium, and if herbage sodium goes below 0.3% (see Table 12.1), the rate of magnesium absorption will fall

*Clinical signs*

One of the functions of magnesium in the body is to act as an electrical suppressant of nerve and muscle activity. The symptoms of deficiency are therefore the reverse of this, that is *excitability*. In the early stages the cow will have an erratic, slightly stiff-legged walk, with her head held high and her eyes wide and staring. If she is suddenly excited, or even if she is driven for any distance, she may fall over and go into *hypomagnesaemic tetany*: her legs will either be stiff and in spasm, or they will be paddling violently. Her head will be straight, her eyelids 'fluttering' if you approach them with your hand and she is likely to be frothing at the lips and 'chomping' with her mouth. The 'wild' eye and frothing are two features clearly recognisable in Plate 6.2. A proportion of cows are simply found dead, the excitement hav-

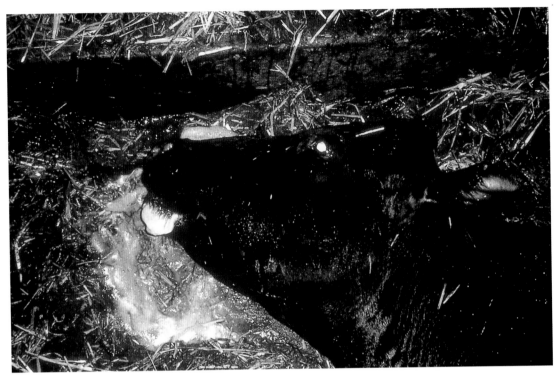

Plate 6.2. Hypomagnesaemia. Note the wild frightened look in her eye and frothing at the mouth.

ing produced heart failure, but even then the presence of extensive struggling and paddling marks on the ground where she has been found lying may give a clue as to the cause of death.

*Treatment*

If hypomagnesaemia is suspected, try to avoid exciting the cow and precipitating a session of tetanic spasms. Magnesium therapy, usually as 400 ml of a 25 per cent solution of magnesium sulphate, should be given immediately. If you have some to hand, administer a bottle *subcutaneously* – if given intravenously it will precipitate a fatal heart attack. At the same time, and especially if the cow is showing spasms, veterinary assistance should be sought. Your vet will be able to administer sedatives such as barbiturates to calm the cow, thus reducing the risk of a heart attack, and will probably give a mixture of magnesium and calcium by slow intravenous injection, monitoring the heart as he does so. He will also want to discuss the relevant control measures for the remainder of the herd.

Following the administration of magnesium and sedatives, the excitability of the cow is soon reduced. She should then be propped upright, putting her legs in the correct sitting position to avoid muscle damage, and drenched with 60–90 g of calcined magnesite, or some similar preparation, to restore intestinal magnesium levels.

*Prevention and control*

Magnesium is not stored in the body and control is based on providing a regular daily intake during the period of risk, that is whenever the cows are grazing lush young pasture. In the UK this occurs especially during May and early June, and can also be a problem in September. Outbreaks of disease are seen particularly following stress, for example on a very cold, wet day, when the cow's energy intake is also reduced. Hypomagnesaemia is also more likely to occur in cows which are mobilising large amounts of body fat and hence there may be an association with fatty liver syndrome. There are numerous methods of improving magnesium supplementation and you will need to choose the system best suited to your own farm routine:

1.  Increase the calcined magnesite level in the concentrate to 60 g in 5.5 kg. Unfortunately this reduces its palatability and may lead to refusal by some cows. Others, particularly those on a higher level of feeding, may scour. However, the main problem is that when ample grazing is available, it is uneconomic to feed high levels of concentrate.
2.  Magnesium supplementation of the drinking water. This is probably the best method of control since the higher-yielding cows who need more magnesium will be drinking more water and will hence receive a higher intake of supplement. Usually a concentrated solution of magnesium acetate is used and this can be added to the water trough by hand, or by means of proportioners. The latter may be fitted to the mains supply, thus medicating the drinking water for the whole farm, or there are simple and relatively inexpensive devices which can be attached to individual water troughs. One such device is shown in Figure 6.6.

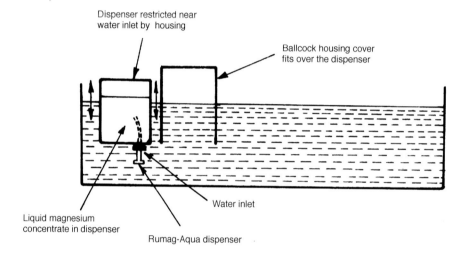

Note: Water flow rate into the trough must be adequate. If the dispenser falls onto its side, it ceases to dispense.

Figure 6.6. The Rumag-Aqua dispenser, a method of adding magnesium to the drinking water.

A much cheaper, but somewhat less accurate, method is to use commercial magnesium chloride, which is approximately 50% pure. A reasonable dose would be 60 g per cow per day, but this of course depends enormously on how much magnesium is being obtained from grazing and other foodstuffs. To obtain the full 30 g per day requirement, a 30 litre cow would need to consume 120 g per day of magnesium chloride. Put the daily amount required by the herd into a fertiliser sack, add some stones and then tie the top. Punch 8–10 holes in the sack, and then place it in the water trough. The magnesium then diffuses into the water. It should be stressed that this is not an accurate method, but by supplementing the drinking water it does mean that all cows receive an additional intake.

3.  Hypomagnesaemia can also be controlled by feeding dry forage (hay or straw) each day before turnout onto the lush grazing of spring or autumn. This is a good practice generally, since it helps to reduce the risk of bloat and milk fever and offsets the reduction in butterfat which often occurs, as well as controlling hypomagnesaemia by reducing the rate of passage of food and preventing high ruminal pH levels. Buffer feeding (also known as storage feeding), whereby cows are fed silage throughout the spring and summer grazing, is an even better preventive measure.

4.  Improve the magnesium content of the sward. This can be done in four main ways, namely:

- Use a clover mixture, since clover has a much higher magnesium content than grass.
- Add calcined magnesite to the soil at the rate of 250 kg per acre. This has an effect only on sandy or low pH soils.
- Avoid using high potassium fertiliser on pastures which the cows are going to graze in spring and also avoid grazing pastures which have had heavy applications of slurry during the winter (both slurry and straw-based manure have high potassium levels). A high potassium content in the soil significantly reduces magnesium uptake by the plants and hence increases the risk of hypomagnesaemia.
- Regular liming maintains the correct soil pH and improves magnesium uptake. A general discussion on methods of increasing soil and pasture mineral levels, and on supplementation in general, is given in Chapter 12.

5.  Pasture dusting: spreading calcined magnesite over the pasture every second or third day, using an artificial fertiliser distributor, works quite well, although it is fairly laborious and entails driving over the grazing. It should be applied at a rate which will provide an intake of 60 g per cow per day.
6.  Free-access high-magnesium minerals will undoubtedly help, but some cows will take far more than they need (probably because they like the taste of the salt added to it), while others will take nothing and be at risk. This is a good example of the fallacy of the statement that 'cows take whichever mineral they need' (for a fuller discussion of this method of mineral supplementation, see Chapter 12).
7.  Magnesium bullets: these are large, cylindrical, metallic objects which, given by mouth, lodge in the bottom of the reticulum where they slowly dissolve, releasing magnesium at a controlled rate each day. Their weight keeps them in place, although in a small proportion of cows they are regurgitated with the cud and these animals are then at risk. Generally two bullets are given to reduce this risk and they supply magnesium to cover a two month period.

Because of the risk of rapid death from hypomagnesaemia, some form of additional magnesium supplementation should always be given when the cows are grazing lush spring pasture. However, one of the problems is defining the period of risk and this can only be done by sampling those cows which are most susceptible, that is, the highest-yielding cows receiving no concentrate. Your vet can take blood samples to check magnesium levels, although analysis of urine is even better. Not only does urine analysis give advance warning of impending hypomagnesaemia, but it also indicates when magnesium supplementation is excessive, in other words, when it can be reduced or discontinued. In this way expense may be saved without putting the cows at risk.

*Winter hypomagnesaemia*
Chronic low-grade hypomagnesaemia has become increasingly common in grass silage-fed dairy herds over the past few years. Although associated production problems have not always been identified, some herds seem to improve in food intake and milk yield when magnesium supplementation is given. Winter hypomagnesaemia is often detected on the metabolic profile test.

## Acetonaemia (Ketosis)

Acetonaemia, which is also called *ketosis* or *slow fever*, occurs in higher-yielding cows in early lactation. To appreciate why the disease occurs and also what causes fatty liver syndrome, we need to understand a little of the biochemistry of the metabolism of the cow. This is given in outline in Figure 6.7.

High-carbohydrate starch type foods, e.g. barley or wheat, are broken down by the ruminal micro-organisms into a simple acid, *propionate*, and this is carried to the liver, where it is used to produce glucose. The main function of glucose is in the synthesis of milk and in fact the rate of milk production is largely determined by the rate of supply of glucose to the udder. This is why glucose is one of the metabolites measured as an indicator of energy status in the metabolic profile test. Propionate has a second

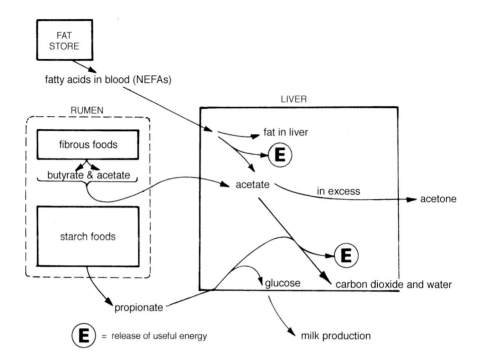

Figure 6.7. Energy metabolism in the cow.

function, however, and that is its involvement in fat metabolism, or more precisely in the release of useful energy (E in Figure 6.7) from fat. The cow in early lactation is unlikely to be able to consume sufficient energy in her diet to meet the needs of milk production and so she sends out an alarm signal to her fat stores. Fat is broken into small blocks, the *fatty acids*. They can also be measured in the metabolic profile test when they are known as NEFAs, i.e. non-esterified fatty acids, and these are carried via the blood to the liver. Once in the liver they are broken down to *acetate* (or acetic acid) and this releases considerable quantities of useful energy E. However, the complete degradation of acetate to carbon dioxide and water with the release of further energy requires the interaction of propionate. The diagram also shows that fibrous foods (hay, etc.) are decomposed by the ruminal micro-organisms into acetate and butyrate. These two metabolites pass directly to the liver; the butyrate is converted into acetate, further increasing the cow's requirements for propionate.

If the cow is not being adequately fed, her total propionate production will be converted into glucose and used for milk production. There is still a signal going out for the mobilisation of fat to produce energy, however, but because there is no further propionate available, fat metabolism cannot proceed beyond the acetate stage, and the excess acetate accumulates in the liver. After a while the liver is unable to store any further acetate, and to dispose of it two molecules of acetate are combined to produce *acetone*. The acetone passes from the liver into the blood, where it acts as an intoxicant to the cow, producing the symptoms of *acetonaemia*. The word literally means acetone in the blood, and it is effectively caused by an inadequate intake of starchy food in a cow which is already mobilising body fat. Other ketone compounds formed from the excess acetate include *acetoacetate* and *beta-hydroxybutyrate*. The latter compound is also used as an indicator of energy status in the metabolic profile test. High blood levels of beta-hydroxybutyrate indicate a dietary energy deficit.

## Clinical signs

Acetonaemia is seen primarily in higher-yielding cows and the first symptom is likely to be a partial or total refusal to eat concentrate, although the cow will probably continue to eat some hay or silage. She then becomes very dull and lethargic, and hence the name slow fever. After a short while, rumination virtually ceases, the dung becomes dry and hard, and milk production falls. In a proportion of cows the acetone can affect the brain and these animals become excitable, froth at the mouth, lick objects excessively or stand with their heads raised and pushed into a corner. The Guernsey cow shown in Plate 6.3 had several relapses of acetonaemia. She was unsteady on her legs and tended to go round in circles, drooling from the mouth and biting at her shoulder. Excessive biting and licking (Plate 6.4) are commonly seen with the nervous form of ketosis. Some cows may even collapse in the parlour, resembling hypomagnesaemia. However, the most common clinical signs are a drop in yield, poor appetite, dullness and constipation, which is the result of excessive fluid loss from the body producing very dry dung.

The best diagnostic sign is the smell of acetone on the breath, which has a 'sharp' scent, like pear-drops. If you are in doubt, try sniffing the breath of a normal cow, then the breath of an affected cow and finally a bottle of nail varnish remover, which is neat acetone!

*Treatment*
Because there are other conditions, for example, displacement of the abomasum (see Chapter 13) which can lead to secondary acetonaemia, you would be well advised to seek veterinary advice for the diagnosis and treatment. The treatment prescribed will most probably consist of three components. Firstly drugs given by injection, to stimulate an increase in blood glucose levels and to boost the rate of liver metabolism generally. These drugs will be of the steroid or glucocorticoid groups.

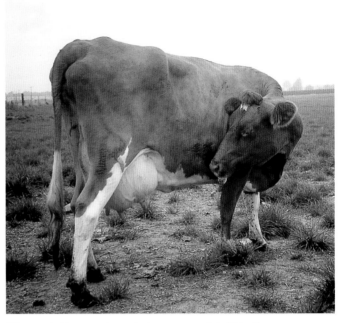

Plate 6.3. Nervous ketosis (acetonaemia). This Guernsey cow walked round in circles, drooling from the mouth and biting her shoulder.

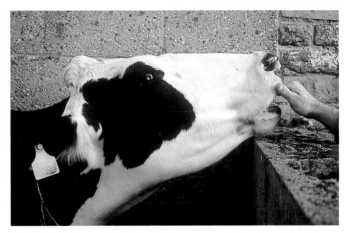

Plate 6.4. Nervous ketosis. This cow was biting herself and would try to eat her owner's hand! Note her sore nose, due to excessive licking, and her glazed eyes. She was almost blind!

Secondly, substances can be given by mouth to boost blood sugar levels and to improve metabolism. Probably the most common are sodium propionate, propylene glycol, and glycerol, which are chemically closely related. Reference to Figure 6.7 shows how propionate can combine with the excess acetate in the liver, allowing its full metabolism to carbon dioxide, water and energy. This will not only reduce blood levels of acetone, but it will also allow the release of considerable quantities of energy from the acetate, and in so doing it overcomes the primary defect of acetonaemia. Glucose will only be beneficial if given by intravenous injection. If given by mouth it is decomposed by the ruminal micro-organisms.

Finally, altering the ration of sick animals and feeding them individually will help. Sometimes affected cows will eat barley, sugarbeet pulp or fodder beet, but not proprietary dairy cake, with its higher protein content. Molasses may also be palatable.

*Prevention*

As acetonaemia is caused by an energy intake which is inadequate to meet the demands of milk production, then clearly prevention and control of the disease are based on maintaining a correct diet. The ration must contain sufficient readily available energy to meet the needs of metabolism as described in Figure 6.7; that is, a reasonable intake of cereal products or proprietary concentrate. If the forage is of poor quality (poor hay or silage), then additional concentrate needs to be fed to balance this and, as a rough guide, the M/D of the overall ration for a high-yielding early lactation cow should not fall below 11.0 MJ/kgDM. Especially dangerous are rations containing excessive fibre levels, silage with poor palatability, e.g. with a butyric fermentation, high nitrogen levels, or diets with a gross excess of protein. These factors can lead to outbreaks of acetonaemia, with quite large numbers of cows affected. If apparently normal cows from such herds were blood sampled, e.g. as part of a metabolic profile, they would have low glucose levels, high acetones and high levels of non-esterified fatty acids (NEFAs) and beta-hydroxybutyrate in their blood.

Acetonaemia can also occur in individual animals and here it may be management which is at fault. Possible causes include inadequate feeding space, so that the smaller cows or heifers get pushed away and do not receive their fair share. Secondly uneven distribution of the daily feeds can lead to some cows being unable to cope, while those with larger appetites can compensate. A third cause is cows which are overfat at calving because excessive fatness leads to reduced appetites in early lactation, thus making them more susceptible to acetonaemia. This may occur as an individual or a herd problem.

Sometimes there is a primary failure of the liver, so that the cow is unable to carry out her metabolic functions correctly. Chronic liver fluke would be a good example, or the fatty liver syndrome which is discussed in the next section. The conversion of propionate to glucose and the complete oxidation of acetate to carbon dioxide and water both occur in the liver cells, and hence liver damage can predispose to acetonaemia.

> Acetonaemia (ketosis) may be caused by
>
> - low starch/energy in the ration
> - unpalatable feeds
> - inadequate feeding space
> - overfat cow at calving
> - secondary to displaced abomasum, etc.

## Fatty Liver Syndrome

The cause of this clinical disorder is very similar to that of acetonaemia. Research has shown that even normal cows can have quite a high proportion of fat stored in their liver cells immediately prior to calving. Then, with the stimulus of milk production, a signal is sent out calling for mobilisation of fat from the fat stores of the body to meet the energy deficit. This was explained in Figure 6.7. When the fat arrives in the liver, there may already be a backlog of acetate and so surplus fat is stored in the liver cells until it can be used. Eventually the amount of fat stored reaches such a high level (up to 60% of the space inside the liver cell) that the liver's normal functions, including acetate metabolism and the conversion of propionate to glucose, are seriously retarded. This means that the rate of acetate utilisation is further reduced and even more fat accumulates. All aspects of liver function are now affected and in the extreme case the cow simply degenerates into a condition of acute liver failure. A lesser degree of fatty liver seems to be common in many dairy herds. One survey showed that in 40% of the cows sampled at one to two weeks post calving, more than one-fifth of the space within their liver cells was occupied by fat.

*Clinical signs*

The severe disease of total liver failure is often precipitated by some other condition, quite commonly an unresponsive case of milk fever. While the cow is on the ground her appetite will be reduced and so she has to mobilise fat from her reserves to her liver to meet her energy requirements. Some animals continue to eat and drink and generally look bright. Others become dull and depressed and, after a day or two, stop eating – these may be the liver failure cases. Their eyes become dull and they cease to notice your approach or any other movements around them. They tend to sit with their heads twisted around to one side, almost touching their hind feet, and they may then start to make small moaning and groaning sounds with each laboured breath. Any movements are uncoordinated and severely affected animals roll over onto their sides and are unable to sit up, even with assistance. At this stage the prognosis is hopeless and no treatment will be of any value. Blood samples taken in the early stages would give very high GOT/AST values, indicating liver damage.

Such severe manifestations of fatty liver are only the tip of the iceberg.

Table 6.2. The effects of fatty liver on fertility and disease incidence.

| | Normal cows (less than 20% fat) | Fatty liver cows (greater than 20% fat) |
|---|---|---|
| *1. Calving to:* | | |
| first ovarian activity | 20 days | 30 days |
| first observed oestrus | 50 days | 70 days |
| services per conception | 1.6 | 2.4 |
| | | |
| *2. Incidence of disease in 17 experimental cows:* | | |
| ketosis | 2 | 5 |
| mastitis | 1 | 6 |
| retained placenta | 1 | 1 |
| cystic ovaries | 0 | 2 |
| milk fever | 1 | 2 |
| | | |
| *Total disease incidence* | 5 (in 9 normal cows) | 16 (in 8 fatty liver cows) |

From Reid I. & Roberts J. (1982), *In Practice* 4 164.

Many cows are now known to be mildly affected, so that various important liver functions are depressed, simply because of the bulk of fat present in the liver cell. Probably the most significant of these is the effect on subsequent fertility. The protein *albumin* is manufactured in the liver. Its rate of production is depressed in cows with fatty liver syndrome and blood albumin levels fall. Research has shown that cows with low blood albumin levels after calving will have a reduced conception rate when they are served later in their lactation. Table 6.2 shows a survey which grouped cows into those with 'normal' levels (<20%) of fat in their liver cells at one to two weeks post calving and those with moderate to severe fatty liver (>20% fat). The difference in the subsequent fertility of the two groups is quite startling. Cows with fatty livers are also more susceptible to infectious disease and to other metabolic disorders. This is clearly demonstrated in the second part of Table 6.2 which shows the incidence of disease in an experiment in which eight cows developed fatty liver and nine cows remained normal.

*Prevention*
Cows should be fit but not fat in late pregnancy and must be fed well in early lactation to avoid excessive weight loss. Diet is therefore extremely important in control and these points have already been mentioned in relation to acetonaemia. Not only do overfat cows (body score 4.0 and above) have excessive fat in their liver cells, but they will also have reduced appetites in early lactation, thus exacerbating their energy deficit. Cows calving in condition score 2.5 to 3.0 are probably ideal. Providing a *small* quantity of the post calving ration for the final one to two weeks pre calving will help. This will acclimatise the rumen microflora to the new diet, and it also helps to compensate for the reduction in feed intake seen in most cows during the few days prior to calving. Those who use the DCAB system (page 160) consider that quite high levels of feed can be given pre calving. Avoid gross overfeeding of concentrates in very early lactation. This can lead to acidosis, with a consequent ruminal atony and depressed food intake.

## Acidosis

Acidosis could be considered as a metabolic disorder, although some would say that it is simply a digestive upset. Cattle fed all-forage rations have a pH in their rumen of around 6.0–6.5, and the products of micro-organism fermentation are acetate (70%), propionate (20%) and butyrate (8%) in approximately the proportions shown. Following a feed of concentrate, that is highly fermentable carbohydrate, certain types of bacteria proliferate to produce lactic acid and this results in a fall in rumen pH. If the acidity reaches pH 5.5, there is likely to be a reduction in rumen motility, in other words the rumen stops contracting (Appendix One). This results in a loss of appetite, especially for forage, and she may not eat anything for one to two hours after a large feed of concentrate.

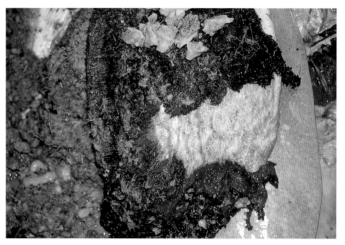

Plate 6.5. Rumen acidosis, in this instance caused by overeating fodder beet. Note the red, inflamed rumen wall and the way in which the black rumen lining is peeling off.

Greater reductions in ruminal pH, for example to pH 5.0, can result in quite severe signs of ill health. The acid rumen inhibits cellulolytic (cellulose digesting) bacteria, and many of the protozoa are killed. This means that only starch fermentation continues, thus making the syndrome worse. When the pH reaches 4.5–4.0 death is likely. The lactic acid concentration in the rumen is so high that the

| The importance of rumen pH | | |
|---|---|---|
| | pH | Effect |
| normal | 6.0–6.5 | good rumen function |
| mild acid | 5.5–6.0 | reduced rumen motility and forage intake; poor cellulose digestion |
| moderate acid | 5.0–6.0 | sick cow; scouring |
| severe acid | 4.0–4.5 | death likely |

rumen wall becomes inflamed and the lining starts to fall off (Plate 6.5). Fluid is drawn in from the circulation by osmosis, blood pressure falls and shock sets in. This is classically referred to as the overeating or starch overload syndrome and is described in detail (as is rumen function) in Chapter 13.

Some of the lactic acid will be absorbed from the rumen and pass into the bloodstream. This produces *metabolic acidosis*. In this example metabolic acidosis is therefore secondary to rumen acidosis. Metabolic acidosis can also be secondary to other syndromes, for example calf scour (Chapter 2). Cows are particularly susceptible to acidosis around parturition. Figure 6.8 shows that all cows have depressed rumen movements at the time of calving. We know this: if you do your late evening check on the calving yard and all the cows are sitting chewing their cud, then you know you can go to bed without worrying!

After calving the rate at which rumination starts to return to normal is considerably affected by diet. Diets high in long fibre promote good rumination. High concentrate diets do not. The cow normally overcomes excess acidity in her rumen through the buffering effects of the bicarbonate and phosphate in her saliva. Saliva is produced when the cow chews the cud, i.e. when she ruminates. Failure to chew the cud will lead to reduced saliva production and the rumen becomes more acid. Increased rumen acidity depresses rumen motility, which in turn depresses food intake and especially intake of the long fibre which is so essential for *stimulating* rumen movements. The whole process of rumen motility and rumen acidosis is intimately connected to the natural depression of rumen movements around the time of calving, and as such it is *essential* that *adequate long fibre* is included in the ration, particularly at the time of calving. This is sometimes referred to as the scratch or tickle factor of the diet. A healthy functioning rumen means a healthy cow.

Straw is probably the best feed to achieve this and it is interesting that many dairy farmers are now feeding increased amounts of straw to dry cows, and are also incorporating 1–2 kg of long chopped straw in the production ration. Rumen acidosis has an effect on lameness, particularly sole ulcers and white line abscess (see Chapter 9). The highest incidence of lameness occurs eight to twelve weeks after calving and this is thought to be associated with the stress of calving.

Probably the worst scenario is seen on those farms where cows are put onto full concentrate immediately after calving, when rumen motility is already in a depressed state. At this stage high concentrate intakes can:

- further depress rumen motility
- this then depresses food, and particularly forage, intake
- if the cow continues to milk, her early lactation energy deficit will be severe. The risk of fatty liver and other post-partum diseases (see Table 6.2) then increases enormously

*Clinical signs*
How would you recognise the presence of acidosis in your cows? The main symptoms are:

- an increased incidence of digestive upsets, for example cows intermittently off-colour and down in milk for a few days
- loose faeces, often with a slightly yellow appearance, and in more extreme cases having a characteristic sickly, foetid smell. Ideally a cow pat should form a discrete,

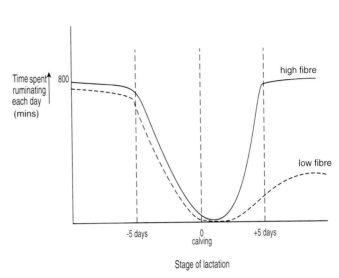

Figure 6.8. All cows show a reduction in time spent ruminating around calving. Increased long fibre diets encourage a more rapid return to normal rumination.

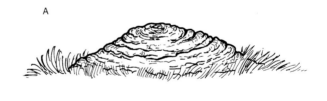

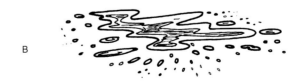

Figure 6.9. A normal dung pat (A) should be well formed, looking almost like a poached egg. Very loose faeces (B), which spread across the floor, can be a sign of acidosis.

solid mass, with a 'poached egg' upper surface, as in Figure 6.9. Very loose dung which spreads across the floor can be a sign of acidosis, although, of course, it can be associated with a whole range of other factors

- increased respiratory rate, with a sweaty matted coat, rather than the sleek smooth appearance we would expect to see in an early lactation cow

- regurgitation of the cud. Dropped cuds (irregular masses of partially chewed fibrous food), approximately the size of a small fist, may be found in the collecting yard or at the front of the cubicles. A typical example is seen in Plate 6.6. The addition of 1–2 kg of straw or hay to the ration, or access to big bale silage, invariably stops this within a day or two

- increased tail-swishing. Some say that acidosis produces acid urine, which in turn leads to an inflamed vagina. The constant tail-swishing can lead to soiling on the back of the cow, as seen in Plate 6.7

- severe acidosis can produce acute laminitis, seen as a cow tender on all four feet. The hooves will be hot and a strong pulse can be palpated in the leg. This will produce an increase in foot problems (sole ulcers and white line abscess) one to two months later

- depressed milk fat levels. Butterfat is formed by joining acetate mol-

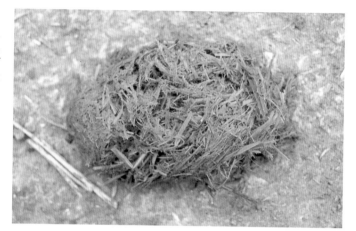

Plate 6.6. Cud regurgitation can be a sign of acidosis.

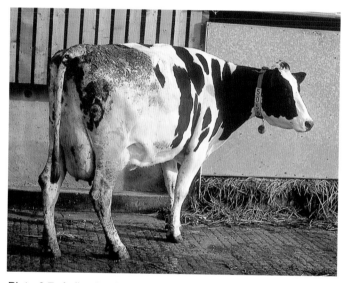

Plate 6.7. A dirty back, as seen in this recently calved cow, can be a sign of acidosis. The dirty back can be due to tail-swishing arising from a vagina irritated by acid urine.

ecules end to end in a long chain (see page 173). If the acid rumen is due to excess concentrate and starch overload, then there will be high levels of propionate in the rumen, but low acetate, and this leads to low milk fat

- depressed fibre digestion. The protozoa (rumen micro-organisms) which are responsible for digesting cellulose are unable to function in an acid environment. In fact in severe acidosis they are killed off altogether, which is why it may take several days for cows affected by 'overeating' to regain their appetite

*Prevention*
The main way of preventing acidosis is to ensure that the ration contains a reasonable balance between starch and digestible fibre and that there is sufficient long fibre/roughage being eaten to stimulate good rumen activity and hence saliva and sodium bicarbonate production. In more detail this can be

achieved by:

- maintaining a minimum of 40% forage in the ration. It is ideal to add 1–2 kg of long-chopped straw to a complete mix. If the straw is chopped too short, it will not provide sufficient stimulation for rumen motility. If it is too long, cows may well leave it at the bottom of the trough. Although straw can be offered on free access, this is by no means as good as mixing it in with a complete ration so that the cow eats the straw *with* the concentrates, which is ideal
- ensuring an adequate balance between starch (e.g. barley and wheat) and digestible fibre (e.g. sugarbeet pulp or cotton seed) in the diet. Although both starch and digestible fibre are sources of energy, the starch ferments much more rapidly in the rumen, promotes propionate production and increases milk protein. Digestible fibre gives a slower and more sustained release. Both are necessary for good digestion. Note the difference between *physical* fibre to promote rumen motility and *digestible* fibre to slow the rate of fermentation in the rumen. It is often said that more attention should be paid to feeding the rumen and less towards feeding the cow. Achieving the correct balance of fibre levels is one way to do this. Medium to high energy foods are available in which the energy source comes mainly from digestible fibre. Examples include sugarbeet pulp, citrus pulp and maize gluten (only about 50% of its energy is digestible fibre)
- spacing the concentrate feeds as evenly as possible throughout the day. This is best achieved in a total mixed ration (complete diet). Feeding systems where high levels of concentrates are fed in the parlour twice daily only are dangerous. There may well be a period of one to two hours of rumen inactivity after each feed. Parlour concentrate intakes in excess of 4.5 kg per feed should be avoided

The type of concentrate chosen and its starch level should depend on the quality of the basic forage. If the forage is already high in fermentable sugars and starch, then a concentrate high in digestible fibre will be needed. If it is a lower quality silage, then a higher starch concentrate will be needed as a 'food source' for those rumen micro-organisms which have to digest the forage.

## Factors Affecting Milk Quality

The quality of milk is not strictly a metabolic disorder, but I have included it in this section because it is strongly influenced by diet and feeding practices. The average composition of typical Holstein– Friesian milk is given in Table 2.1. The main components are:

water 87.5%
butterfat (BF) 3.8%
solids not fat (SNF) 8.6% = 3.2% protein (2.6% casein, 0.6% albumin + globulin)
                                                        4.7% sugar (lactose)
                                                        0.7% ash (minerals, including calcium)

To a certain extent the levels of fat and protein for a lactation are established during the first six to ten weeks after calving. If milk quality is poor at this stage, then it is quite difficult to achieve an improvement later in the lactation and it may not be until the following year that full correction occurs. Total yield is similarly affected.

Diet is probably the major factor affecting milk quality. Fibrous foods (e.g. hay and silage) are degraded by the ruminal micro-organisms to produce acetate, and butterfat consists of long chains of acetate molecules joined end to end. On the other hand, the rate of production of milk protein, which is also synthesised in the udder, is dependent on the availability of glucose, and therefore on the level of propionate production from starchy foods in the rumen (see Figure 6.7).

Inadequate long fibre or excess concentrate in the ration leads to low butterfat levels. If silage is young and of a very high digestibility, the provision of 1–2 kg of hay or straw is beneficial. This applies especially when turning out to lush grazing in the spring or autumn. A minimum of 2 kg of long fibre is required for the average cow.

Conversely, diets with inadequate energy or excess fibre lead to low milk protein. This is common in herds fed hay or poor-quality silage, unless the ration is supplemented with sugarbeet, potatoes, barley or some other energy source, although fodder beet seems particularly beneficial. Surprisingly it is the protein fraction of the milk protein which is reduced with low energy rations. Inadequate dietary protein, especially insufficient undegradable protein, can reduce milk protein, but has less effect than the energy content of the ration. Ruminal acidosis can also affect milk quality as described in the previous section.

Protected fats, that is fats which have been treated to prevent them being broken down by the ruminal bacteria, can be added to the ration up to about 1 kg per cow per day, or about 7% in the concentrate. They pass directly into the small intestine, where they are absorbed and then used by the udder to produce butterfat. They will produce a rise in butterfat, but if too much protected fat is included, milk fat and protein levels will fall. By coating both the rumen micro-organisms and the particles of food with a thin layer of oil, high dietary fat levels have an overall inhibitory effect on rumen function. The fat content of the *total diet* should not rise above 4.5%. This is particularly the case if unsaturated fats (oils) are being used.

Part of the effect of nutrition on milk quality is determined during the dry period. Cows which calve down in poor condition may suffer a depression of around 0.1% protein and 0.2% butterfat and this can persist throughout the lactation. You should aim to calve the cows fit but not fat, that is at a body score of 2.5 to 3.0. Higher than this can lead to fatty liver.

Before leaving the effects of diet on milk quality, it ought to be pointed out that some of the factors which lead to high yields will automatically lead to a reduction in quality. Part of this is simply due to the dilution of milk, although payment systems over the past few years in the UK have placed increasing importance on quality, partly because a greater proportion of milk is being used for manufacture rather than liquid sales.

The main diseases affecting milk quality are parasitism and mastitis. Fluke, worms and even a very heavy louse infestation will all reduce butterfat and milk protein, although the most common is the effect of fluke on milk protein. Mastitis leads to a decrease in lactose and a reduction in milk casein, although overall milk protein may remain constant because the reduction in casein is counteracted by increased globulins. For example, a herd with a cell count of 750,000 cells/ml is probably losing 0.5% lactose, 0.4% casein, 0.3% butterfat and yields will be depressed by 750–900 litres per annum (see Table 7.2). The control of cell count is covered in Chapter 7.

Both butterfat and, to a much lesser extent, milk protein are inherited characteristics, so breeding can have a significant long-term effect. Bulls should be chosen with a high milk-quality performance and poor cows should not be used for breeding. As the genetic variation in butterfat is much greater than for protein, breeding for improved protein status is likely to produce a slower response than breeding for butterfat. Milk quality is generally highest in heifers, falling with increasing age to about the fifth lactation, when it remains approximately constant. It is also lowest at peak yield (probably a dilution effect), although the improvement in quality in later lactation is greater in pregnant than in non-pregnant animals. A large number of cows reaching peak yield in November, combined with the final batch of late calvers being dried off, is a common cause of a reduction in milk quality in autumn-calving herds. Aiming for a well-fed, young herd, paying attention to mastitis and parasite prevention and keeping a tight control on breeding and fertility should all help to maintain a satisfactory milk quality status.

*Chapter 7*

# MASTITIS AND CONDITIONS OF THE TEAT AND UDDER

Mastitis continues to be a major cause of economic loss to the national dairy herd and I suspect that, combined with teat injuries, it is one of the greatest aggravations to the herdsman. Mastitis also has welfare implications for the affected cow. Although the incidence of infections caused by *Staphylococcus aureus*, *Streptococcus agalactiae* and *Strep. dysgalactiae* has decreased and the national mastitis cell count has fallen, this has been matched by a rise in the number of cases caused by *Escherichia coli* and *Strep. uberis*, known as environmental mastitis.

A Mastitis Surveillance Scheme carried out on 144 herds in England from 1994 to 1996 showed that an average herd of 100 cows would have 43 cases of mastitis each year, defining a 'case' of mastitis as one quarter affected on one occasion. There is, of course, tremendous variation in the severity of mastitis, ranging from a few clots needing only one course of treatment, to an acute case in which the cow dies. However, the average cost of a case of mastitis, based on the antibiotics used, milk discarded, reduction in quality and the reduced milking potential and increased cell count of the cow for the remainder of the lactation, has been estimated at approximately £90 for each case at 1998 values. Even at 35 cases per 100 cattle per annum, with approximately 2.6 million cows in Great Britain, this is a cost to the national herd of £82 million per year or £31 for every cow in your herd! Other surveys have shown an incidence of over 50 cases per 100 cows per year, which means that the overall cost would rise to £45 per year for every cow in your herd, viz an average of £4500 every year lost in mastitis alone for a 100 cow herd!

**Mastitis, Yield and Milk Flow Rates**

Milk yields have increased considerably over the past 35 years. Approximate UK average figures increased from 3320 litres per cow in 1960 to 5500 litres in 1996. In addition, 'easy' milking cows have been selected to achieve faster parlour throughputs.

Both factors lead to more open teat ends and therefore an increased risk of mastitis. For example, it has been shown that over the past 40 years milk flow rates from the teat end have doubled from 0.8 kg to 1.6 kg per quarter per minute, and this increased flow rate has produced a *twelve-fold increase* in susceptibility to mastitis. The situation is still changing and as yields increase, milk flow rates will rise and it is likely that susceptibility to mastitis will increase even further. This does not mean that the incidence of mastitis will increase, of course, but it does mean that we need to learn to understand the disease and to house, manage and milk our cows in such a way that mastitis is minimised. It is the understanding of mastitis that this chapter sets out to give.

## MECHANISMS OF MILK SYNTHESIS

The structure of the normal teat and udder is shown in Figure 7.1. Milk is produced by the gland cells lining the alveoli deep in the udder and it is stored in the alveoli, their ducts and in the udder cistern between milkings. The average composition of milk is given in Table 2.1. Its components are derived from metabolites carried in the blood and it is said that 500 litres of blood must flow through the udder to produce each litre of milk. The gland cell synthesises a globule of milk fat in its cytoplasm and then extrudes it out into the alveolar space. As the globule passes through the cell membrane, it becomes coated with a thin layer of protein, and in this way the fat and some of the protein components of the milk are formed (see Figure 7.2). Mastitis can damage the cell membrane, and fat globules may then be

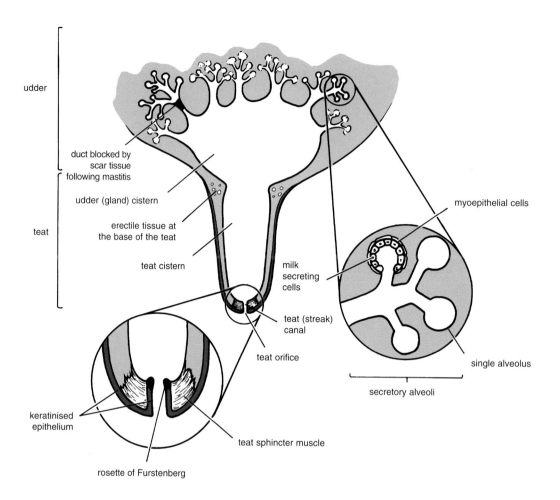

udder

duct blocked by
scar tissue
following mastitis

teat

udder (gland) cistern

erectile tissue at
the base of the teat

teat cistern

teat cistern

milk
secreting
cells

myoepithelial cells

single alveolus

secretory alveoli

teat (streak)
canal

teat orifice

keratinised
epithelium

teat sphincter muscle

rosette of Furstenberg

Figure 7.1. The structure of the udder
and teat.

passed with an incomplete protein
covering. In this form the fat can
decompose, a process known as *lipolysis*, and this is why cows with mastitis often produce milk which has a
bitter taste. The majority of milk protein (casein) is similarly synthesised
in the alveolar cell cytoplasm and
extruded into the alveolar space. Lactose (milk sugar) is produced by combining one molecule of glucose with
one molecule of galactose and is
extruded from the cell in a similar
manner.

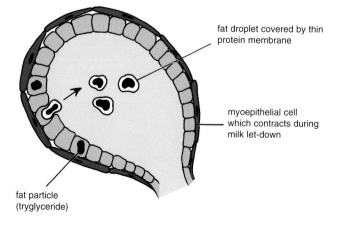

fat droplet covered by thin
protein membrane

myoepithelial cell
which contracts during
milk let-down

fat particle
(tryglyceride)

Figure 7.2. The synthesis of milk fat droplets in the alveolus.

# THE CONTROL OF MILK PRODUCTION AND LET-DOWN

Nutrition and genetics are clearly the greatest factors affecting the level of milk production, and as is explained later in the chapter, mastitis can also influence yields. This short section deals primarily with the hormonal and managemental factors involved.

The induction, or start, of lactation is controlled by a hormone called *prolactin* which is produced by the pituitary gland, situated at the base of the brain. Chapter 8 will discuss the factors which maintain high levels of progesterone during pregnancy. Immediately prior to parturition, blood progesterone levels fall. This allows prolactin levels to rise, and prolactin then produces the changes in the udder tissue needed to start milk production. In many species milk yield is maintained by high levels of circulating prolactin, and the higher the level of prolactin, the greater will be the level of milk production. This is not so in the cow, however, where the continuation of milk yield appears to be controlled by a combination of growth hormone (BST) from the pituitary gland, thyroxine, produced by the thyroid gland in the neck (see Plate 12.3), and steroids from the adrenal glands situated beside the kidneys.

*Bovine somatotrophin (BST)*
BST is a natural growth hormone secreted by the pituitary gland, a small organ situated at the base of the brain. High yielding cows have higher levels of BST circulating in their blood than lower yielders and cows at peak more than late lactation animals. Being a simple protein in structure it can be synthesised by means of biotechnology, viz by injecting the gene into bacteria, inexpensively producing large quantities which can then be injected into cows to boost their yields. BST alters the cow's metabolism so that a greater proportion of her food is used for milk production, thus making her more efficient.

At the dosages suggested, yields will be increased by around 10–20% or 4–6 litres per day for an average early lactation cow. This is approximately the same effect as that gained by milking three times a day (see page 178). Some four to six weeks later there will be an associated increase in food intake and dry matter appetite capacity and this will further increase her efficiency. In trials carried out to date, there have been no adverse effects on either the health or longevity of treated cows. BST is detectable in minute quantities in the milk of normal cows, and cows under treatment do not have detectably higher levels. (This is despite the fact that tests are very sensitive – sufficient to detect the equivalent of one second in 32 years!)

BST is totally harmless to man. Being a protein hormone it is destroyed in the intestine by the normal processes of digestion and even if it was accidentally self-injected there would be no adverse effect. Massive doses were even once used for the treatment of dwarfing in man, but with no beneficial results, since the growth hormone required for man has a different structure.

However, even with all these assurances of safety, there could still be considerable consumer resistance to the thought of drinking milk from 'hormone treated' cows. In addition, the product has to be given by regular intramuscular injections, which some people might consider unacceptable. There could also be problems with pedigree breeding programmes, since careful surveillance would be needed to compare BST-treated with normal cows. As of May 1999 the product has not been licensed for use in the EU, although it is used in many states in the United States.

*Milk let-down*
When milk has been synthesised, oxytocin, yet another hormone produced by the pituitary gland, is needed to eject the milk from the udder. Oxytocin causes the contraction of small muscle-like myoepithelial cells surrounding the alveoli, shown in Figure 7.1. This forces the milk down into the ducts and hence into the udder cistern and then to the teat cistern, where it is ready for withdrawal by the calf or the milking machine.

The overall process is known as milk let-down, and oxytocin is released from the pituitary gland by what is known as a reflex action, that is in response to a *consistent* stimulus which the cow associates with milking. This stimulus may be udder-washing or foremilking, but neither is necessary. The cow can be trained to produce milk let-down (in response to oxytocin) simply by entering the parlour.

One point is important, however. The stimulus for oxytocin release *must* be the same at every milking. If the proper stimulus is not provided, or if it is inhibited, then milk stays in the alveoli and as little as

50% of normal production may be obtained. Oxytocin has a very short duration of action – approximately 20 minutes. If the milking machine is not applied soon after the teat fills, the myoepithelial cells will relax, the alveoli enlarge once again and milk will be drawn back into the udder. It is absolutely vital that a constant routine is established in the milking parlour therefore, so that the cow knows precisely when the unit will be applied and she can train herself to let-down accordingly.

In addition this whole process can be inhibited by the action of the hormone adrenalin, which is produced by the adrenal gland. Adrenalin is sometimes known as the 'flight or fight' hormone: in man it causes a thumping heart, cold hands and sweating, all of which are associated with fear. Anything which disturbs the cows – unusual noise, strangers, rough handling etc. – will lead to adrenalin release and may interfere with milk let-down and therefore overall production. It is adrenalin which produces the defaecation associated with excitement – a phenomenon I expect every stockman will have witnessed! Treatment of milk let-down failure is discussed at the end of this chapter.

*Milking frequency*
Frequency of milking can have a marked effect on milk production. If cows are milked once a day, yields will fall by some 40%. The majority of farms milking twice daily do so at intervals of fourteen hours and ten hours. Trials suggest that only in the highest yielding herds does this produce significantly lower production than precise twelve-hourly milking.

However, increased frequency of milking does increase yields and hence the interest in automatic milking. Cows could then go through the milking system as frequently as they wish and yields would rise even further. Changing from two to three times daily milking leads to increased yields of:

- 10–15% in cows
- 15–20% in heifers

Because of the flatter lactation curve produced, three times daily milking has to be continued to the end of lactation to obtain its full beneficial effect.

It is not the pressure of milk within the udder which limits further milk production, but the presence of an *inhibitor protein* in the milk which reduces further milk synthesis. Increased frequency of milking leads to more frequent removal of the inhibitor protein and more milk is produced. There are two stages to this:

- Initially the existing milk-producing cells simply work harder and more efficiently.
- After one to two months of frequent milking, *more* milk-producing cells form, that is there is an overall increase in productive tissue within the udder.

By more frequent flushing of the teat canal, three times daily milking also *decreases* the incidence of mastitis, and is something to be considered as welfare-friendly in high yielding herds.

*Residual milk*
Machine stripping, that is additional manual pressure applied to the cluster at or towards the end of milk flow, may lead to a secondary release of oxytocin but it may also train cows to 'hold back' some milk for this period. For this reason, and to reduce the risk of teat end impacts (page 192), machine stripping should not be done. For the average yielding cow, leaving *small* quantities of milk (e.g. 1–2 litres) in the udder is not too important in terms of overall yield, and if on one occasion a cow leaves the parlour only half-milked you will certainly not lose any more than a small part of the next milking's production, and possibly nothing if she is not a particularly high yielder. If a cow is consistently undermilked however, for example if only 60% of the milk is withdrawn for seven to ten days, then this will result in a lowering of production. This effect can even be seen in an individual quarter, for example a quarter badly affected by teat end damage.

*The dry period*

At the end of lactation the old milk-producing alveolar cells die off and are replaced by new tissue during, and especially towards the end of, the dry period. A dry period of six to eight weeks is ideal, and if the cow is not dried off at all, the next lactation may be as much as 30% lower. Situations such as this can occur when a bull is run with the herd continually and no pregnancy testing is carried out. In addition to having a very short or non-existent dry period, some cows may conceive so soon after calving that both their 305 day lactation and their annual production will be depressed.

## TEAT AND UDDER DEFENCES AGAINST MASTITIS

Before discussing practical aspects of mastitis control, the natural defence mechanisms of the teat and udder will be examined. This will enable the reader to appreciate more fully the reason why he is carrying out certain procedures in the milking parlour. The section is subdivided into teat defences and udder defences.

### Teat Defences

The teat has a number of ingenious defence mechanisms aimed at preventing the entry of bacteria and reducing the chances of mastitis (Figure 7.1). The outer layer of teat skin, called stratified squamous epithelium, has a lining of dead cells, all impregnated with a hard, inert material called keratin, and this does not easily support bacterial growth. Only when the teat is cracked or chapped can large numbers of bacteria grow on the surface of teat skin. Secondly the physical tightness of the teat sphincter muscle keeps the streak canal firmly closed and this helps to prevent bacterial entry. Third, the streak canal is also lined by kera-

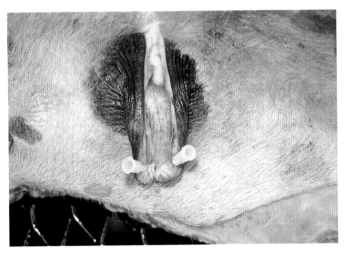

Plate 7.1. Section through a teat showing the interlocking folds of keratinised epithelium of the sphincter.

tinised epithelium (Plate 7.1), the superficial dead cells of which attract, and trap bacteria which may be invading. When milk flows out, both bacteria and dead cells are flushed away from the udder. Perhaps most interesting of all, the epithelial lining around the teat end and through the streak canal contains lipids and proteins which have specific antibacterial activity. These protein molecules are even positively charged so that they can attract negatively charged bacteria towards them before damaging their membrane and destroying them. In addition, the lipid surface lining of the teat canal acts as an extra 'seal'. At the end of milking the teat sphincter contracts and this pushes the opposing surfaces of the teat canal together, thereby either expelling any residual milk, or at least breaking the milk column up into small 'lakes'. There is then no longer a solid column of milk through which bacteria can track back into the teat, ie any 'wick' effect has been eliminated. These small residual lakes of milk can be removed by foremilking before the clusters are attached at the next milking. If the teat canal has been damaged the lipid seal may not be complete, and any serum oozing from the cracked teat canal would act as a nutrient for invading bacteria.

The inside of the teat cistern is lined with a similar type of epithelium (but it is not keratinised) and this provides a further defence against certain types of bacteria, although others may be able to establish colonies in this area.

*Teat closure and mastitis*

At the end of milking the small sphincter muscle around the tip of the teat canal (see Figure 7.1 and Plate 7.1) contracts, thus closing the teat. This considerably reduces the chances of bacteria entering the teat between milkings. Under the stimulation of milk let-down (provided by either the calf or the milker), engorgement of erectile tissue around the base of the teat makes it become turgid and holds it open. It then fills with milk and the teat sphincter relaxes to allow milk to flow.

The pressure required to force bacteria back up through the teat canal is therefore much less during milking than between milkings. Approximate pressure figures required are:

– 15 kPa before milking
–   5 kPa during milking
–   3 kPa at the end of milking
– 15 kPa 30–40 minutes after milking, when the sphincter has closed again
(kPA = kilopascal, a measure of vacuum. One inch of mercury (Hg) is equivalent to 3.33 kPa)

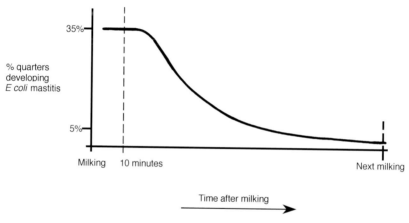

Figure 7.3. The importance of teat sphincter closure and *E. coli* mastitis. Thirty-five per cent of the teats which were exposed to a culture of *E. coli* in the first ten minutes after milking developed mastitis, whereas this fell to only 5 per cent when the culture was applied one hour before the next milking.

Figure 7.3 shows the effects of applying a culture of *E. coli* to the teat end. If applied 10 minutes after the end of milking, 35% of quarters developed mastitis, whereas this fell to only 5% of quarters if the culture was applied one hour before the next milking. The practical implications of this are that cows should be kept standing, in a *clean* environment, for at least 30 minutes after milking. If they walk through a dirty cubicle passage and then lie down with their feet against their udder while the teat ends are still open, the risk of mastitis can be enormous.

The increasing openness of the teat sphincter, leading to increased susceptibility to mastitis, was referred to on page 175. When called to treat severely ill cases of down-calving mastitis, often the affected cow is a very easy milker with a very open teat end. Milk may flow out easily, but unfortunately bacteria can get in equally as easily! We must therefore milk and manage our cows in such a way as to minimise this ever-increasing risk.

In summary, the defence mechanisms of the teat to counteract bacterial invasion include

● Keratinised squamous epithelium is a hostile environment for bacterial multiplication.
● Contraction of the teat sphincter between milkings closes the canal.
● An inner lipid layer completes the seal.
● Specific lipids and proteins have antibacterial properties.
● The surface layers of keratin which adhere to invading bacteria are flushed away at the next milking.

## Udder Defences

Even when bacteria have penetrated the many defences of the teat, it is by no means certain that they will become established in the udder to cause mastitis. Probably the most effective means of eliminating recent invaders is the milk flow itself: the majority of bacteria entering the udder are simply flushed back out again. For those which remain there is a range of very effective defence mechanisms within the udder to deal with them. These mechanisms are:

- intrinsic defences in milk
- macrophages in milk
- neutrophils from the blood

*Intrinsic defences*
Milk contains a range of bacterial inhibiting systems. For example, lactoferrin is present in the dry cow and prevents *E. coli* multiplication; lactoperoxidase is probably important in the control of *Streptococcus uberis*; immunoglobulins in milk coat the surface of bacteria and render them more susceptible to phagocytosis by macrophages and neutrophils.

*Macrophages*
Macrophages are large cells present in the milk which are capable of engulfing and destroying bacteria. This is known as the process of phagocytosis and was described in Chapter 1, Figure 1.3. A cow with a high cell count has an increased number of macrophages and neutrophils in her milk. Although macrophages assist in the control of infection and provide the primary line of defence, they are not the major 'attack force'. This consists of the neutrophils, or to give them their full name, polymorphonuclear cells, PMNs.

*Neutrophils*
Neutrophils are white cells which can pass from the blood into the milk in huge numbers in response to an alarm signal sent out by the macrophages. An analogy could be made between the 'bobby on the beat' (macrophages) and a 'rapid reaction force' (neutrophils).

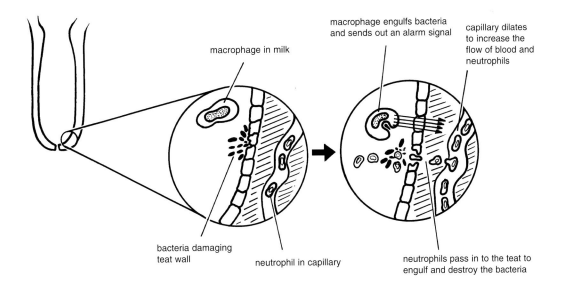

Figure 7.4. The response of the teat to bacterial invasion. This reaction can also take place in the udder cistern and ducts.

The 'alarm signal' consists of a combination of waste products, produced as the macrophages destroy bacteria, plus toxins released by the multiplying bacteria themselves. *E. coli* is an especially active producer of toxins. This is why in some cows we see an extreme udder response to *E. coli* infections. The sequence of events following release of the alarm is shown in Figure 7.4 and is as follows:

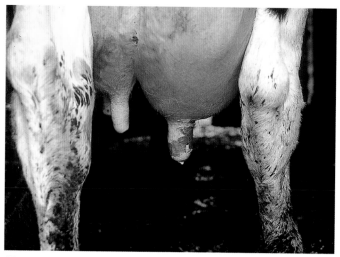

1. Mammary blood vessels including capillaries in the teat wall dilate to carry more blood (and therefore neutrophils) to the udder. This is why a mastitic cow may have a hard, hot, swollen and painful quarter (Plate 7.2).
2. The cells lining both the teat wall and the capillaries move apart, so that neutrophils can pass through into the milk. This also allows leakage of serum, which is why in many cases of *E. coli* mastitis the 'milk' appears brown-coloured, like serum.
3. Once into the milk the neutrophils rapidly locate and then destroy the invading bacteria. This produces more 'signals' and further amplifies the alarm. After a severe bacterial

Plate 7.2. Swollen quarter, typical of mastitis. The teat has been damaged.

invasion of the udder the neutrophil response can be so effective that almost all the white cells are drained out of circulation and blood counts may fall to almost zero! At the same time the cell count of milk may rise from a background level of around 100,000 ($10^5$) per millilitre to as high as 100 million ($10^8$) per millilitre within a few hours. In this case the majority of the cells would be neutrophils – and if milk from just one mastitic quarter were to enter the bulk tank, the bulk milk cell count would rise dramatically!

Although the whole process can be in operation in as little as four hours from the entry of *E. coli*, cows vary enormously in the rate at which their neutrophils can mount a counter-attack, and also in the ability of their neutophils to kill bacteria. In one experiment, some cows were able to destroy 98% of the *E. coli* infused into a quarter in as little as six hours, whereas other cows destroyed only 80%. This variation in activity, which is probably genetic, is seen at any age and at all stages of lactation, so heifer calves could be blood sampled to assess their ability to withstand mastitis infection. Research is even being carried out on bulls by taking a sample of their blood and monitoring the response of their neutrophils to chemo-taxin and *E. coli* attack. In this way it may be possible one day to predict those bulls that will produce daughters with a rapid neutrophil response to *E. coli*; that is those which are able to easily counteract *E. coli* mastitis.

*Stage of lactation and response to infection*
Numerous surveys have shown that the highest incidence of mastitis occurs around the time of calving and this is particularly true for coliform infections. In some ways this finding is rather surprising, because the freshly calved cow has high levels of antibody in her colostrum and this might make you think she would be more resistant, rather than more susceptible. There seems to be something about the freshly calved cow which reduces her ability to mount a good response to infection. This is demonstrated in Figure 7.5. Figure 7.5a shows a good response in a mid lactation cow. There is a rapid rise in neu-trophils and the *E. coli* are quite quickly eliminated from the udder. The herdsman sees this clinically as a cow with a hard, hot and swollen quarter, probably producing a brownish, watery secretion. The cow

may well have a raised temperature and be off-colour, but if a milk sample is taken, it could well be sterile: the inflammatory response mounted by the cow was so effective that all the bacteria were eliminated in six to eight hours and the herdsman is simply seeing the residual damage caused by the *E. coli*.

Contrast this with the situation in Figure 7.5b, which is a freshly calved cow. For some reason she was unable to mount a good neutrophil response. The *E. coli* continue to multiply unchecked and huge numbers are present in the udder. (If this quarter was milked into the tank, bulk milk TBC would soar!) There is no swelling or hardness in the quarter because the cow has been unable to mount an inflammatory response, and initially there are probably very few changes in the milk, but she will be very sick, probably scouring, unable to rise and with sunken eyes. These changes are produced by the release of endotoxin from the bacterial cell walls. Even the use of antibiotics will have a limited effect: the cow needs treatment for generalised shock, since many of her body organs will be affected by endotoxin.

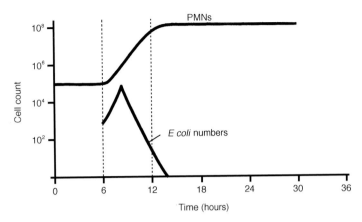

Figure 7.5a. Good neutrophil response in a mid lactation cow can lead to rapid elimination of *E. coli*.

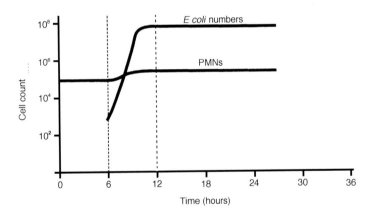

Figure 7.5b. The poor cellular response seen especially in some freshly calved cows allows E. coli to multiply to very high numbers in the udder (compare this with the good response shown in Figure 7.5a). Provided the cow survives, bacterial numbers may remain high for several days.
From Hill, A. W. (1981) *Res Vet Sci*, 31, p. 107.

---

The major factors which influence the effectiveness of the teat and udder at controlling invasion by mastitis bacteria are:

● the quality of teat skin, especially at the teat end: poor-quality cracked skin predisposes to bacterial growth
● the openness of the teat canal
● the speed at which neutrophils can pass from the blood into the udder
● the ability of those neutrophils to engulf the bacteria in milk
● the nature of the invading organism: does it produce toxins (*E. coli*) or does it have adhesive properties (*Staph. aureus*)?
● stage of lactation: the freshly calved cow is particularly bad at mounting a response against *E. coli*

*Response to Staphylococcal and Streptococcal Mastitis*

Staphylococci and streptococci invade the deeper parts of the gland and evoke a similar neutrophil response, although much less intense. These organisms differ from *E. coli* in that they have *adhesive* properties. Because they stick onto the inside of the udder tissue, they are much more difficult to eliminate, even though macrophages and neutrophils kill some of them.

It is important to remember the following:

- Staphylococci and some streptococci produce *persistent* infections. Persistently infected cows then act as a reservoir of infection for other cows.
- *E. coli* does not have adhesive properties and does not persist in the udder. Other cows are therefore *not* reservoirs of infection for *E. coli*, its major reservoir being the environment.

With staphylococcal and streptococcal infections the smaller udder ducts may become blocked with clumps of bacteria, neutrophils and general debris (Figure 7.1). By this stage the alveoli will no longer be producing any milk. The blockage may become almost permanent, and it will then be difficult for antibiotics to penetrate the foci of bacteria trapped inside. Some bacteria will periodically leak out during the course of the lactation, however, to evoke an inflammatory response in adjacent alveoli. This is seen clinically as a recurrent case of mastitis, but even if no clots are evident the cow will be intermittently shedding bacteria in her milk and will therefore be a danger to others. A cow with a chronic *Staph. aureus* infection often has a hard and swollen quarter, as shown in Plate 7.3.

With the virtual elimination of *Staph. aureus* from many farms, *Strep. uberis* is now becoming a more common cause of chronic recurrent mastitis. Although it probably starts

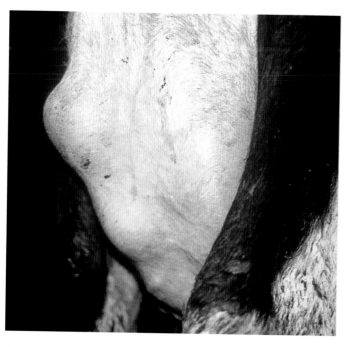

Plate 7.3. Swollen quarter typical of chronic *Staph. aureus*. This cow consistently showed a cell count of 3 million.

as an environmental organism, chronic *Strep. uberis* infections should undoubtedly be classified in the 'contagious' category. Natural antibody defence mechanisms within the udder are relatively poor at eliminating *Strep. uberis*, and many strains of the organism appear to be able to resist phagocytosis by macrophages and neutrophils. Why penicillin appears so ineffective against such strains remains unknown, because all strains are sensitive to penicillin on the plate test (treatment is discussed in detail in a later section).

## WHAT IS MASTITIS?

Any word ending in '-itis' denotes inflammation, and 'mastitis' means inflammation of the mammary gland. Usually an infection is involved, although the inflammation can be the result of bruising. Externally the inflammation may be seen as heat, pain or swelling of the quarter. The cow may or may not be off-colour and, of course, there are changes in the milk.

*Diagnosis by clinical signs*

The extent and nature of the clots in clinical mastitis are often more of a reflection of the response of the cow to infection, rather than the type of bacteria present. It is not possible to be sure which bacteria are causing mastitis simply by the appearance of the milk and the degree of illness of the cow. 'Ordinary' white, flaky clots (Plate 7.4) may be caused by staphylococcal or streptococcal infections, although they may also be caused by a mild *E. coli* infection. The brown-tinged fluid with no clots (Plate 7.5) is typical of an acute *E. coli* infection in a cow which is mounting a good defence against that infection. The blood-tinged gassy secretion of gangrenous mastitis (page 221) is usually caused by *Staph. aureus*, although *E. coli* is occasionally involved.

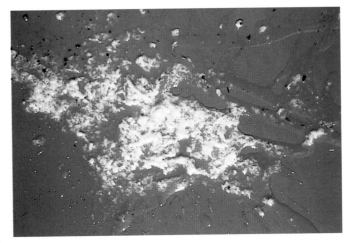

Plate 7.4. It is not possible to be sure which organism is causing mastitis simply by the appearance of the milk. These typical clots could be caused by staph or strep infections, or by a mild *E. coli*.

*Mastitis definitions*

A variety of terms are applied to the different stages of mastitis. They are:

Clinical – an infected quarter where clots, swelling, heat, pain or other signs of mastitis are evident

Subclinical – the quarter is infected, shedding bacteria and therefore a danger to other cows, but there are no outward signs of mastitis and nothing to tell the herdsman that infection is present. In any herd there will be far more subclinical than clinical infections

Clinical mastitis may be seen in a variety of forms, namely:

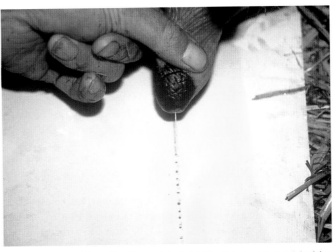

Plate 7.5. Mastitic milk. Brownish fluid like this is most probably caused by an *E. coli* infection.

Acute – a severe infection, but probably only lasting for a short period of time
Chronic – a less severe infection, but one that persists for a long period
Peracute – the most severe infection

## THE CONTROL OF MASTITIS

When penicillin was introduced in the 1940s it was assumed that with such an effective treatment, mastitis would soon be eliminated. This proved not to be the case. In fact mastitis is an interesting condition because many of the control methods which we can apply to other diseases are simply not relevant. For example:

- *Eradication* will never be possible because there are so many different sources of infection, many being normal bacteria in the environment.
- *Vaccination* does not work well because there is a wide range of bacterial serotypes involved and because immune systems in the udder are relatively poor.
- *Antibiotic treatment* cannot be relied upon to eliminate infection because chronic foci exist which antibiotics are unable to penetrate.
- *The breeding of resistant cows* has achieved some success, but is a very slow process.

The basis of mastitis control is therefore *herd management*, specifically aimed at reducing the level of bacterial challenge at the teat end and thereby reducing the rate of new infections. Mastitis can never be eradicated. However, if milking routines and hygiene techniques are improved so that the spread of infection is reduced, the number of new cases will decrease. This must be done within economic constraints: it is undoubtedly more cost-effective to accept a low level of infection within a herd than to spend large sums of money trying to eliminate the last few cases.

For mastitis therefore, all control measures are aimed at *prevention*, and as with any other infectious disease, the preventive measures can be subdivided into a number of different stages. For mastitis these are:

1. Control the *source* of infection. Sources of mastitis bacteria are:

- from other cows, either within the udder or on the teats. These are known as *contagious* mastitis organisms and are spread from cow to cow *during* the milking process
- from the environment, for example straw, sawdust, bedding or faeces. These are known as *environmental* organisms and are transferred from the environment onto the teats *between* milkings
- from flies. This applies specifically to summer mastitis, which is discussed in a separate section on page 216

2. Control the *vectors* which *transmit* infection from the source to the teat end.

- for contagious mastitis, vectors are anything – hands, gloves, cloths, machine liners – which repeatedly touches the cows' teats during the milking process
- environmental mastitis vectors are less precise, but they include anything which can splash infection onto the cows' teats and any milking machine factor (for example, teat end impacts) which can force environmental bacteria up through the teat canal

3. Maximise the *natural defence* mechanisms of the teat and udder, for example maintaining teats and especially teat ends in good condition and ensuring that nutritional status (including vitamin E/selenium) is good and stress is minimised. (Chapter 1 explains how stress reduces the immune response.)

These three major preventive measures summarise all the important points in the control of mastitis. The remainder of the chapter will be spent in examining the different aspects of mastitis control and how the above factors can be applied on a practical basis.

As stated above, there are three major types of mastitis infection. The organisms involved in each group are:

*Contagious mastitis organisms*
These are infections contracted from other cows and transmitted during the milking process. The common examples are:

- *Staph. aureus* (sometimes referred to as coagulase positive staphylococci). Found within the udder and on teat skin, especially if the skin is dry, cracked or chapped
- *Strep. agalactiae*, found only in the udder
- *Strep. dysgalactiae*, especially common on damaged teat skin; it is also involved in the summer mastitis complex

- some strains of *Strep. uberis*
- mycoplasma

*Environmental mastitis organisms*
These infections are present in the bedding and general environment and are transferred onto the teats between milkings. These include:

- coliforms, including *E. coli, Pseudomonas, Klebsiella, Pasteurella, Enterobacter* and *Citrobacter*
- *Strep. uberis* (most strains)
- bacillus species
- yeasts and fungi

*Summer mastitis*
This is a fly-transmitted infection of dry cows caused by a range of bacteria; see page 216.

With such a variety of causes of mastitis, and such a wide variation in the epidemiology of the organisms involved, there can clearly be no one single mastitis control programme applicable to every farm. The various control measures available are discussed under the following headings:

- the milking routine
- the milking machine
- milking the mastitic cow
- post milking teat disinfection
- dry cow therapy
- the environment and mastitis

## THE MILKING ROUTINE AND MASTITIS CONTROL

During the milking process contagious organisms may be transferred from cow to cow and environmental organisms which have become deposited on the teat end may be forced up through the teat canal to cause mastitis. The milking routine is therefore vitally important in the control of mastitis and will be discussed in some detail.

### Teat Preparation

It is essential to adopt and maintain a constant routine for the cow in order to stimulate milk let-down. If cows are nervous entering the parlour or if there is some other change in their routine, then let-down may be inhibited. This could possibly lead to teat end damage, especially if the machine is applied one to two minutes before the teat fills with milk. It will certainly have the effect of reducing milking speeds.

*Wash or dry wipe*
Teats may be washed. This should be done with warm running water containing 250 ppm hypochlorite or 60 ppm iodine as a sanitiser. The supply tank providing the warm water must be covered with a lid to prevent contamination with dust and debris. *Pseudomonas* mastitis can be a particular problem with dirty header tanks.

Buckets and cloths are particularly liable to transmit infection and must never be used. Even if there is a high level of sanitiser or disinfectant in the water, it must be remembered that it takes up to *30 minutes* for a disinfectant to work against *Staph. aureus*. It would be totally impractical to soak a cloth for that length of time. The disinfectant in the cloth cannot possibly destroy, say, the staphylococci from the outside of the teat of one cow before the next cow is wiped. Similarly, paper towels impregnated with antiseptic and sold for multiple use must be very dangerous.

It is the *teats* which should be washed, rather than the udder, and after washing, the teats *must* be dried, using individual paper towels. If the teats are not dried, there will be a small drop of dirty water at the teat end and when the unit is applied, this could be forced up into the teat, especially if there are vacuum fluctuations. In addition, excess water running off a wet udder may collect around the top of the liner, as in Plate 7.6, where it could be sucked into the milk and be the potential cause of increased TBCs and/or environmental mastitis. Washing and drying the teats is clearly important in reducing the TBC (total bacterial count) of milk (see page 214).

Provided that the teats are clean and the TBC is low, an increasing number of herds have discontinued washing. The action of entering the parlour and being given concentrates is sufficient to stimulate the cow's milk let-down, and omitting the washing certainly reduces milking time. There may be a small decrease in yield for the first few days after

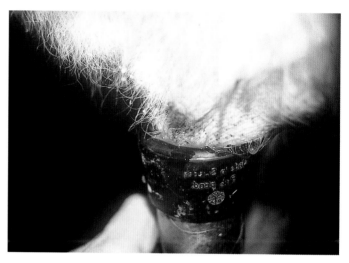

Plate 7.6. This clearly shows the effect of washing the teats (and udder in this case!) and not drying. The pool of dirty water on the top of the liner mouthpiece will soon be sucked into the milk and could easily be propelled into the teat by vacuum fluctuation, causing teat end impacts.

washing has been discontinued, but this is only temporary. The mastitis risk is also reduced, but there is an increased possibility of sediment and other contamination which might contravene the Milk and Dairies Regulations.

An intermediate between the two extremes, and probably the best procedure, is to use a 'dry wipe'. This removes the dust and debris from the teat pre milking, it provides some stimulation for let-down and it also enables a physical check to be made for the presence of mastitis. Alternatively use a medicated teat wipe for each cow. This cleans and disinfects both the cow's teats and the milker's hands between cows.

Of course, if the teats are obviously dirty, then they will have to be washed, but because washing removes the normal layer of protective fatty acids and also the 'natural' bacteria from teat skin, unnecessary washing is undoubtedly detrimental. When the teats dry off they lose some of their natural elasticity and pliability, and this can exaggerate teat chapping. The answer is clearly to house and manage cows so that they keep clean and teat washing is not required.

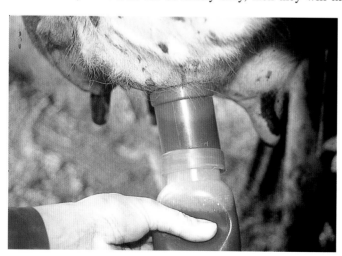

Plate 7.7. Pre milking teat disinfection is the ultimate step in producing a clean teat prior to milking and will reduce significantly the incidence of environmental mastitis.

### Pre milking teat disinfection
The 'ultimate' step in producing clean teats prior to milking is to dip the teats in an iodine solution before milking, as shown in Plate 7.7. Special low iodine (0.1%) solutions with a high free (3–4 ppm) iodine content have been formulated for the 'rapid kill' effect required of a pre dip and these are the best products to use.

Diluted post dip solutions may not achieve this rapid action and are probably best avoided. The dip (or spray) must be left on the teats for a minimum of 30 seconds and then wiped off immediately prior to the application of the cluster.

Because of its higher concentration and disinfectant properties, pre milking disinfection is by far the best way of cleaning teats. It should be carried out as the final stage of teat preparation, after washing, drying and foremilking. Trials have shown that it can *halve* the incidence of environmental mastitis, and those people who use the technique say it also reduces TBCs and improves teat skin quality, which in turn reduces liner slip (see page 192). Pre dipping has an indirect effect against contagious mastitis, but its main effect is against environmental infections.

A comparison of the effects of pre and post dipping is given on page 200.

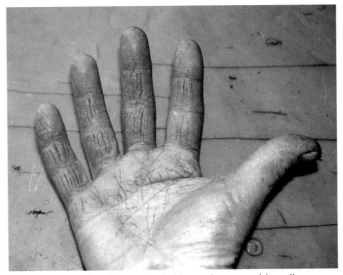

Plate 7.8. Hands with cracked skin, as here, could easily harbour bacteria.

## Use of Gloves

Mastitis organisms may be present on the skin of the teat or within the udder and these may contaminate the milker's hands when he is washing the udder or stripping the foremilk for evidence of mastitis. Cracks and chaps in the milker's hands may be harbouring bacteria and these may be a source of *Staph. aureus* mastitis infection. Whatever the origin of the bacteria on the milker's hands, they represent a potential source of danger to the next cow to be handled.

The danger can be reduced by wearing rubber gloves. Not only are they less likely to harbour bacteria, but they are less likely to transmit

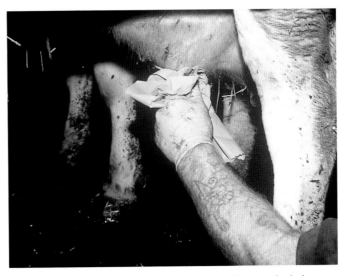

Plate 7.9. Dry wiping with a paper towel. Latex surgical gloves are becoming very popular for milkers, due to improved comfort. To be effective, they must be regularly cleaned during milking.

infection from cow to cow. However, for gloves to be effective they *must* be cleaned, for example by dipping them into a bucket of hypochlorite or by rinsing in teat dip and wiping dry on a paper towel. Ideally, this should be done between cows, or at least between batches of cows, and certainly after handling a high cell count or mastitic cow. Plate 7.8 shows a typical cracked hand which could easily harbour bacteria and would be very difficult to clean. Compare this with the surgically gloved hand in Plate 7.9. This type of glove is becoming very popular. They are comfortable to wear and cheap enough to use a new pair at each milking. Gloves are particularly important in reducing the transfer of contagious infection.

## Mastitis Detection

The early detection of clinical cases of mastitis is extremely important for three reasons:

- Affected cows can then be milked after the rest of the herd, or perhaps with a separate cluster, thus avoiding the risk of transferring infection.
- Prompt treatment can be given, thus reducing the risk to other cows as well as increasing the prospects of full recovery.
- Infected milk can be discarded: if it passes into the bulk tank, not only may this contravene the contract with the dairy marketing company, but it may also cause a massive increase in the cell count and the total bacterial count of the milk.

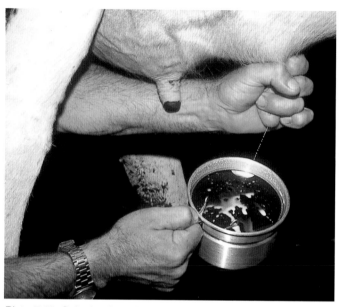

Plate 7.10. Stripping foremilk into a strip-cup for mastitis detection. Some say that milk splashing onto the black examination plate creates an aerosol which could infect other teats.

The best way of detecting clinical mastitis is by stripping foremilk into a strip-cup (Plate 7.10), but this is clearly a very onerous task. Simple stripping onto the floor of the parlour during the washing/wiping process is a useful alternative to the strip-cup Although mastitis is not so easily detected by this method, and there is the risk of spreading mastitis organisms into the environment, it does eliminate the risk of an infective aerosol splashing back up from the strip-cup onto clean teats and contaminating them.

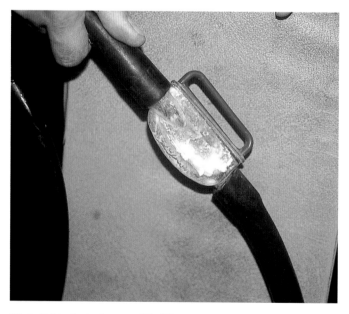

Plate 7.11. An in-line mastitis filter.

### Checking foremilk

Although there are many advantages in checking foremilk, there are some potential disadvantages. In an average herd where there are only 35 cases of clinical mastitis per 100 cows per annum, the herdsman would have to strip almost 8000 teats to detect one case of mastitis! At this rate the risk of transmitting mastitis bacteria from teat skin and subclinical carriers by repeated handling of teats must be close to the risk of mastitis spreading by failing to detect a case quickly enough. This is one reason why an increasing proportion of people no longer foremilk. However, if yours is a herd with a high cell count and a high incidence of contagious mastitis, then I would certainly recommend foremilking.

*Automated mastitis detection*

Electronic systems based on changes in the electrical conductivity of mastitic milk are available, or in-line filters can be fitted, as shown in Plate 7.11. The disadvantage of both systems is that the milk has already entered the bulk tank by the time the mastitis has been seen. Even milk from a single mastitic quarter can increase both the TBC and cell count of bulk milk. In-line filters may also have the disadvantage that they disrupt milk flow through the long milk tube. However, they are an extra method of mastitis detection and provided that *they are checked regularly* and examined after every cow, then they can provide a useful addition to the mastitis control programme. Of course they would not detect the 'watery' *E. coli* mastitis where there are no clots present.

## THE EFFECT OF THE MILKING MACHINE

The milking machine can affect mastitis in several ways. For example

- in the way the milker uses the machine
- by the machine acting as a vector in spreading infection from cow to cow
- because inherent faults in the machine produce teat end damage or teat end impacts

These aspects are discussed in the following sections.

### Unit Alignment

Once the udder is prepared, the cluster is attached and milking proceeds. It is important that the unit hangs evenly on the udder. This ensures that:

- all four quarters are milked at the same rate
- it is comfortable for the cow
- there is no liner slip, and hence teat end impacts (see next section) are minimised.

A unit with poor alignment is shown in Plate 7.12. The weight of the long milk tube is distorting the positioning of the cluster. An increasing number of parlours now install support arms so that this does not occur. A typical example can be seen in Plate 7.13. The unit is suspended very evenly from the udder. Old cows with pendulous udders, where the suspensory ligament has ruptured (as in Plate 7.14), are particularly liable to suffer from liner slip and should therefore be culled.

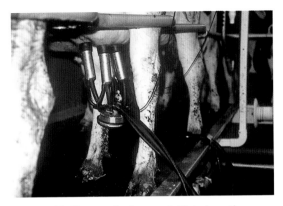

Plate 7.12. Poor unit alignment. Note how the weight of the long milk tube is pulling at the hind quarters.

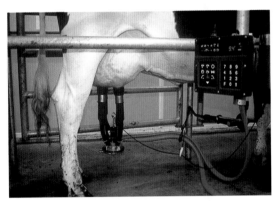

Plate 7.13. Perfect unit alignment is achieved with this support arm.

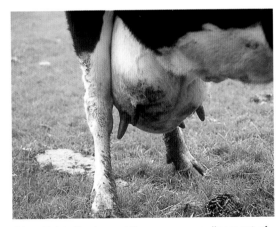

Plate 7.14. Rupture of the suspensory ligament of the udder. This can lead to liner slip and teat end impacts.

## Liner Slip and Teat End Impacts

One of the most dangerous aspects of any milking machine in the causation of mastitis is the presence of liner slip and teat end impacts. Teat end impacts are defined as a reverse flow of milk hitting the teat end. When vacuum is applied to the pulsation tube, the liner starts to open to extract milk from the teat (Figure 7.6). The vacuum at the end of the teat now reaches a peak. If in some way air leaks into the liner (right), milk will flow back through the claw to hit the other teat end (left) at speeds of up to 40 mph. This momentary reverse flow of milk from the claw produces an *impact* and of course it can easily carry with it infection from one of the other quarters. Admittedly many of the bacteria would be washed away again by the flow of milk from the teat itself, but some are not, and research has shown that milking plants producing a high number of impacts have far more mastitis.

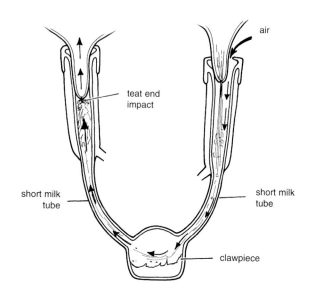

Figure 7.6. Teat end impacts (left) are caused when air enters between the teat and the liner (right), leading to an imbalance of pressure between the teat end and the clawpiece.

Teat end impacts can be increased as a result of faulty milking techniques. If air is allowed to enter the liner beside the teat, then milk rushes up from the clawpiece. This can occur if the cows are nervous and restless, perhaps because they have sore teats or possibly because the unit has already been left on too long. It can be the result of badly fitting liners which slip during milking, or it can occur when the cow is being machine stripped.

A teat end impact is a reverse flow of milk which can hit the teat end at speeds of up to 40 mph. Impacts are important causes of mastitis, often in association with:

- liner slip
- poor unit alignment
- excessively wet teats
- vacuum fluctuations within the plant
- machine stripping
- nervous or restless cows
- poor udder conformation, including rupture of the suspensory ligaments
- poor timing of ACR
- claws of insufficient volume or with blocked air-bleeds

*Machine stripping*
Machine stripping should not be carried out. There is ample evidence to show that leaving the last 1 or 2 litres of milk in the udder has no effect on total lactation production, whereas the accidental inlet of air while machine stripping will produce teat end impacts and predispose to mastitis. For a similar reason, that is to avoid impacts, the vacuum should always be switched off before removing the cluster. Many modern parlours have automatic cluster removers (ACRs) and provided they are correctly adjusted, they will be beneficial in leading to a reduction in mastitis.

*Vacuum fluctuation*
Probably the worst feature of the plant for producing teat end impacts is excessive vacuum fluctuation, especially if the fluctuation is at the teat end. Vacuum fluctuations in the whole plant are usually the result of a faulty regulator valve; for example one milking plant inspection service

reported that poorly maintained vacuum regulators, leading to excessive vacuum fluctuation, were by far their commonest finding. The regulator should be cleaned at least once a week. Any dirt or corrosion means that it may 'stick' and this can lead to fluctuating vacuum. Another common cause of fluctuation was inadequate vacuum reserve of the pump and this occurred particularly when an existing parlour was enlarged or if vacuum-operated feeders or gates were added, but the same vacuum pump was used.

*Claw air-bleeds*

An important feature of the clawpiece is the presence of a small air-bleed, a hole approximately 0.8 mm in diameter, which allows the entry of air. The reason for this is that a mixture of air and milk will flow more evenly along the milk tube and away from the claw. If the air-bleed is blocked, milk leaves the claw in 'plugs' and this leads to excessive vacuum fluctuation at the teat end. Even with an air-bleed, claws can get clogged when milk flow rates are high, so there has been a trend in recent years to increase the internal volume of the claw.

A full discussion of all the causes of vacuum fluctuation would be outside the scope of this book; high-level recorder jars and even the nature of the pipe runs can have quite an effect. More detailed information is given in *Mastitis Control in Dairy Herds* which is listed in the Further Reading section.

I think it is sufficient for the reader to understand the significance of teat end impacts, their relation to mastitis and the way in which vacuum fluctuations can produce them. It is then up to him to call in the specialist on milking machine function for the twice-yearly test or as a check when problems occur.

*Teat shields*

One of the ways of preventing teat end impacts is by means of teat *shields* or *deflectors*, fitted into the base of the liner. An example is shown in Figure 7.7. The reverse squirt of milk is now deflected towards the sides of the liner so that teat end impacts under force cannot occur. Reverse *flow* can still occur, however, and the end of the teat may still get bathed in infected milk.

An alternative and much more effective system is to fit non-return valves. With these it is impossible for milk from one teat to pass across the claw to infect other quarters, and after a carrier cow is milked, only one teat liner will be contaminated. Trials have shown a 15% reduction in new infection rates when using teat shields and a 25% reduction in clinical mastitis with the ball valve claw (a, Figure 7.8). Other manufacturers have fitted a non-return valve into the liner (b) (Check-ball

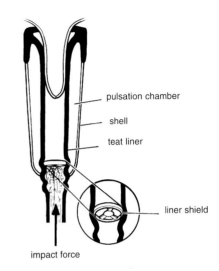

Figure 7.7. Liner shields help to reduce the effect of impact forces.

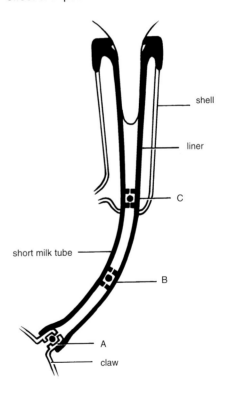

Figure 7.8. Reflux of milk from one quarter to another can be prevented by ball valves in the claw piece (A). Valves may alternatively be fitted in the liner (B) or inserted into the short milk tube (C).

by Alfa-Laval) or into the short milk tube (b) (Hydramast by Deosan). Diagrams of these systems are shown in Figure 7.8. Although these are much cheaper designs, the closing of the valve is not gravity assisted and as yet there is no significant data available on their benefits.

*Hydraulic milking*
It was found that not only did non-return valves reduce new infection rates, but, by eliminating the air-bleed from the claw, they almost totally changed the principles of milk extraction from the teat to a process known as hydraulic milking. Figure 7.6a shows that during conventional milking, milk is drawn from the teat by the milk pump vacuum after the pulsation vacuum has risen sufficiently to open the collapsed liner. With a ball valve present in the claw, however, when the pulsation vacuum rises to open the liner, the valve remains closed (Figure 7.9B), thus cutting off the milk pump vacuum from the teat end. It is now the opening of the liner under the pulsation vacuum produced in the shell which creates a vacuum *inside* the liner and in this way milk is drawn from the teat end. The milk pump vacuum is used to remove the milk and

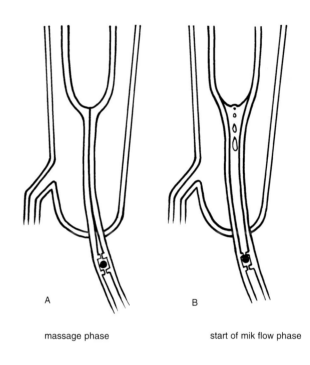

A        massage phase

B        start of mik flow phase

Figure 7.9. Hydraulic milking. (A) Massage (rest) phase: liner is collapsed but the teat remains bathed in a small quantity of milk. (B) Extraction phase: the ball valve initially remains closed. Application of pulsation vacuum opens the liner and this draws the milk out from the teat. When the liner is full the ball valve opens and milk is drawn away.

this occurs only when the liner is fully open and full of milk, and during the early stages of liner collapse (at the 'rest' phase of the pulsation cycle – Figures 7.9 and 7.10). During ball valve milking, therefore, liners and short milk tubes are continually flooded, the teat is continually bathed in milk and the forces on the teat end are applied through a column of milk and not by air. This is why the process is known as *hydraulic milking*.

Extremely high vacuum levels (up to 90 kPa) are reached at the teat end during hydraulic milking, and unless the machine is carefully adjusted, this could have an adverse effect on the teats. Milking speeds are considerably faster when compared to conventional milking systems. In addition, the continually flooded liners make electronic measurements for milk yields, mastitis, heat detection and the like much simpler and more accurate than with the air/milk mixture which would be present in a conventional system. If automatic cluster removal is required with hydraulic milking, then an air-bleed is needed in the claw, but used only immediately prior to cluster removal. Not all systems have been successful, however, and advice should be taken before installing hydraulic milking plants.

## The Importance of Pulsation

The teat is a very sensitive structure and if it is to function correctly and act as a reasonable barrier to the entry of mastitis organisms, it must be maintained in a healthy state. Pulsation during milking allows proper blood flow around the teat and if the pulsators do not allow sufficient rest, teat end damage as in

Plate 7.15 could occur. Figure 7.10 (top) shows the curve produced by a good pulsator. The vacuum outside the liner (in the pulsation chamber – see Figure 7.7) rises quite rapidly to induce milk flow and then falls to zero to rest the teat. The liner has now collapsed and blood flow is being restored. Figure 7.10 (bottom) shows a pulsator which barely reaches atmospheric pressure and certainly gives no rest period. This is bound to cause teat damage. Pulsators can also be adjusted to give varying periods of milking time to massage time (A:B in Figure 7.10). A ratio of 60:40 (milking:massage) is generally satisfactory. Higher than this (e.g. 70:30) produces a faster milk flow rate but may allow insufficient rest and can cause teat end damage. More details are given in *Mastitis Control in Dairy Herds*.

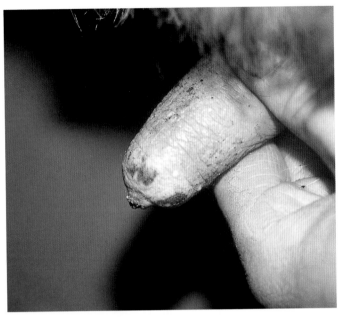

Plate 7.15. Haemorrhage and hyperkeratosis of the teat end are often associated with a machine fault.

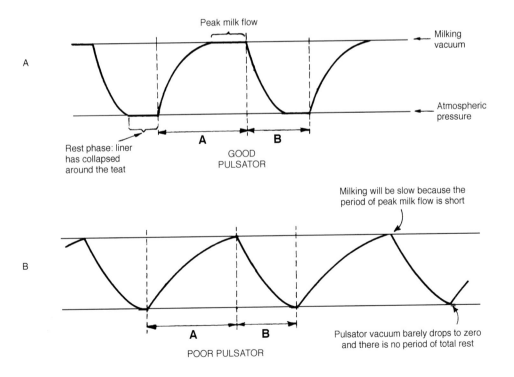

Figure 7.10. The pulsation curves of good (top) and bad (bottom) pulsators. The pulsation ratio is the ratio of A:B, viz. milk flow: massage periods.

## Removal of the Cluster at the End of Milking

Before the cluster is removed from the cow, the milk line vacuum *must* be switched off and sufficient time must elapse to allow the vacuum reservoir in the claw to be vented. If this is not done, there are two possible dangers:

- Air introduced beside one teat, while the other three are still under vacuum, will produce teat end impacts.
- If the cluster is pulled off *before* the vacuum is vented, this puts enormous strain on the teat end. Plate 7.16 shows a teat from a herd where badly adjusted ACRs meant that the cluster was being removed while still under vacuum. The amount of damage and hence the risk of mastitis are enormous. As claw volume has increased over recent years, the problem has increased, because larger volume claws act as a greater reservoir of vacuum which must be vented before removal.

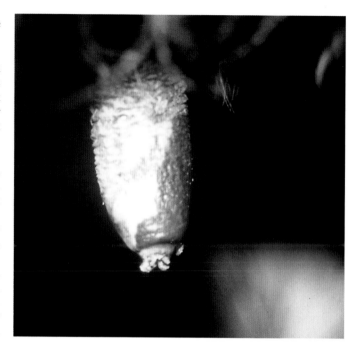

Plate 7.16. Severe teat sphincter eversion (hyperkeratosis) associated with poorly functioning ACR.

Cows which kick when the ACR is being pulled off, as in Plate 7.17, are obviously uncomfortable. Both the ACRs and teat ends need checking. Similar teat lesions can be caused by too high a vacuum, excessive fluctuation of the vacuum, or simply by excessively worn liners.

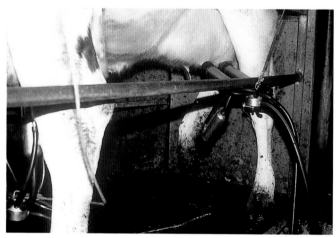

Plate 7.17. Cow kicking as the ACR pulls the cluster from the teats. It is likely that there is insufficient delay between vacuum shut-off and the ACR pull.

## Liners and Other Rubberware

Worn liners lose their elasticity, resulting in poor pulsation and reduced milking speeds, and they may also cause teat end damage. Plate 7.15 shows a teat with both haemorrhage and hyperkeratosis (protrusion of the sphincter) at the teat end. The hard, dry and cracked skin not only promotes bacterial multiplication, but it also reduces the defence mechanisms of the teat canal and will predispose to the entry of infection and mastitis and to blackspot (Plate 7.35 and page 223).

Cracked liners are difficult to clean, and they are likely to transmit mastitis bacteria and to cause high

TBCs. Rough liner surfaces, due to a buildup of milkstone, as in Plate 7.18, can cause teat chafing and predispose to mastitis. If the short milk tubes or short pulsation tubes are cracked or split, this can lead to either teat end impacts or have a serious effect on pulsation. Both predispose to mastitis.

Poorly fitting liners can also be dangerous. If they are too large they may fall off, or they may allow air to suck in, producing teat end impacts and slow milking. If they are too small, they constrict both blood flow and milk flow and increase teat end damage. Liners should be soft-mouthed so that they hang on teats of varying sizes without causing problems.

Most manufacturers recommend that rubber liners should be changed after every 2500 milkings, or at six months, whichever comes first. If they are allowed to become old or worn, when air enters the pulsation chamber during the rest or massage phase (to restore blood flow – see Figure 7.9a), the liner slaps against the side of the teat, producing pain and teat damage.

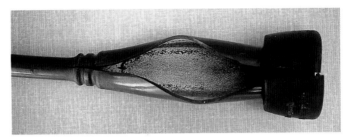

Plate 7.18. Severe milkstone buildup, as in this liner, can transmit mastitis and increase TBCs. It may lead to teat damage.

The most important considerations when using the milking machine are:

- unit alignment
- teat end impacts
- vacuum fluctuations and inadequate vacuum reserve
- inadequate claw bleed; small-volume claws
- poor pulsation and other factors leading to teat end damage
- poorly fitting and infrequently changed liners
- worn and cracked rubberware

This pain may reduce let-down and lead to overmilking and further teat end damage.

The herdsman should regularly check that the oil level in the vacuum pump is adequate and that the belts are tight; that the vacuum regulator is functioning properly and is regularly cleaned; that all pulsators are operating correctly; and that leaking, cracked and worn rubbers are replaced. A regular twice-yearly check on machine function, combined with routine maintenance, is essential.

In summary then, even the normal milking machine is a major factor in transmitting mastitis organisms, and when it is not functioning correctly the risks are considerably greater.

## Overmilking

At one time it was considered that overmilking was a major cause of mastitis. However, it is well known that 60% of the milk comes from the hind quarters. Assuming that milking speeds are equal in the hind and fore quarters, the fore quarters must milk out first and it is therefore likely that fore quarters are regularly overmilked. However, most mastitis comes from the *hind* quarters, so presumably overmilking is not an important cause of mastitis, *provided* that the milking plant is working well.

This conclusion has been acted on by one milking parlour manufacturer. By creating a more 'gentle' milking routine of very soft liners, a rapid pulsation speed of 70 cycles per minute and a 50:50 milk flow:massage pulsation ratio, the manufacturer has dispensed with ACRs and said that it does not matter how long the units are left on. Experience to date indicates that the system works well. Individual cow milk flow rates are slower, but parlour throughput (cows per hour) is kept high by milking larger numbers of cows per batch. This more 'gentle' milking system could be an important step forward to compensate for the increased mastitis susceptibility of our current higher flow rate cows (page 175).

## MILKING THE MASTITIC COW

When a cow subclinically infected with mastitis (and particularly staphylococcal mastitis) goes through the parlour, the liners will become contaminated with bacteria. As a result, staphylococci will be transmitted to the next six to eight cows to be milked through that cluster. Great care needs to be taken to avoid this cross-contamination, especially when milking cows under treatment or those cows with high cell counts. Ideally when such cows enter the parlour they should be milked through a separate cluster and into a dump bucket, as in Plate 7.19. This has the following advantages:

- The cluster can be left soaking in a bucket of hypochlorite or similar, so that there is a longer time for disinfection before it is next used.
- The milk is transferred straight into a dump bucket and hence there is no risk of antibiotic or mastitic milk being accidentally transferred into the bulk tank.

A similar system can be used to take colostrum from freshly calved cows, but one word of warning; DO NOT transfer the cluster from a mastitic cow directly onto a fresh calver without first disinfecting it. You do not want to infect her at the start of lactation.

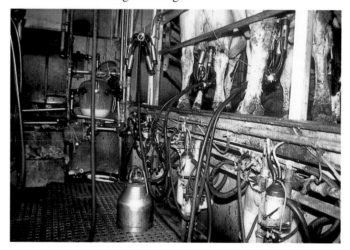

Plate 7.19. A dump bucket used for milking mastitic cows. This must also have a separate cluster which should be cleaned after use.

### Cleaning of Clusters between Cows

As mentioned above, when a cluster is removed from a cow the liners may be contaminated by mastitis organisms which have arisen from either the teat skin or the infected milk of a subclinically infected animal, and these organisms may be transmitted to the next cow to be milked. One way of reducing the spread of mastitis is to clean the clusters between each cow by flushing with water; by dipping them into hypochlorite and then flushing; or by pasteurisation (that is circulation with water at 85°C). Only pasteurisation has any great effect. There is no doubt that a combined disinfection and heat treatment of clusters would reduce significantly the spread of mastitis organisms, but at the moment it is not included as a routine in a 'package' of mastitis control measures in the UK, partly because of the cost (hot water) and partly because of the time involved (allowing the disinfectant to act).

This is a good example of how the practical costs and problems of a mastitis control procedure outweigh its advantages. However, if you are faced with a herd outbreak of staphylococcal/streptococcal or mycoplasma mastitis it would be an excellent control measure to put into operation in the short term, even if you only did it after removing the clusters from clinical cases or from cows which had had mastitis earlier in their lactation. Even better, of course, would be to put all known infected cows into a separate group and milk them last, or to use a separate cluster for known infected cows.

## POST MILKING TEAT DISINFECTION

Even the most careful milking routine is likely to have produced some transfer of bacteria during the milking process. Although a few bacteria may have already penetrated the teat canal (due to teat end impacts), the majority will still be on the skin of the teat and teat end. Disinfecting the teats after milking

– post dipping – eliminates the majority of these bacteria. It is a *vital step* in mastitis control and should be carried out on every cow at every milking.

*Chemicals used*
Most dips are formulated to persist for only two to three hours, but this is quite sufficient to exert their bacterial-killing action. Chlorhexidine possibly persists for slightly longer (four to six hours). There are five basic types of material used for post dips:

● hypochlorite – not less than 10,000 ppm (1%) and preferably 40,000 ppm (4%) available chlorine
● iodophor – not less than 5000 ppm (0.5%) available iodine
● chlorhexidine – not less than 5000 ppm (0.5%) chlorhexidine gluconate
● quaternary ammonium compounds (QUATs)
● dodecyl benzene sulphonic acid (DDBSAs)

Hypochlorite is the cheapest and may be adequate for use in the summer. However, it quickly loses its potency if it gets dirty from the cows splashing mud or slurry onto their teats, or from milk contamination in the teat dip cup. This is why any remaining dip should be discarded at the end of each milking and the cups should be washed. The other chemicals are less affected by contamination and in addition they can be mixed with *emollients*, that is substances like glycerine or lanolin which improve the condition of the teat skin. Concentrations of 10% glycerine or 2.5% lanolin are used, although these can be increased if chapping is a severe problem. Very high concentrations of emollients, that is above 15%, will reduce the bacterial killing action of the dip, however, and as bacteria growing deep in the crevices of the skin tend to make the chaps worse, a balance is needed between the emollient and bacterial-killing effects. If hypochlorite is to be used with an emollient, it should be added immediately before milking to avoid excessive inactivation of the disinfectant.

*Barrier dips*
Barrier dips attempt to achieve prolonged action and therefore provide some protection against environmental infections. These commonly combine a disinfectant, a gel and a solvent, often isopropanol. The isopropanol permits rapid drying of the teat, leaving a barrier film of gel over the teat end. Although products are continually improving, one of the disadvantages of some persistent dips is their sticky nature and the thick residual film of gel which has to be removed before the next milking or it will clog the milk filters. Dirt and debris can also adhere to sticky teats and will need to be removed at the next milking.

*Dipping or spraying*
Teat disinfectants are applied by dipping the teat into a cupful of liquid or by spraying. On average, teat dipping uses approximately 10 ml of dip per cow per milking, whereas spraying will use 15 ml.

Several different types of cup have been devised, the best probably being an anti-spill cup, an example of which was shown in Plate 7.7. Make sure the cup is deep enough to accommodate the whole length of even the largest teat (approximately 12 cm). If the cup is too full, immersion of the teat results in wastage of dip, whereas insufficient dip means that the teat

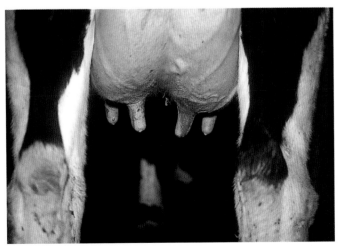

Plate 7.20. Poorly applied spray can lead to only partial teat cover and can predispose to mastitis.

does not get adequately coated. The whole teat needs to be covered with dip, because cracks can occur at any point on it.

Provided spraying methods are carried out conscientiously, they give a reasonable coverage to the teat and the spray material is always clean. However, it is easy to coat only half the teat as in Plate 7.20 and disinfectants with a high emollient content cannot be used. Sprays also use more ingredients and are therefore more expensive. Automated sprays, situated at the exit to the parlour and activated by a photo-electric cell as the cow passes, have not always proved successful. They use up to 25ml per cow per milking. Teat disinfection is most effective if it is carried out as soon as the teat-cups are removed, ideally within 30 seconds, so that a film of dip covers the inside

| A comparison between pre dipping and post dipping | | |
|---|---|---|
| | *Pre dip* | *Post dip* |
| When applied | Immediately before cluster application | Immediately after cluster removal |
| Must it be wiped off | Yes | No |
| Speed of action | Must be rapid | Not important |
| Main effect against | Environmental mastitis | Contagious mastitis |
| Effect on: | | |
| Cell count (SCC) | Limited effect | Decreases SCC |
| TBC | Decreases TBC | Limited effect |
| Season of use | Housing and other periods of environmental challenge | Whole year |

of the streak canal as the sphincter is closing. This cannot be achieved by most automated methods. Post milking teat disinfection has three important functions:

- It kills bacteria transferred from an infected cow via the milker's hands or the machine, and in so doing it prevents the establishment of a bacterial colony at the teat end.
- If mixed with an emollient it keeps the teats supple and prevents chapping and other lesions which can harbour *Staph. aureus* and *Strep. dysgalactiae*.
- Teat chaps with bacteria growing in them are slower to heal and so the antiseptic properties of teat disinfectants also promote the healing of teat lesions.

The overall effect of teat disinfection is to halve the rate at which new infections become established, and as such it is of considerable long-term benefit.

## Potential Disadvantages of Post Milking Teat Disinfection

Post milking teat disinfection has no effect against *existing* infections. For example, in one post dipping trial a 50% reduction in *new* infections led to only a 14% reduction in *existing* infections over a 12 month period. Therefore the concurrent *removal* of existing infections by treatment, by dry cow therapy and by culling is important if mastitis incidence is to be decreased. Post milking teat disinfection alone cannot be expected to result in a rapid reduction of cell count or mastitis incidence.

There is even some evidence that in low cell count herds with a high incidence of clinical mastitis, post dipping increases the incidence of coliform mastitis, especially in heifers. In a Dutch study of five herds over an eighteen month period, two quarters of each cow were post dipped, whereas two quarters were left undipped. The undipped quarters showed:

- a 23% increase in clinical *Staph. aureus* mastitis (as would be expected)
- a 75–80% increase in subclinical coagulase negative staphylococcal and *Corynebacterium bovis* infections
- but a 41% *decrease* in clinical coliform mastitis

It was suggested that the presence of *C. bovis* at the teat end in some way prevented coliform infections. Clearly it would not be sensible to discontinue post dipping totally. However, if faced with an outbreak of coliform mastitis in freshly calved cows (and the majority of environmental mastitis occurs at this stage of lactation), a temporary stop to post dipping (or at least a stop for the first four to six weeks of lactation) might be a useful control measure. However, as yet there is no proof that this is a practical option.

## DRY COW THERAPY

By removing any reservoir of infection from the udder, dry cow therapy plays an extremely important part in the control of contagious mastitis. Treatment of mastitis during the dry period has several advantages over treatment during lactation.

Although clots and clinical signs may disappear, probably *half* the cows treated for mastitis during their lactation remain carriers. This is especially true for staphylococcal infections. In addition there will be a second group of animals which pick up infection but never show any clinical signs – they go straight into the subclinical phase. Both groups provide an important reservoir of infection for the other cows in the herd, and both are best treated during the dry period, when the udder tissue regresses. This is known as *dry cow therapy*.

Special long-acting antibiotic preparations can be used because there are no problems with milk-withholding periods. Treatment during the dry period is also far more effective than when the cow is milking. It is an especially important opportunity to eliminate chronic *Staph. aureus* infections and the dry cow antibiotic used should therefore be chosen with this organism in mind.

Table 7.1 shows that for clinical cases of *Staph. aureus* treated during lactation, viz when clots are seen, the response to intramammary antibiotics can be as low as 25%. This is a particularly low figure, however, and if infections could be treated early, if possible at the high cell count subclinical stage, response rates would be higher. With dry cow therapy, response rates are much higher, and even with *Staph. aureus* reach 65%. This figure applies to younger animals.

Table 7.2 shows that if the staphylococci become well and truly established in the udder, as they would in an older cow, then even in the dry period response rates may be as low as 33%. In such instances, culling remains an important option for control. The table also demonstrates how important it is to prevent infection from becoming established. If heifers are milked hygienically and given dry cow therapy at the end of each lactation, it should be possible to prevent chronic infections from becoming established.

Many new infections are picked up soon after drying off and these can cause mastitis either in the dry period or in the next lactation. For example, in one trial, 25% of quarters were infected in cows being dried off. Although 5% of these quarters eliminated their infection naturally, another 10% became infected during the dry period, so that at calving 30% of quar-

Table 7.1. Response to treatment (% bacteriological cure rates).

| Bacteria | Lactation | | At drying off |
|---|---|---|---|
| | Clinical | Subclinical | |
| Strep. agalactiae | 85 | > 90 | > 95 |
| Staph. aureus | 25 | 40 | 65 |
| Strep. dysgalactiae | 90 | > 90 | > 95 |
| Strep. uberis | 70 | 85 | 85 |

Adapted from Dodd, 1978.

Table 7.2. Response of *Staph. aureus* infections to treatment during the dry period. First and second lactation animals respond much better than older cows.

| Lactation number | Number of cows treated | % response to treatment |
|---|---|---|
| 1–2 | 51 | 63 |
| 3–5 | 99 | 37 |
| > 5 | 40 | 33 |
| Total 190 | Average 43 | |

From Meany, W. J. (1992), *Proc BCVA* 1991–92, p. 211.

ters were infected. Dry cow therapy increases the number of quarters which lose their infection during the dry period and it also reduces the rate at which new infections become established. Various trials have shown that cows are *fifteen to twenty times* more likely to contract infection during the first two weeks of the dry period and for the two weeks prior to calving. This is discussed further on page 206. Management of cows before calving and maintaining a clean environment at this stage is therefore extremely important. Pre calving teat dipping may also help.

There has been a suggestion by some that continued use of dry cow therapy reduces udder infections to such a low level that it lowers the cow's resistance to *E. coli* mastitis. This theory has not been conclusively proved or disproved. My advice to the reader would be to continue with dry cow treatment for all cows. I suspect that the advantages far outweigh the disadvantages. It is doubly important during July to September, when there is a risk of summer mastitis (see page 216).

At drying off, milking should be discontinued abruptly, even at yields of 20–25 litres per day. This is because once a day milking or, even worse, alternate day milking leads to an increased risk of mastitis (see page 178) and to a massive increase in cell count. Probably the worst procedure is to leave the cows for four or five days and then give 'one last milking' before inserting the dry cow tubes.

Dry cows should be removed from the milking herd. This avoids the risk of milking a cow which has been given antibiotics and eliminates the stimulation of a let-down which might otherwise encourage further milk production.

Points to note regarding dry cow therapy are:

- It is an important means of removing reservoirs of infection from the herd.
- It helps prevent new infections during the dry period, including summer mastitis.
- Its main effect is against contagious mastitis.
- Tubes should be administered hygienically and gently.
- Dry off abruptly and remove dry cows from the milking herd.
- It is much more effective than treatment during lactation.
- There is no cost of discarded milk.
- The risk of bulk milk antibiotic contamination is reduced.

## THE ENVIRONMENT AND MASTITIS

A well-functioning milking machine and a correct milking routine are extremely important in the control of both contagious and environmental mastitis. Teat end impacts in particular can force environmental bacteria through the teat canal during milking. However, there are some important aspects of mastitis control which are peculiar only to environmental organisms. Because the environment is the source of infection, transmission of infection by the milker and milking machine is less important, although the machine will obviously have some influence via teat end impacts. Pre dipping is a very important control measure, but dry cow therapy and post dipping are generally ineffective.

Environmental infections are deposited on the teat between milkings and so control of environmental mastitis must be based on:

- reducing the challenge from the environment
- thoroughly cleaning the teats before milking
- maintaining the natural defences of the teat sphincter

The two most common environmental infections are *Strep. uberis* and coliforms including *E. coli*.

*Streptococcus uberis*
This organism is found in the mouth, vulva, teats and faeces of the cow, as well as in the environment. It is particularly associated with straw bedding and straw yards. Typically *Strep. uberis* will produce a hot, hard and swollen quarter and the cow may be off-colour and have a raised temperature for 24 hours, but

she is by no means as sick as with a severe coliform infection. Most cases respond well to penicillin therapy, although there has been a recent increase in the number of chronic recurrent cases, with no obvious reason for their failure to respond to treatment. They may be caused by a different strain of *Strep. uberis* and as such can be categorised as a contagious organism. Pre dipping is usually very effective in the control of new *Strep. uberis* infections.

### Coliforms, including E. coli

The problem starts with the cow's own faeces. Each gram, a quantity no bigger than your little fingernail, contains between one and ten million *E. coli* bacteria and this figure can be even higher for an early lactation cow fed on a high concentrate/low fibre ration. Systems must therefore be designed and managed so that they result in the minimum contact between the cow's teats and her faeces. This is why coliform mastitis normally declines dramatically in the summer months – the cows are no longer crowded and so there is a reduced risk of faecal contamination.

### Environmental factors

Some of the factors which can reduce the incidence of environmental contamination and hence *E. coli* mastitis are as follows. Cubicle passages should be scraped at least twice daily, preferably during milking and before the cows are dispersed. If permitted, cows tend to lie down immediately after milking and if they can walk back along clean passages they are less likely to carry contamination onto the cubicle beds. Ideally they should be excluded from the cubicles until 30 minutes after milking to allow the teat sphincter to close fully (see Figure 7.3). Cubicle beds should also be clean and fresh bedding

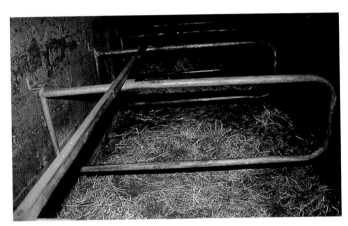

Plate 7.21. Badly soiled cubicles predispose to mastitis.

applied daily. Wet and soiled material (as in Plate 7.21) should be removed at least twice a day before scraping the passages; then if necessary fresh bedding should be applied before the cows return from milking.

### Cubicle design

Make sure that the cubicle dimensions are correct for the size of your cows, so that they are comfortable and dung in the passage and not on the bed. Cubicle comfort is discussed in detail in Chapter 9. Earth, ground limestone or sand floors may be used in cubicles. They have the advantage of being more comfortable than concrete, but the disadvantage is that urine pooling at the rear of the bed can leave a wet area for the udder and predispose to mastitis (Plate 7.21). Concrete bases are more common, presumably because they are more easily managed – they are certainly not more comfortable! A rear lip may help to retain bedding, which improves comfort, but it may also prevent drainage of muck and urine, again leading to mastitis.

### Bedding

The choice of bedding material must be a compromise between comfort, cost and hygiene. Sawdust can be a dangerous source of coliforms, including *Klebsiella*, and this is particularly the case if it gets damp during storage. Coliform levels in bedding and on teats in Table 7.3 were much higher with sawdust than with shavings or straw. Other workers have shown that sand as cubicle bedding supports an even lower coliform population, although it may be less comfortable, more abrasive on the teats and can cause problems when handling the slurry. Chopped straw, applied fresh daily with a straw chopper into a lip-less cubicle, seems the best alternative, although straw supports the survival of *Strep. uberis*, and these infections are very common in straw yards. A small quantity of slaked lime sprinkled onto the beds twice weekly acts as both a drying agent and a disinfectant (Plate 7.22).

A word of warning, however: the level of *E. coli* in bedding material is not necessarily related to the degree of visual soiling. Unused sawdust may already contain high coli numbers if it has been allowed to get wet. It is the *dampness* of the bed as much as the degree of faecal soiling which affects the overall coliform numbers, and this is why slaked lime is beneficial. Care is needed, however, because excess lime can damage the teats.

Even after fresh bedding is added, *E. coli* numbers soon build up and then remain constant (unless the bed gets wetter or dirtier) irrespective of how long the cows are housed. The practice of thoroughly clearing out

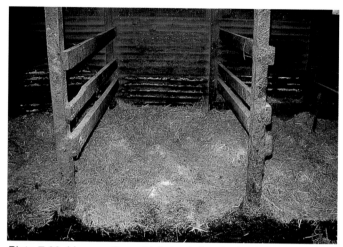

Plate 7.22. Lime on the cubicle beds has both drying and disinfectant properties.

Table 7.3. The coliform populations supported by different types of bedding, and their effect on the coliform numbers obtained from a teat swab.

|  | Total coliform count in cubicle bedding | Mean no. of coliforms obtained from a teat swab |
|---|---|---|
| sawdust | $52.0 \times 10^6$ | 127 |
| shavings | $6.6 \times 10^6$ | 12 |
| straw | $3.1 \times 10^6$ | 8 |
| From Rendos, Eberhart & Kesler, *J Dairy Sci* 58 1492. | | |

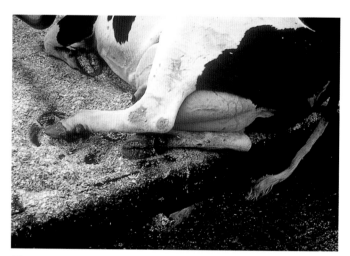

Plate 7.23. Milk leaking from the udder, as in this cow, is particularly dangerous, as the mixture of milk, faeces and bedding supports high levels of coliform bacteria.

the cubicles and re-bedding them during the winter period has little to recommend it therefore, unless additional efforts are made with regard to cleanliness after the re-bedding. Ideally cubicles and straw yards should have clean bedding added every day. The mixture of milk, faeces and bedding which is sometimes seen where the cow has been lying is especially dangerous (Plate 7.23). Milk provides nutrients for *E. coli*, and the cow's udder warmth, so that bacterial numbers can multiply to very high levels, for example one thousand million *E. coli* per gram ($1000 \times 10^6$) in the very area where the cow's teats are lying. This is at least 100 times higher than the level found in faeces, and 20 times higher than the levels shown for sawdust in Table 7.3. As early lactation cows are not only the most susceptible to *E. coli* mas-titis but they also have the highest faecal *E. coli* levels and are the animals most likely to be leaking milk, it is a good idea to keep them in a separate group. They can then have their cubicles cleaned and re-bed-ded at least once a day, the passages scraped twice daily, and they can be pre dipped.

Overcrowding should be avoided. Cows which are packed together, rushed through passageways or simply have inadequate space are more likely to get faecal contamination of the teat ends. Overcrowding can also lead to inadequate ventilation and increased humidity, both of which may predispose towards a buildup of *E. coli*.

*Calving boxes*
Calving boxes should be kept as clean as possible. The dry cow is almost completely resistant to *E. coli* mastitis, but there is some evidence that infections contracted during the dry period, and especially during the final two weeks, remain dormant in the udder until after calving. At calving the cow is at her most susceptible to coliform mastitis. Cleanliness of the calving boxes and during the late dry period is therefore essential and if faced with a severe outbreak of down-calving mastitis, consider calving outdoors. Many farms have inadequate calving facilities, and the practice of having a single calving yard, used by the whole herd during the calving season, should be discouraged. Ideally each cow should have its own box, where the straw bedding should be kept meticulously clean and dry (see also page 206). The shorter the period of winter housing, the less will be the risk of *E. coli* mastitis. There are more outbreaks of environmental mastitis, and often of greater severity, if October and November are warm and humid, and this is particularly so in cows which have been housed since August.

*Straw yards*
Straw yards should be designed so that they are wide and shallow (as shown in Figure 7.11), rather than long and narrow. Long and narrow yards get badly soiled by the cows walking to and fro, and this is especially the case if the water trough is sited at the rear of the yard. Ventilation is vital: cows produce around 55 litres of water each day from urine, faeces, skin and breathing, and unless there is good

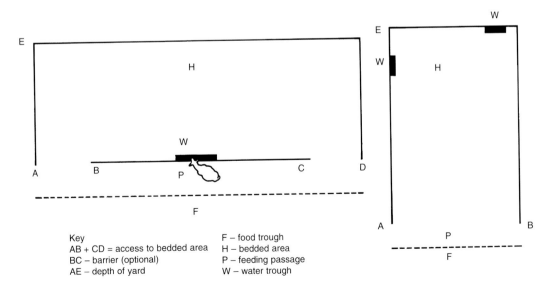

Figure 7.11. Design of straw yards: long, narrow poorly ventilated yards with badly placed water troughs should be avoided (right). A more useful design is shown on the left.

ventilation, the whole building 'drips' (Plate 7.24), predisposing to bacterial growth. If you are unable to see the rear of the building on a winter's morning because of condensation, then the ventilation is inadequate! Straw yards should be cleaned out at least every six weeks; otherwise the heat produced by the accumulation of soiled bedding increases humidity and predisposes to mastitis.

*The importance of new infections in the dry period*

Although the presence of lactoferrin in the udder of the dry cow prevents the multiplication of *E. coli*, it is now known that many new infections of

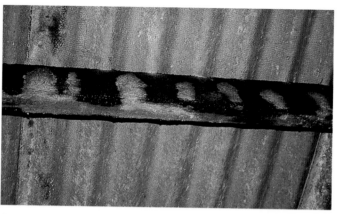

Plate 7.24. Condensation dripping from the roof onto the cubicle beds, as in this picture, is conducive to environmental mastitis. It also suggests inadequate ventilation.

the dry cow lie dormant in the udder to cause post calving mastitis. For example, a UK study by Bradley and Green showed that in 700 non-lactating quarters in dry cows sampled for *E. coli*

- 81 quarters cultured positive for *E. coli*, and of these 14.8% developed clinical coliform mastitis during the next lactation.
- 619 quarters cultured negative for *E. coli*, and of these only 1.8% developed clinical coliform mastitis in the next lactation.

Cows becoming infected during the dry period are therefore eight times more likely to develop coliform mastitis than those not infected, and DNA finger-printing studies showed that it was exactly the same organism contracted during the dry period which caused the post calving mastitis. Some of the cases of acute coliform mastitis are of course new infections contracted during lactation, but the importance of dry period infections is surprising. Of the total number of clinical *E. coli* mastitis cases seen during lactation

- 4.5% are thought to be contracted during the first half of the dry period.
- 65% are thought to be contracted during the second half.
- Only 30.5% of cases are new infections picked up during lactation.

The importance of this in terms of dry cow hygiene and management, the use of teat seals and the use of a dry cow therapy antibiotic that gives protection against *E. coli* is obvious.

## TREATMENT OF MASTITIS

The correct procedure for handling the mastitic cow was discussed on page 198. This section describes the options available for treatment.

When a milker first encounters a case of mastitis, he will have relatively little idea which organism is causing the mastitis and what the likely outcome of this particular case will be. He has to make immediate decisions. For example, is treatment worthwhile? There is a body of opinion which says that antibiotic treatment of clinical mastitis is not worthwhile because:

- Many cases are coliforms, many of which will resolve spontaneously.
- Treatment of staphylococci produces a poor bacteriological response, with only 25–40% success rate in some cases.

However, I would not subscribe to this conclusion. Whilst there is some logic in the two points above, I think that on balance antibiotic therapy is cost-effective because:

- Early treatment including first-time staphylococcal infections in heifers produces quite a good cure rate. This is shown in Tables 7.1 and 7.2. It is only older cows and long-standing infections which have such a low bacterial cure rate as 25–40%.
- Mastitis control is largely a numbers game, aimed at reducing bacterial challenge. Even if the bacteria are not totally eliminated, a reduction in their numbers should help to control spread.
- If antibiotics only contribute to saving the life of an occasional acute coliform case, they will soon pay for themselves.

## Choice of Antibiotic

The choice of antibiotic for treatment should be decided after discussion with your vet, although it needs to be a broad-spectrum product, effective against staphylococci, streptococci and coliforms. He will know the type of problem on your farm and should be able to prescribe a suitable drug, although you will know the products which seem to give a better response. The technique of administering intramammary antibiotics is described on page 209. As a general rule, streptococci are always sensitive to penicillin. However, a proportion of staphylococci (viz those which produce penicillinase) will not be, in which case the synthetic penicillins (e.g. cloxacillin) or antibiotic combinations (e.g. amoxycillin and clavulanic acid), or specific penicillinase resistant antibiotics (e.g. erythromycin, novobiocin and framycetin) will have to be used. *E. coli*, *Pseudomonas* and *Klebsiella* are totally resistant to penicillin, and other drugs such as the tetracyclines, cephalosporins or amoxycillin must be employed in their treatment. I think it is important to have only one, or at the most two, preparations in routine use on your farm.

## Taking a Milk Sample for Bacteriology

The initial choice of drug should depend on the results of a bacteriological examination of mastitis samples and the herdsman should routinely take his own milk samples for mastitis. Cleanliness is vital of course, to avoid getting false results. A good routine for milk sampling is as follows:

- Wash and dry the teat.
- Discard the first four to five squirts of milk: they may contain bacteria which have been growing in the teat canal, but which are not causing mastitis.
- Rub the end of the teat five to ten times with a swab soaked in methylated spirits.
- Only then should you open the sample bottle, keeping the lid facing downwards and the opened bottle almost horizontal. This prevents particles of dust and bacteria dropping into the bottle.

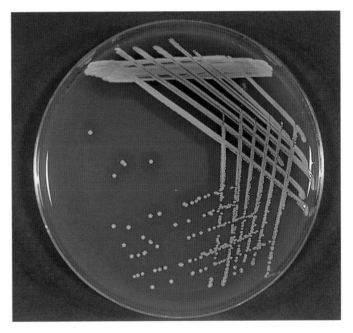

Plate 7.25. *Staph. aureus* growing on a blood agar plate. Each small dot in the centre of the plate is a colony, containing many millions of bacteria.

- Finally, with the bottle between the horizontal and a 45° angle, squirt in one jet of milk and replace the cover immediately.
- Label the bottle with your name, the identity of the cow, the date and the quarter sampled.

The sample should be taken to the laboratory as soon as is reasonably possible, although a delay of up to 24 hours is acceptable, provided that it is stored in a refrigerator. At the laboratory the milk is smeared across a blood agar plate and left to grow in an incubator at 37°C for 24–48 hours. Bacteria can be seen growing as small white clumps and sometimes their appearance alone is sufficient to identify them. Plate 7.25 shows typical colonies of *Staph. aureus*. To confirm their identity, however, they should be stained and examined under a microscope.

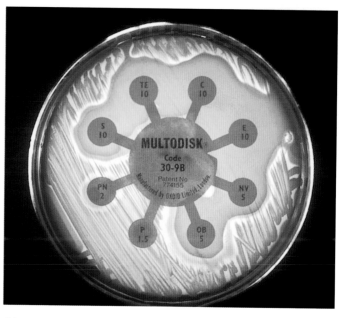

Plate 7.26. Antibiotic sensitivity testing. Penicillin (P 1.5) and ampicillin (PN 2) would not be effective against this strain of *Staph. aureus* because bacteria have grown up to the edge of the antibiotic discs.

## Antibiotic Sensitivity Testing

Antibiotic sensitivity tests are performed by covering a second blood agar plate with a suspension of bacteria and then placing on small paper discs, each impregnated with a different antibiotic. After a further 24 hours incubation this second plate is examined. If the bacteria have grown up to the edge of the paper disc, then the antibiotic contained in it is not killing them. If there is a 'zone of growth inhibition' around the disc, however, then that antibiotic *may* be effective for treating the cow. Plate 7.26 shows a typical example. This strain of *Staph. aureus* is sensitive to all drugs tested except penicillin (P 1.5) and ampicillin (PN 2).

## Factors Affecting Treatment Efficacy

There are many other factors which can affect a drug's action, such as the ease with which the product can penetrate the udder, the concentration achieved and the persistence of the drug in mammary tissue following administration. Often the small ducts leading to the alveoli (Figure 7.1) are blocked with pus and debris and the antibiotic is simply unable to penetrate to the site of the infection. Although the clots disappear, the cow is left with a focus of infection in the udder. She is then a *chronic carrier*, or we may say that she has a *subclinical infection*. This situation is especially common following *Staph. aureus* infection, although it can also occur with *Strep. agalactiae* and *Strep. dysgalactiae*.

Certain strains of staphylococci and *Strep. uberis* may even continue to live after they have been engulfed by the neutrophils or macrophages of the udder (see Figure 7.4). Whilst inside these cells they are protected from the action of antibiotics. When the macrophage dies, however, the bacteria are released and can start multiplying again. This is another cause of the chronic carrier cow, and of mastitis which seems unresponsive to treatment. As we have already seen, subclinically affected cows are a risk to themselves in that the mastitis may recur or spread to another quarter, and they are also a danger to the other cows in the herd.

The main reasons for the poor response of *Staph. aureus* to treatment are:

- Many strains of *Staph. aureus* are resistant to penicillin and ampicillin (although all are sensitive to cloxacillin and cephalosporins).
- *Staph. aureus* can remain alive even when engulfed by macrophages. When inside these cells, it is protected from many antibiotics (tylosin, tilmicosin and fluoroquinolones may penetrate).
- In chronic infections, parts of the udder become walled off by fibrous tissue, so that antibiotics cannot penetrate.
- In milk, some strains of *Staph. aureus* become surrounded by a 'slime' capsule, which renders them resistant to phagocytosis.

## Inserting an Intramammary Tube

Whether for the treatment of mastitis or for dry cow therapy, infusing an intramammary antibiotic is probably one of the most frequent veterinary tasks that the herdsman has to perform. Cleanliness and gentle handling are essential; otherwise infections such as *E. coli* or yeasts can be introduced into the udder. Only special iodine preparations (see page 220) are effective against yeasts and many dry cow tubes do not have any effect against *E. coli*.

If dealing with a case of mastitis, thoroughly strip out the quarter, possibly leaving it for five to ten minutes, and then strip it again. Stripping is an excellent way of removing the bacteria and toxins. If they are not stripped out, the cow has to remove them by absorbing them into her system, and this can increase the severity of the illness. Oxytocin injections improve milk let-down.

If the teats are very dirty, they should be washed *and* dried. Next rub the end of the teat five to ten times with a piece of cotton wool soaked in methylated spirit, alcohol or antiseptic. Only at this stage should you remove the protective cap from the nozzle of the antibiotic tube – many herdsmen find that their teeth are the best way of doing this!

Holding the teat in one hand, bend it slightly so that the orifice is pointing towards you. If the orifice is not clearly visible, draw a few drops of milk to act as a marker. Holding the tube in the other hand, gently touch the nozzle against the orifice (Plate 7.27) and then slowly slide it in. If the cow is nervous, use an anti-kick bar or get help from a second person rather than risk contaminating the tube and introducing infection. It is only necessary to insert the tip of the tube into the teat canal, as in Plate 7.27. Excess dilation of the canal can lead to cracking of its keratin lining and will predispose to mastitis. Withdraw the tube and, holding the tip of the teat between your thumb and forefinger, use the other hand to work the antibiotic up into the udder. Finally

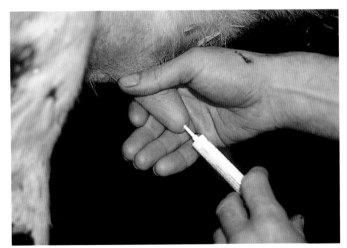

Plate 7.27. Inserting an intramammary tube. Cleanliness and gentle handling are essential.

apply teat dip and then record the cow number, date of administration, quarter affected and medication used. If it was a lactating cow, make sure that she is distinctly marked so that she can be identified and her milk discarded at the next milking.

## Other Mastitis Treatments

In addition to antibiotic tubes, a wide range of other treatments has been suggested for mastitis. Antibiotics may also be given by injection and there is considerable evidence that a combined course of tubes and injections is more effective than tubes alone. This regime is used particularly for recurrent cases and sick animals, and as the cost of antibiotics is relatively small compared with the cost of discarding milk and further cases of mastitis, many people use the combined treatments as a routine. Some antibiotics, e.g. tylosin, achieve high concentrations in the udder following intramuscular infection and have been recommended for treatment of high cell count cows.

Severely ill animals need treatment for shock. This can take the form of anti-inflammatory and anti-endotoxin drugs such as flunixin and/or fluid therapy. If a cow is sick and will not drink, then fluids need to be given. The easiest way of achieving this is by mouth, for example gently running fluids from the spout of a watering can into the side of the mouth. Initial oral dosing with sodium bicarbonate may induce closure of the oesophageal groove (see Chapter 2), thereby ensuring that the fluids are delivered directly into the abomasum where absorption is likely to be better. Fluids may also be given intravenously. Intravenous hypertonic fluids, e.g. 2–3 litres of 7.2% sodium chloride, will often stimulate the cow to drink.

Continual stripping is important. This removes both bacteria and toxins and, by flushing the udder, promotes healing. Oxytocin will assist this process. If the cow has a hard, hot, swollen and painful udder she is highly unlikely to let her milk down properly. An injection of oxytocin as she enters the parlour will produce milk let-down two or three minutes later, and the milk and toxins can then be stripped from the quarter. Some people suggest the use of oxytocin alone, without additional antibiotic therapy. Whilst this may well work in a proportion of cases, it is likely that overall a better resolution of the infection will be obtained if antibiotics are administered. Topical treatments such as Cai-pan Japanese peppermint can be rubbed into the surface of the affected quarter. This probably helps the healing process by providing a massaging effect and feeling of warmth, both of which are likely to improve milk let-down and increase the feeling of well-being in the cow.

Remember that the cell count of an individual quarter stays high for at least two weeks after treatment, even if the treatment was successful at eliminating the bacteria. If possible, therefore, try to discard the milk for longer than the antibiotic withdrawal period demands, or possibly feed the milk to calves. This could be significant in reducing herd cell counts.

## MASTITIS RECORDS AND TARGETS

I am a firm believer in recording the incidence of all types of disease on a farm but it is particularly important for mastitis. General disease monitoring and how this is co-ordinated with veterinary advisory visits and general farm involvement is discussed in Chapter 8.

If you have a problem of increasing cell counts or a high incidence of mastitis, talk it through with your vet. It would probably be worth getting him to come along at milking time one day to watch. It is surprising how an extra pair of eyes can help. It may be that the cows are uncomfortable when being milked or they have an excessive degree of teat end damage, both being an indication of machine induced problems. Perhaps you are not applying the post milking teat spray evenly, or there is some way in which infection is being inadvertently transferred from cow to cow. A combination of observation, bulk milk bacteriology and analysis of records can solve the majority of problems.

The type of recording system used is not too important, but you *must* carry out the following procedures:

● Record every case of mastitis, giving the cow, date, quarter affected and tubes used.
● Record repeat treatments, so that chronic carriers are easily identified. Table 7.4 shows two types of recording systems. In the top method it is obvious that cow 42 has had several attacks in the left hind quarter. The same information is present on the second chart, but it is by no means so obvious. It is even better to keep whole lifetime records of individual cows, and the information can be used for culling and even selection decisions.
● Periodically analyse the records to calculate your own mastitis performance.

| Cow | date | quarter | date | quarter | date | quarter | date | quarter |
|---|---|---|---|---|---|---|---|---|
| 79 | 22.2 | LH | | | | | | |
| 42 | 25.2 | LH + RH | 3.4 | LH | 15.5 | LH + RF | 23.7 | LH |
| 83 | 2.3 | LF | | | | | | |
| 14 | 15.3 | LF | 17.6 | RF | | | | |
| 27 | 12.5 | RH + LH | | | | | | |
| 176 | 25.6 | RH | | | | | | |
| 9 | 3.7 | LF | | | | | | |
| 17 | 14.8 | LH | | | | | | |
| 101 | 21.8 | RH | | | | | | |

| Cow | date | quarter |
|---|---|---|
| 79 | 22.2 | LH |
| 42 | 25.2 | LH + RH |
| 83 | 2.3 | LF |
| 42 | 3.4 | LH |
| 14 | 15.3 | LF |
| 27 | 12.5 | RH + LH |
| 42 | 15.5 | LH + RF |
| 14 | 17.6 | RF |
| 176 | 25.6 | RH |
| 9 | 3.7 | LF |
| 42 | 23.7 | LH |
| 17 | 14.8 | LH |
| 101 | 21.8 | RH |

Table 7.4. Two types of annual mastitis records. The system on the left most easily identifies the problem cows as all information relating to the same cow is recorded on one line. In the chart to the right separate cases of mastitits in the same cow are not related back to each other as they are in the first chart.

A case of mastitis is defined as one quarter affected once. Hence a cow calving down with mastitis in all four quarters represents four cases of mastitis. Recurrence rate is defined as the percentage of cases which need *one or more* repeat treatments during a recording period. In Table 7.4 there is only *one* repeat treatment, namely cow 42 in her left hind quarter (although this quarter was treated four times). The total number of cases of mastitis is sixteen, so the recurrence rate is one divided by sixteen = 6.25%. Using these definitions, suggested target figures are:

- mastitis rate: 30 cases per 100 cows per year
- herd incidence: 20% of cows affected per year
- recurrence rate: 10%
- tube usage: 4.5 tubes per milking cow

These are target figures. Unfortunately, many herds have a considerably higher incidence of mastitis than this, and more effort should be put into mastitis control. If there is a mastitis problem in the herd, records can also be used to help differentiate between environmental and contagious organisms (see page 186). For example, in the classic case, an outbreak of *environmental* mastitis produces:

- a high mastitis rate
- a high herd incidence
- a low recurrence rate
- a low cell count but sometimes a high TBC

On the other hand, a typical *contagious* mastitis problem may produce:

- a high mastitis rate
- a lower herd incidence
- a high recurrence rate
- a high cell count but probably a low TBC

In practice the distinction is not always quite so clear and many herds will have a combination of both contagious and environmental mastitis.

Mastitis records should be examined just prior to drying off. Cows which have had four or more cases in one quarter in a lactation should be considered for culling or, if not, at least for some additional therapy, for example a course of tubes and injections just before drying off, or perhaps a second dose of dry cow tubes two weeks after the first.

## SOMATIC CELL COUNTS

The cell count, or somatic cell count (SCC) of milk, is a measure of the number of cells present in the milk. Most of the cells present are macrophages, a type of white cell which responds to mastitis infection. There are also lower numbers of neutrophils and epithelial cells. The cell count is therefore an indication of the degree of inflammation within the udder, or the amount of mastitis infection present. Cell count results are usually expressed in thousands, so a cell count of 250 means that the milk contains 250,000 cells per millilitre.

*Effects on manufacturing*
All dairy companies in the UK pay a premium for milk with a low cell count. Within the EU it has been illegal since July 1997 to use milk with a cell count of over 400,000 for either liquid sales or manufacturing. This is because milk with a high count is less valuable for manufacturing, due to:

- a decreased casein content. It is the casein in the milk which coagulates during manufacture to produce cheese, yoghurt etc
- increased levels of plasmin. Plasmin is an enzyme which degrades casein, continuing to act even after pasteurisation and refrigeration
- increased levels of lipase. Lipase can inhibit yoghurt starter cultures and may also lead to taints in manufactured products

The combination of these factors can lead to as much as a 15% reduction in manufactured yield if poor-quality milk is used.

*Effects on yield*
Cows with increased cell counts also have reduced milk yields. For example, Canadian work has shown that for every 100,000 increase in cell count above 200,000, yields decreased by 2.5%. This is shown in Figure 7.12.

The importance of cell counts is that they give an indication of the level of chronic infection in an udder. An acute infection with *E. coli* normally leads to a rapid increase in cell count due to the large numbers of neutrophils entering the udder, as shown in Figure 7.4. However, because *E. coli* infections rarely persist, cell counts quickly return to normal. On the other hand, staphylococci, *Strep. agalactiae* and *Strep. dysgalactiae* all have adhesive properties. This means they may persist in the udder, producing continuous high cell counts. This is especially the case if they have not been treated adequately.

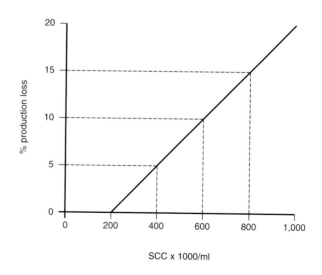

Figure 7.12. Effect of herd cell count on milk production: milk yield drops by 2.5% for every increase in cell count of 100,000 above a base figure of 200,000.
Adapted from Philpot, W. N. (1984), *Veterinary Clinics of North America Food Animal Practice*, 6.

## Individual cow SCCs

Because of this variation in the effects of contagious and environmental organisms, *no action* should be taken on the basis of a single sample from a cow showing a high cell count. At least two, and preferably three, monthly samples need to be taken from that cow before we can be sure that a chronic infection is present. Many other factors, not related to mastitis, can also increase the cell count of an individual cow.

These include age (heifers generally have lower counts), stage of lactation (counts are high in early and late lactation), milking frequency (once daily or alternate day milking leads to an increase), very low yields and stress, for example testing for tuberculosis.

## Herd cell counts

If the herd has an elevated cell count it is likely that there will be a penalty on milk sales and that yields will be depressed. Action needs to be taken and a range of steps is possible. No action may be taken on a single high monthly herd figure, but if the problem continues, monthly individual cow cell counts will be needed. It may be that only two or three cows with a very high cell count are having an enormous effect on the bulk sample and if their milk is discarded (or fed to calves), then the herd count will return to normal.

An alternative to cell counting is the California Mastitis Test (or CMT), which uses the chemical sodium dodecyl lauryl sulphate to detect high cell count milk. After discarding four to five squirts of foremilk, milk from

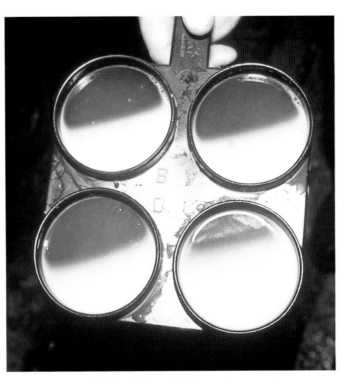

Plate 7.28. The California Mastitis Test, a simple parlour technique to detect high cell count. Milk from affected quarters turns gelatinous.

each quarter is drawn into a tray divided into four separate dishes (Plate 7.28). An equal volume of reagent is added and the tray (or paddle, as it is often called) is slowly and gently rocked from side to side, so that the milk can be examined as it flows across the dish. If the milk turns gelatinous, or even totally solidifies, then it has a high cell count. The test is only a guide to the level of cell count, but it is reasonably accurate. For example, one survey showed that bacteria could be cultured from:

– 85% of CMT positive milks
– but only 15% of CMT negative milks

The great advantage of the CMT test is that it is cheap, easy to perform and the results are immediate. However, as with cell counts, the test needs to be positive three times at monthly intervals before any action is taken. Even before cell count or CMT results are available, it would be worth discarding the milk from any known chronic recurrent mastitic cows or quarters to see if that helps to reduce the bulk milk count.

## Reducing herd cell counts

After individual cow cell counts or California Mastitis Tests have been carried out, or even while waiting for the results, there is a range of other measures which can be considered to reduce herd cell counts.

These include:

- Use bacteriology on high cell count cows. Table 7.1 shows that if the infection is *Strep. agalactiae*, it should be possible to treat successfully, even during lactation. Sometimes whole herd treatments are carried out. Known as blitz therapy, this needs careful planning with your vet.
- Check the milking routine and especially the efficacy of post milking dipping. If contagious infection is present in the herd, meticulous post dipping is vital.
- Check that dry cow therapy is being given to all cows.
- Ensure that cows are being dried off abruptly and that no cows with yields below 10 litres are being milked. Gradual drying off and very low yielding cows both increase cell counts. For example, in one trial a group of late lactation cows had a mean cell count of 237,000. When not milked for two days this increased to 540,000, and when left for a further four days this increased to 7,600,000, with one cow reaching 15 million!
- Monitor mastitis and ensure that all clinical cases are detected and that their milk is discarded, not added to the bulk tank.
- Make sure that milk from freshly calved cows is discarded for at least four days: colostrum has a high cell count. This includes heifers.
- Discard milk from aborted cows and heifers. The first milk from a dry cow or heifer that has aborted may have a cell count of 6 to 8 million! She needs to be milked to stimulate production, but milk for the first week should be discarded or fed to calves.
- Discard milk for longer after treatment. Following experimental infection it may take up to *thirty* milkings for milk from the infected quarter to fall below 400,000, even though treatment may have been effective and the clots disappeared within a few days.
- Try treatment of the infected quarter. Drugs such as tylosin accumulate in the udder, and may be effective if the mastitis has not been present for too long.
- Dry off the offending quarter and continue to milk the cow on three. There is some evidence to show that longer dry periods lead to improved spontaneous recovery.

As soon as two or three sets of monthly cell counts are available, action can be taken on individual problem cows, the main options being

- cull
- dry off early
- feed the milk to calves
- treat (do not expect a high success rate)

The problem with all except the first two options is that by continuing to milk high cell count cows there is a risk of spreading infection to other animals via the milking machine.

## TOTAL BACTERIAL COUNT (TBC) OF MILK

Whereas *cell count* measures the number of cells present in milk and is an indicator of mastitis infection, the total bacterial count (TBC) is a measure of the number of bacteria present. Dairy companies pay a premium for milk with a low TBC and impose penalties or even reject milk with high TBCs. Bacteria in milk usually originate from one of three major sources:

- mastitis
- dirty teats
- the milking plant

Milk from a single case of mastitis, especially if *Strep. uberis* or *Strep. agalactiae* is involved, may be sufficient to increase the bulk milk TBC from 10,000 to 70,000 bacteria per millilitre. Mastitis is a common cause of wildly fluctuating TBCs, especially in herds where mastitis detection is poor and the milk from affected cows enters the bulk tank. *Staph. aureus* produces relatively low numbers of bacteria and is unlikely to be involved.

Dirty teats, especially if splashed with faeces, will lead to an increase in the *coliform* count of milk and may be sufficient to incur TBC penalties. Teats which are washed but not wiped commonly lead to high TBCs. Teats with chaps, cracks and generally poor teat skin condition support increased bacterial populations and may also be involved. A change of teat dip to a higher emollient product may be required.

An inadequately cleaned milking plant is probably the most common cause of raised TBCs and this leads to an increase in the *thermoduric* or *laboratory pasteurised* count of bulk milk. Details of plant cleaning techniques and the investigation of problem herds can be found in *Mastitis Control in Dairy Herds*. The most common problems are inadequate use of chemicals, inadequate volumes of hot water and inadequate water temperature. Ideally 18 litres of hot water per milking unit are needed for circulation cleaning. With the move towards larger bore milking equipment (used to improve vacuum stability), water requirements have increased. Air injectors may also be needed to produce a swirling effect in the milk transfer line; otherwise the wash-up water runs along the bottom of the line, leaving an accumulation of cheesy material impacted onto the top of the pipe. If TBCs are increasing in your herd, remove the ends of the milk transfer lines and look inside with a torch. On occasions I have seen enormous quantities of stale, coagulated milk stuck to the roof of the pipe. Worn rubberware with a rough surface, as in Plate 7.18, is much more difficult to clean and may be involved. Check that the wash cycle is correct. Most circulation systems involve an initial rinse to waste with warm water, circulation at 60–70°C for five to eight minutes, then a flush through with cold water, perhaps containing a low level of hypochlorite. If the solution becomes too cool, perhaps because it was left circulating for too long, then some of the milk soil is deposited back on the pipes and TBCs may increase.

Finally, check that refrigeration is adequate. Faulty cooling can lead to multiplication of all types of bacteria, giving an increase in TBC, thermoduric and coliform counts. When faced with TBC problems, submit a bulk milk sample to a laboratory for a differential bacterial count. If thermodurics are high, the problem is poor plant cleaning. Raised coliforms indicate poor teat preparation, and the presence of *Strep. agalactiae* suggests mastitis is involved. A high *Staph. aureus* count could indicate the cause of an elevated cell count, but is unlikely to contribute significantly to TBCs. Increased *C. bovis* (page 220) could indicate poor post-dipping and *Strep. dysgalactiae* poor teat skin condition.

*Bactosan*

In many countries bacteriological counts are now carried out electronically using a system such as Bactoscan. A dye which stains all living bacteria is added to the milk. The milk is then passed through a machine which counts the coloured particles. Bactoscan figures give higher results than standard cultural methods of TBC, because Bactoscan includes all bacteria present, whereas by culture only those organisms which grow at a specific temperature on a particular growth medium are counted. Psychrotrophs, dust organisms present on the teats of housed cattle especially, can lead to a high Bactoscan result when TBCs are acceptable. Pretreatment of milk also allows Bactoscan to count all bacteria, whereas with cultural techniques staphylococci and streptococci, which exist in clumps and chains respectively, may be counted as colonies (i.e. groups of bacteria) and not as individual organisms.

As of January 1998 in the UK, a TBC of over 20,000 bacteria per millilitre and a Bactoscan count of over 100,000 incur penalties, and some dairy companies pay an additional premium for milk with a TBC below 10,000/ml. It is likely that stricter limits will be imposed in the future.

## ANTIBIOTIC RESIDUES IN MILK

One of the more expensive aspects of mastitis is the milk which has to be discarded from cows under treatment. There are several reasons why milk contaminated with antibiotics should not be sold. These are:

1. *Public health.* Some people are allergic to antibiotics, especially the penicillins, and even fatalities have been known to occur. If, in this health-conscious age, milk gains a public reputation for containing antibiotics, liquid sales could decline quite rapidly.
2. *Interference with manufacturing.* Antibiotics can destroy the bacterial cultures used in yoghurt and cheese manufacture.
3. *Legality.* In the UK it is a contravention of both your contract with the dairy company and of Public Health (Trading Standards) Regulations to sell milk contaminated with antibiotics.

Since 1997 the maximum permissible level of antibiotic in milk in the EU has been 0.004 i.u. per millilitre. The test is based on the addition of penicillin-sensitive bacteria to milk and monitoring their growth. Other types of antibiotics (e.g. neomycin) and certain sulphonamides are less easily detected. Most test failures are simply due to not discarding the milk for the recommended length of time following intramammary antibiotic treatment. This may be deliberate or accidental, e.g. cows under treatment were not easily or accurately identified, or inadequate records meant that the herdsman or relief milker was not sure when he could start to re-use milk from a treated cow. Ideally mastitis cows should be milked after the rest of the herd or using a separate cluster fitted onto a bucket or a churn which is kept in the pit. If cows under treatment have to be milked into the jars, the jars should be drained and then rinsed with clean water before continuing onto the next cow. Even then, leaking fittings can allow enough antibiotic milk into the bulk tank to lead to a test failure.

The other common reason suspected for test failures stems from dry cow therapy. The contract with most dairy companies states that milk should be withheld for the first four days after calving, and if this is not done there is a risk of antibiotic contamination. Cows which calve early pose a particular problem especially if dry cow therapy has been administered in the preceding three to four weeks.

Table 7.5. Reasons suggested for antibiotic test failures.

| Reason | Percentage |
|---|---|
| Poor records or none | 32 |
| Not withholding milk for the full period | 32 |
| Calving early/short dry period | 15 |
| Accidental transfer of milk | 14 |
| Prolonged excretion | 12 |
| Contamination of recorder jars | 9 |
| Withholding milk from treated quarters only | 8 |
| Lack of advice on withholding period | 6 |
| Mechanical failure | 6 |
| Recently purchased cows | 3 |
| Milking through jars | 1 |
| Use of dry cow preparation during lactation | 1 |

Survey of farmers in 1981. From J. Booth, *In Practice*, July 1982.

Table 7.5 shows a list of reasons suggested by farmers as to why their milk had failed the test. The figures add up to more than 100% because several farmers gave more than one reason for a test failure. Poor records and inadequate withholding periods seem to be the main causes. Most dairy company contracts state that all milk should be discarded from a cow under any form of antibiotic or oestrogen therapy. However, very occasionally individual cows produce natural inhibitors usually in association with udder injury, colostrum or mastitis. They then fail the test, but no antibiotic is present.

# SUMMER MASTITIS

This is a condition seen especially in pregnant cows and heifers, although it can also occur in non-pregnant animals, young calves and occasionally even in steers. The first sign that something is wrong may be that the animal is standing apart from the others and perhaps she is walking rather stiffly. Careful examination of the udder shows that one or more of the quarters is hard, hot, swollen and, especially in a heifer, it will be very painful, so take care when handling her. If milked, a yellow, custardy material is produced which normally has a foul smell, although the absence of the smell does not completely rule out summer mastitis. Another characteristic, and one which is often not mentioned, is that the teat sinus becomes thickened. Squeeze and roll one of the other teats between your thumb and forefinger: you will find it feels soft and empty. In the quarter affected by summer mastitis the teat seems thicker, as if it has a fibrous cord through the teat cistern. Heifers are especially affected in this way. Sometimes heifers calving down with a blind quarter have a similar thickening of the teat and I suspect that these have had a low-grade summer mastitis which was not detected (see page 228 for a further discussion of blind quarters).

   In the early stages the affected animal will be running a high temperature, due to septicaemia and toxaemia. Untreated cases may abort or even die, while others may develop a permanent arthritis from infection localising in the joints. It has been shown that even if the calves of affected animals are born alive, they will probably be stunted and have a reduced viability.

*Cause*
There are four bacteria involved*:

- *Actinomyces (Corynebacterium) pyogenes* (85%)
- *Peptococcus indolicus* (62%)
- *Streptococcus dysgalactiae* (24%)
- a micrococcus (22%)

*It is interesting that two other bacteria, namely *Bacteroides melaninogenicus* and *Fusobacterium necrophorum*, both of which cause foul-of-the-foot, are commonly isolated from cases of summer mastitis in Denmark and The Netherlands, but are rarely cultured from cases in the UK.

The percentages shown express the number of times each organism was cultured from clinical cases of summer mastitis in a UK survey reported in 1988. Pure cultures of any one of these bacteria applied to the teat end will not produce disease, but mixed cultures will, especially using *Peptococcus* and *A. pyogenes*. Infection is transferred to the teat end by females of the sucking fly *Hydrotaea irritans*, also known as the sheep-head fly. *H. irritans* lives near woods, small copses and around wet ground, with sandy soils rather than clay being preferred. The adult fly deposits its eggs in the earth in October and these overwinter to emerge in June or July the following year. The adults roost in trees and bushes from where they fly out to feed. There is only one generation of adults each year and they are found during July, August and September. These are therefore the three worst months for summer mastitis and disease occurs most commonly when the weather is warm and humid, with humidity being the most important factor. This is because high winds (above 20 km per hour) and heavy rain inhibit the activity of the flies.

   Although it carries infection, *H. irritans* probably cannot cause disease on its own. There must first be damage to the end of the teat, either by biting flies, or by the cow walking over sharp grass, thistles or thorns, or even by licking her own teats excessively. *H. irritans* then comes to feed on the small drops of blood or serum oozing from the tip of the teat and in so doing transmits summer mastitis infection.

   Summer mastitis seems to affect the fore teats more often than the hind teats, possibly because the tail is more effective at removing flies from hind teats. Animals with hairy udders are less commonly affected, whereas cows which are easy milkers are particularly susceptible. Presumably this is because it is easier for infection to penetrate their teat ducts.

*Treatment*
Unfortunately, by the time summer mastitis has been noticed, the quarter has usually already been lost and treatment is mainly aimed at reducing the illness in the animal, thereby preventing abortion.

Occasional quarters do recover, however, especially if the cow or heifer calves soon after. Your vet will probably use penicillin, given both by injection and as tubes into the quarter, although some say that it is pointless applying any intramammary treatment.

Summer mastitis is effectively an abscess in the udder and, as such, *drainage* is vital. It is best achieved by regular stripping preferably several times each day until the quarter dries up, although as this can take several weeks and may be painful to the animal, some farmers prefer to have the end of the teat amputated to allow natural drainage. The

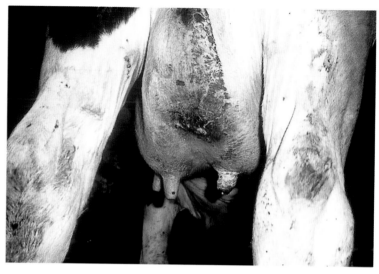

Plate 7.29. Summer mastitis. In this advanced case infection has burst through the rear of the udder. Note the swollen, painful teat.

affected animal should be removed from the group and kept separate to prevent infection from spreading.

Even after treatment, many animals are left with a focus of infection in their udder and this may burst out some time later, particularly after calving. A typical example is shown in Plate 7.29, where the shrivelled teat is still discharging pus, despite the fact that the udder has burst.

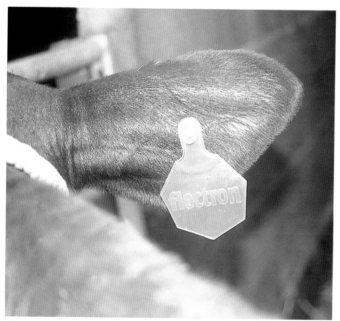

Plate 7.30. A fly repellent ear tag. The insecticide from the tag should flow over the whole body (except the teats) in the natural skin oils.

*Prevention*

Prevention consists of two parts, dry cow therapy and fly control.

**Dry cow therapy** Dry cow antibiotic gives good protection, but it persists for only three weeks, so a second or even third infusion may be necessary for cows with a long dry period. However, with such cows additional care needs to be taken to avoid antibiotic contamination of the milk after calving. Dry cow tubes can also be given to heifers, especially if they are 'bagging up', although there should be at least four weeks before calving to avoid antibiotic problems.

The only difference in technique is that the tip of the dry cow tube is placed against the outside of the heifer's teat sphincter, rather than through the streak canal as you would normally do for a cow. For both cows and heifers it is essential to clean the end of the teat first, so as to avoid introducing other infections.

**Fly control** In dairy herds fly control has several advantages in addition to preventing summer mastitis. If the cows are irritated by flies they tend to bunch together in the shade rather than graze and this will reduce their milk production. They may be restless when being milked and perhaps kick off the clusters, or, even worse, they can tear their teats when kicking at flies. This is particularly common in older cows with pendulous udders and close to calving, because there is often a drip of colostrum on the end of the teat which attracts the flies. In heifers fly control is an important preventive measure against New Forest eye (see Chapter 4).

By far the best method of fly control for summer mastitis is to apply insecticide directly onto the udder every one to two weeks. It is easily applied once the heifers or cows have been rounded up.

Alternatively chemicals which claim to give protection against flies for between two and eight weeks can be applied by knapsack sprayer or using a spray race. More popular are pour-on preparations in which a low volume of persistent insecticide applied along the animal's back is absorbed and spreads all over the skin.

As the favourite landing place for *H. irritans* is along the animal's abdomen and on its udder, this is the important area to cover with fly repellent. It is simply not sufficient to spray insecticide over the animals' backs and then feel pleased that fewer flies are seen on their heads and shoulders. The fly is attracted by any discharge and very large numbers will be seen on the end of an affected teat.

Another possibility is a large plastic ear tag (Plate 7.30) which has been impregnated with an insecticide, usually a pyrethroid. As the animals groom themselves they wipe the tag across their coat and the natural oils in the skin (the sebum) dissolve the cypermethrin, to give a complete body covering. There is a flow of body oil passing over the skin of the animal, especially from the shoulder backwards, and a complete coating of insecticide is achieved within 12 hours of applying the tag. Unfortunately this flow of sebum does not continue onto the teats, and this is probably one reason why experience with the tags has shown that they reduce fly numbers but do not control them totally and some cases of summer mastitis will still occur, even when a tag is used in each ear.

Another method of keeping flies away from the teat is to cover the ends with a permeable micropore plaster as in Plate 7.31. This can be left on for three weeks and does not seem to irritate the teats. First clean the teats with surgical spirit and allow to dry. Then spray on the adhesive, allowing 30 seconds for it to dry, before wrapping the tape twice round the teat, making sure that there is an overlap of 10–15 mm at the sphincter. The overlap can then be squeezed together to form a seal. Take care not to apply the tape too tight; otherwise blood flow may be restricted. Although this is clearly more laborious and more expensive than using other repellents, it is generally considered to be effective. The same tape can be used in the repair of teat wounds.

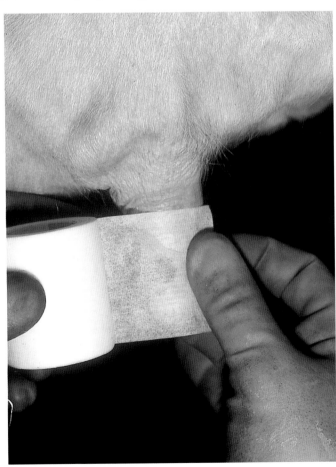

Plate 7.31. Permeable teat tape used to cover the teat end and protect against summer mastitis. It can also be used to aid healing of cut teats.

Finally, try to avoid grazing heifers and dry cows near woody or wet areas during the summer months. If you have had a bad outbreak of summer mastitis in a particular field in one year, you know it must be a good breeding place for *H. irritans* and should therefore be avoided in future years.

## UNCOMMON CAUSES OF MASTITIS

We have dealt with the common causes of mastitis and their control, but there are a few odd infections which may not fit into the standard pattern. A word of warning however: by definition these infections are not particularly common and if you have a difficult mastitis problem in your herd it is more likely that environmental or contagious organisms are involved. I will list the names of the unusual infections and give a few notes on their significance.

### Corynebacterium bovis, Staphylococcus epidermidis and micrococci

These three can be dealt with as a single group. They rarely cause clots or any other clinical signs, but they can lead to a high cell count. They are controlled by teat dipping and dry cow therapy. *C. bovis* is sometimes used as an indicator of suboptimal post milking teat disinfection. If there is a high *C. bovis* count in the bulk milk, extra attention needs to be paid to post dipping techniques. However, all three organisms may have some protective effects against coliforms (see page 200).

### Mycoplasma

There are at least three species of mycoplasma which can cause mastitis in cattle. *M. bovigenitalium* is a relatively mild condition. *M. californicum* gives a chronic hard quarter with a dramatic decline in yield, thick clots almost like pus and an extremely high cell count (5–10 million). Affected animals are not sick in themselves, and both milking and dry cows can be affected. *M. bovis* causes the most severe syndrome. Although the changes in the udder may be similar, the cow is often seriously ill. She may abort, get pneumonia or develop an inflammation and swelling in the joints, producing extreme lameness. The fetlocks are the most commonly affected and although no treatment seems to alleviate the condition, many cases resolve on their own after three to four weeks. Lameness and mastitis are not necessarily seen in a herd at the same time.

Treatment of mycoplasma mastitis is difficult, since the organisms are not bacteria and only a few antibiotics (erythrocin, tylosin, spectinomycin and oxytetracycline in very high doses) are effective. Intramammary therapy is of very limited value and treatment needs to be by injection for several days. Teat dipping and parlour hygiene are extremely important in control. This is one instance where pasteurisation of the clusters between cows (see page 198) would be worthwhile.

### Yeasts

Yeasts are another group of non-bacterial infections which can cause mastitis. They produce changes similar to mycoplasma, although the cow invariably has a significantly raised temperature. Yeasts are common in the environment, and this is the source of infection. They may be introduced when infusing intramammary antibiotic against a normal bacterial mastitis if careful aseptic precautions are not used, and they are totally unresponsive to antibiotics. Success in treatment has been reported from the infusion of 60–100 ml of a mixture of 1.8 g of iodine crystals in 2 litres of liquid paraffin, plus 23 ml ether, into the quarter once daily for two to three days, ensuring that it is thoroughly stripped out at the next milking. Concurrent administration of intravenous sodium iodide or oral potassium iodide may improve the response in refractory cases.

### Leptospira hardjo

Leptospirosis causes a rise in temperature, the cow may be off her food and the small amount of milk present is rather thick, almost like colostrum. One of the most prominent clinical signs is the sudden and massive drop in yield, with all four quarters affected, and hence the names milk drop syndrome or flabby bag are sometimes used. Treatment with streptomycin is generally effective, although the cow may take several days to recover. There is a good vaccine available and you should ask your vet if it is worthwhile for your herd. The disease is dealt with in more detail in Chapter 13.

## Pseudomonas

*Pseudomonas* normally leads to a slightly thickened quarter and white lumpy clots in the milk which would be indistinguishable from staphylococcal/ streptococcal infections. The bacteria can grow *inside* the udder cells, however, and this largely protects them from the action of antibiotics which tend to be mainly in the extra-cellular fluid surrounding the tissues and only reach low concentrations inside the cells. Response to treatment is therefore very poor. Many cases continue for days or weeks, or they may appear to recover but then recur a few days later. A proportion of cows develop chronic illness and weight loss. *Pseudomonas* can grow in the header tank which feeds the udder washing equipment and also in improperly cleaned milking machines. These are the most probable sources of infection where no antiseptic is being used, or if the plant cleaning routine is inadequate.

In freshly calved cows *Pseudomonas* can cause a very severe or even fatal mastitis and the symptoms of this are identical to an acute *E. coli* infection (described on page 183).

## Klebsiella

This organism can also cause a very severe mastitis, with udder changes similar to those caused by *E. coli* in the fresh calver. Treatment is often unsuccessful. The infection is associated with sawdust as cubicle bedding, especially if the sawdust was damp and heated up before it was used.

## Bacillus Species

*Bacillus licheniformis* causes a mild mastitis with a chronic thickening of the quarter. Even though the organism should be sensitive to most antibiotics, including penicillin, some cases can be surprisingly difficult to treat. Cases often occur when cows are allowed to lie outside on waste fermenting maize silage. *B. licheniformis* infections ascending into the vagina may also cause endometritis ('the whites', see Chapter 8) and poor fertility. *Bacillus cereus* is classically associated with brewers' grains and can cause an acute, gangrenous mastitis.

## Gangrenous Mastitis

At first the affected quarter feels cold to the touch, the 'milk' drawn from the teat will be dark red in colour and often mixed with gas, and the teat skin may start to blister, as in Plate 7.32. Some cows are very sick, while others appear surprisingly bright, alert and healthy. The former are best slaughtered. If the infection is allowed to progress, the tissue of the quarter may literally fall out (Plate 7.33), and although some cows eventually recover, the healing process can be quite lengthy, with an open festering sore being present for several months. *B. cereus*, *Staph. aureus* and *E. coli* can

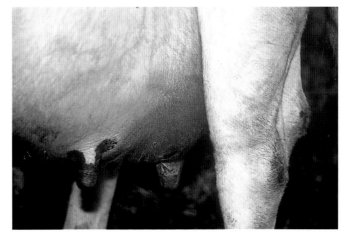

Plate 7.32. The cold, black lower area of the hind quarter and crinkled skin over the teat are typical of gangrenous mastitis. The blood on the cow's leg has been discharged from the teat.

all cause gangrenous mastitis. Most probably a dramatic loss of udder immunity causes the problem, rather than a particularly virulent strain of infection. For example, if an antiserum against bovine neutrophils is infused into the udder of a chronically affected *Staph. aureus* carrier cow, all of her neutrophils will be removed and the cow will die from peracute gangrenous mastitis within a few days.

## DISORDERS OF THE TEAT AND UDDER

Mastitis is defined as infection of the mammary gland. There are a few other conditions affecting the teat and udder which are worthy of note. Most of these are associated with physical damage, but a few are infectious.

### Milking Machine Damage

The milking machine may damage teats by faulty pulsation, worn liners or improper use, for example removal of clusters while they are still under vacuum. A certain amount of swelling (oedema) of the teat end (Plate 7.34) is a normal feature and is seen immediately the cluster is removed, but the teat sphincter should be smooth and not prolapsed. Plate 7.15 showed how milking machine damage could lead to eversion of the teat sphincter, often referred to as hyperkeratosis. There was also haemorrhage on the teat caused by excessive vacuum fluctuation. An advanced case of hyperkeratosis, associated with poor ACR function, was also shown in Plate 7.16. As a healthy sphincter is an important part of the defences against mastitis, teats with hyperkeratosis will be more prone to mastitis and will have increased cell counts.

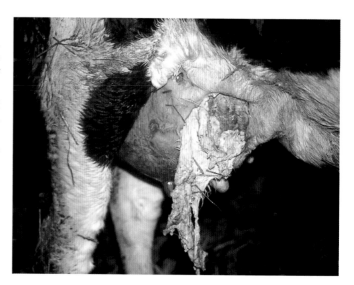

Plate 7.33. Tissue discharging following a gangrenous mastitis. This cow should be culled.

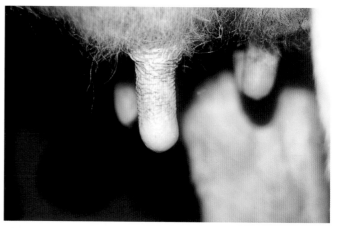

Plate 7.34. Mild oedema or ballooning of the teat end, as in this cow, is a normal feature following removal of the milking machine.

### Blackspot

Blackspot is the term used to describe a particularly severe teat sphincter sore, usually consisting of a combination of an ulcerated area plus necrotic (dead) tissue, as in Plate 7.35. The 'pull' of the milking machine twice daily must retard healing and the damage to the teat canal obviously predisposes to mastitis.

Blackspot has no single cause. It usually starts with trauma, either by the milking machine or from crushing of the teat end. Secondary infection by the bacterium *Fusobacterium necrophorum* then develops. Chilling by cold and wet weather exacerbates the condition.

Resting the teat, for example discontinuing milking for one or two weeks, or using a teat cannula (Plate 7.36) will help to improve healing, but both can lead to mastitis. If a teat cannula is used, make sure that a small quantity of antibiotic is deposited in the teat canal at the end of each milking for the four or five days following removal. The main risk of mastitis is after removing the cannula, presumably because the teat canal will have been badly stretched and its bacterial defence mechanisms will no longer be functioning. If you continue milking, remove the machine from that quarter as soon as possible. Teat dipping and antiseptic creams help to promote healing, as do ointments containing organic acids, which remove dead tissue. Some people have reported success using hypochlorite dips.

## Cut Teats

Sometimes herds experience 'outbreaks' of deep gashes in their teats. The cut may run halfway round the teat or more; it is often at the lower end towards the sphincter and it may penetrate into the canal. A typical example is shown in Plate 7.37,

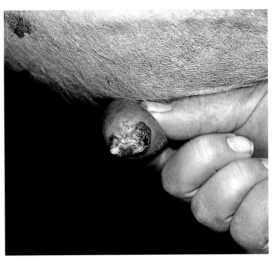

Plate 7.35. Blackspot is severe teat end damage caused by trauma and secondary bacterial infection.

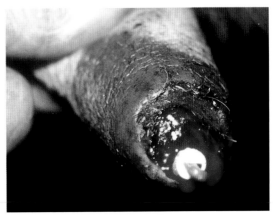

Plate 7.36. A teat cannula used to allow milk to flow through a damaged teat end. The red plug can be removed to allow milk to flow.

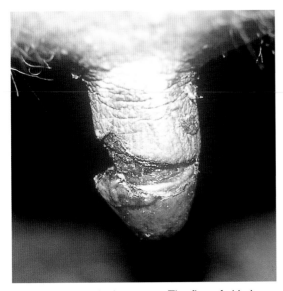

Plate 7.37. A typical torn teat. The flap of skin is pulled downwards each time the unit is removed, making it very uncomfortable for the cow. Amputation of the flap promotes surprisingly rapid healing.

and I know that the sight of this fills any herdsman with gloom. Teats which are split through the canal, as in Plate 7.38, are much more difficult to treat and often develop mastitis.

You will obviously need your vet to attend to the damage, but it may be worth looking at a few of the possible causes. The cut is most probably caused by the teat being stepped on, either by the cow itself, or by another cow. To try to prevent further cases you should look at possible overcrowding, cows being rushed about, poor cubicle design, insufficient cubicle numbers, inadequate dunging passage width, slippery floors and insufficient loafing areas leading to high stocking densities. It is also possible that you have a high proportion of older cows with pendulous udders, where the teats are more at risk.

Treatment is by suturing or by amputating the skin flap. Alternatively the wound can be taped over using a special adhesive plaster and aerosol spray (Plate 7.31). Although it is traditionally thought to be important to continue milking the teat because of the risk of mastitis, I think that mastitis is far more likely if a teat cannula is used (as in Plate 7.36). If the affected teat is simply left for one to two weeks, without being milked at all, this will promote much more rapid healing and most of the milk production from the teat will be

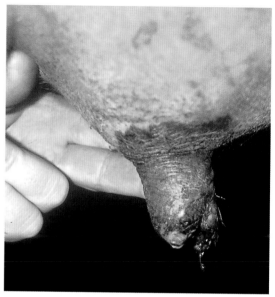

Plate 7.38. There is no specific treatment for a split at the teat end. Infuse a small quantity of antibiotic daily and remove the milking machine quickly. The split may eventually heal.

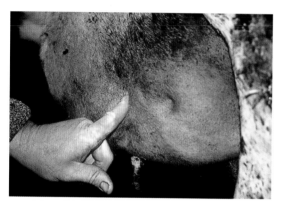

Plate 7.39. Udder oedema or 'nature' is detected by pushing your finger into the udder. If a depression remains after removal, this indicates oedema.

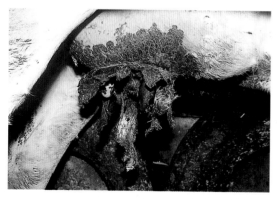

Plate 7.40. Necrotic dermatitis is seen in freshly calved heifers and is often a consequence of excessive oedema. The teat skin becomes very hard and dry.

regained later. Make sure that milk from at least the first two milkings after resuming milking is discarded, as after two weeks the milk will have a very high cell count.

## Udder Oedema and Necrotic Dermatitis

Oedema is the name given to fluid accumulating under the skin. It can be detected by pushing your finger into a swollen udder, then removing it. If a depression is left, the udder swelling is caused by oedema (Plate 7.39). At calving, udder oedema may be referred to as 'nature'. It is caused by factors such as overfeeding, inadequate exercise and excessive salt or mineral intakes during the one to two weeks prior to calving. If severe, the oedema can restrict blood flow to the udder and teat skin to such an extent that the skin dies. This leads to the condition of necrotic dermatitis. Initially the affected skin will feel very hard and dry, and some areas may eventually fall off, leaving large sores.

Occasionally heifers may be so badly affected that they are almost impossible to milk. A typical example is shown in Plate 7.40. Sores may develop between the udder and legs (Plate 7.41), or in older cows between the quarters at the front of the udder

(Plate 7.42). These sores are very slow to heal. The best treatment is to wash with antiseptic solution, cleaning the area and removing all dead tissue, and then to dry and liberally apply an emollient such as glycerine. In the early stages, bathing the udder in a concentrated solution of warm Epsom salts may help to remove the oedema and restore blood flow.

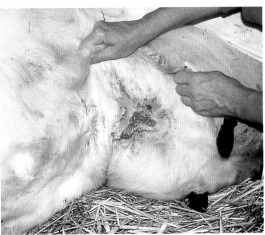

Plate 7.42. In older cows sores at the front of the udder are often first detected by their pungent smell!

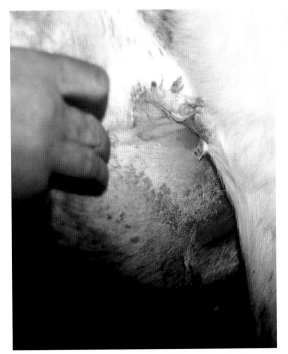

Plate 7.41. Sores may develop between the leg and udder, especially in freshly calved heifers.

## Pseudocowpox

This is a paravaccinia virus and is probably the most common of the infectious teat lesions seen in cows. Typically it consists of irregular circular or horseshoe-shaped areas of small haemorrhagic spots, as in Plate 7.43. There may be normal skin in the centre of the lesion. Sometimes the blister which precedes these changes may be noticed.

As it is a virus infection, there is no specific treatment, although teat dip will help to prevent secondary bacterial infection and if mixed with an emollient it will promote healing. Hypochlorite also has a non-specific viral-killing action if in direct contact with the virus, although of course it

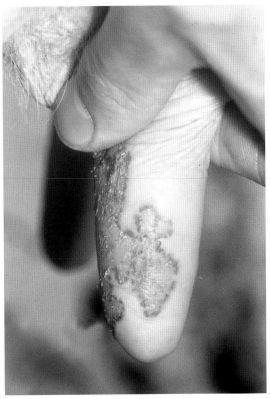

Plate 7.43. Pseudocowpox is a viral infection, seen as irregular circular shapes on the teat skin. It is not particularly painful. (Courtesy D. Weaver.)

is difficult to use with emollients (see page 199). If you have a severe outbreak you would be wise to milk the affected cows last to reduce the rate of spread of infection. Usually there are only a few cases in each herd, often in recently introduced heifers, because these have little or no immunity. Immunity to pseudocowpox is relatively short-lived anyway, and because of this some herds may experience waves of infection and disease every six to twelve months.

Gloves should be worn to prevent the development of *milkers'* nodules, small warts on your hands and fingers which are caused by the virus. The virus is closely related to, if not identical with, the orf virus which causes scabs on the lips and nose of sheep and which can also affect man.

### Bovine Herpes Mamillitis

This is another virus infection, fortunately much less common, because the disease is very severe. Large and very painful blisters develop on the teat and they may be so sore that milking is virtually impossible. When the blisters burst, a raw scabby area is exposed (Plate 7.44) and this may take two or three weeks to heal. Cannulas may have to be used for milking. Heifers are most susceptible, and even the skin of the udder may be affected. At this stage it looks similar to a severe photosensitisation, but affecting only the teats and sometimes the skin of the udder. I have known freshly calved heifers to be so badly

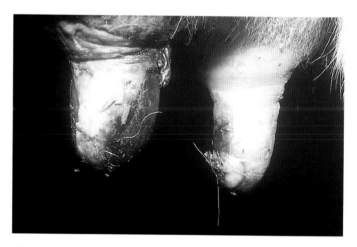

Plate 7.44. Bovine herpes mamillitis is a much more severe viral infection which leads to teat blistering.

affected that they have had to be culled because they were impossible to milk. Luckily immunity is good, lasting four or five years, and herd outbreaks are relatively rare.

Teat dipping and separation of affected animals are the only useful control measures. Use an iodine teat dip, since iodine kills the virus. Disease is seen mainly from July to December, with September and October being the peak months, and most cases occur soon after calving. Even in a herd outbreak it is unusual for more than 10% of the cows to be affected, although the virus may persist in carrier cows for many years before becoming reactivated.

### Udder Impetigo

This is seen as small pustules, like weeping sores, over the skin at the back of the udder. It is caused by a staphylococcal infection and responds well to simple treatment with topical antibiotic or antiseptic cream. The teats are not affected.

### Teat Warts

Warts are another virus infection and again it is heifers which are by far the worst affected, this time yearlings and in-calvers. Warts may appear as fleshy lumps (Plate 7.46) or they may be of the feathery type. Feathery warts (Plate 7.45) are the easiest to deal with because most of them can be quite easily pulled off and the teat dressed with an antiseptic cream or teat dip. With either type of wart you can ask your vet to send a specimen to a laboratory to have an *autogenous vaccine* prepared. The vaccine, which can be injected either into or under the skin, is probably only 30% effective, but sometimes heifers are so severely affected that any help is welcome. The virus is thought to be transmitted by flies, so attention to fly control (described on page 219) is important.

Body warts may also occur, with the head, neck (Plate 10.15) and belly (Plate 7.46) being particularly badly affected. They occur mainly in cattle one to two years old and most cases spontaneously recover during the next summer at grazing. If the warts become so large that they ulcerate and develop a secondary bacterial infection, a vaccine can be prepared and this is much more effective than vaccines against teat warts.

Both types of warts can sometimes be prevented by mixing heifers with cows when they are younger, viz during their first grazing season.

## Teat Chaps

This is the name given to cracks and splits in the teat skin. They become infected with bacteria which makes them sore, and of course they act as reservoirs of infection of the mastitis organisms *Stap. aureus* and *Strep. dysgalactiae*. The best treatment is teat dip or an ointment which has both antiseptic and emollient properties. Chaps occur particularly in the spring and autumn, when cows have to walk through muddy gateways and when there are cold winds. Teat skin does not have the sebaceous glands found elsewhere in the body. This means that when dry, the normal pliable and elastic properties of the skin are soon lost, its keratin layer cracks, and chaps soon form. This is one reason why pre milking teat washing is being discontinued, especially in herds which do not dry teats afterwards.

## Milk Let-down Failure

Milk let-down, that is the expulsion of milk from the glands where it is produced (Figure 7.1) into the teat, is stimulated by the hormone oxytocin.

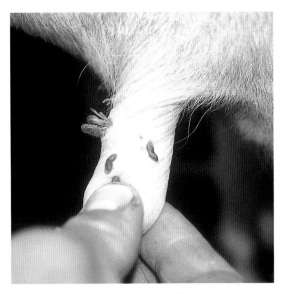

Plate 7.45. Feathery teat warts. These are caused by a virus infection and are most commonly seen in heifers.

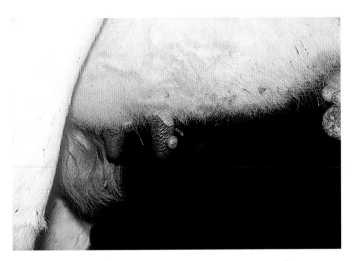

Plate 7.46. 'Fleshy' teat warts are also caused by a virus.

In some cows the normal activities of entering the parlour, feeding and udder preparation do not seem sufficient to stimulate oxytocin release, and virtually no milk is given. This can be particularly true with heifers which are apprehensive or nervous, because the hormone adrenalin acts as an antagonist to oxytocin. The problem can be approached in two ways. First, careful and gentle handling may overcome the heifer's fears and, second, injections of oxytocin can be given two to three minutes before the milking machine is applied. In practice you would probably use both methods. When you have established the dose of oxytocin required to produce let-down, try slowly decreasing it over a few days until the heifer's own behavioural reactions take over.

Sometimes cows which are being suckled, or are suckling others, stop letting down their milk. Provided you can identify the culprit, most cases can be controlled with an anti-suckling nose plate (as in

Plate 7.47), which covers the cow's mouth and prevents her getting hold of a teat. It is said that group-housed calves which are allowed to suckle each other during rearing are more likely to suckle as adults. Ideally calves should be penned individually until well after weaning.

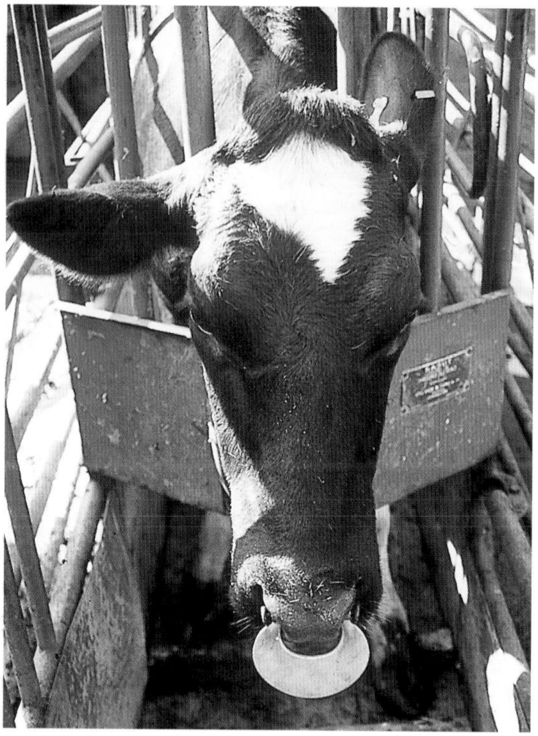

## Blind Quarters

This is a condition seen primarily in heifers, and would not be noticed until the first milking. The udder appears normal, but no milk can be drawn from the teat. I have experienced three separate categories of this condition. The first, and by far the most common, is the presence of a membrane across the top of the teat, producing a permanent barrier between the teat cistern and the gland cistern (see Figure 7.1). The teat feels normal but it does not fill with milk during let-down. The teat is anaesthetised and a long cannula (often called a teat siphon) is inserted through the teat sphincter. Often the cannula can be forced through the membrane to allow milk to flow. Making a series of holes in this way can occasionally resolve the blockage, but many eventually heal over again.

The second cause of a blind quarter is a blockage at the teat sphincter. The teat feels full of milk, but it cannot be drawn out. This is the easiest condition to deal with. With the teat anaesthetised, a small knife (called MacClean's knife) with a disc blade just below the guide tip is forced up through the sphincter as shown in Plate 7.48. It is then rotated through 180° and pulled back out again. This produces two transverse cuts, and once milk starts to flow, it usually continues very successfully, although it may be best to infuse intramammary antibiotic into the teat end after each milking for the first few days as a mastitis preventive. The same procedure can also be used to dilate the teats of cows or heifers which are very slow milkers, provided the sphincter is normal. If the slow milking arises from a crushed teat or some other abnormality, however, I have not found the knife particularly successful.

The third cause of a blind quarter is summer mastitis. The heifer will already have had the infection, quite possibly unnoticed, and may well have recovered without treatment, but the teat is left permanently damaged. It feels as if there is a thick fibrous

Plate 7.47. An anti-suckling nose plate. Some plates also have protruding spikes, which discourage the cow doing the suckling.

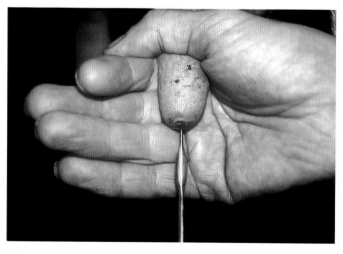

Plate 7.48. A MacClean's teat knife, used to dilate the teat canal of a 'tight' (slow) milker and also to remove teat 'peas'.

core running up through the teat cistern. This is easily detected by rolling the teat between your finger and thumb and comparing the affected teat with a normal one. There is no treatment.

## Blood in Milk

It is not uncommon for cows to calve down with blood in their milk, and I have always felt that it is more common in animals which have very tight oedematous udders or sometimes following a difficult calving when the udder may have been bruised by the cow's own leg movements. Sometimes the blood has formed clots and then the diagnosis is easy. At other times it is mixed with colostrum, and it may be very difficult to decide if there is an acute mastitis present. Looking for a raised temperature, heat and pain from the quarter and general signs of health should distinguish between the two conditions, but if you are in any doubt I would strongly recommend that you infuse a tube of antibiotic. I know of no drugs which are consistently effective against blood in milk, and the only action is not to milk the quarter or to relieve it only lightly so that the back pressure from the milk stops the blood flow. There is some evidence that cows will develop a 'light' quarter, that is they will not milk as well, after they have had blood in their milk.

## Pea in Teat

Sometimes milk flow from the teat is obstructed by a small lump which floats around in the teat cistern but acts like a valve as soon as milk is drawn from the sphincter. This is called a 'pea'. Examples are shown in Plate 7.49. The red-coloured 'peas' are very like blood clots, which suggests that they could be a consequence of blood in milk, with milk salts, fat and udder cells then adhering to the blood clot in the more mature (cream-coloured) cases. 'Peas' can occur at any stage of lactation, but are most commonly seen during the first three months after calving, when the cow is at peak yield.

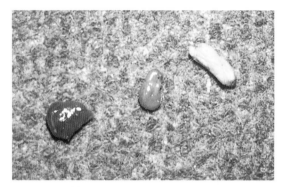

Plate 7.49. Examples of teat 'peas'. Some are quite soft, like a blood clot, which suggests this could be their origin.

Small peas may be squeezed out manually, perhaps by first crushing them inside the teat, using your finger and thumb. However, in the majority of cases the sphincter has to be dilated with a MacClean's knife (Plate 7.48) to facilitate removal. Alternatively, use a pair of special forceps inserted through the canal to crush the pea and then pull it out in pieces. Sometimes the pea is attached to a membrane growing out from the wall of the teat cistern, or it is the membrane itself which is causing the blockage. Although milk flows easily through a cannula, as soon as the teat is drawn by hand the membrane obstructs the teat streak canal. I have never found any successful way of treating such cases.

*Chapter 8*

# FERTILITY AND ITS CONTROL

After feeding, fertility is the factor which has the greatest effect on the economics of dairy farming. Maintenance of good fertility is to a large extent governed by management, and this means that the individual farmer or herdsman has a very important part to play in its control. First let us look at the economics. The *calving interval*, the overall measure of herd fertility, is the period between one calving and the next and should be 365 days, that is exactly one year.

At 1998 UK values, agricultural economists quote a loss of up to £3.50 per cow for each *day* that the calving interval is extended beyond 365 days. Figures such as these, cited in abstract, often have relatively little meaning, however, and the following gives an idea of how the amount is calculated. I would urge the reader to insert current day values and local prices in order to calculate a truly accurate cost.

## COSTS OF A MISSED HEAT

Take a rather mediocre cow giving 5840 litres in a 305 day lactation, with a calving interval of 365 days. Averaged out to include her 60 day dry period, this gives a potential milk production of 5840 divided by 365 = 16 litres per day. Other assumptions are:

- milk price of 22p per litre
- concentrate price of £130 per ton (13p per kg)
- a high level concentrate use of 0.3 kg/litre over the whole year, namely 0.3 x 5840 = 1.75 tons per year. This high value relative to the cow's yield is used to compensate for the additional forage which a milking cow eats compared to a dry cow
- a calf value at birth of £73.00

Using these figures it can be calculated that:

- cost of producing 1 litre of milk
    = concentrate cost per kg x concentrate use per litre = 13 x 0.3 = 3.9p per litre
- gross profit margin per litre of milk
    = milk price minus concentrate cost per litre = 22 – 3.9 = 18.1 p per litre

Our simplified example assumes that the maintenance costs and overheads of the cow – grazing, forage, utilities, finance, labour etc. – will remain constant, whether or not she is pregnant, that the profit comes from milk production and that there are no savings or increases in production associated with an extended lactation. (This is not entirely true of course.) Every day over 365 days that she does not become pregnant is therefore a day of lost production. In our example this becomes:

lost production
= 16 litres/day at a margin of 18.1p per litre
= 16 x 18.1p
= 289.6p per day lost margin

Even the calf is worth 20p per day (£73 divided by 365) over the year, so the overall cost is:
289.6 + 20 = 309.6p per day

In practical terms an individual cow rarely loses time on a daily basis: she either conceives or does not conceive and so the cost of a missed heat or a failure of conception is measured in 21 day cycles:

cost of a 21 day cycle = 309.6 x 21 = £65.02

This figure is slightly lower than the value of £3.50 per day (£73.50 per 21 day cycle) quoted earlier, because it does not include the additional costs of disturbance of the calving pattern, higher replacement rates and other factors.

I would also urge the reader to try different levels of yield. A cow giving 7300 litres in her 305 day lactation, for example, could be losing a potential margin of 382p per day, or £80.22 per 21 day cycle, at 1998 values. There is a tendency by some to allow high-yielding cows a longer calving interval because, it is said, they are milking so well that you will never get them in calf and anyway they will keep producing at a high level later in lactation. As Figure 8.1 shows, however most milk is given at peak lactation and a cow which has two 'peaks' over an 18 month period will perform much better than a cow which was left unserved because she was a high yielder. This is an extreme example, but it illustrates the point very well. In addition, cows which do not get back in calf quickly often end up by having a longer dry period and may get overfat. One survey showed that for every one day increase in calving interval, lactation length increased by only 0.6 day; i.e. 40% of the increased interval was in the dry period.

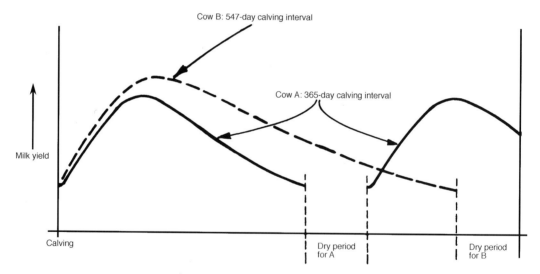

Figure 8.1. The effects of calving interval on milk yield. Cow A had a 365 day calving interval and therefore achieved two peak yields in an 18 month period. Although cow B peaked at a higher level and milked extremely well, her overall milk production was lower.

## Extended Calving Intervals

If cows continued to milk, did not have extended dry periods and did not get overfat before the next calving, there would certainly be some benefits from extended calving intervals. One obvious advantage is a reduction in disease. Most of the common health problems of dairy cows – mastitis, milk fever, ketosis, calving problems, retained placenta, suboptimal fertility and even lameness – are associated with calving and the early lactation period. If the calving interval was, say, extended by 3 months, from 12 to

15 months, this could result in a potential reduction in disease costs of as much as 25% (3 months in 12 = 25%). This is only an option for all year round calving herds and would have to be carefully managed. Perhaps it could result in improvements in cow welfare, and as a result it is likely that longevity and overall lifetime production might also improve.

For a 15 month calving interval cows would need to be served at 6 months into lactation. By this stage they would be well past peak and one would expect an improvement in fertility. However, anyone reading this needs to carry out a very careful economic appraisal of their own system before embarking on any changes. If herd fertility is good and disease incidence is low, the benefits will not be so attractive and even in a herd with health problems there may well be more economic ways of improving the situation.

## THE COMPONENTS OF THE CALVING INTERVAL

The calving interval is defined as the period between one calving and the next and it is an overall measure of fertility status. There are several distinct stages however and these need to be identified before we can discuss the factors affecting fertility.

Take calving as the starting point. After calving, the cow must overcome any uterine infections. She must then begin her ovarian cycles, to come on heat and ovulate every 21 days, and she must cycle regularly without any abnormalities. In a herd using artificial insemination she has to be seen to be bulling so that she may be presented for AI, and this is known as *heat detection*. After service the egg must be fertilised and then the developing embryo must attach itself or *implant* onto the wall of the uterus. These two processes of fertilisation and implantation are together known as conception. Good conception rates, that is avoiding large numbers of repeat services, are very important in fertility management. Once the foetus has become established in the uterus, there is still the possibility of early foetal death or, at a later stage, abortion, defined as the premature expulsion of the calf. A successful calving should result in the production of a live calf, so the final hurdle is the elimination of stillbirths.

Each of these factors will be dealt with in detail later in the chapter, but to enable a better understanding of the processes involved, some of the physical and hormonal changes associated with the oestrous cycle are described.

---

Components of a successful calving interval are:

- elimination of uterine infection
- commencement of ovarian activity and establishment of regular oestrous cycles
- visual observation of oestrus, i.e. heat detection
- fertilisation
- embryo recognition leading to implantation of the placenta onto the uterine wall
- minimising embryo deaths
- avoiding abortions
- production of a live calf

---

## THE OESTROUS CYCLE

This is the name given to the sequence of physical and hormonal events which culminate in the behavioural signs of the cow being 'on heat' or 'on bulling', or 'in oestrus', approximately every 3 weeks.

*Puberty* is the age at which an animal becomes sexually mature; that is when oestrous cycles begin. In heifers the onset of puberty can vary from as little as 6 to as much as 18 months old, with nutrition being the most important determining factor.

### Physical Changes

Figure 8.2 and Plates 8.1 and 8.2 give the basic anatomy of the cow's reproductive tract. It was also shown in detail in Plate 5.1. At birth, the ovary contains all the eggs the cow will need for her reproductive life (some 75,000 eggs are present in each ovary!) and from puberty onwards one egg is passed down into the uterus every 21 days, interrupted only by pregnancy and a short period of ovarian inactivity in early lactation. When it is ready to be shed, the egg is contained in a small fluid-filled sac on the surface of the ovary called a *follicle*.

At the end of oestrus the follicle bursts and releases the egg into the oviduct. This is known as ovulation (see Figure 8.3). The egg then passes down to the junction of the oviduct and uterus, and this is the point where fertilisation may take place.

Immediately after ovulation, glandular tissue begins to form in the base of the ruptured follicle and it grows until there is a mass protruding from the surface of the ovary. This structure is called the *corpus luteum*. It is sometimes known as the 'yellow body' because of its colour, or simply abbreviated as 'the corp'. It is clearly seen in Plates 8.1 and 8.2. This structure can be felt from day 4 or 5 onwards, and it is what your vet is feeling for when he is assessing whether or not a cow is cycling. From its shape and size he will also be able to give you some idea of how many days past the previous bulling the cow is at the time of examination and this will help you to know when to watch for her next heat. If the cow conceives, the corpus luteum remains in the ovary for the whole of pregnancy. However, if she does not conceive it decreases in size from days 16–18 onwards and this allows the development of a second follicle, as shown in Plate 8.2.

As the follicle expands and

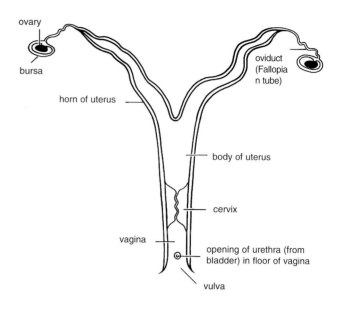

Figure 8.2. The reproductive tract of the cow.

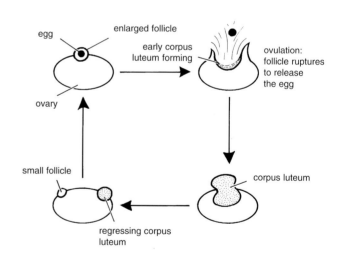

Figure 8.3. Changes in the ovary during the oestrous cycle.

matures in preparation for ovulation, it produces increased quantities of the hormone *oestrogen*. It is the action of oestrogen in the body which causes the physical changes associated with oestrus including, for example, enlargement of the vulva, passage of the 'bulling slime' and, of course, mounting behaviour. In fact waves of follicles develop and regress throughout the oestrous cycle, with some cows having two wave cycles and others three wave cycles. A three wave cycle denotes the fact that there is increased follicular activity on the ovary on, for example, days 8, 13 and 22. A two wave cycle would have follicles at days 10 and 21 only. In each case it is *only* the follicles at days 20–22 which rupture to release the egg.

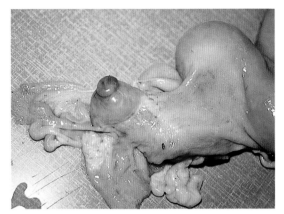

Plate 8.1. An ovary showing a corpus luteum approximately 7 days after ovulation. The convoluted tube on the left is the oviduct (fallopian tube).

Each time there is a new wave, 2–3 follicles on the ovary increase in size, a process known as recruitment. These follicles produce an increase in circulating blood oestrogen and the cow may show slightly more interest in other cows in oestrus, although it is unlikely that she will stand to be mounted. At day 21 one of the follicles ovulates and all the other follicles undergo atresia, that is they regress back to normal size and may be selected (recruitment) for another follicular wave in the future. As one might expect, cows experiencing three wave cycles have an oestrous cycle 1 to 3 days longer than cows with two wave cycles. This helps to explain the variable cycle length in some cows. Two wave cycle cows show a better response when GnRH is used on repeat breeders (page 272).

A few days after ovulation the corpus luteum begins to produce the hormone *progesterone*. This has almost the opposite effect to oestrogen. Progesterone suppresses the signs of heat, suppresses the release of the hormones FSH and LH from the

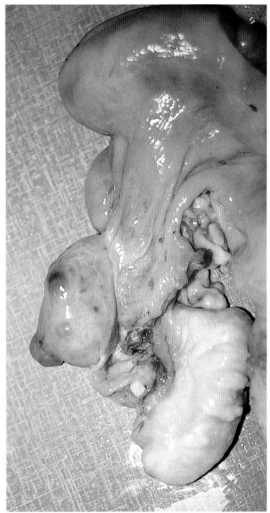

Plate 8.2. As the corpus luteum decreases in size progesterone levels fall, allowing the development and maturation of the next follicle. The plate shows an orange corpus luteum protruding from the left of the ovary and a dark grey, fluid-filled follicle in the centre.

pituitary gland (thereby inhibiting the start of the next cycle, Figure 8.4), and prepares the uterus to accept the fertilised egg, known as the ovum.

After 16 to 18 days and in the absence of pregnancy, the wall of the uterus produces the hormone *prostaglandin* (PG). This passes to the ovary and 'dissolves' the corpus luteum (Figure 8.5). Considering that it is quite a large structure, the corpus luteum regresses surprisingly rapidly: in as little as 3 or 4 days. As the corpus luteum regresses, progesterone levels fall, allowing the release of hormones from the brain to initiate the next cycle.

## Hormonal Changes

The two major hormones acting on the ovary are:

follicule stimulating hormone (FSH)
luteinising hormone (LH)

Both are produced and stored in the anterior pituitary gland at the base of the brain, although once produced their release is controlled by hormones from the hypothalamus, as shown in Figure 8.4. Both hormones are needed to stimulate follicular development, but LH has additional functions in that it leads to ovulation and it also promotes the growth of the corpus luteum. Measurements of LH in the blood of a freshly calved cow show quite low activity: perhaps one 'pulse' is released into the bloodstream every 6–8 hours. However, as follicles get closer to maturation (under the influence of FSH) the frequency of the LH pulses increases to once every 30 minutes.

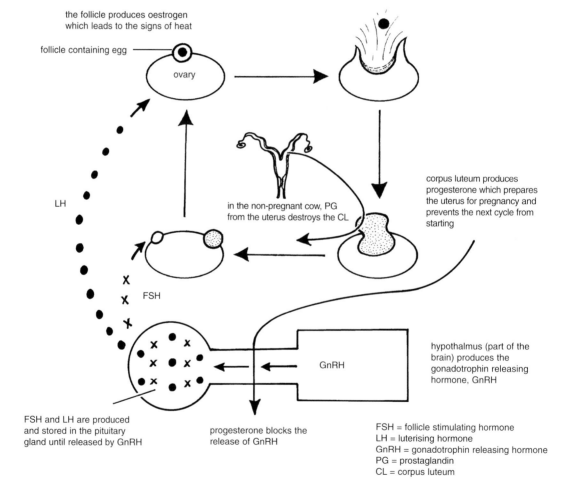

Figure 8.4. Hormonal changes during the oestrous cycle. Progesterone produced by the corpus luteum inhibits the release of GnRH from the hypothalamus. When progesterone levels fall, GnRH releases LH and FSH from the pituitary, and the next cycle starts.

This rapid pulse release is extremely important in the development of the next crop of ovarian follicles and it is interesting that it is inhibited by factors such as:

- a suckling calf (and so beef cows are slower to come on heat after calving than dairy cows)
- negative energy balance (typical of the early lactation cow at peak yield)
- progesterone from the corpus luteum
- placental steroids produced in late pregnancy

The release of LH and FSH into the bloodstream (and therefore to the ovary) is controlled by yet another hormone, namely GnRH, gonadotrophin releasing hormone. (FSH and LH are called gonadotrophins because they influence the growth of the gonads.) GnRH is produced in the hypothalamus, and its action is inhibited by progesterone. Towards the end of a normal oestrous cycle the sequence of events, shown in Figure 8.4, is as follows:

- FSH and LH accumulate in the pituitary gland, but cannot be released because progesterone produced by the corpus luteum is blocking the action of GnRH.
- In the absence of pregnancy, the uterus produces prostaglandin around day 16.
- Prostaglandin dissolves the corpus luteum, progesterone levels fall and GnRH becomes activated.
- FSH and LH are released from the anterior pituitary gland and pass to the ovary to stimulate the development of the next crop of follicles.

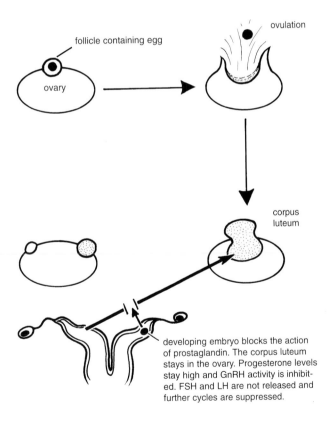

## Recognition of Pregnancy

In much the same way as the full-term calf tells the cow it is ready to be born (see Chapter 5), it is the embryo which sends out a signal to inform the cow that she is pregnant. This signal is a protein, known as bovine trophoblastin (bTb), and it is similar in structure to interferon. The signal inhibits production of prostaglandin by the uterus and so in the pregnant cow this leads to the following sequence of events (see Figure 8.5):

- The foetus inhibits the release of prostaglandin from the uterus.
- The corpus luteum remains in the ovary and progesterone levels stay high.
- High progesterone levels inhibit the action of GnRH, thereby preventing the release of LH and FSH, so that the next ovarian cycle does not start.

Figure 8.5. In the pregnant cow the developing embryo releases a signal (above) which inhibits uterine release of prostaglandin. In the non-pregnant cycling cow the uterus produces prostaglandin from day 16. This dissolves the corpus luteum, thereby initiating the next cycle.

If the corpus luteum is removed for some reason, for example by injecting prostaglandin or cortisone, progesterone levels fall and the cow will abort.

## Action of Fertility Cycle Drugs

Many of the hormones which we have described are also available as injectable preparations and you may find it interesting to know which types of drugs your vet uses for fertility treatments.

*Oestrogen*
Oestrogen can be used to stimulate ovarian function in cows which have not started cycling after calving and also as a treatment for endometritis. It has two disadvantages, however. Firstly there is a danger of cystic ovaries developing after treatment and secondly the cow may only show the *behavioural* signs of oestrus, without going through any of the ovarian changes which lead to pregnancy.

*FSH and LH*
FSH and LH are commonly used to stimulate ovarian activity, or GnRH can be given to stimulate the release of FSH and LH which is naturally produced. LH can also be used as a 'holding injection' on the day of service to ensure that ovulation occurs and on day 12 post service to reduce embryo death. This is described in more detail on page 272.

*Prostaglandin*
Prostaglandin, either the natural hormone or a synthetic product, is an extremely commonly used drug. When given by intramuscular injection it causes the dissolution of the corpus luteum, progesterone levels fall, GnRH becomes activated, FSH and LH are released and the cow comes into oestrus 3–4 days after injection. These changes can be followed in Figure 8.4. Prostaglandin can only act if there is a corpus luteum in the ovary, however, and the corpus luteum is only sensitive to prostaglandin during days 5–15 of the cycle.

One word of caution: prostaglandin will lead to the regression of the corpus luteum whether or not the cow is pregnant, and if given to a cow at less than 150 days or more than 250 days of pregnancy, it is highly likely that she will abort. Your vet will therefore want to carry out a rectal examination of the cow prior to the administration of the drug and you should also check your records to ensure that there is no possibility of the cow having been served in the preceding 6 weeks, since pregnancies of this age or less may not be detectable by rectal examination. Prostaglandin is also used in the treatment of endometritis (page 266).

*Gonadotrophin releasing hormone*
GnRH is used primarily in the treatment of cystic ovaries and to improve conception rates. Its action and uses are described on pages 242 and 272.

*Progesterone releasing devices*
A variety of devices that maintain a continuous level of progesterone circulating in the cow's system are on the market. This has the effect of blocking GnRH, as in Figure 8.4, and in so doing it prevents the release of LH and FSH, preventing the start of a new cycle. When the device is

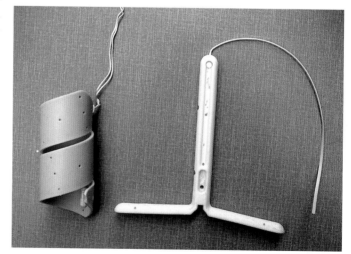

Plate 8.3. Progesterone releasing devices, a PRID (left) and CIDR (right).

removed after 10–12 days, blood progesterone levels fall, GnRH becomes activated and sufficient LH and FSH will have accumulated to initiate ovarian activity, inducing a fertile oestrus two days after the device has been removed. The most common devices are shown in Plates 8.3 and 8.5.

A PRID (progesterone releasing intravaginal device) consists of a progesterone impregnated silicone rubber coating around a metal coil. The coil is inserted into the vagina, with the string protruding from the vulva (Plate 8.4) for easy removal after 12 days. The small gelatine capsule at one end (Plate 8.3) contains oestradiol. This dissolves naturally soon after insertion of the PRID and acts by removing any remaining corpus luteum. One disadvantage of the PRID is that it sometimes produces a vaginitis, with copious quantities of purulent material discharging from the vulva following its removal. However, although this looks unsightly, it does not seem to affect conception rates.

A CIDR (controlled internal drug release) consists of a nylon T-shaped spine covered by progesterone impregnated silicone (Plate 8.3) with a small plastic tail which is left protruding through the vulva. The CIDR is said to cause less vaginitis, but it has no oestradiol capsule, so prostaglandin injections are often given just prior to CIDR removal.

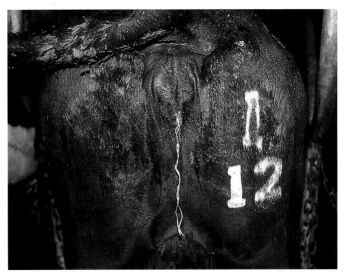

Plate 8.4. A PRID is removed after 12 days by pulling on the string, which can be seen protruding from the vulva.

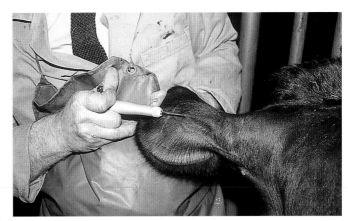

Plate 8.5. Progesterone releasing devices can also be implanted under the skin of the ear, as with this CRESTAR.

The CRESTAR is a progesterone implant which is placed under the skin of the ear, as shown in Plate 8.5. A single dose of oestradiol is given by intramuscular injection at the time of implantation and this helps to remove any remaining corpus luteum. After 9–10 days a small scalpel cut is made in the overlying skin and the implant is squeezed out. The cow comes on heat 48 hours after removal.

CRESTAR implants probably give the best heat synchronisation and as such the manufacturers state that only one insemination is required after removal, whereas for PRID and CIDR, inseminations on two consecutive days, or at observed oestrus, are recommended. There is also no risk of vaginal infections with a subcutaneous implant.

Failure of the progesterone releasing devices can be caused by:

- Persistence of a corpus luteum in the ovary. The use of oestradiol with the PRID and CRESTAR should minimise this and an injection of prostaglandin is recommended when using a CIDR.
- Insertion of the device when the cow is very close to oestrus. In a small proportion of such animals

there is then a corpus luteum in the ovary when the implant is removed 10–12 days later and she fails to come on heat.

● Refractory anoestrous cows. Cows which are very thin or stressed in some other way sometimes totally fail to respond. In such extreme cases it may be better to wait until they start regaining weight before the device is administered.

If the device is left in place for significantly longer than 12 days (to allow all luteal tissue to regress naturally), the prolonged period of progesterone may depress subsequent conception rates. An alternative system, therefore, is to inject prostaglandin 1 day before the device is withdrawn, for example, inject on day 9, withdraw on day 10 (that is, a shortened period) and serve on day 12. This is obviously more expensive, but it does produce better synchronisation and more successful conception rates.

Both prostaglandin and the PRID can be used to synchronise the onset of oestrus in groups of cows or heifers, thus allowing fixed-time AI and eliminating the need for heat detection. This will be covered in more detail later in the chapter.

## Embryo Transfer

Many of the drugs mentioned above are used during embryo transfer. This is a technique to increase the number of offspring from a cow of exceptional genetic merit. An embryo is an egg or ovum which has been fertilised. In the normal cow only one follicle ovulates, producing one ovum each time the cow comes on heat (possibly two for twins). However if a large dose of FSH (usually in the form of pregnant mare serum gonadotropin, PMSG) is given daily for 2–3 days before oestrus, then the number of ova shed from the ovary will be increased. This is known as *superovulation*. After fertilisation by AI, the resulting embryos can be flushed from the donor cow by means of catheters fed into her uterus, separated out and placed singly into recipient heifers. Table 8.1 gives a typical schedule for embryo transfer. There are many alternatives.

The embryo is very fastidious in its requirement for uterine environment and because of this it is *essential* that it is transferred into a recipient which is at the same stage of the oestrous cycle as the donor. This means that the recipients must be observed to be in standing oestrus within 24 hours of the donor, and preferably less. This synchronisation of heats is achieved by using prostaglandin or progesterone releasing devices (PRDs). To ensure that the donor *releases* the large number of ova following superovulation, an injection of GnRH is given on the day of the insemination. Flushing of the donor to remove the embryos from her uterus is usually carried out 6–7 days after insemination. Each

| | Event/treatment | |
|---|---|---|
| Day | Donor | Recipients |
| 0 | Bulling | |
| 2 | | Insert PRD |
| 10 | Inject FSH/PMSG | |
| 11 | Inject FSH/PMSG | Inject prostaglandin |
| 12 | Inject FSH/PMSG | Remove PRD and inject prostaglandin |
| 14 | Observe for heat late pm | Observe and record heats |
| 15 | Inseminate Inject GnRH | Observe and record heats |
| 22 | Flush embryos | Transfer embryos |

PRD = a progesterone releasing device.

Table 8.1. A typical schedule of events for embryo transfer. The time of day for some injections will be precisely specified.

embryo must be carefully examined under a microscope before it is transferred into a recipient. Some eggs will not have been fertilised (that is, they are still ova and have not developed into an embryo). Some embryos may be degenerating and are not suitable for transfer. The transfer into recipients may be carried out surgically, by an incision through the flank and by depositing the embryo directly into the uterus, or non-surgically by passing a catheter through the cervix. Surgical transfer may give slightly better results but is more expensive.

What results can be expected? The great variable is the response of the donor to superovulation treatment, so the number of embryos recovered may vary between none and 25. However, an overall average result, for example, for non-surgical transfer, would be eight embryos recovered, six suitable for transfer and resulting in three established pregnancies. This may not seem a lot, but of course the donor cow is not yet pregnant. She can either be flushed again for a further crop of embryos or inseminated in the usual way. Flushing should not have any adverse effect on her subsequent fertility.

Embryos can be stored for long periods of time in liquid nitrogen. This overcomes the variable response to superovulation because once the embryos are frozen, a suitable number of recipients can be synchronised for transfer at a later date.

## Cystic Ovaries

In Figure 8.3 we saw that the normal follicle ruptured to release the egg (the process of ovulation) and this was followed by the growth of the corpus luteum. Sometimes, however, instead of rupturing, the follicle continues to enlarge and this forms an ovarian cyst (see Figure 8.6 and Plate 8.6). Cystic ovaries are classically subdivided into two types, follicular and luteal cysts, depending on their development and which hormone they produce. However, this is probably an artificial subdivision, in that there is good evidence that at least a proportion of cows have cysts which intermittently produce either oestrogen or progesterone, while other cows develop cystic ovaries which resolve spontaneously. This is particularly common in early lactation. Although a cow with irregular heats should always be checked, do

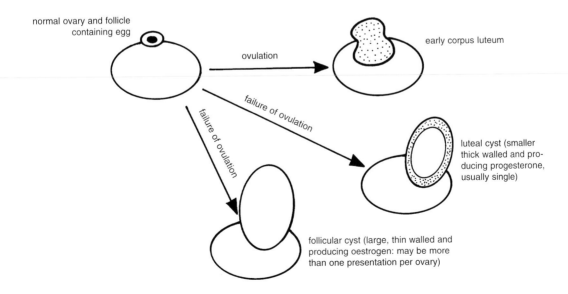

Figure 8.6. The development of cystic ovaries.

not be too surprised if no abnormalities are found.

*Follicular cysts*

If oestrogen is produced, the cow is said to have a follicular cyst and she shows signs of excessive oestrous behaviour. The cow is sometimes said to be nymphing, or we say that she has become a nymphomaniac. These cows will come into oestrus at irregular intervals, perhaps every 8–12 days or even more frequently, and they may stay on heat for 3–4 days instead of the normal 12–18 hours. They may also become active whenever any other cows in the herd are bulling. If left untreated, they develop a very high tail head and their pelvis may creak as they walk, due to oestrogen relaxing the supporting ligaments. Eventually masculinisation develops and the cow starts roaring and pawing the ground like a bull.

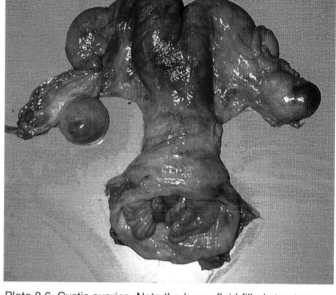

Plate 8.6. Cystic ovaries. Note the large, fluid-filled structures present in both ovaries. Some cysts can be many times larger than this.

*Luteal cysts*

In some cows a layer of progesterone producing luteal tissue may grow on the inside of the cyst wall and this is known as a luteal cyst (Figure 8.6). The progesterone produced by the luteal cyst blocks GnRH activity, ovarian cycles cease and the cow is never seen on heat. She is now in the true state of *anoestrus*, which simply means without ovarian activity.

The differentiation between follicular and luteal cysts is not always an easy matter. Only the extreme forms have been described. Intermediate stages occur and in other instances follicular cysts develop into luteal cysts which may then recover spontaneously. Differentiation may influence treatment. Follicular cysts are typically larger and have thinner walls than luteal cysts. The best diagnosis can be obtained by using milk progesterone tests (see page 244). Luteal cysts can be treated with prostaglandin; follicular cysts with LH, GnRH or a combination of LH and progesterone. Progesterone releasing devices should be effective against both types.

*Causes of cystic ovaries*

Normally about 4% of cows develop cystic ovaries each year, although in some herds they can become quite a problem. The condition is partly inherited – I can remember treating a cow and two of her daughters for cysts on one farm on the same day! In Sweden, cystic ovaries once occurred in 10% of all cows, so they introduced a careful selection policy to ensure that bulls used for breeding were not derived from cows which had had cystic ovaries. This reduced their national incidence to 5%, much the same as the current level in Great Britain.

Stress is thought to be another factor involved. It causes a variety of hormonal upsets. It has been suggested that a cow under stress does not produce enough GnRH in the brain (Figure 8.4) and this leads to an inadequate release of FSH and LH. A follicle is produced and the cow comes on heat, but there is insufficient LH to cause ovulation.

Nutrition has also been suggested as a cause of cystic ovaries, particularly in high-yielding cows underfed at peak, but to my knowledge there is no direct proof of this. There have been anecdotal suggestions that cows given excess amounts of high starch concentrates immediately after calving, for example when they are offered peak intakes within the first week post-partum, may also be more susceptible to cystic ovaries. This could be related to acidosis and fatty liver, as shown in Table 6.2. Cows with fatty livers have been shown to have much higher levels of circulating prostaglandin than normal cows, and this could interfere with their oestrous cycles and subsequent fertility. Manganese deficiency may be involved, and factors such as B-carotene deficiency and the presence of certain oestrogenic toxins in the food are all possible predisposing causes.

## Failure to Cycle

Most cows have started some oestrous cycle changes in their ovaries by 2–3 weeks after calving, although the first *visible* heat may not be seen until 4 or 5 weeks. However, a few cows remain with inactive ovaries until 60 days or more after calving and you will need to get your vet to attend to these. They are true anoestrous cows. He will carry out a rectal examination to make sure that there are no abnormalities on the ovary and then he will give a suitable treatment, most probably a progesterone releasing device. The hormones FSH and LH are responsible for the initiation of ovarian cycles and follicular development and, as described previously, the frequent pulsatile release of LH is particularly important.

Failure to cycle is most commonly seen in first calved heifers which have lost excessive bodyweight during the first few weeks of lactation – in other words, it occurs as a result of underfeeding. It is also seen in suckler cows and in this case the continued presence of the calf seems to inhibit ovarian activity. Stress, leading to increased levels of cortisone, may also be involved, since this inhibits the pulse releases of GnRH required to initiate ovarian cycles. Possible causes of stress are described in Chapter 9.

In some high-yielding cows (about 3%) ovarian cycles start but then stop again. The commonest cause of cows not *seen* bulling is poor heat detection, but the possibility that the cow has stopped cycling should not be overlooked and you should get your vet to check for this. The syndrome is referred to as the 'long low progesterone' or 'anovulatory' phase and its importance has been identified by means of serial milk progesterone sampling (see Figure 8.12). Sometimes such cows are said to be hovering: they may often appear to be close to bulling and show interest in other cows in oestrus, but will not stand to be mounted themselves. As such they show behavioural similarities to cows with cystic ovaries.

## PREGNANCY DETECTION

It is vitally important that the herdsman knows not only *if* the cow is pregnant, but also *when* she became pregnant. Many of the management decisions throughout lactation – observation of heat, insemination, drying off date, calving pattern, fulfilment of milk quota, etc. – are based on a knowledge of an accurate conception date and therefore calving date. Methods of pregnancy detection include:

- the cow fails to return to oestrus
- milk progesterone testing
- ultrasonic scanning
- bovine pregnancy associated glycoprotein (bPAG) testing
- rectal palpation
- testing for oestrone sulphate in milk
- external abdominal palpation

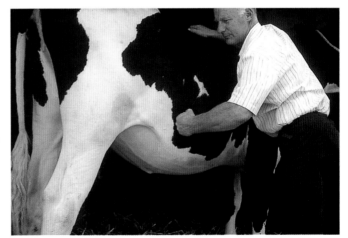

Plate 8.7. Late pregnancy can sometimes be detected by pushing your fist firmly in and out of the lower abdomen, in a swinging action. The calf is felt as a hard structure, bumping against your fist.

Failure of the cow to return to oestrus is the most common and the most important method, although it is not discussed in the following. External abdominal palpation can be used from approximately 7 months of pregnancy onwards. It should be possible to ballot the calf by gently but firmly pushing your fist in and out of the lower flank area, as in Plate 8.7.

## Milk Progesterone Tests

In Figures 8.3 and 8.4 we saw how the corpus luteum is present in the ovary between one heat and the next and that it produces the hormone progesterone. Progesterone circulates in the blood and passes into the milk and measurements of *milk* progesterone levels can be very useful in several areas of fertility control. Figure 8.7 shows the milk progesterone of a cow which had her first heat at 30 days after calving. When she is on heat there is no corpus luteum present in the ovary and so milk progesterone levels fall to zero. Levels rise to a peak during the middle of the next cycle and then return to zero 21 days later (now 51 days after calving) at the following oestrus. Figure 8.8 shows the same cow, but this time she was successfully inseminated at day 51. Because pregnancy was established, the corpus luteum stayed in the ovary and she did not come on heat at day 72. The dot-

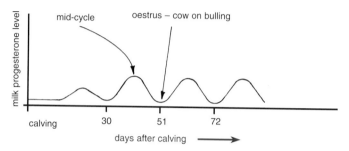

Figure 8.7. Milk progesterone in a normal cycling cow.

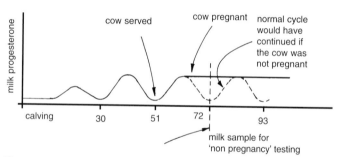

Figure 8.8. Milk progesterone levels in pregnancy.

ted line shows how the cycles would have continued if the insemination had not been successful. This is the basis of the *milk progesterone pregnancy test*. A milk sample is taken 24 days after insemination – at 24 days because the cow could well return to service at 21–24 days and there is no point in sending a milk sample to the laboratory at day 21, only to find that the cow comes bulling 1 or 2 days later. Even if she came on heat at day 19–21 but was not observed, milk progesterone levels would still be low at day 24.

A high milk progesterone level at 24 days after service suggests pregnancy whereas a low level indicates that the cow is not pregnant, and that she was on heat at 19–24 days but that oestrus was not observed. The accuracy of the test is very good for cows which are *not* pregnant (i.e. low progesterone levels), but only 80–85% of the cows which had high progesterone values will be pregnant when examined manually at 8 weeks after service. Because of this many prefer to call milk progesterone an indicator of *non-pregnancy*.

Some of the reasons for the false positive results are given in Figures 8.9, 8.10 and 8.11. The first cause is early embryonic death (Figure 8.9). The cow was pregnant when she was milk sampled at 24 days after service, but she then lost her calf and came on heat 54 days later. Irregular return intervals such as these are a good indicator that early embryonic death has occurred.

A second cause of false positive results is incorrect heat detection. In Figure 8.10 the graph shows the cow's normal cycles. The cowman missed her heat at day 51, but mistakenly thought she

| Causes of high progesterone 24 days after insemination |
| --- |
| ● pregnancy |
| ● poor heat detection |
| ● persistent corpus luteum |
| ● luteal cyst |
| ● pyometra |

was bulling at 65 days so had her served. Unfortunately he also missed her true heat at 72 days and so he took a milk sample 24 days after serving her. Of course by this stage the cow was in the middle of her next cycle, so the milk sample came back with a high progesterone level, a 'positive' result, but we know that the cow could not have been pregnant. Because his heat detection was poor, the cowman missed both of the true heats at days 51 and 72.

This type of situation is more common than you may think. Surveys have been carried out in which all cows presented for AI have been milk sampled. If they are truly on heat the progesterone levels should be zero. In fact results have shown that around 10–15% of cows presented for AI are *not on heat*. Clearly the conception rate of these cows will be zero and this shows how heat detection and conception rates are closely linked. Herds with a high proportion of *negative* milk progesterone results (viz returns at 21 days were not observed and so the cow was milk sampled at 24 days) are likely to have a poorer conception rate, as well as a larger number of false positive milk progesterone results.

The third category of false positive results covers factors *other than pregnancy* which hold the cow in mid cycle, that is maintain the corpus luteum in the ovary. Pregnancy is obviously the main reason for a 'persistent' corpus luteum, but a type of uterine infection known as a *pyometra* (see page 266) and a luteal cyst can have the same effect. Sometimes the cow simply stays in mid cycle for no apparent reason (Figure 8.11), and this may be called a persistent corpus luteum, or simply prolonged luteal activity.

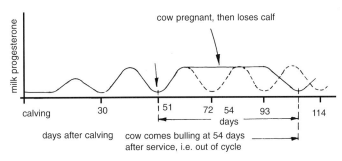

Figure 8.9. Milk progesterone and early foetal death.

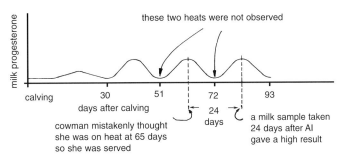

Figure 8.10. Milk progesterone and poor heat detection.

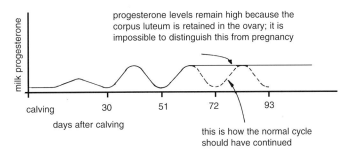

Figure 8.11. Milk progesterone and retained corpus luteum.

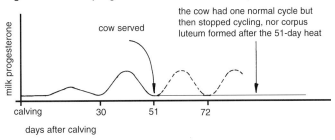

Figure 8.12. Long low progesterone or anovulatory phase.

On other occasions a cow may start cycling and then stop, but without any corpus luteum in the ovary. This would give the long low milk progesterone or anovulatory pattern shown in Figure 8.12. It will not confuse the milk pregnancy test, however, because the result of low progesterone, that is 'not pregnant', will be correct anyway. These cows are often referred to as hovering, that is they are very close to oestrus but do not ovulate (see also page 243). I find it a particularly frustrating syndrome to deal with when doing fertility work. The cow is presented as 'not seen bulling'; on examination I diagnose 'close to bulling' or 'follicle left/right ovary', yet in 2 weeks time when she is presented again, she is at exactly the same stage of the cycle. Nothing has changed. A progesterone releasing device will probably be inserted for treatment and 2 weeks have been wasted. It would be very useful if hovering cows could be diagnosed at the first examination.

Numerous whole herd milk progesterone serial samplings have been carried out in the UK and the incidence of the various oestrous cycle abnormalities assessed. Approximate percentages are:

- 10% not cycling by 60 days post-partum
- 4% persistent corpus luteum (range 2–6.5%)
- 4% hovering (range 3–5%)

In one of these surveys, cows which were hovering had mean yields higher than the remainder of the group: 6627 litres versus 5203 litres, suggesting that perhaps the condition is induced by the stress of higher yields.

*On-farm kits*

There are now a variety of kits available for on-farm testing, the majority of which are based on colour change. There is relatively little advantage in doing your own progesterone testing for pregnancy at 24 days, because you do not need the result until 12–15 days later, that is when the cow is due to come back on heat. There are, however, two occasions when on-farm testing is ideal. These are:

- testing at 18–19 days after the previous service to see which cows are *about* to come on heat. Some systems have even recommended a 'blind' service on the basis of two low progesterone readings on alternate days
- as a method of heat detection. If a cow is at 21 days past her last heat or service and you are not sure whether she is bulling or not, a milk progesterone will help. A high progesterone says that she is not on bulling

## Ultrasound Scanning

The scanner consists of a probe which is inserted into the cow's rectum (Plate 8.8) and, by palpation, passed over each horn of the uterus. The probe emits a beam of ultrasound which, after reflection off tissues of varying density, is collected by the same head and transformed into a picture on the screen. Soft tissues such as the walls of the rectum, uterus, blood vessels and the corpus luteum are seen as grey/white areas. Denser fluid – blood inside arteries and veins, uterine fluid, the fluid in cystic ovaries and urine within the bladder – is seen as dark areas. The screen of the ultrasound scanner therefore shows a black and white TV picture of the uterus and surrounding tissues in cross-section. The wall of the uterus is light in colour, the uter-

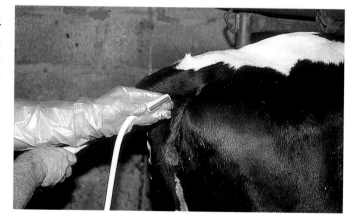

Plate 8.8. Rectal examination using an ultrasound probe can detect pregnancy from approximately 30 days post service.

ine fluid dark and the developing embryo is light (Plate 8.9). It is a video and not a still photograph and so the foetal heartbeat can be seen – often as early as at 30 days of pregnancy!

Several types of scanner are available. Some have a fixed beam (linear scanners) and others a beam which waves to and fro, like a searchlight (sector scanners). Different levels of magnification are also available, depending on whether you want to see small objects (for example, early bovine pregnancy or ovarian follicles), or larger structures (such as scanning the abdomen of a dog externally for pregnancy or intestinal obstruction).

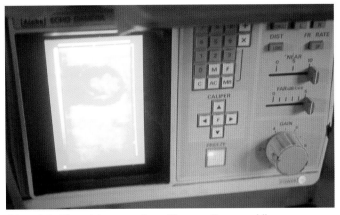

Plate 8.9. The picture produced by an ultrasound linear scanner. The wall of the uterus (light colour), uterine fluid (dark) and developing embryo (35 days old) are shown.

The main advantages of the scanner are:

- Pregnancy can be diagnosed at an early stage, for example from 30 days onwards.
- Ovarian structures – follicle, cyst, corpus luteum – can be more accurately visualised than by rectal palpation.
- Early embryo death can be detected, seen as white 'snowflakes' in the uterine fluid.

The disadvantages are:

- Cost. An average machine was priced at £8000 in 1998.
- The equipment is cumbersome. It is not always easy to find somewhere safe and convenient to position the scanner at the correct height beside a cattle handling system. Cattle, expensive equipment and electricity extension cables are not always a good mix!
- Low lighting is required. It is absolutely *vital* that the screen is in an area of low light intensity, preferably in a building. If in bright sunlight, accurate examination of the screen is virtually impossible.

Even the early pregnancy diagnosis has some disadvantages. Because the rate of natural embryo loss is higher in early pregnancy, a greater proportion of cows diagnosed as pregnant at 30 days will lose their embryo than if pregnancy was diagnosed later. This is particularly the case in problem herds, where embryo losses are high. However, there is still a big advantage in pregnancy checking prior to 6 weeks, because cows suspected *not* pregnant can be treated, or simply watched much more carefully, and then served again at 42 days.

## Bovine Pregnancy Associated Glycoprotein (bPAG)

This protein is only produced by the developing embryo and unlike milk progesterone tests, cows can be sampled for pregnancy at any stage of the cycle. Blood samples are taken from 35 days of pregnancy onwards and the test is highly accurate. However, bPAG is also present in the immediately post-partum cow and ideally animals should be more than 100 days after their previous calving before testing for their next pregnancy, which somewhat limits the usefulness of the test.

## Rectal Palpation

Pregnancy can be detected by rectal palpation from 6 weeks of gestation onwards and from 5 weeks in heifers with small compact uteri. Animals which are very fat are much more difficult to examine. When palpating through the rectal wall, the first step is to compare the size of the two uterine horns. The pregnant side is larger and at 6 weeks the placental membranes may be felt enclosing a bag of fluid. It is most important to distinguish this uterine enlargement from a pyometra or simply failure to return to a normal size following a previous pregnancy. At 8 weeks the calf can be felt, approximately the size of your thumb nail, and by 12 weeks cotyledons are developing.

Assessing the stage of gestation gets less accurate as the pregnancy advances. From 4 months onwards the foetus often drops down into the abdomen and can no longer be palpated, so that stage of pregnancy can only be assessed by the size of the cotyledons. This is not particularly accurate. In late pregnancy, probably from 8 months onwards, the calf becomes palpable again and the stage of gestation is assessed by calf size and position. This is also not particularly accurate. A very small calf may be diagnosed as a 7 month pregnancy, only to be born 2 weeks later – as I know from personal embarrassment!

The advantages of a manual rectal examination are that it is accurate, that in heifers especially, pregnancy can be detected from 5 weeks onwards or even less, that an assessment of the stage of pregnancy can be made, and that if the cow is not pregnant possible reasons why can be given by examining the ovaries. The risks to the cow are minimal, and abortion will occur only if the very young calf (8 to 10 weeks pregnancy) is grasped and squeezed between the finger and thumb. This is almost impossible to achieve accidentally.

Although often discussed, to my knowledge there is absolutely no evidence that rectal palpation leads to any higher rate of embryo loss than scanning and recent research has confirmed this. There will be a low natural loss following both methods, and in both instances herds with a fertility problem will have a higher rate of loss.

## Oestrone Sulphate

Oestrone sulphate is a hormone produced only by the pregnant uterus. Significant quantities can be detected in the milk from 120 days of pregnancy until calving. The test is very accurate and has the advantage over milk progesterone that milk samples do not need to be taken on a specific day. It cannot be used for early pregnancy detection, however.

## HEAT DETECTION

'Heat' or 'on bulling' is the expression given to the behaviour shown by the cow when she is in oestrus, that is when she has a mature follicle in her ovary and is about to ovulate. In herds using artificial insemination it is vital that heat detection is accurate and for this we need to know the signs of heat. These can be roughly divided into early, mid and late.

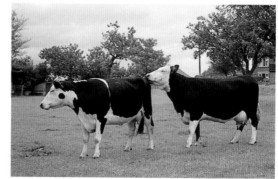

### Early signs of heat
The cow becomes restless, perhaps standing apart from the main group; she may be looking around in the parlour instead of eating her concentrate, and her yield will be down. She may lick or sniff the urine and vulva of other cows or simply rest her chin on another cow's back as shown in Plate 8.10. Sometimes there is playful head to head bunting and nudging behaviour. A proportion of cows will become very noisy, perhaps moving towards a gate or fence, calling to other cattle in the distance. In all the activities where two cows are involved, it could be either cow coming on heat. In the

Plate 8.10. Heat detection: chin resting could be a sign that either cow is in the early stages of heat. In this instance both cows were on heat.

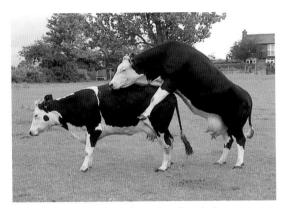

Plate 8.11. Heat detection: standing to be mounted is the best sign of heat. It is the underneath cow which is on heat, although the cow doing the mounting may be either a few days before or after bulling.

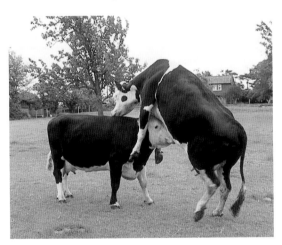

Plate 8.12. Heat detection: mounting head to head. In this case it is the top cow which is on heat.

early stages, the cow may try to jump others, but she will not stand to be mounted.

*Mid signs of heat*

Standing to be mounted is the most sure and positive sign of heat (Plate 8.11) and you should always look for this. It is the cow standing underneath which is on heat. The exception to this is when the two cows are mounting head to head, in which case it is the top cow which is on heat (Plate 8.12). All the early signs of sniffing, nudging and chin resting may still be present, possibly slightly more intensely, and they are often a preliminary to mounting. You may see some enlargement of the vulva and later slime will be passed, known as the bulling string. This is often seen hanging from the vulva, particularly when the cow is sitting in the cubicles. The mucus is produced in the uterus, and released as the cervix opens when oestrus approaches. If you do not see the slime itself, look for signs of clear tacky mucus stuck around the tail at the level of the vulva, as in Plate 8.13.

---

Some common signs of heat

- standing to be mounted – the most important single sign
- attempts to mount other cows (which run away)
- rub marks on tail-head
- sweaty coat and muddy flanks
- behavioural changes, yield drop, bellowing
- mucous discharge ('bulling string')

---

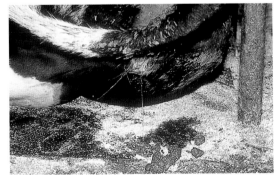

Plate 8.13. Heat detection: a flow of vaginal mucus is known as the bulling string.

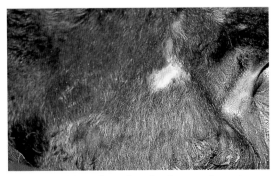

Plate 8.14. Heat detection: fresh raw rub marks each side of the tail head are a sure sign that the cow has been on heat.

*Late signs of heat*

The cow will now be less restless and will no longer stand to be mounted by others. You should be able to see the marks where she has been ridden however, for example areas of raw skin on the tailhead (Plate 8.14) or on each side of the tail, and there may be muddy marks down her flank. If you see fresh blood on the tail or mixed with the bulling string, you could well be too late: she may have been on heat yesterday or even the day before. Some say that blood on the insemination catheter is a sure sign that the cow will return to service. This is not true, although it may indicate that she was inseminated fairly late in heat.

## Measurement of Heat Detection

There are two ways of measuring heat detection, namely:

- efficiency of detection
- accuracy of detection

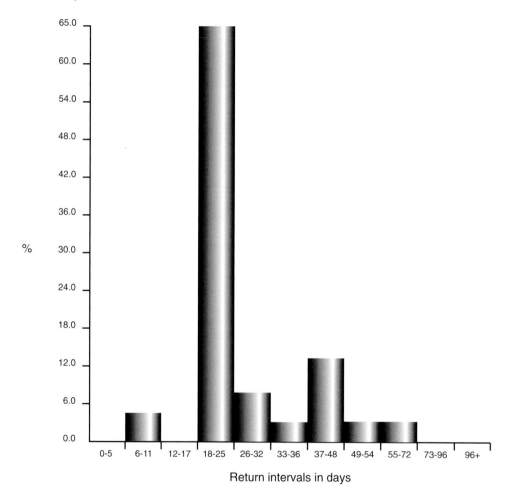

Figure 8.13. Heat detection accuracy and efficiency. This is a good herd, with a high percentage of returns at 18–25 days.

*Efficiency of detection*
This is a measure of how good you are at spotting heats. Assume that you have an autumn calving herd, that you intend to start serving on 5 November and that on that date there will be 50 cows eligible for service. By 26 November (21 days later) you have served 40 cows. Assuming that all 50 cows were cycling normally:
    heat detection efficiency = 40 out of 50 = 80%
Compared to many large herds this is very good: 60% is an average figure and although 40% is poor it is by no means uncommon. However, even in our good herd, 10 heats were missed. If each lost heat costs £65.00 (see page 232), this means a potential loss of £650.00 in only 50 cows.

*Accuracy of detection*
Of the 40 cows submitted for AI in the above example, accuracy of detection measures the number which were actually on heat. Even in an above average herd, only 37 of the 40 cows presented for AI may have been in oestrus:
    accuracy of detection = 37 out of 40 = 92.5%
Put another way, 3 cows (7.5%) presented for AI were not on heat and clearly their conception rate would be zero. Modern computer systems such as DAISY use the interval between serves (the inter-service interval) as a measure of both efficiency and accuracy of heat detection. Examples are given in Fig-

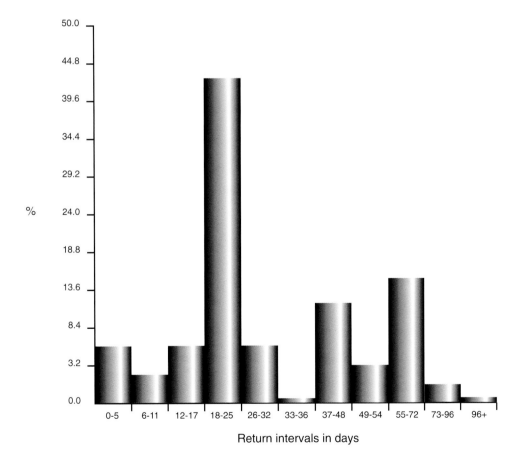

Figure 8.14. Heat detection accuracy and efficiency. A poor herd, with too many returns at 5–17 days, 26–36 days, 37–48 days and 55–72 days.

ures 8.13 and 8.14. Figure 8.13 shows a good herd. The majority of returns (65%) were observed at 18–25 days, with only a small peak (10%) at 36–44 days. The herd in Figure 8.14 obviously has problems:

- Too many cows were served at 5–17 days after the previous service. This could be due to inaccurate heat detection or a high incidence of cystic ovaries or hovering cows.
- Only a small peak (43%) were served at 18–25 days.
- Excessive numbers were served at 26–36 days. This could be inaccurate heat detection or embryo loss.
- Small peaks at 37–48 days and again at 55–72 days indicate that some cows were missed at 21 or both 21 and 42 days and suggests poor efficiency of detection.

*Why is heat detection such a problem?*
People such as Dr Esslemont and colleagues from Reading University have watched cows continuously, 24 hours a day, for 45 days or more. They found that most cows came bulling 40 days after calving, but for some of them heat periods were very short. This was particularly so in the dark, cold days of winter. For example, they found that although the average heat period lasted for 15 hours there were numerous problem areas as highlighted in the following:

- 20% of cows were on heat for less than 6 hours, with some for as little as 2 hours.
- There was an average of 20 minutes between mounts.
- 20% were mounted less than 6 times during their heat period.
- A larger proportion came on heat during the night, especially between 10 pm and 5 am.

Detection rates improved as lactation advanced, because the first one or two cycles after calving produced shorter heat periods. This is demonstrated numerically in Table 8.2.

If a cow came on heat at 11 pm she might well have finished by 5 am, so heat detection would be almost impossible. This is most likely to happen towards the end of the breeding season, when cows are being served earlier after calving and when there are fewer cows in oestrus. Heat periods are then even shorter. The problem is compounded by the fact that around 5% of pregnant cows also show heat and stand to be mounted.

| Cycle no. | No. cows | % detected |
|---|---|---|
| 1 | 96 | 12 |
| 2 | 96 | 31 |
| 3 | 96 | 40 |
| 4 | 82 | 52 |
| 5 | 53 | 64 |

Fonseca, Britt, McDaniel, Wilk & Rakes. (1983), *J. Dairy Sci.* 66 1128. Cycles were monitored by assay of progesterone in blood samples collected twice weekly. Detection percentages refer to the proportion of cows that were detected by standing oestrus.

Table 8.2. Rate of heat detection during the first 5 cycles after calving.

This is discussed in more detail on page 264, where possible courses of action are suggested.

*Improving heat detection*
You can do more for your overall herd fertility by improving heat detection than by any other single action. Because inaccurate heat detection leads to poor conception rates, improvements in heat detection not only get cows served sooner, but by being more accurate they also improve conception rates. Some of the more important factors are as follows:

**Observation** Careful and regular observation is the essential ingredient of good heat detection. Everyone on the farm should be on the look-out for cows on heat and the herdsman should set aside specific times of the day for heat detection. As the average interval between mounts is 20 minutes this should be the minimum period he spends watching. Twenty minutes may seem a very long time to stand watching and waiting in the middle of a busy day, but if it is compared with the £65 cost of possibly missing a heat, it will be time well spent.

More cows come on heat at night, so go and have a look round last thing in the evening, before you go to bed, and again first thing in the morning, before you start milking. This may not be a particularly welcome thought in the cold and dark of winter, but it can pay dividends. The best time for observation is when the cows are resting. Most of them will be lying down cudding and some may be at the silage face. It is the small group of 3–4 cows standing away from the others which should attract your interest. Watch them carefully.

When cows are being moved, for example, brought in for milking or put in a separate yard for scraping out or feeding, they are less likely to show oestrous behaviour. Admittedly some cows will be seen at this stage, but many will be more interested in the next feed than they are with mounting. This is why problems of heat detection sometimes occur in herds which are milked 3 times a day or fed late at night. The cows know that whenever they see the herdsman they are going to be fed or moved and so mounting activity decreases as soon as he arrives.

For similar reasons it is a good idea to have continuous low level lighting for the cows. There is some evidence that this increases both heat activity and conception rates. In addition, if the light is already on, there is even less disturbance to the cows when the herdsman comes in to check for heats.

**Identify the buller area** On many farms there is a small corner of the yard, perhaps halfway between the cubicles and the outside feeding area, where a group of cows congregate when one of them is on heat. This is known as the 'buller group' or the 'buller area' and if you can identify a favourite haunt such as this it makes heat detection much easier. This facility can be improved still further if a bull is penned adjacent to it. The presence of a bull not only draws cows on heat to one area, thereby increasing the manifestation of heat, but he also stimulates the early resumption of ovarian cycles after calving. Table 8.2 shows that heat detection gets easier with each cycle after calving, so the sooner the cow has her first cycle, the easier it will be to detect her on heat when she is ready to be served.

The other aspects of observation include almost any change in the cow's normal behaviour. She may come into the parlour last rather than with an earlier group. Her milk yield is likely to be down – one survey in New Zealand showed that cows which had a 25% reduction in yield at one milking followed by a 25% compensatory increase at the next were highly likely to be in oestrus, and these changes were sufficient to make insemination worthwhile. Cows on heat may stand away from the feeding area and bellow over the gate, and when in the parlour they may be restless, shuffling their feet, looking around and not eating their food.

**Minimise ill health and deficiencies** Healthy cows are more likely to show signs of heat than animals which are thin due to underfeeding or disease. Lameness is especially important: cows with bad feet spend far more time lying down and are bound to be difficult to catch bulling. Similarly, ruminal acidosis and other digestive upsets giving abdominal discomfort are likely to suppress the signs of heat, so correct feeding, particularly providing adequate fibre, is also necessary. Some say that specific mineral and trace element deficiencies can lead to poor heats, sometimes called 'silent heats'. For example, calcium, phosphorus, manganese and iodine have been suggested. While there may not be any conclusive proof of this, there are so many hormonal changes involved in the oestrous cycle that it must be logical to provide a properly balanced ration and thus avoid nutritional stress.

**Housing** Adequate loafing areas and good floor surfaces can also play a part. Overcrowding has been mentioned as a factor increasing the incidence of both lameness and environmental mastitis, and I am sure that cows which are packed into small, poorly ventilated and often purpose-built cubicle houses which give very little room for movement are much more difficult to spot when on heat. I like to see at least one open yard for a loafing area, somewhere where the 'buller group' can become active, without the risk of treading on the teats of other cows. This is one advantage of having the feeding area reasonably separated from the cubicles or bedding area.

The type of floor surface in the yard is also important. One trial compared cows on a dirt yard (which gave them a firm footing) with cows on concrete. Those on the dirt yard were seen standing to be mounted 50% more frequently (3.7 vs 2.5 mounts per 30 minutes) than those on concrete, and they were also in standing heat for longer (13.8 hours versus 9.4 hours). Results are shown in detail in Table 8.3.

|  | Type of surface | |
|---|---|---|
|  | Dirt | Concrete |
| No. cows | 69 | 69 |
| % in heat > 12 hr | 86 | 12 |
| Duration of heat (hr) | 13.8 | 9.4 |
| Mounts per 30 min | 3.7 | 2.5 |
| Stands per 30 min | 3.8 | 2.7 |

Britt, Scott, Armstrong and Whitacre (1986), *J. Dairy Sci.* 69 2195.

Table 8.3. Influence of foot surface on expression of oestrus in Holstein cows.

Floor surface also affects the accuracy of heat detection. For example, another trial looked at the proportion of cows submitted for AI which were not on heat. On dirt yards there was only a 3% error, but the error rate increased with concrete yard surfaces; 10% were incorrectly observed in alleyways, while the worst error was in cubicles. Of the cows submitted for AI on the basis of having been seen standing to be mounted in cubicles, 25% were not on heat! Cows mounted while in a cubicle cannot get away, of course, so they are bound to appear to be 'standing'. This is further proof that a quiet inspection last thing at night, looking for cows in the 'buller area', is by far the best method of heat detection.

**Increased activity of other cows** If a cow fails to show heat it is assumed that she had a 'weak' heat – but possibly it was simply because other cows failed to mount her. It has been shown that the majority of 'mounting' cows are, in fact, close to coming on heat themselves, and if our bulling cow is the only one on heat and all the other animals are in mid cycle, then she will be ridden relatively few times. For example, in a group of heifers, when only one animal was on heat and no others were close to bulling, standing to be mounted was seen only 2–3 times per hour. However, if two heifers were on heat (or one was on heat and one was about to come on), then standing was seen 7 times an hour. This has important practical implications for the smaller farmer, who is more likely to have only one cow on bulling at any one time. The ideal group size for effective heat detection is 30–40 cycling, non-pregnant animals. Injecting a steer or barren cow with hormone to make them continually sexually active would make an ideal heat detector, but this is rarely done.

**Oestrus synchronisation** Grouping cows to come on heat together and in so doing increasing the oestrous activity of each cow is, in my opinion, one of the main reasons for using prostaglandin and other heat synchronisation systems at routine veterinary visits. Cows not seen bulling are one of the most common examinations requested. By using a heat synchronisation treatment, not only

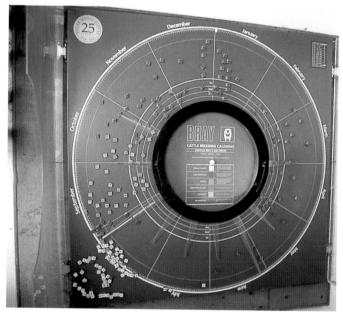

Plate 8.15. A breeding calendar is an excellent system of assessing the status of a herd. If you suspect a cow is bulling, check the calendar to see if she was 'on' 3 weeks previously.

do they come on heat sooner (possibly saving £3 per day), but heats will be stronger, thus improving both heat detection and conception rates. Details of oestrus synchronisation methods are given in a later section.

**Records** Records play a vital role in heat detection. If you have a visual display board like the one in Plate 8.15 you can see which cows should be on heat over the next few days and they can be watched especially carefully. It also helps with the 'buller group'. The herdsman may see three cows in a 'buller group'. He records their numbers on a pad and in the office he finds that only one of them was due on heat: one had just calved and the other one was already pregnant. He now needs to go back and watch the suspect cow much more carefully.

**Cow identification** You may see a cow jump when she is too far away for you to be sure which cow it is. Clear markings, preferably at both the front (ear tags or collars) and rear (freeze-branding) of the cow, make mistakes less likely. This is particularly important if you look at the cows last thing at night and have to leave a message for someone to keep the cow in for AI on the following day, or if you want other farm staff to assist with heat detection.

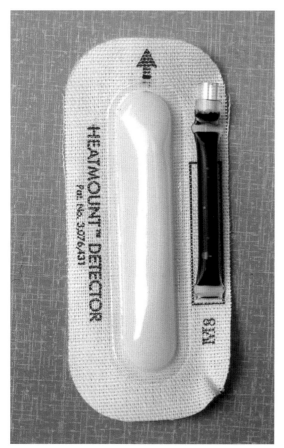

**Regular veterinary visits** Although not specifically aimed at heat detection, routine fertility visits play an important part (see page 277 for a fuller description). Cows which have not yet been seen on heat are identified for special attention, whereas others can be confirmed as pregnant and need not be watched so closely.

**Heat detection aids** There are a few devices which can be used to help you identify a cow on heat. I think the best of these is the Kamar heat mount detector. This consists of a small clear plastic tube (Plate 8.16) with a fine hole in the constriction at the front end. It is enclosed in an opaque plastic shield fixed to a piece of cloth and the device is glued to the tail-head of the cow, making sure the arrow is pointed forwards. If the

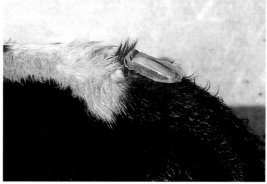

Plate 8.16. A Kamar heat mount detector consists of a tube of dye contained in a plastic outer cover. The dye is squeezed out of the very fine hole at the front end of the dye tube.

Plate 8.17. A positive Kamar. This cow is on heat: the plastic cover has turned red, the cloth surround is soiled brown and the cow's coat is sweaty with the hair standing on end.

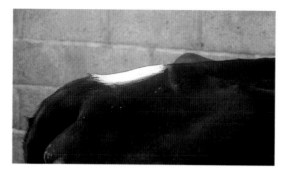

Plate 8.18. Tail paint can also be used for heat detection. When the cow is mounted, the paint cracks or is rubbed off altogether.

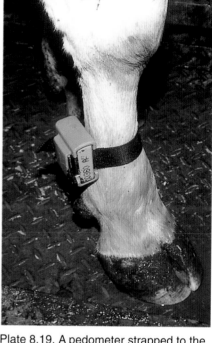

Plate 8.19. A pedometer strapped to the cow's leg measures her movements. A sensor at the entrance to the parlour leads to a computer printout (Figure 8.15) which gives the activity of the cow between milkings.

cow walks under a rail the ink in the inner tube is pushed to the back but cannot escape. If she is mounted by another cow, however, the weight and thrusting action of the mounting cow force the dye forwards, through the fine hole at the front of the tube and into the outer casing. The white opaque plastic then turns a brilliant red colour, as shown in Plate 8.17, indicating that the cow is on heat. False positives do occur, for example due to an oestrous cow mounting a Kamar cow when she is not in a position to escape. The plate probably shows a definite oestrus, however, because the sides of the Kamar are dirty and the hair on the cow's tail arch has been rubbed forwards.

Tail paint is used in a similar way. A thick layer of paint is applied as a band along the tail-head (Plate 8.18) so that it flattens the hairs of the coat which run backwards. The paint dries and hardens, but when the cow is mounted, it cracks up, or is rubbed off altogether. With the paint, therefore, you have to remember which cows were marked and then act as soon as the paint has gone, whereas the appearance of a bright red Kamar is much more obvious.

Pedometers, devices which are strapped to the cow's leg to register movement, are becoming more popular with the increasing computerisation of the milking parlour. An example is shown in Plate 8.19. As the cow enters the milking parlour she passes across a sensor which off-loads the information about her activity since the previous milking. This is then summarised in the printout shown in Figure 8.15. Day 0 is today's date, so cow 770 was bulling 3 days ago, when there was a big increase in pedometer activity (and also a reduction in yield), and 21 days ago).

With any device you must remember that it is only an *aid* to heat detection: you should consult your records to see if the cow is supposed to be on heat and then look carefully to see if she is showing any other behavioural signs or rub marks.

The other two heat detection aids worthy of note are closed-circuit television cameras, so that the cows can be watched from the comfort of your kitchen or living-room, and sniffer dogs. Apparently dogs can be trained to sniff out and identify cows on heat: perhaps they could also sort the bulling cows from the others and phone the AI!

## SYNCHRONISATION OF OESTRUS

As the words suggest, synchronisation of oestrus means that the oestrous cycle is manipulated so that all the cows or heifers in a group come bulling at the same time, and they can then all be inseminated on the

**COW 770**

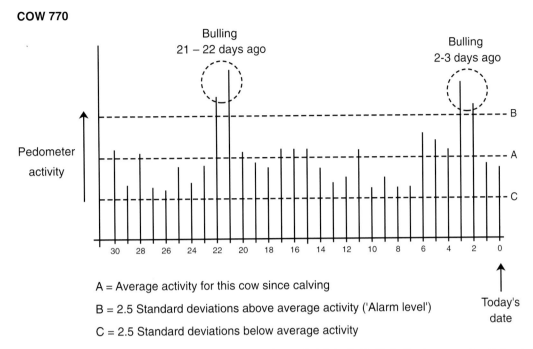

Figure 8.15. Heat detection using the pedometer shown in Plate 8.19. Note the increased activity at days −3 and −21.

same day. Synchronisation therefore removes the need for heat detection. It can be a very useful technique for heifers. If they are running outside, insemination on one day makes handling much easier, and batch calving can also be a big advantage. Using Holstein–Friesian semen means that an additional group of Holstein–Friesian heifer calves may also be available, and this is especially useful in an expanding herd. The two main products used in synchronisation are prostaglandin and progesterone releasing devices.

## Prostaglandin (PG)

Prostaglandin (PG) acts only if the cow is cycling normally and when she is between days 5 and 15 of her cycle. An injection of PG dissolves the corpus luteum, progesterone levels fall and the cow comes bulling 3 or 4 days later. The hormone sequence is shown in Figure 8.4. Unfortunately the period between administration of PG and oestrus is not precise. This is partly due to the variation in response caused by the presence or absence of mid cycle follicular waves. The use of GnRH 2 days after the prostaglandin injection, followed by AI on the third day, has been shown to improve the synchrony between prostaglandin injection, ovulation and AI and will give better conception rates.

Two injections of PG are needed to synchronise oestrus in a group of cows or heifers, the second being given 11 days after the first. The reasons for this are shown in Figure 8.16 and are as follows: At any one time the cows will be at varying stages of their cycle, from 0 to 21 days, so following the first injection only those at 5–15 days of their cycle will respond, to come bulling 3–4 days later.

The second injection for synchronisation is given 11 days after the first, and Figure 8.16 shows the various stages of the cycle which the cows will be spanning at that stage. Cows which were originally at 0 and 4 days will now be at 11 and 15 days of their cycle respectively. Cows which responded to the first injection came bulling in 3–4 days, so after 11 days they will be 7–8 days into their next cycle (11 − 3 = 8 days). The cows which were originally at 16 days did not respond to the first injection, but came bulling naturally 5 days later, so after 11 days they are 11 − 5 = 6 days into their next cycle. Similarly, those cows originally at 21 days will be 10 days into their next cycle. From this it can be seen that 11 days after the first injection, all of the cows in the group will be between 6 and 15 days of their cycle and are therefore sensitive to prostaglandin. Following the second injection they will all come bulling within 3 or 4 days and the group can be inseminated on both days.

An alternative is to give one insemination after 78–80 hours. Although this may result in a very small reduction (e.g. 3–4%) in conception rate, it is probably much less than the cost of an additional insemination.

The above describes the standard

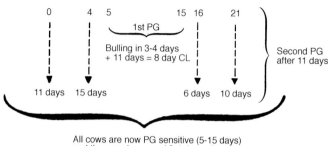

Figure 8.16. Prostaglandin synchronisation of heat.

way of using prostaglandin for synchronisation, but there are several alternatives. For example, in a group of randomly cycling heifers, at any one time half will be between days 5 and 15 of their cycle and therefore sensitive to prostaglandin. Consequently, if the whole group is injected on day 1, half will come bulling on days 4 and 5 and with careful heat detection they can be served. Continue serving on sight until day 11. All unserved animals can then be given a second injection. These animals should come on heat on days 14 and 15 and again can be served on sight, perhaps with the additional use of Kamars. It is best to discuss the system most suitable for your herd with your vet.

## Progesterone Releasing Devices (PRDs)

The various types of progesterone releasing devices (PRDs), their mode of action and their site of insertion (intravaginal or subcutaneous) were described on page 238. The cost of a PRD is approximately the same as two injections of prostaglandin (PG). The PRD is more difficult and therefore more expensive to administer; however, only one veterinary visit is required, since the herdsman normally removes the PRD, whereas two visits are required with prostaglandin. On a cost basis, therefore, the two treatments are approximately equal. Prostaglandins act only on cows which are already cycling, whereas a PRD will also stimulate ovarian activity and may cure any cysts present.

Probably the best synchronisation is achieved by a combination of PG and PRD, that is by injecting PG one day before the PRD is removed. Remove the PRD, wait one day and serve the following day. Intravaginal PRDs may cause a white, foul-smelling discharge in a proportion of animals. This is of vaginal and not uterine origin, and it is due to irritation by the PRD. It does not seem to have any effect on conception rate even though it looks rather unpleasant, and in most cases the discharge disappears a few days after the PRD has been removed. Occasional animals develop a severe vaginitis and the PRD has to be removed early.

## Effective Synchronisation

Whichever system is used, there will be a small proportion of animals which fail to synchronise. The problem is worse with cows, because their normal cycle lengths are much more variable. Only 90% of normal cows have cycle lengths of 18–24 days. In other words, 10% of quite normal cows have cycles of less than 18, or more than 24 days. The enthusiastic reader might like to substitute these cycle lengths for those in Figure 8.16 and see for himself how a proportion will then fail to synchronise! If you are *sure* that a cow is standing to be mounted 1 or 2 days after she has already received a double AI, then she *must* be inseminated for the third time, because she clearly failed to respond to the synchronisation process.

Synchronisation of oestrus has provided a useful opportunity to study some of the factors affecting conception rate. Very good results are possible, but to ensure good fertilisation and implantation, it is essential to ensure that the animals are on a rising plane of nutrition from 4 weeks before insemination, until 3 weeks after. Grazing heifers, or those on hay or silage, should be supplemented with 1.5–2 kg of barley or other cereals, and early lactation feeding of dairy cows needs to be such that weight loss over this period is minimised. Stress should definitely be avoided, so the idea of inseminating the heifers when

Table 8.4. Comparing the theoretical performance of normal observation and synchronisation in 100 cows at the start of the service period.

| | Heat detection rate (%) | Conception rate (%) | Cows pregnant after 3 weeks |
|---|---|---|---|
| Observation and AI | | | |
| Good heat detection | 80 | 60 | 48 |
| Poor heat detection | 50 | 60 | 30 |
| Synchronisation and AI | 95 | 55 | 52 |

they are being handled for worming or tuberculin testing is definitely not on; neither should they have their ration suddenly changed (for example, with housing) part way through the treatment.

When synchronisation was first introduced, a few people expected it to be a cure-all; insufficient attention was paid to husbandry, poor results were obtained and the technique fell out of favour. Because of the problems of heat detection, however, it can be an excellent way of starting the service period to get good batch calving, and trials have shown that it is cost-effective to do this. Table 8.4 shows the theoretical performance of 100 cows with good heat detection (80%) and conception (60%) rates. Even then, only 48 cows (100 x 0.8 x 0.6) would be pregnant at the end of 3 weeks. If synchronisation was used, there may be a small proportion of cows which fail to respond (say 5%) and conception rates may fall slightly (again, say 5%) but the overall performance at the end of 3 weeks is significantly better. If heat detection was poor (say 50%), then Table 8.4 shows that the benefits of synchronisation are considerably greater. In fact if heat detection was poor, conception rates would also be poorer for the reasons given on page 264, and so even fewer than 30 cows would be pregnant after 3 weeks.

*Use of synchronisation in heifers*
One of the most important aspects of maintaining a tight calving pattern is to introduce heifers into the herd at the start of the calving period. With the almost unavoidable problems of early lactation weight loss, it is only too easy to let cows 'slip' around the year a few weeks, and it is therefore logical to introduce heifers into the herd in a tight batch as early as possible. Oestrous synchronisation helps to achieve this. In addition, if Holstein–Friesian semen is used, the heifers will produce a valuable extra crop of heifer calves. These calves are being born at the very start of the calving season so that when they are introduced into the herd 2 years later they will be well grown, better able to compete with the cows and will probably get back in calf faster in their first lactation. Although calves from heifers may be smaller, there is good evidence to suggest that most of the size difference is made up during rearing. One survey showed that heifers reared from heifers gave more milk than heifers reared from cows:

| *Average first lactation of* | *Litres* |
|---|---|
| heifers from heifers | 4800 |
| heifers from first calvers | 4500 |
| heifers from second calvers | 4400 |

These yields are very low if compared to the modern Holstein–Friesian heifer, but the figures serve to emphasise the point. The difference is considerably more than would be expected from the normal rate of genetic improvement, although the reason is unknown.

Provided the bull is carefully selected and the heifers are well grown (see Chapter 5), there are no more problems calving heifers at 2 years than when they are older. In fact, almost the reverse is true in that it is the bigger heifer which can attain a higher forage intake that is more likely to get overfat and

| | Age at Calving 2 years old | 3 years old | 3+ years old |
|---|---|---|---|
| % calving problems | 16 | 13 | 22 |
| % calf mortality | 12 | 12 | 28 |
| % conception to first service | 69 | 55 | – |
| % *not* conceiving | 5.5 | 11.4 | – |
| **Lifetime production** number of lactations (i.e. average life in a herd) | 4.00 | 3.84 | 3.78 |
| total milk production (litres) | 18,708 | 17,927 | 17,621 |

Adapted from Esslemont, Baille and Cooper, *Fertility Management in Dairy Cattle.*

Table 8.5. Heifers calving at 3 years old have more calving problems, are more difficult to get back in calf in their first lactation and have an overall lower lifetime production than 2-year-old calvers.

produce an oversized calf, especially if she is fed concentrates pre calving in addition to liberal intakes of grass. Table 8.5 shows that not only does the older heifer have more calving problems, but she also has poorer subsequent fertility and an overall lower lifetime production than a heifer calving at 2 years old. If proven bulls are used, there is also a good argument that obtaining an additional crop of Holstein–Friesian heifer calves from heifers is increasing the rate of genetic selection by one generation. However, as the heritability of milk production is only 45%, it may be more profitable always to introduce well-grown heifers into the herd at the start of the calving season rather than trying to get a Holstein–Friesian calf from a late calver just because she is a high yielder.

## CONCEPTION RATES

So far we have dealt with ovarian cycles and the importance of heat detection. Having served our cow, we hope that she will become pregnant. The proportion of cows which hold to service is known as the conception rate. This may be expressed as the conception rate to first service, the conception rate to all services, or inversely as the number of services per conception. A very good figure would be 65% conception to first service, although 55% is probably average for the national herd and figures of 40% or less are by no means uncommon. The past 10–15 years have seen a fall in conception rates worldwide.

| 100 eggs shed | Losses |
|---|---|
| 95 fertilised ova | 5 fertilisation failure |
| 70 survive to 21 days | 25 early embryonic mortality |
| 60 survive to 45 days | 10 implantation failure/ embryonic mortality |
| 55 cows calve | 5 abortions/deaths/culls |
| **Total calvings 55** | **Total losses 45** |

Table 8.6. The fate of 100 bovine eggs in a herd with good fertility.

These are conception rates, however, and they will be significantly higher than final calving rates. Research has shown that if you take 100 cows a few days after insemination, almost 95% of the eggs shed will have been fertilised and are developing as embryos, but many of these die in the early stages so that by 21 days the number of living embryos has fallen to 70%; that is, 25% have been lost already, and 25% of the cows will return to service. By the stage of manual pregnancy testing at about 45 days, a further 10% of embryos will have been lost partly due to failure of implantation at 30–35 days, and only 60% of the cows are likely to be detectably pregnant to the first service. Allowing a 5% loss from abortion culls and deaths this gives an eventual calving rate of 55%. The stages are shown in Table 8.6. In poor fertility herds losses will be very much higher than this.

## CAUSES OF LOW CONCEPTION RATES

Causes of poor conception rates will be discussed under the following headings:

  Poor embryo recognition
  Serving too soon after calving
  Poor heat detection
  Timing of insemination
  Endometritis
  Fatty liver
  Genital and other infections
  Stress
  Poor handling facilities
  Operator technique
  Semen quality
  Nutrition

### Poor Embryo Recognition

The cause of this high rate of early embryonic loss described in the preceding section has been the subject of much speculation and research. It would appear that at least part of the problem is that although conception has occurred, the cow fails to *realise* that she is pregnant. In such a case, a cascade of hormonal changes is then put into place which starts the next cycle – and a viable embryo is eliminated. The hormonal changes are described in Figures 8.4 and 8.5, which should be used in conjunction with this section. From approximately 12 days of pregnancy onwards, before the placenta attaches to the wall of the uterus, the embryo produces a protein known as bovine trophoblastin (bTb). This acts as a signal, telling the cow she is pregnant. If, for some reason, the signal is not received by the cow, then at day 16–18 the uterus produces prostaglandin, the corpus luteum is dissolved and the next cycle begins.

Possible reasons why the signal is not received include:

● a 'weak' signal from the embryo, caused by low bTb production
● the uterus is not in a receptive state and does not 'hear' the signal

Embryos which are small and underdeveloped certainly produce poorer signals. This has been clearly demonstrated by embryo transfer work: the larger the embryo (at a fixed age), the better the conception rate. Small embryos could result from a poor uterine environment, poor timing of AI (due to aging of the semen or ova before fertilisation occurred) and poor semen storage.

Some embryos are genetically non-viable. In other words, if these embryos were to develop into a full-term calf, the calf would be so badly deformed that it could not live a normal existence. Early embryonic mortality is therefore a method of eliminating such calves in the early stages and this must be an advantage to the survival of the species. Older cows have a higher rate of genetic abnormalities and embryonic mortality than heifers. It is worth comparing this with women, where there is an increased incidence of certain genetic birth defects with age, and where up to 30% of miscarriages are thought to be due to chromosomal abnormalities.

Failure of the uterus to receive or react to the signal is a more common cause of embryo loss. Once again this could be due to any one of a number of factors, some of which are discussed in more detail later in the chapter. Examples include:

- serving the cow too soon after calving, before the uterus has recovered from the previous pregnancy and therefore before it is in a receptive state
- uterine infections which can produce inflammation of the wall of the uterus, making it less receptive to the embryo signal
- stress

Stress for dairy cows is a difficult area to define. It will encompass many aspects of feeding, management, disease and housing, which are discussed in more detail on page 268. In relation to embryo recognition, stress can be compared to extraneous 'noise', so that the cow is unable to 'hear' the very faint signal produced by the embryo. A happy and contented cow, which is sitting quietly, is much more likely to be able to 'hear' a faint signal than an animal which is concurrently receiving many other sensory inputs from pain, hunger, fear or discomfort. Practical causes of poor conception rates are given in the following section. Some will have a direct influence on maternal embryo recognition and have been mentioned already.

Table 8.7. A theoretical comparison of the overall calving to conception (C–C) interval of 100 cows where serving started at 50 days after calving and achieved a 60% conception rate (top group), with another 100 cows served from 34 days onwards and achieving only a 40% conception rate.

| | No. cows served | No. cows conceiving | Mean C–C interval | No. cows not pregnant |
|---|---|---|---|---|
| 1st service at 50 days | 100 | 60 | 60 | 40 |
| 2nd service | 40 | 24 | 81 | 16 |
| 3rd service | 16 | 10 | 102 | 6 |
| 4th service | 6 | 4 | 123 | 2 |
| 5th service | 2 | 1 | 144 | 1* |

**Mean C–C** 72.7 days (= 353.7 days CI)

| | | | | |
|---|---|---|---|---|
| 1st service at 34 days | 100 | 40 | 44 | 60 |
| 2nd service | 60 | 24 | 65 | 36 |
| 3rd service | 36 | 14 | 86 | 22 |
| 4th service | 22 | 9 | 107 | 13 |
| 5th service | 13 | 5 | 128 | 8 |
| 6th service | 8 | 3 | 149 | 5 |
| 7th service | 5 | 2 | 170 | 3 |
| 8th service | 3 | 1 | 191 | 2* |

**Mean C–C** 72.3 days (= 353.3 days CI)

* These cows would be culled as infertile.

Although the mean calving intervals (CIs) are almost identical, the first group is the preferred situation because its spread of calvings for the next year will be much tighter and there are far fewer services per conception (1.7 compared with 2.5 for the second group).

## Serving Too Soon after Calving

If cows are served too soon after calving, conception rates will be lower. This is thought to be due to the uterus not having settled down properly after the previous pregnancy and not being ready to accept the embryo for implantation. Figure 8.17 shows that you need to delay service until 70 days post calving in order to achieve the best conception rates, and if you serve at 35–40 days, conception rates may fall to 40%. As an approximate rule of thumb, the conception rate achieved is likely to be numerically equal to the number of days from calving to service. For example:

*Conception rate of cows served after*

    20 days = 20%
    30 days = 30%
    40 days = 40%
    50 days = 50%
    60 days = 60%

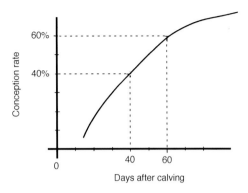

Figure 8.17. Conception rate varies with the interval from calving to first service.

It is, of course, no use waiting until 100 days and hoping for 100%!

Under average farm conditions I would recommend that cows are served after 50 days. The overall measure of fertility is the average period from calving to conception, since calving to conception plus gestation length (281 days) gives the calving interval (CI), and the gestation length is constant.

Table 8.7 shows that if you begin with 100 cows you get almost the same overall calving to conception (C–C) interval by starting the service period at 34 days and accepting only a 40% conception rate, as you do by waiting until 50 days post calving to get a 60%+ conception rate. Assuming that it takes 21 days to serve all the cows in a group, if the serving of 100 cows is started at 34 days post calving, then the average calving to first service interval (and calving to conception interval for those which hold to service) will be 44 days. Similarly, if serving is started at 50 days post calving, then the average calving to first service interval will be 60 days (viz 50 + (21 divided by 2) = 60).

Table 8.7 assumes that the conception rate remains constant throughout the service period in both groups and that heat detection efficiency is 100%. However, if the 40% conception rate is due entirely to serving too soon after calving, then by the second service the conception rate may have risen towards 60% and the figures will not be strictly accurate. The table also shows that one normal cow would need 5 services starting at 50 days post calving, whereas 3 cows would need 8 services starting at 34 days. Although the calving to conception intervals are very similar, the 50 day starting point is the preferred result, because it will give a tighter calving pattern the following year, there will be fewer culls and there will be fewer insemination fees. For example 1.7 inseminations were required for each conception in the first group, but this rose to 2.5 services per conception by starting at 34 days. If your herd already has a poor conception rate, however, you may be forced to start serving at less than 50 days, although there is then a risk that this may depress conception rates even further. Similar data is shown in Table 8.8. Although conception rates (services per conception) were poorer at 40–60 days, days open (calving to conception) were better.

There is a danger of being *too* concerned about conception rates. If you are doing your own AI and using inexpensive semen, then the important thing is to get the cow pregnant, so if you suspect that the cow is bulling, she is best served – even if it means that she is served again 2 days later when her true heat occurs. The exception to this rule comes when cows have been served already, since AI could then abort an existing pregnancy. This is discussed in the next section.

The *submission rate* is the proportion of cows eligible for service – namely those within the service period window – which are actually served. Submission rates are an important measure of fertility and often used in the analysis of data from problem herds.

Table 8.8. Influence of interval from calving to first service on reproductive traits of Holstein cows.

| | Days from calving to first insemination | | | | | |
|---|---|---|---|---|---|---|
| Reproductive trait | <40 | 41–60 | 61–80 | 81–100 | 101–120 | >120 |
| Con. rate 1st serv. | 47 | 45 | 60 | 56 | 63 | 69 |
| Services/conception | 2.1 | 1.9 | 1.7 | 1.6 | 1.6 | 1.4 |
| Days open | 78 | 87 | 97 | 115 | 126 | 154 |

From Britt (1977), *J. Dairy Sci.* 60 1345.

## Poor Heat Detection

The way in which poor heat detection affects fertility was explained in detail in the milk progesterone section on page 245.

On average, 10–15% of cows presented for AI are not on heat. It is interesting that data gives similar figures from the UK and from North America. Clearly the conception rate of these cows is zero. But even worse: if they are presented as a 'repeat' service, an incorrect insemination may abort an existing pregnancy. Abortion is less common if the incorrect AI is at 3 weeks and consequently some cows calve 3 weeks early, viz to the earlier service date. However, at 6 or 9 weeks or later, the larger placenta has expanded into the body of the uterus and incorrect insemination is much more likely to cause abortion.

The problem is compounded by the fact that about 5% of cows show standing heat when they *are pregnant* and it is impossible for the herdsman to know whether or not a bulling cow is pregnant. Unless he has already had her checked for pregnancy, he is almost certain to have her inseminated, thus running the risk of aborting an established foetus. If you are unsure whether a cow is bulling or not, the following options are open to you:

If heat detection is poor,

- many cows are not seen bulling and therefore are not served. Heat detection efficiency and submission rates are then both low

- a higher proportion of cows presented for AI will not be on heat, so heat detection accuracy influences conception rates

- Ask your vet to examine her for pregnancy.
- Carry out an on-farm milk progesterone test. A low progesterone means that the cow is in oestrus.
- Let the bull serve the cow. If she is pregnant, natural service will do no harm.
- Use AI, but inseminate into the cervix only. If she *is* in oestrus, there may be a 5–10% decreased chance of conception, but if she is not in oestrus, intracervical insemination will not abort an existing pregnancy.

## Timing of Insemination

If you see a cow bulling this morning, should she be inseminated today or tomorrow? I would recommend that the cow is inseminated on the *same* day as she is seen on heat and not the following day. We have already noted that standing heat is a very variable period, lasting from 3 to 30 hours. There is a sharp rise in LH release from the pituitary gland 1–2 hours *before* the onset of true standing heat and ovulation seems to occur approximately

30 hours later, that is 30 hours *after* the LH surge, irrespective of how long heat lasts. For most cows ovulation occurs 6–18 hours *after* the end of standing heat. The optimum service time is towards the end of standing heat, which is 12–24 hours pre ovulation and 12–18 hours after the LH surge. To predict the timing of ovulation, it is therefore much more important to know when heat starts than when it ends. There are two other important factors to consider in the timing of insemination:

- Once shed, the egg remains viable for only 6–8 hours, whereas semen can survive in the uterus for up to 36 hours.
- Once in the uterus, semen has to undergo a process of changes known as *capacitation* before it is ready to fertilise the egg. This takes 4–6 hours. The semen also has to swim from the cervix along the uterus to the end of the oviduct to fertilise the egg.

For these two reasons it is better to have the sperm ready and waiting for the egg from ovulation.

When you see a cow standing to be mounted, you may not have any idea of whether she is just starting heat or just finishing, or how long heat will last. The only sure way is to have her inseminated, so that the semen is ready and waiting for ovulation to occur. This is particularly important if you are using an inseminator service which only calls once every 24 hours and you cannot specify the time of day. Also, in some areas you cannot call after 10 am for AI service on the same day.

For those doing DIY AI, the best advice would be to serve 12 hours after heat is first seen; that is the 'am–pm' method, whereby cows seen in the morning are inseminated in the afternoon and vice versa. On 24 hour inseminator service, if a cow served in the morning is still standing very late at night, or particularly the following morning, then she should be served again. The following gives an example of two possible scenarios. Let us assume that

- Two cows were seen bulling at 8.00 am one morning (day 1).
- One cow (ST) was just starting her heat and the other (E) just ending.
- Both cows were standing to be mounted for the average heat period of 15 hours.
- Ovulation for both cows occurred 24 hours after the onset of heat (viz approximately 26 hours after the pre ovulatory LH surge).
- They must be served by an AI inseminator at 10.00 am on either day 1 or day 2.
- The egg lasts for only 6 hours after ovulation, semen for 36 hours after insemination.

|  | Cow ST (heat starting) | Cow E (heat ending) |
|---|---|---|
| Heat started at | 8.00 am day 1 | 5.00 pm day 0 |
| Ovulation | 8.00 am day 2 | 5.00 pm day 1[1] |
| Egg dead by | 2.00 pm on day 2 | 11.00 pm day 1 |
| AI at 10 am on |  |  |
| day 1 | OK | OK |
| day 2 | OK[2] | too late |

1 Cow E had been on heat for 15 hours at 8.00 am on day 1, which means that her heat started at 5.00 pm on day zero and ovulation therefore occurred 24 hours later at 5.00 pm on day 1 (i.e. 9 hours after she was first seen on heat).

2 Fertility here may not be very good because the semen will only just have time to undergo capacitation. (Insemination at 10.00 am and capacitation by 2.00 pm, just as the egg is dying.)

This example shows how many complex factors have to be considered when trying to decide a simple issue like the timing of AI. If cow E had a heat period for longer than 15 hours, then ovulation and egg death would have occurred even sooner. A further complicating factor is that you cannot specify the time of day when the inseminator will call. For both cows the timing of AI on day 1 would make no difference. However, if cow ST was inseminated at 2.00 pm on day 2 instead of 10.00 am, this would also be too late. The bull only serves a cow when she will stand to be mounted and the advice given above, namely to inseminate a cow during or soon after standing heat, is simply trying to mimic nature.

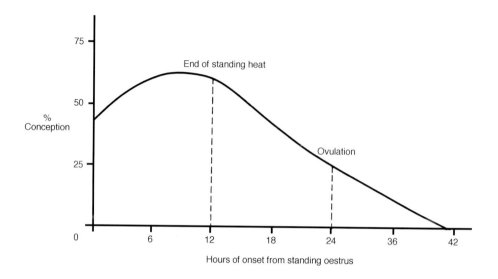

Figure 8.18. The effect of timing of insemination on conception rates. This cow was in standing oestrus for 12 hours and ovulated 12 hours later.

Figure 8.18 also shows how poor timing of insemination leads to reduced conception rates. Although cows served early or late in oestrus may conceive, their chances of doing so are much less, and the best conception rates are obtained by serving a cow when she is actually in standing heat. Figure 8.18 shows that there is a greater reduction in conception rate by serving too late rather than too early.

## Endometritis

Sometimes also known as 'the whites' or 'dirty' cows, this is an infection of the inner wall of the uterus (endo- = inside; -metr- = uterus; -itis = inflammation of). When a cow is on heat the cervix opens and the uterus contracts, expelling the bulling string, so if there is any discharge present, this is the time when it is most likely to be seen. In more severe cases there may be a continual discharge, visible as white mucoid globules on the tail or at the vulva (Plate 8.20). Sometimes the uterus is full of pus but no discharge is produced. This is called a *pyometra*.

Prostaglandin is the treatment normally used for pyometra. It brings the cow into oestrus, thus emptying the uterus. At the same time the increased levels of circulating oestrogen associ-

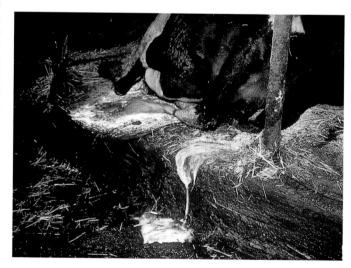

Plate 8.20. Endometritis ('the whites') can be seen as a vaginal discharge from cows lying in the cubicles.

ated with oestrus boost the activity of the bacterial-fighting cells which are lining the uterus and this prompts a more rapid 'cleaning up' process. Sometimes injections of oestrogen (oestradiol) are used to produce a similar effect.

One study showed that if all cows were injected with prostaglandin at about 2 weeks after calving, their subsequent conception rates would be improved. This is not often carried out as a routine in the UK, although if you

Causes of endometritis include

- retained placenta
- dirty calving boxes
- unhygienic, premature assistance with calving
- difficult calvings
- calves born dead
- overfat cows at calving (fatty liver)
- poor bodily condition at calving, or excessive weight loss post calving

had a problem it could be an option which your vet might suggest. Other options include the use of intrauterine pessaries or oxytocin injections 12–24 hours after calving. There can be no doubt that cows 'dirty' with endometritis subsequently have a much reduced fertility. Another survey monitored 180 endometritis cases from 24 farms and found that compared with 'clean' cows in the herd, 'dirty' cows

- had a lower first service conception rate (33% vs 53%)
- needed more services per conception (2.6 vs 1.8)
- overall took 20 days longer to get back in calf. At a cost of £3.40 per cow per day, this represents an average loss of £68.00 per cow, in addition to the cost of treatment!

It was also found that cows receiving their first treatment reasonably soon after calving had better fertility than those treated later. This is shown in Table 8.9, where early treatment of endometritis cases improved the calving to conception interval by 21 days (107 days versus 128 days), a considerable economic benefit. Prompt and effective treatment is therefore essential and I would suggest that cows are examined at between 14 and 28 days after calving. Unless they are obviously 'dirty', cows are best left for the first 2 weeks after calving before checking, because many early discharges will clean up spontaneously without treatment.

There is a range of factors which can lead to uterine infections and a high incidence of endometritis. One of the most common is retained placenta, particularly if it is not treated correctly. (Retained placenta, its causes and treatment are described in Chapter 5.) Not all cows with retained placenta subsequently develop endometritis, however, and it is only those cows with endometritis which are difficult to get back in calf. Retained placenta on its own may have relatively little adverse effect. Endometritis may also be associated with some of the many factors which lead to an increased incidence of retained placenta, namely overfat cows, excessive interference, twins, mineral or trace element imbalances, even though the incidence of retained placenta is normal.

Clean calving boxes are very important. During normal birth, uterine contractions push the calf's legs and nose part way through the vulva. When the cow then relaxes, the calf falls back into the abdomen – and of course draws air back in with it. If the bedding is very dirty, then the air will be heavily contaminated with bacteria, these will pass into the uterus and endometritis may develop.

Some authorities are so convinced of the importance of hygiene that they even recommend washing the hind quarters of a cow before calving

| Timing of first treatment | Number of cows | Calving to conception (days) | Services per conception |
|---|---|---|---|
| **EARLY** (less than 28 days after calving) | 74 | 107 | 3.22 |
| **LATE** (more than 56 days) | 44 | 128 | 3.21 |

From Anderson (1984).

Table 8.9. Endometritis is known to lead to poor fertility, but the effect is even worse if treatment is delayed.

and wrapping a bandage round her tail to prevent aspiration of infection during the birth process. Similarly, if you are assisting with a calving, *make sure that you are clean*. Wash your arms and the cow's vulva with soap and water before examining her, and if (or when!) faeces fall onto your arm, make sure you wash them off before going back into the uterus. Clean calving ropes are obviously essential.

Even the choice of bull has an effect. A large bull giving difficult calvings will lead to a higher incidence of endometritis. One of the greatest risk factors for endometritis is in fact a stillborn calf. Any factor leading to stillborn calves (for example, overfat cows, poor sire selection, excessive interference) increases the risk of endometritis. Causes of stillbirths are discussed later in this chapter.

Underfeeding and excessive weight loss in early lactation can lead to increased endometritis, especially in heifers. Presumably this is because the stress of underfeeding decreases their resistance to infection and, in addition, ovarian oestrous cycles which would naturally clear up the endometritis fail to start.

In summary, inadequately treated endometritis leads to poor conception rates and can be caused by a range of factors.

## Fatty Liver

This is described in Chapter 6. Cows with fatty liver have low albumin and glucose levels in their blood and their conception rates will be reduced. They are also more susceptible to retained placenta, uterine infections and cystic ovaries, and this may have a secondary effect on conception rate, as shown in Table 6.2.

## Genital and Other Infections

Poor conception rates caused by specific genital infections with such organisms as *Brucella abortus*, *Trichomonas foetus* and *Campylobacter* (previously known as *Vibrio*) are fortunately less common in Britain nowadays. However, as bulls are being used more often in dairy herds, particularly as 'sweepers' at the end of the service period, the possibility of campylobacteriosis should not be overlooked. Your vet will need to take special samples of vaginal mucus or washings from the bull's prepuce to check for this organism.

Leptospirosis, BVD, IBR and *Neospora* are all infections which can cause poor conception rates. The effects of leptospirosis and BVD are particularly pronounced and are dealt with elsewhere in this book.

## Stress

Social stress in cows is an interesting condition but as it is rather difficult to define, a few examples are needed. It is quite easy for a cow introduced into a small herd of 40–50 others to come into contact with each one of them and soon establish her own position in the 'pecking order'. The chances of getting to know 250–300 cows over a few days is much less, however, and the situation becomes almost impossible if cows are being taken in and out of the herd all the time. In this situation our cow will be continually meeting new faces and possibly having to fight to establish her superiority (or otherwise) to them. This is a clear example of stress, and it is becoming increasingly apparent that if group size goes above 100 cows or if group composition is constantly changing, then the cows will be adversely affected.

Unless food is freely available, group feeding can be a high stress situation. For example, if cows are given a mid day feed there may be a 200% variation in individual food intake, and this can be even greater if trough space is inadequate.

Heifers probably suffer most from stress. They are regularly reared in a separate group, having only to compete with animals of their own age and size. After they calve, their world almost falls apart. There will be discomfort around the perineum (vulva and vagina) from calving and perhaps soreness due to an enlarged or oedematous udder. They have been transferred into a large and strange group of much bigger and aggressive animals, namely the main dairy herd. They have often come from soft ground (pasture or straw yards) onto a hard and slippery floor (concrete). They are made to stand for long periods of time, waiting to be milked, or waiting for their turn to feed. The diet will have changed dramatically and if access to forage is poor, for example, because trough space or access to self-feed silage is inadequate, they may well develop acidosis from eating excessive concentrate in the parlour. The buildings are often overcrowded. There may be no loafing area, nowhere to get adequate exercise and so they stand almost motionless on hard concrete. They may have never seen cubicles before, so lying times are reduced and this causes intense laminitis/coriosis and later lameness. Even when they do learn to use the cubicles, the shed may have passageways with blind endings and no escape routes, so that the heifers feel too intimidated to enter. In a few instances the herdsman himself (and his dog?!) may increase their sense of alarm by rough handling, rushing them when walking on rough or slippery concrete, driving them with tractors or ATV bikes and packing them tightly into the collecting yard for milking.

The net result of all this stress is that lameness (especially), mastitis, displaced abomasum and other diseases become more common, compounding the stress further in individually affected animals.

Can we be surprised that heifers sometimes do not perform well? Yields are certainly better if they are kept in separate heifer groups for their first lactation, which must be an indication of reduced stress.

I have obviously painted the worst possible scenario in order to emphasise the point, but it serves to demonstrate the many potential areas for improvement. Stress reduces fertility by increasing endometritis, delaying the onset of ovarian cycles, increasing embryo mortality and reducing conception rates. It also increases the animal's susceptibility to disease and reduces its milk production.

## Poor Handling Facilities

A stress factor which can affect both cow and operator is poor handling facilities. If the inseminator has to chase your cow around the yard and then stand her in the front of a herringbone parlour where she can wriggle from side to side, you cannot expect him to do a perfect job. The cow should be well restrained, ready and waiting for him and preferably left with an adequate supply of food and water. It is not an easy task to pass the insemination catheter through the cervix and into the uterus. The cow needs to be on the same level as the inseminator and restrained so that she cannot move forwards or sideways. If the cow is excessively excited and stressed, this may upset her hormonal mechanisms so that ovulation or fertilisation may fail to occur anyway.

## Operator Technique

It is possible that even the best trained inseminator can develop faulty techniques, leading to reduced conception rates. For this reason and for on-farm inseminators especially, it is important to consider

● regularly attending retraining sessions
● monitoring performance, especially if it is possible to compare your own performance with other inseminators working in the same herd

## Semen Quality

Poor-quality semen can originate from poor semen storage (for example, a flask low in liquid nitrogen), poor thawing techniques (water too hot), poor handling (semen allowed to cool excessively prior to insemination) or a bull with suboptimal fertility. The latter could be temporary, for example, following an illness, or it may be that the bull has inherently poor fertility. Any of these factors will obviously affect conception rates.

## Nutrition

Eating is probably the most important activity of the dairy cow, because without food she cannot milk or grow. Many aspects of feeding can have an effect on fertility and some have been mentioned already, for example:

● Inadequate feeding space can cause stress and lead to an increased incidence of early embryonic mortality, as well as causing difficulties with heat detection.
● General underfeeding and weight loss in early lactation may be associated with uterine infections.

- An energy deficit in overfat cows immediately after calving may lead to fatty liver syndrome.
- Excess calcium or inadequate magnesium intakes during the dry period can cause an increased incidence of milk fever and this in turn may lead to more endometritis and reduced conception rates.
- Acidosis caused by a forage:concentrate imbalance can lead to laminitis and subsequent lameness, and lame cows are more difficult to detect on heat.

Earlier in this chapter we saw that the physical and hormonal changes in the ovary associated with oestrus are extremely complex. The hormonal balance needed to maintain pregnancy is equally as intricate. It is likely that minerals and trace elements affect only minute aspects of these events and so it would therefore be illogical, if not naive, to expect nutrition to have a precise and consistent effect on overall fertility. The exact relationships have yet to be established and my own approach to a herd fertility problem is to examine the diet and to correct as many of the abnormalities as possible. This may seem rather unscientific, but fertility control is a dynamic process. At any one time it is influenced by a wide variety of factors and if we can help the cow to overcome some of her nutritional imbalances, then she may well cope with the remainder and the herd can once more return to reasonable fertility. These are general comments. There are certain aspects of nutrition which are more positively correlated with conception rate, however, and which need to be discussed in a little more detail.

> Effects of nutrition on fertility
>
> - direct: inadequate energy balance may depress conception rates
> - indirect: adverse nutrition increases the incidence of disease, and the disease has an adverse effect on fertility. Examples include lameness, fatty liver and milk fever
> - specific: deficiency of a single trace element or vitamin may adversely affect fertility

*Energy balance*

It was once well accepted that conception rates improve if cows and heifers are served on a rising plane of nutrition. This is very difficult to achieve in early lactation. Figure 8.19 shows how milk yield reaches a peak well before the cow achieves her maximum appetite capacity and so some weight loss is bound to occur. The problem is more acute with first-calved heifers which not only have to compete with older cows for food, but also need an additional allowance for growth. This occurs at a time when they are changing their front teeth (Plate 13.1), making eating even more difficult. If nutrition is adequate, weight loss may have stopped by the time the cow is ready to be served and there may even be some weight gain. This is especially true by the second or third service if the cow repeats.

These traditional views have become modified following the introduction of flat-rate feeding and from what has become an almost classic experiment by Ducker. Using 100 heifers, he divided them into two groups which were fed high or low both before and after calving. He found that heifers which were fed at a high level in order to gain weight at the time of service had a reduced fertility, whilst those losing weight got back into calf quite well. The higher-fed heifers had higher yields and this depressed fertility. This is almost certainly why herds practising flat-rate,

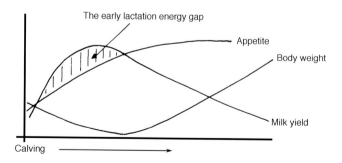

Figure 8.19. In early lactation milk yield peaks before a cow reaches her maximum dry matter intake. The energy gap leads to weight loss.

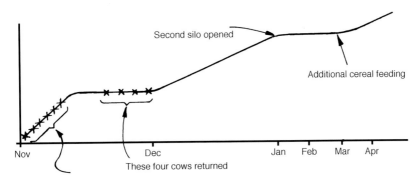

Figure 8.20. A Cu-sum graph of conception rate.

lower concentrate feeding do so well. It produces a much flatter lactation curve and, as changes in body-weight are by no means as extreme, fertility seems to be better. This is only an observation, however, and I know of no trial work producing any conclusive proof. It is likely that the most important factor is to avoid any extremes of weight change.

Energy balance can be measured in a variety of ways. Conventionally the quantity and quality of the food being eaten are compared with the cow's requirements for milk production and a diet balance sheet is prepared. Secondary checks are always worthwhile, however, and measurements such as bodyweight loss, body condition score, the bulk milk protein content and betahydroxy butyrate and blood glucose levels in the metabolic profile test (see Chapter 6) will all help in the assessment of energy status. Energy balance may affect those cows in a herd which were being served when there was just a short-term problem.

Figure 8.20 is a Cu-sum graph of conception rate. The cows are arranged in order of service date along the horizontal axis, the bottom of the graph. Starting from zero in November, if a cow conceives the plot moves up one square. If the next cow does not conceive, the plot moves along one square, but remains horizontal. In some systems Cu-sums are arranged so that conception moves up one square and failure moves down one square. A horizontal plot then denotes a 50% conception rate. In Figure 8.20 a line with a 45° slope represents a 100% conception rate. The distance for November and December is much greater than for February and March, because far more cows were served in the first 2 months. The overall graph shows a serious fall in conception rate for cows served during late January and early February. This was because when the second clamp was opened, the silage was much poorer and there was an overall fall in energy intake. Additional cereal feeding introduced in late February improved the conception rate of the cows served in March and April.

*Protein balance*
There is increasing evidence that high protein diets (often fed to boost yields) lead to depressed conception rates. This is particularly the case with high levels of rumen degradable protein (RDP) such as urea and lush autumn grazing, and also when there is a concurrent energy deficit. Diets high in UDP (undegradable or rumen by-pass protein) do not appear to have the same deleterious effect. As overall dietary protein intakes have increased over the past ten years, this could be one reason why conception rates have been falling.

*Minerals and trace elements*
Dairy farmers spend millions of pounds each year on mineral and trace element supplements, with phosphorus probably coming top of the list. Specific and consistent associations between minerals and fertility are virtually impossible to prove. We have already seen the massive range of other non-nutritional factors which can affect fertility and which can confuse the results of feeding trials. Deficiencies of copper, manganese, cobalt, iodine, phosphorus and selenium have all been associated with poor conception rates and the calcium-to-phosphorus ratio in the diet is also said to be important. Details of the levels required and of the effects of deficiencies and excesses are given in Chapter 12.

Deficiency of vitamin A impairs fertility, and several workers have shown a relationship between B-carotene (a vitamin A precursor) and conception rates. The position with regard to vitamin E and selenium is less clear. Deficiency in rats causes sterility, but no relationship has ever been *proven* in dairy cows. If your herd has an inadequate vitamin E status, however, it is most sensible to provide additional supplementation. There is some evidence that inadequate vitamin E/selenium status leads to increased placental retention and endometritis, and endometritis definitely affects subsequent fertility.

## THE REPEAT BREEDER COW

Over the years a good deal of effort has been expended in investigating the repeat breeder cow, that is the cow which has been served 5, 6 or even 7 times and continues to return to service every 21 days. However, Table 8.7 shows that in a 100 cow herd with a good conception rate (60%), you would expect 2 cows to need 5 services before they conceived, whereas in a herd with a poor conception rate (40%) 13 'normal' cows may need 5 services or more before conceiving. Many of the repeat breeder cows are therefore simply normal animals which, by chance, have not conceived. Having said this however, there will be a proportion of repeat breeders which do have problems and it would be worth getting them examined to see if there are any abnormalities which can be treated. Examples of problems found include:

- endometritis
- thickening of the fallopian tube or adhesions of the bursa to the ovary
- ovarian cysts, which occasionally are present in the normally cycling animal
- pregnancy: although this is very rare, I have examined occasional repeat breeders which were pregnant!

### Adhesions

Adhesions of the bursa to the ovary could be due to stretching or tearing at calving, metritis or rough handling of the ovaries on rectal palpation. (Manual removal of the corpus luteum or manual cyst rupture can lead to haemorrhage and subsequent bursal adhesions.) A bursa which is fused to the ovary may not be able to function properly, so that any eggs released at ovulation drop into the abdomen, rather than pass down the fallopian tube. This would obviously lead to a repeat breeder.

### Use of GnRH

For repeat breeders, one product which has been trialled extensively and which seems to be beneficial in cows is GnRH. GnRH can be injected at one or both of the following times:

- at service, as a 'holding' injection: expect a 6–7% improvement in conception rate (Table 8.11)
- at 12 days after service: expect a 9–12% improvement in conception rate (Table 8.10)

At service, GnRH acts by ensuring that the egg is released from the follicle, to give better synchronisation of insemination with ovulation (luteinising hormone, LH, may also be used).

| Triallist | No. of cows in trial | Improvement in pregnancy rate over controls |
|---|---|---|
| MacMillan | 225 | 11.5% |
| ADAS | 660 | 12.0% |
| Sheldon | 1040 | 9.4% |

Data from Hoechst.

Table 8.10. The effect on first conception rates of GnRH given 12 days after service.

| | | | Pregnancy rate (%) | | |
|---|---|---|---|---|---|
| | No. of herds | No. of cows | Controls | Treated | Improvement (%) |
| First service | >60 | 11,048 | 53 | 59 | 6% |
| Repeat services | 81 | 3,608 | 42 | 49 | 7% |

Data summarised from reviews by Mee et al. (1990) and Stevenson et al. (1990).

Table 8.11. The effect of GnRH at the time of insemination on the pregnancy rate of cows.

At 12 days after insemination (the timing is critical) GnRH works by prolonging the life of the corpus luteum and in so doing it increases the length of the cycle. This means that the embryo will be a few days older before the cow considers producing prostaglandin from her uterus to start the next cycle. By being slightly older, the embryo can produce a stronger signal and this may be sufficient to 'alert' the cow to her pregnancy and 'cancel' the next cycle. After the injection of GnRH at 12 days, the cow will have a slightly longer (1–2 days) cycle length. In fact, if repeated injections are given every 3 days, many cows will not come on heat at all!

The use of GnRH is particularly good if the cows are stressed, for example following inseminations carried out just after turnout to grazing. Results show a 9–12% improvement in conception rates after the first service (Table 8.10), and in one trial this increased to 13% for cows at their second service and almost 30% at their third service. The number of animals involved at the second and third service was quite small, however, so the data needs to be interpreted with caution. Others have shown that the use of GnRH or LH at both service and at 12 days post service produces a better result in problem herds, viz where conception rates are inherently low.

**Use of Embryos**

An alternative approach is to implant an embryo into a repeat breeder cow. This would work even if the fallopian tubes were blocked or there were bursal adhesions present. The technique has become a practical possibility using embryos frozen in ethylene glycol, because these can be thawed in a single step, in much the same way as frozen semen. (Originally embryos were frozen in glycerol and had to be thawed in several stages.) Sometimes two embryos are placed in each cow, in the hope that twins will give double the amount of embryo 'signal' (bTb) and thus improve chances of conception. Initial results suggest a 50% conception rate, so with relatively inexpensive embryos and no sophisticated equipment needed, the technique becomes a practical possibility.

**Dosing Individual Cows**

A wide range of mineral, multivitamin and 'nutrient boost' products have been tried, some with apparent success. By all means try using them, especially if they are inexpensive, but do your own trial to monitor their performance. They may or may not work in your particular situation.

## ABORTION

One of the final hurdles in our components of the calving interval (see page 233) is the maintenance of pregnancy to full term to allow the birth of a normal live calf. If early foetal death occurs, it is most likely that the foetus will be reabsorbed in the uterus and nothing is seen. If the calf is expelled from the uterus at any stage of pregnancy before full term, then this is called an *abortion*.

The age of the aborted calf in days can be estimated by the distance from the crown of its head to its rump (or anus), using the formula:

age = 2.5 x (crown to rump length in cm + 21)

Most abortions are expelled from the uterus soon after foetal death and appear to be quite fresh. However, sometimes all of the placental fluids are reabsorbed and the calf becomes dry and chocolate-brown in colour. This is known as a *mummified foetus* and an example is shown in Plate 8.21. Mummified calves will often remain in situ, with some being expelled several months later – for example a 3 month old calf at 7 months of gestation – while others remain in the uterus and the cow simply fails to give birth.

Even with brucellosis eradicated, the average abortion rate for cattle in Britain in 1998 remains at approximately 4%. This is based on the number of abortions reported and checked for brucellosis by the Ministry of Agriculture, however, and so the actual abortion rate might be somewhat higher. The incidence of abortion with twins is much higher than with single births. Some herds definitely experience a much higher rate than 4%, and it always seems worse when several cows abort over a short period of time.

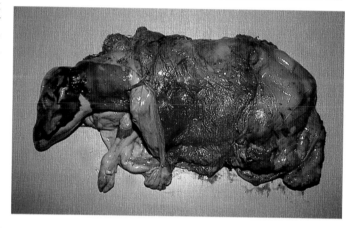

Plate 8.21. A mummified foetus may die in early pregnancy, although it may not be expelled from the uterus for several months.

In some countries (including the UK) the law obliges you to report all cases of abortion to the Divisional Veterinary Officer, so that samples can be taken to eliminate the possibility of brucellosis.

Most of the diseases causing abortion are dealt with in detail elsewhere in the book. They include:

- brucellosis, Chapter 11
- IBR (infectious bovine rhinotracheitis), Chapter 4
- BVD (bovine viral diarrhoea), Chapter 4
- leptospirosis, caused by *Leptospira hardjo*, Chapter 13
- salmonellosis, especially *S. typhimurium* and *S. dublin*, Chapter 11
- any peracute fever, such as summer mastitis, Chapter 7
- *Bacillus licheniformis*

Diseases discussed in this chapter are:

- mycotic abortion (Aspergillosis)
- *Neospora caninum*
- chlamydia
- Q fever
- listeriosis

Aspergillosis is the most common fungal cause of abortion. It is a mould with a green/grey colouring which is often seen growing on silage. A typical example was shown in Plate 1.1. Suspect food should therefore not be fed to late pregnant animals.

*Neospora* is thought to account for some 20–40% of all bovine abortions. A protozoan parasite, *Neospora caninum* originates in dogs, and one Canadian study showed a strong association between the presence of dogs on the farm and the number of cows which blood tested positive to *Neospora*. Little is known about its method of spread. The organism probably multiplies in the gut, spreads throughout the cow's body and passes to the uterus, where it then invades the developing foetus. Infection may cause abortion, mummified calves or calves born alive with brain incoordination (cerebellar hypoplasia, see Plates 1.8 and 1.9). The presence of *Neospora* cysts in the brain was one of the early diagnostic tests. Both monensin and decoquinate, drugs used against *Toxoplasma*, a related organism in sheep, have been used for treatment, as yet with unproven success. Once infected, cows can remain carriers and either abort every year or give birth to a calf congenitally infected with Neospora, which may then abort in later life.

Chlamydia and Q fever are both members of the Rickettsia family, that is organisms which share properties of both bacteria and viruses. They are mainly associated with tick infested areas (see Figure 13.7), and both have been known to cause abortion.

*Listeria monocytogenes* more commonly produces abortion in sheep than cattle but can cause a brain infection in both species. The infection may originate from big bale silage.

Less is known about the causes of mummified calves. Possible factors include:

- BVD
- *Neospora*
- genetics (very occasionally particular sires will produce a high incidence in their offspring)
- stress in early pregnancy (proven in pigs but not in cattle)

Farmers tend to be more careful when handling heavily pregnant cows and this is probably a good thing in order to avoid teat and leg damage. I suspect that fairly severe mishandling is necessary to cause abortion.

## STILLBORN CALVES

If there is a high incidence of stillbirths, the first step in the investigation must be a careful examination of the records. Were the majority of cases associated with a particular sire, with twins, with heifers or with older cows? For example, if twinning is significantly higher than the normal rate of 4–5%, this could be the sole cause of the problem.

Iodine has been strongly implicated in the perinatal weak calf syndrome, which has caused stillbirth rates as high as 30% in Ireland. Investigation of iodine deficiency by means of blood samples and foetal goitre weights is discussed in Chapter 12. Selenium/ vitamin E deficiency may produce 'slow calvings' in heifers, but this has not been well proven. For example, some heifers seem to start calving and then proceed no further, so that by the time assistance is given, the calf is already dead. Similarly, a high incidence of milk fever in cows could be involved. In both cases it must be worth blood sampling a few animals to confirm that selenium, calcium and magnesium status is adequate. To get a true assessment of calcium/milk fever status, samples need to be taken from the cow at calving.

Examine the calf to see if it died before (prepartum) or during (intrapartum) birth. The presence of meconium (foetal dung, see Chapter 5) on the calf's coat or in its ears, trachea or stomach indicates that it was alive at

Potential causes of stillbirths include:

- poor sire selection, producing oversized calves
- heifers and cows which are either extremely fat or excessively thin at calving
- poor stockmanship, including excessive disturbance and assistance given too early
- twins
- physical calving problems: leg back, breech etc.
- deficiencies such as iodine, selenium/ vitamin E, vitamin A
- abortion and premature calving
- maternal problems, e.g. a high incidence of milk fever
- salmonella, summer mastitis and other toxaemias

the start of the birth process, but because it became short of oxygen, it defaecated into the amnion (inner water bag) when struggling for breath. Intrapartum stillbirths are the most common. Prepartum deaths can be associated with salmonella, so laboratory culture of a few stillbirths can be worthwhile.

Many of the physical and management factors associated with calves born dead are described in Chapter 5, which should be read in conjunction with this section.

## PREVENTIVE MEDICINE AND HERD FERTILITY MANAGEMENT

Because preventive medicine programmes in dairy herds are usually based on a regular fertility visit, this is a good opportunity to introduce the subject. I like to define preventive medicine as *'the routine implementation of common sense husbandry'*.

No new technical information is needed, but rather a different approach to disease control in general, that approach being towards prevention rather than treatment. For some conditions, for example blackleg, vaccination is the preventive measure and the disease can be completely eliminated, although infection remains in the soil and in the intestine of the animal. Most other conditions are far more complex, however, and the level of farm performance needs to be continually monitored if progress is to be made. Mastitis and fertility are good examples of this. Mastitis will never be eradicated and so preventive programmes must be devised to reduce the incidence of the condition to economically acceptable levels, such as those suggested in Chapter 7.

We can only assess the effectiveness of our preventive programmes if we actually record and monitor mastitis incidence and fertility, and I believe that this is one of the functions of your vet. Not only should he be advising you on the appropriate mastitis control measures for your herd, but he should also make sure that you are *recording* those cases of mastitis which do occur and that periodically the overall incidence of mastitis in your herd is assessed by an *analysis of the records*, so that you can compare your performance with other herds. This is commonly available for subclinical mastitis using cell counts, but it needs to be expanded to include clinical cases.

Herd fertility control should be tackled in a similar way. Your vet should be able to advise you on the type of records needed and make sure that a regular analysis of those records is carried out. You can then see if you need to put additional effort into fertility control. Calculation of a range of indices including conception rates, submission rates, heat detection efficiency and accuracy (Figures 8.13 and 8.14), and Cu-sums (Figure 8.20) are all important in achieving this.

### The Costs of Disease

The concept of monitoring margin over concentrates and other criteria before making financial decisions has been well accepted and a similar approach should be instigated for animal disease. Before spending money on disease prevention measures we need to know:

- the cost of an average case of a particular disease
- the incidence of that disease in your herd

The subject has been extensively researched in the UK and much of the following is taken from an analysis of herds using the DAISY recording system. The cost of disease may be subdivided into two components, namely direct and indirect costs.

Direct costs: drugs used, reduced milk sales during illness, milk discarded during therapy, vet and herdsman's time involved in treatment

Indirect costs: increased risk of a fatality, increased risk of other diseases and a possible adverse effect on fertility and on long-term productivity

For many diseases the indirect costs are greater than the direct costs. For example, some typical figures quoted by Esslemont for the cost of a single case of disease are given in Table 8.12.

The striking feature of these figures is the very high costs of disease and the fact that for most conditions the indirect costs are greater than the direct ones. These figures represent the cost of a *case* of a particular condition. For example, even in a good herd the incidence of lameness and mastitis is 25 and 35 cases per 100 cows per year. This gives total annual costs for a 100 cow herd of £6150 (25 x £246) for lameness and £6405 (35 x

| Disease | Direct costs | Indirect costs | Total cost |
|---|---|---|---|
| Retained placenta | £83 | £215 | £298 |
| Milk fever | £59 | £165 | £220 |
| Mastitis | £118 | £65 | £183 |
| Lameness | £93 | £153 | £246 |
| Endometritis | £70 | £91 | £161 |

Esslemont, 1995 UK values.

Table 8.12. Estimated per cow costs of a case of disease.

£183) for mastitis and include an allowance for repeat treatments. The cost of a single case would be less than this. The figures are based on average cases of lameness and mastitis. If there was a high incidence of sole ulcers or of peracute coliform mastitis in your herd, then the figures could be double. Veterinary costs (fees and drugs) represented only a small proportion of the total costs of disease, for example, 14% of the cost of a case of lameness. So although a farmer may think that veterinary costs are high when dealing with an outbreak of lameness, the total costs of the problem will be very much greater.

It should be emphasised that these are one author's estimate and 1995 figures and the reader is urged to substitute current day values when reading this text. The effect of releasing milk quota, which could then be used elsewhere, has also not been included. This would reduce disease costs.

## Use of Records

The on-farm monitoring of disease incidence is therefore an essential part of maintaining profitability. Not only will records indicate when the incidence of a condition is becoming excessive, but they may also help to identify the cause of the disease. Examples of how records can be used to distinguish between environmental and contagious mastitis were given in Chapter 7. Other good examples of on-farm performance monitoring are heat detection analysis (Figures 8.13 and 8.14) and the Cu-sum plot (Figure 8.20). The Cu-sum is very simple and yet it gives a good check on conception rate. Fluctuations in fertility will undoubtedly occur: if possible the causes of these fluctuations should be identified, so that preventive measures can be introduced to prevent their recurrence.

This is an area where computerisation has a great deal to offer. For example, we have seen already that poor conception rates may be due to a variety of factors and unless we have a fairly sophisticated means of analysing herd fertility data, it may be impossible to identify which of the factors is a problem in your particular herd. If you are choosing a computer system, make sure that it offers the facility of an in-depth analysis of data, as well as a routine monitoring. It may be important to know whether poor conception rates are related to a particular bull, or serving too soon after calving, or previous cases of endometritis, or the average interval between services, or the accuracy of heat detection, and so on. The records are then used in a *diagnostic capacity*.

I have given several examples of what I think the vet ought to be doing in terms of preventive medicine programmes, so what part should the farmer be playing? First it is important that records are kept and that they are accurate. It is obviously pointless spending time monitoring performance data if the basic records are incorrect. Second, you need to allow your vet to visit the farm regularly, perhaps every 2 weeks, learning what the problems are and how they have been tackled so far.

To give an idea of what I mean, I will briefly describe the system we have used for farms in our own veterinary practice. The DAISY computer programme is now used both for construction of action lists and analysis of health and fertility data, although a non-computerised manual system to construct action lists proved successful for many years.

There are three basic fertility examinations carried out, namely:

- A post calving examination is made to check that there is no residual endometritis. This is performed at between 2 and 4 weeks after calving because many discharges will clear up without treatment by 2 weeks post calving. The examination simply consists of washing the vulva and then inserting a gloved hand into the vagina to check that the cervix is closed and that there is no gross evidence of pus in the cervical mucus. Some vets use a speculum and simply look at the cervix.
- Cows not seen bulling by 40–50 days post calving are examined to make sure they are cycling normally and that there are no cysts.
- Pregnancy diagnosis is performed 5–7 weeks after the last service date.

Cows which have been cycling irregularly, those which have been served more than 3–4 times but have not conceived, and those previously diagnosed as pregnant but which the herdsman suspects may have been bulling may also be presented for examination.

The list of cows sent to the farm in advance of the visit has two important uses. Firstly it compels the farmer to spend a few minutes going through his own records, deleting 'non-bulling' cows which have since been served, and cows due for a pregnancy check which have returned to service. Secondly the list reminds him that the visit is due. The discipline of having to check through the herd records every 2 weeks in itself makes a big contribution to improving overall fertility. Problem cows are regularly identified and as such are watched much more carefully.

For a routine visit system to be successful, it should cause the minimum of disturbance to the cows and to the farm routine and, if possible, I like to carry out fertility examinations immediately after morning milking.

Because your vet is checking cows on a routine basis, he can get an immediate idea of whether there is a problem with endometritis, or if too many normal cycling cows have not been seen on heat. This would then be verified by consulting the records. He is in a good position to suggest corrective measures. It may be that he will need to take samples, for example blood samples for a metabolic profile to check energy, protein or mineral status. Because he is attending on a routine basis, it is much easier to follow up at the next fortnightly visit with the results and any corrective measures needed. After a further 2–4 weeks the records may show if the necessary improvement was achieved.

In addition to carrying out fertility examinations, the routine visit is a good opportunity to check a few of the cows which have had troublesome feet, or maybe a group of weaned calves which are a bit loose and not growing as well as they ought. You may also want to talk about worm control in the young stock, or about a new animal health product which has been recently launched on the market.

Mastitis is such a complex subject that it is best to schedule a special discussion period at least once a year, perhaps just before afternoon milking. The records are examined to see what the current herd mastitis status is like and this in itself may give an idea of what to look for. There may be a high incidence of environmental cases for example, or possibly an excessive number (more than 20%) of treated quarters have needed repeat treatment, suggesting a chronic staphylococcal problem. If it is the winter the cubicles are checked for comfort and cleanliness. Finally, in the parlour the milking routine is monitored, as are milking speeds and hygiene procedures such as teat dipping and udder washing, and teat ends can be examined and scored immediately after cluster removal. The whole visit may take an hour or more, but it is an excellent opportunity for the herdsman to discuss mastitis problems and for the vet to check that none of the standard routine control measures are being overlooked. With mastitis costing an average of £31.00 for every cow in your herd, this is time and money well spent.

These are all aspects of preventive medicine. The overall concept is to reduce the effects of disease to economically acceptable levels by a regular assessment of performance as seen both in the records and in the cows themselves. It requires enthusiasm and trust on the part of both the farmer and his vet, but it is the way that veterinary services will progress in the future; that is, in the routine implementation of common sense husbandry.

## CHAPTER 9

# LAMENESS AND FOOT TRIMMING

Lameness is not only a major economic problem, but it is also a major welfare issue – for both the cow and the herdsman! There are few conditions which regularly produce as much pain and distress to the dairy cow and few conditions where the herdsman has to spend so much time and effort on routine prevention, in other words, hoof trimming. If we could learn to house, feed and manage our cows better, much of this effort would not be needed.

Lameness is also an expensive disease. In 1998 Esslemont estimated that foot problems cost the United Kingdom dairy herd £90 million each year, which is just under £30 for every cow in the national dairy herd. An individual case of lameness was estimated to cost between £25 and £300, depending on whether it was a simple case of digital dermatitis or a more complicated sole ulcer in an early lactation cow. As a high proportion of lameness occurs in early lactation and as lame cows are more difficult to get back in calf, reduced fertility is a major contributor to the cost of lameness.

The incidence of lameness in the United Kingdom remains high, with almost 25% of the national herd being treated each year. Compare this with mastitis, where around 20% of cows are affected each year. A UK survey carried out in the late 1970s showed that leg disorders accounted for only 12% of all lameness and these were mainly calving injuries. This means that 88% of lameness was associated with the foot. Of these, 86% were in the hind foot, with the outer claw most likely to be affected (85%).

This chapter describes the structure of the foot, what happens during overgrowth and an approach to hoof trimming. It then deals with the many causes of lameness and their control. Clearly only a condensed description can be given in a single chapter, and readers requiring more detailed information, with colour photographs and diagrams, are advised to consult the book *Cattle Lameness and Hoofcare*.

## THE STRUCTURE OF THE FOOT

The bovine claw consists of three main components (Figure 9.1 and Plate 9.1). Moving inwards from the outer casing these are:

- the hoof
- the corium
- the bones

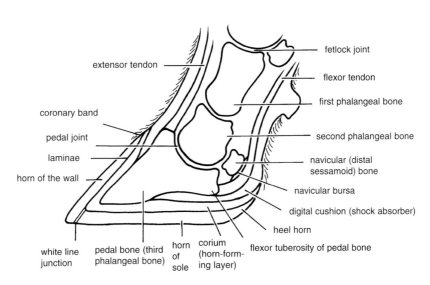

Figure 9.1. The structure of the foot, showing the hoof (wall, white line, sole and heel), the corium and the bones.

## The Hoof

The hoof consists of four parts: the wall, the sole, the white line and the heel. The wall is equivalent to the human finger-nail and is produced at the coronary band, that is the skin–horn junction at the top of the claw, shown in Figure 9.2. Once produced it flows down over the outside of the wall at approximately 5 mm per month. As the distance from the coronary band to the toe in the average cow is around 75 mm, this means that it can take 15 months (75 mm divided by 5 mm = 15) for

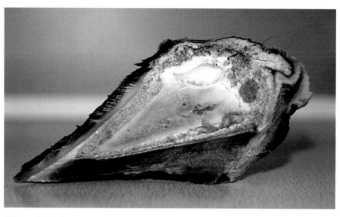

Plate 9.1. A cross-section of the hoof, showing horn of the wall, white line and sole, surrounding the corium and pedal bone.

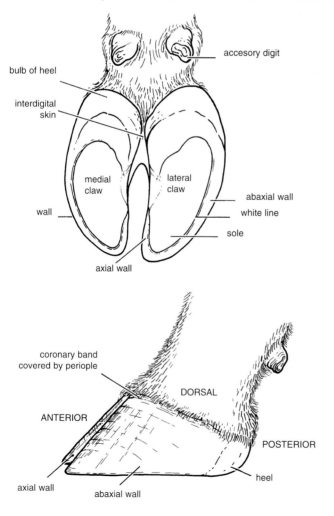

Figure 9.2. Diagram of right hind foot viewed from the bottom and the side, giving the nomenclature of its surfaces.

new horn to come into wear at the toe. Towards the heel the average distance from the sole to the coronary band is only 30–40 mm (Figure 9.7), so horn produced at this point comes into wear more quickly. The coronary band is covered by the periople, which produces a smooth, waxy protective covering to the wall of the hoof. Damage to this leads to sandcracks.

The sole of the hoof is produced by the corium of the sole. The sole would be equivalent to a second 'nail' growing from the tip of a human finger. Where the wall joins the sole there is a 'cemented' junction known as the white line. This is clearly shown in Plate 9.1 and Figure 9.1. The white line runs from the heel along the outer (abaxial) wall of the hoof to the toe and then back for the first third of the inner (axial) wall (Figure 9.2). Because it is a cemented junction the white line is a point of weakness. Whereas the wall and the sole consist of tubular horn (equivalent to concrete with steel reinforcing bars), the white line is more like cement. It has no tubular horn, it is less mature than the horn of the wall and it contains less keratin. All three factors make it much weaker and much more prone to injury.

The heel, or bulb of the hoof, consists of much softer horn and is produced by a continuation of the periople running from the coronary band. As it is a soft structure it expands and contracts during locomotion. This acts as both a shock absorber and a pump, thus allowing blood from the foot to be pumped back up the leg. Consequently if heifers (especially) spend too long standing still, the blood in the foot becomes 'stale' and this can result in poor horn formation. Alternatively excess trauma to the heel can sometimes produce a haematoma (blood blister), which causes lameness.

## The Corium

The corium is the sensitive structure of the foot. A stone or nail penetrating the hoof causes pain and lameness only when the corium is compressed or penetrated. The corium is also a support tissue, carrying blood and nutrients to both the hoof and the pedal bone. When the corium is penetrated the foot may bleed. In addition to providing a nerve and blood supply, the corium is modified at various parts of the foot to provide three other important functions. These are:

- horn formation – by the papillae
- support for the hoof wall – by the laminae
- shock absorber and blood pump – by the digital cushion

*Horn formation*
Plate 9.2 shows the corium after the hoof has been removed. In the pale, cream-coloured area below the coronary band area and beneath, the corium is modified to form large numbers of finger-like projections

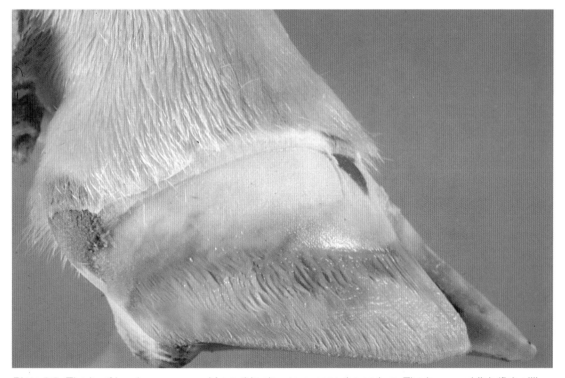

Plate 9.2. The hoof has been removed from this claw to expose the corium. The lower reddish 'fish gill' area is the laminae of the corium, the upper pale pink section the papillae (courtesy Dr. P. Ossent).

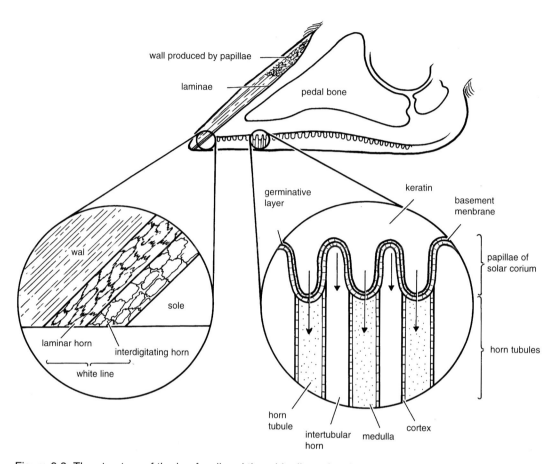

Figure 9.3. The structure of the hoof wall and the white line, showing details of horn formation.

known as the papillae. These are so small that they cannot be seen in Plate 9.2. The papillae extrude the tubular horn which eventually matures and hardens to form the hoof wall. Papillae are also found on the sole, where they extrude the horn of the sole. This is shown in detail in Figure 9.3. The corium also produces the cemented horn of the white line, but this time there are no papillae present, so there are no horn tubules and the horn is weaker.

*Support for the wall*
As the wall of the hoof provides weightbearing and protection for the foot, it has to be firmly attached to the underlying corium. However, at the same time it must be able to both move down over the foot and act as a shock absorber. The remarkable incorporation of these diverse functions is achieved using a series of interlocking leaves known as the laminae. These are clearly shown as the pink area in the lower part of the claw in Plate 9.2. Equivalent leaves are also present on the inside of the hoof wall (Plate 9.3) and these interdigitate with the laminae of the corium. A cow with laminitis has inflammation of the laminae. The increased blood flow, heat and swelling which this produces within the confined space of the hoof leads to intense pain and may distort the growth of the hoof. Although often referred to as laminitis, it is very rare that the laminae alone are affected. In most cows the whole of the corium will be inflamed, producing changes in the wall, sole and white line. The condition would therefore be best described as coriitis or coriosis.

The movement of the hoof wall down over the laminae has been compared to one piece of corrugated cardboard (the wall) moving down over a second stationary piece (the laminae of the corium).

This is shown diagrammatically in Figure 9.4.

*Shock absorber and blood pump*
Within the heel the corium is impregnated with fat, fibrous tissue and elastic material to form the digital cushion. The front portion of the digital cushion extends forward to run under the rear edge of the pedal bone, as shown in Figure 9.1. Because the heel horn is flexible, the digital cushion becomes compressed during weightbearing. When no longer weightbearing, the elastic tissue restores the cushion to its original shape. This regular expansion and contraction is important for both blood flow and shock absorption. If the corium becomes bruised or inflamed, due to excessive weightbearing or coriosis/laminitis respectively, the elastic and fat will be replaced by scar tissue. The function of the digital cushion (shock absorber and blood pump) will then be impaired.

## The Bones

There are really only two bones within the hoof, the pedal bone and the navicular bone. These are technically referred to as the third phalangeal bone and the distal sessamoid bone respectively. The pedal joint (distal interphalangeal joint), which is the junction between the second and third phalangeal bones, is also just within the hoof capsule, as can be seen in Plate 9.14 and Figure 9.1. Infection within this joint produces severe lameness.

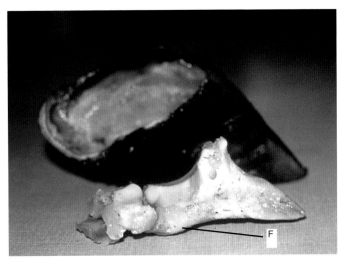

Plate 9.3. The pedal and navicular bones viewed from the inner aspect. Laminae can be seen on the inside of the hoof wall, and the flexor tuberosity F is clearly visible.

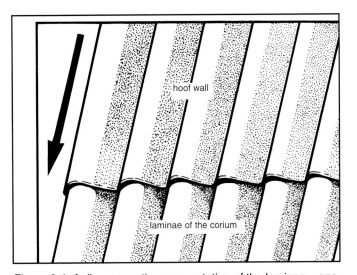

Figure 9.4. A diagrammatic representation of the laminae – one sheet of corrugated cardboard running over the other.

The navicular bone acts as a support structure, improving leverage by pushing the flexor tendon towards the heel as it runs down the leg and attaches to the base of the pedal bone. The padded area between the flexor tendon and navicular bone is known as the navicular bursa (Figure 9.1).

Although the pedal bone is weightbearing around its entire outer edge, its base is arch-shaped on its inner border. This is shown in Plate 9.3. The projection at the rear end of the pedal bone marked F in Plate 9.3 is the point of attachment for the flexor tendon. This projection is therefore called the flexor tuberosity. Compression of the corium between the flexor tuberosity of the pedal bone above and the hard horn of the sole beneath is an important part of the pathogenesis of sole ulcers and is referred to again on page 293. The corium feeds the bone as well as the hoof, so inflammation of the corium may also result in bone deformities.

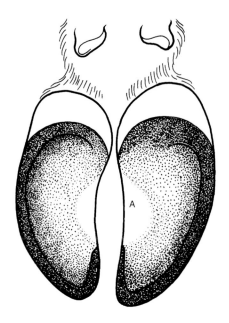

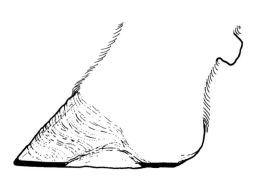

Figure 9.6. An axial (inner) view of the claw, showing weightbearing at the toe and heel, but not in the central sole area.

Figure 9.5. The correct weightbearing surfaces of the foot are the darker shaded areas. Note how the whole area of the toe is weightbearing.

## CORRECT WEIGHTBEARING

As the primary objective of hoof trimming is to restore the foot to its correct shape, it is important that we first examine the normal foot and then the distortions which occur with overgrowth.

The correct weightbearing surfaces of the foot are indicated by the shaded areas in Figure 9.5. They consist of the heel, plus the wall of the hoof which runs from the heel forwards to the toe and

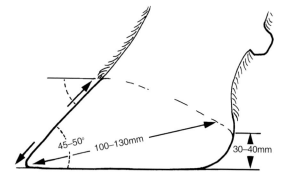

Figure 9.7. The approximate dimensions and angles of a normal claw.

then back for the first 25–30% of the interdigital space. Weight should be taken on the wall, the white line and an area of the sole adjacent to the white line, so that the whole of the toe is weightbearing. However, the central sole area, marked A in Figure 9.5 and positioned immediately beneath the rear inner edge (the flexor tuberosity) of the pedal bone, should not be weightbearing. This is shown in Figure 9.6. To optimise weightbearing within the foot, the anterior wall of the hoof from coronary band to toe should be 70–80 mm long and form an angle of 45–50° with the horizontal of the sole. These dimensions are shown in Figure 9.7. Note that the foot has a good heel height and that the accessory digits are well above the ground.

# HOOF OVERGROWTH

The size and shape of the hoof at any one time will be a balance between the rate of growth and the rate of wear. As one might expect, there are a variety of factors which influence both processes. For example, horn *growth* is faster

- in young animals
- with high concentrate feeding
- with more exercise
- on rough surfaces

The rate of wear is increased by factors such as:

- wet conditions underfoot, leading to softer horn which wears faster
- excessive walking
- hard and/or abrasive floor surfaces

*Overgrowth at the toe*
The horn of the wall is generally harder than the horn of the heel, so although both may grow at the same rate, horn is worn away more slowly from the toe than from the heel. This results in overgrowth *occurring primarily at the toe*. The additional horn at the toe lifts up the front of the foot and the front wall then forms a more shallow angle, decreasing from 45° to 30° or 20°, or even to the horizontal. In extreme cases the front wall becomes concave and the toe is lifted off the ground (Plate 9.4). These changes are shown in Figure 9.8. Internally the pedal bone is rotated backwards, thereby putting even more pressure on its rear edge and further increasing the risk of sole ulcers.

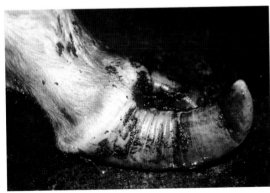

Plate 9.4. Gross claw overgrowth. There is no longer any height of heel and the toe does not make contact with the ground.

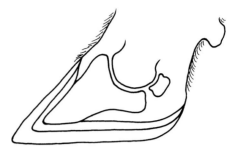

A – normal hoof shape

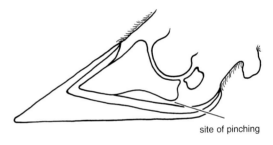

site of pinching

B – overgrowth at the toe

Figure 9.8. Overgrowth at the toe produces a backward rotation of the pedal bone, so that the corium becomes pinched between the pedal bone above and the horn of the sole beneath.

The pedal bone remains the same size, irrespective of the degree of overgrowth. In this respect the hoof is very different from the cow's horn. As the horn grows out from the cow's head the bone inside the horn elongates at an equal rate, as shown in Plate 9.5. This does not happen with the pedal bone.

*Overgrowth of the lateral wall*
In some animals the outer wall of one claw grows faster than the inner and starts to curl under the sole. This produces a corkscrew effect at the toe, as shown in Plate 9.6. Corkscrew claw may be a genetic trait, or can be a result of coriosis/laminitis.

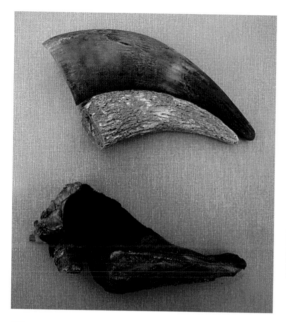

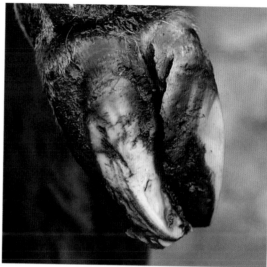

Plate 9.6. Overgrowth of the wall, curling under the sole, makes the central sole area weightbearing.

Plate 9.5. A comparison of a bovine horn with the foot. The bone continues to grow inside the horn but in an overgrown foot the bone remains a constant size.

*Overgrowth of the sole*

A ledge of horn may also grow out from the sole, as in Plate 9.7. This may be so pronounced that it becomes the major weightbearing point of the foot – even though it is immediately beneath the rear edge of the pedal bone and in an area where we want to minimise weightbearing.

*Disparity of claw size*

The outer claw of the hind foot often becomes much larger than the inner claw. There is no single reason for this and suggested causes include: poorer suspension of the pedal bone within the outer claw, leading to pinching of the corium and stimulating the growth of horn; a greater variation in load-bearing on the outer claw compared with the inner claw when the cow is walking; a leg conformation in which the hocks point inwards and the toes outwards; excessive engorgement of the udder at calving, forcing the legs apart; and the fact that the hind feet are the major *propelling* force of the cow during locomotion, pushing her forwards, whereas the front feet are the major *weightbearing* structures. In front feet the position is reversed: the inner claw becomes bigger than the outer claw.

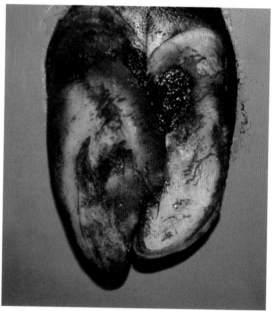

Plate 9.7. Overgrowth of the sole can also lead to weightbearing at the sole ulcer site.

Hoof overgrowth may produce
- lifting of the toe
- corkscrew toe
- a ledge of horn from the sole
- disparity in claw size

## Effects of Overgrowth

The cumulative effects of overgrowth at various parts of the foot lead to distortion of foot shape, disruption of gait, discomfort when walking and a predisposition to diseases such as sole ulcers. If you have any doubt about this, try walking on your heels and see how it feels! Foot trimming attempts to correct these defects and to restore the foot to its correct weightbearing surfaces.

# FOOT TRIMMING

Much has been written about different approaches to foot trimming. To a certain extent the procedures used must be a matter of personal preference. Points to consider are:

- lifting the foot
- equipment used
- claw trimming technique

## Lifting the Foot

I prefer the cow to be standing, with her leg securely tied at both the hock and fetlock. With my head well above hock level (Plate 9.8) I am able to look downwards across the sole surface of both claws and can visualise how the weightbearing surfaces of the foot should make contact with the ground. If the leg was also secured at the fetlock (which it is not in Plate 9.8), the foot would be more firmly fixed in position and I find this makes hoof trimming both easier and safer. Like trying to hammer a nail into a flexible branch, if the foot is not securely fastened, trimming it is much more difficult.

Others prefer to have more freedom of movement around the cow's leg and so use the Wopa box type of crush, shown in Plate 9.9. If large numbers of cows have to be examined I can see the attraction of using the mobile rotating crush shown in Plate 9.10, which remains attached to the truck while in use. The cows entered the crush easily, were tipped over onto their sides using a hydraulic pump, the legs were strapped into position using hydraulic belts and most of the foot trimming was done using electric sanding discs. I tried trimming like this with a knife and did not like it, but it is probably something to which you would grow accustomed.

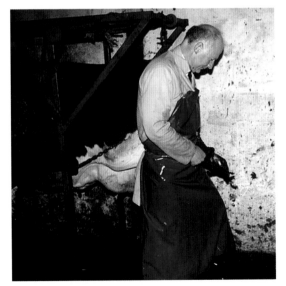

Plate 9.8. With the cow in a standing position, it is possible to look across the sole and visualise the weightbearing surfaces.

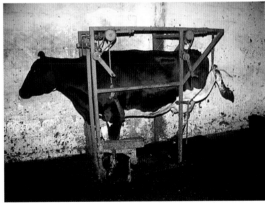

Plate 9.9. A Wopa box gives freedom of access around the foot, but does not restrain the foot as well as tying at the fetlock does.

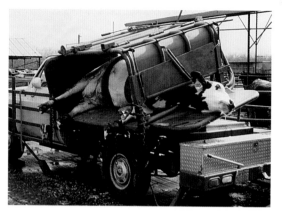

Plate 9.10. A rotating table makes handling the cows much less strenuous for the operator.

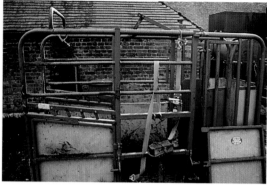

Plate 9.11. If your crush does not have a belly strap, the use of a lorry belt or even a rope under the chest helps to restrain the cow.

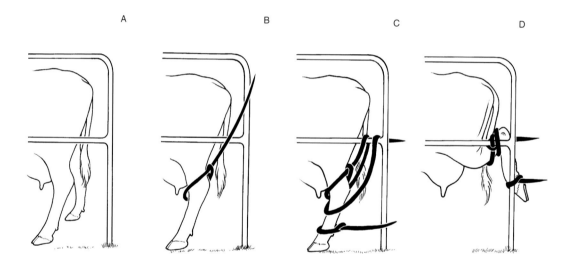

Figure 9.9. A system of using two ropes to lift the hind leg of a cow and tie the fetlock securely to the vertical bar at the rear of the crush.

In conventional crushes a mechanical winch for lifting the foot is ideal, but make sure that the ratchet is secure, so that it does not fly open when the cow kicks. Belly belts help in restraint, especially for the front feet. If your crush does not have a belt, simply use a rope or a belt from the side of a lorry, as in Plate 9.11. If using ropes to lift the hind leg, attach the first rope around the hock with a slip knot (B), and then run it twice around a horizontal bar of the crush to produce a pulling action (C). Place a second rope around the fetlock. By pulling the fetlock rope backwards, the cow will kick, making it easy to lift and tie the hock firmly to the horizontal bar using the first rope and tie the fetlock to the vertical with the lower rope (D). This is shown diagrammatically in Figure 9.9. Whatever system is chosen, the cow should be securely restrained for safety of both animal and operator.

## Equipment Used

Again, this is a personal choice, based on what you get accustomed to. If knives are used they *must* be kept sharp. I prefer to place both hands on the knife, as in Plate 9.12. The knife should be held at a slight angle, as shown in Figure 9.10. It thus passes diagonally through the hoof in a slicing/sawing action, moving down towards the toe and out towards the wall at the same time. A direct push to the toe can be much more difficult. Some people use electric sanders. While these may be safe in skilled hands, there is a greater risk of over-trimming the sole (causing lameness) and of failing to get a good claw shape. Concern has also been expressed about the possible adverse effects of overheating the horn during cutting.

Gloves are useful, both for increasing the speed of hoof trimming and for safety reasons. I also like to wear an arm protector (Plate 9.13) to reduce soiling and grazing of my fore-arm as it slides over the edge of the hoof at the end of a cutting stroke.

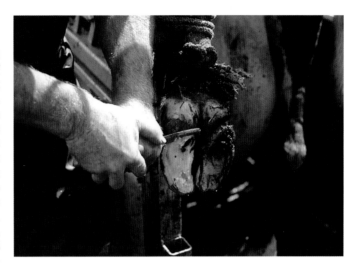

Plate 9.12. Using both hands on the knife gives a good controlled cutting stroke. It would be better if the knife was held slightly diagonally.

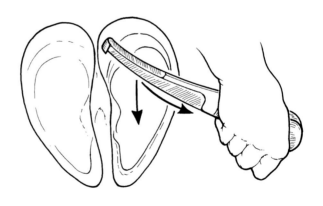

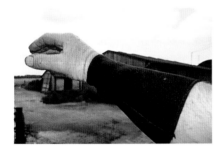

Plate 9.13. An arm protector makes foot trimming more comfortable.

Figure 9.10. Trimming is made easier by holding the knife at an angle and pushing it through the hoof in a slicing action.

## Trimming Technique

Although the technique described in the following is a four stage process, the stages are not necessarily discrete steps and in reality one part of the trimming process merges with another.

### Cut One
Cut the overgrown toe back to its correct length, which is approximately 75 mm from the coronary band to the toe, or one handspan. When learning to trim, it is probably better to actually measure the distance.

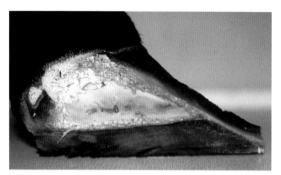

Plate 9.14. Hoof trimming: after Cut One the toe is still too high and the wall no longer makes contact with the ground.

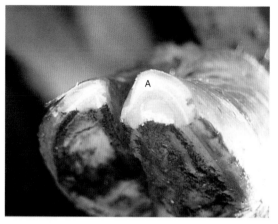

Plate 9.15. Hoof trimming: the white line (A) can be seen running across the square end of the toe after Cut One.

After Cut One the cow is left with a so-called square-ended toe, as in Plates 9.14 and 9.15. In Plate 9.15 it can be seen that the white line now passes across the end of the toe at A and that the wall of the hoof is no longer weightbearing at this point. Although the wall is now the correct length, the toe is still too high and the front angle of the wall remains too shallow. This is demonstrated in Figure 9.11.

*Cut Two*
The next stage is to remove the excess horn from beneath the toe, thus bringing the front wall back to a more upright position, as shown in Plate 9.16. The horn to be removed in Cut Two lies beneath the line AB (Figure 9.11), which is a line joining Cut One to the base of the heel. The first part of Cut Two can be performed by removing part of the wall using hoof clippers (Plate 9.17), but later stages should be carried out with a hoof knife, continually checking the area of the sole for signs of softening. A softening of the horn should not occur, but if it does then you *must* stop. You will have only a few millimetres of horn before the corium is penetrated and exposure of the corium in this area of the foot can lead to quite severe and protracted lameness.

   It is *vital* that Cut One does not make the hoof too short. This scenario is shown in Figure 9.12. Because Cut One was too short, a line drawn from the top of Cut One to the bottom of the heel (AB in Figure 9.12) would lead to penetration and exposure of the corium at the toe, and this would produce severe lameness. If you are unlucky enough to significantly expose the corium at the toe, I would recommend immediate application of a Cowslip or similar shoe to the sound claw (see page 319).

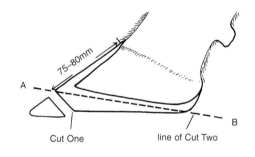

Figure 9.11. Hoof trimming. Cut One: Trim toe to 75–80 mm. Cut Two: remove excess sole horn beneath AB, i.e. mainly from the toe, thereby bringing the front wall back to 45°.

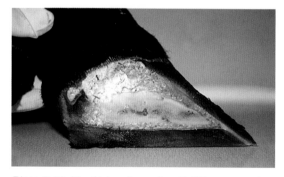

Plate 9.16. Hoof trimming: after Cut Two, correct weightbearing is re-established.

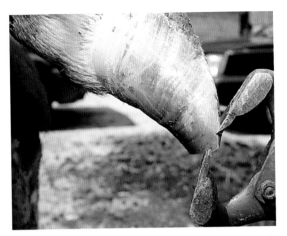

Plate 9.17. Hoof trimming: Cut Two can be started using hoof trimmers.

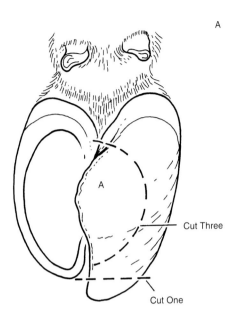

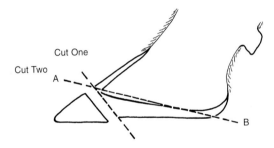

Figure 9.12. Hoof trimming. If Cut One is made too short, Cut Two can penetrate the corium at the toe.

## Cut Three

Cut Three consists of dishing the inner sole surface of both claws (Figure 9.13), so that weight-bearing beneath the flexor tuberosity of the pedal bone is minimised. Any large overgrowths of sole horn, as in Plate 9.7 and Figure 9.13A, have to be removed to achieve this. Cut Three also slightly increases the space between the digits. This makes impaction by dirt and foreign bodies less likely, decreasing the incidence of diseases such as foul, interdigital dermatitis and interdigital skin hyperplasia (corns).

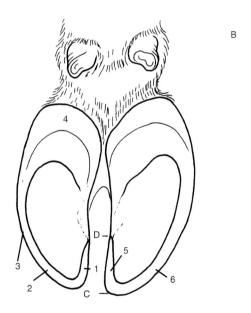

Figure 9.13. Hoof trimming. Cut Three: Remove any overgrowth (A) of the sole, so that weightbearing returns to the correct surfaces and away from the sole ulcer site. When hoof trimming is complete, points 1, 2, 3 and 4, and 1, 2, 5 and 6 should be on the same horizontal planes.

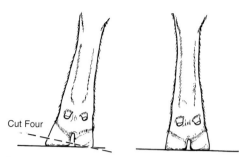

Figure 9.14. Hoof trimming. Cut Four: Trim the outer and inner claws back to an even size, thus bringing the cow back to an upright position (right). This normally involves trimming additional horn off the lateral claws of the hind feet and off the medial claws of the front feet.

*Cut Four*

The final stage is to trim the two claws back to approximately the same size. This usually means removing additional horn from the outer claw of hind feet and the inner claw of front feet, bringing the legs back to the upright position, as shown in Figure 9.14. This produces more even weightbearing.

*General points*

When trimming is complete, points 1, 2, 3 and 4 on Figure 9.13B and points 1, 2, 5 and 6 should all be on the same horizontal plane, to provide adequate weightbearing. The two claws should also be of equal size and their two sole surfaces on the same horizontal plane. Removal of the inner wall CD (Figure 9.13B) is a common mistake made by

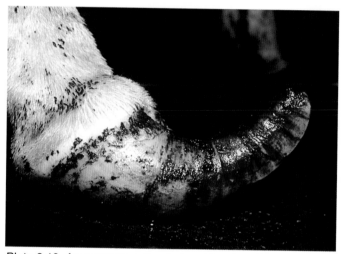

Plate 9.18. An overgrown claw before trimming. Note the concave front wall and the swelling above the coronary band, both indicative of a previous coriosis/laminitis.

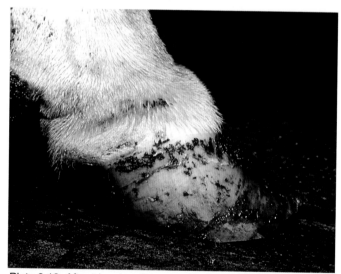

Plate 9.19. After trimming: the concave wall has been removed and the sole makes reasonable contact with the ground (although I should have filed it off to give it a more pleasing appearance!).

some herdsmen who feel that the toes should not be touching once trimming is complete. This is a fallacy. If the wall CD is lowered, the claw will be seriously destabilised, causing it to rotate inwards and allowing overgrowth of the lateral wall, as in Plate 9.6. In the worst case excessive removal of the inner wall might expose the corium, leading to severe lameness.

I prefer not to remove any heel horn unless it is badly under-run, other than as part of Cut Four. If the heel is only slightly pitted, I would leave it alone, since removal of the heel could lead to backwards rotation of the pedal bone and so predispose to sole ulcers (Plate 9.24).

Probably the best time to trim feet is at drying off, and any cow which is lame or overgrown should be trimmed. As many of the management and feeding 'insults' leading to lameness occur at the time of calving, it seems sensible to have feet in optimum shape at this stage. If claws do become accidentally overtrimmed, lameness is less likely after drying off because dry cows do not usually have to do as much walking as milkers.

If feet are allowed to reach the stage of overgrowth shown in Plate 9.4, the tendons become stretched and it is unlikely that they will return to the upright position in a single trimming session. This cow could well be damaged for life. However, it is surprising how much can be achieved in a single trimming. Plates 9.18 and 9.19 show a before and after sequence of a fairly badly overgrown claw. Although the toe is not quite making contact with the ground in Plate 9.19, the improvement is obviously considerable.

# FOOT CONDITIONS CAUSING LAMENESS

The majority of conditions causing lameness affect the foot and of these, sole ulcers and white line disease are the most common. In this section lameness in the foot will be subdivided into:

Sole ulcers and white line diseases

Other conditions affecting the hoof: nail penetration, sandcracks and others

Conditions of the skin: foul, digital dermatitis, corns and mud fever

Conditions of the bones and joints

# SOLE ULCERS AND WHITE LINE DISEASE

As the causes of sole ulcers and white line disease are very similar, these two conditions will be dealt with in the same section. A knowledge of the pathogenesis (the internal changes) leading to sole ulcers and white line disease will help us to appreciate the structure and function of the foot and is described in the following section. This knowledge also considerably improves our understanding of the control measures necessary.

## Coriosis (Laminitis)

On page 281 we saw that the horn of the sole was produced by the corium of the sole. Therefore, if the corium becomes damaged or inflamed, horn formation is likely to be changed in some way. Although, as mentioned previously, we often refer to 'laminitis' as meaning inflammation within the foot, in many instances it is either the whole corium which is inflamed, or just the corium of the sole. The term 'coriosis' is therefore more likely to be correct.

Inflammation and damage to the corium can be the result of a range of things, for example:

● trauma
● infection
● nutrition and metabolic disorders
● toxins

However, the overall result will be the same, namely altered horn production.

### Sole haemorrhage and bruising

Inflammation of the corium leads to increased blood flow. This produces congestion in some areas, with pooling of blood and poor oxygenation leading to tissue damage and poor horn formation in others. The whole process results in the corium becoming much more fragile. In the early stages serum (fluid)

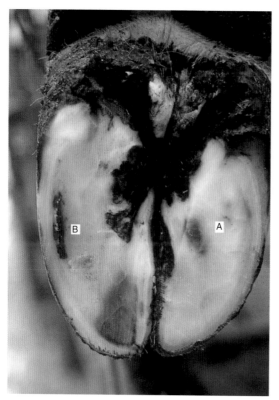

Plate 9.20a. Coriosis: blood released into the horn is seen on the surface of the sole one to two months later. On this foot there is haemorrhage at the ulcer site (A) and the white line (B).

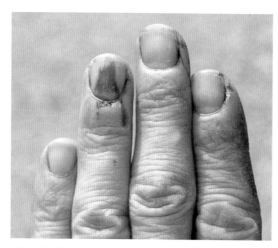

Plate 9.20b. Coriosis: a bruise on a finger (here caused by the author foolishly putting his hand into a cow's mouth without a gag!) grows down along the nail in an identical manner to sole bruising.

leaking from the blood vessels within the inflamed corium is mixed with the horn of the sole as it is being formed. In more advanced cases, rupture of the capillaries produces a mixture of horn and blood. The sole is 5–10 mm thick, so with horn growing at 5 mm each month, it will take one or two months for this deformed and damaged horn to reach the surface. A typical example is shown in Plate 9.20A. There is blood mixed with the horn at both the sole ulcer site A and in the white line B. On the sole adjacent to B especially, the horn has a yellow appearance, due to leakage of serum into the horn. Note that the *wall* of the hoof adjacent to B is still a good, white colour. This horn is considerably older, having been produced at the coronary band several months previously, and so far has not been affected.

Haemorrhage on the sole, seen in Plate 9.20A, is often referred to as bruising. This may be a correct term, although it should always be remembered that the 'bruise' was formed by an insult one or two months previously, when the horn now on the surface of the sole was being produced. As such, bruising of the sole cannot be implicated as a recent cause of lameness.

The effect of mixing serum or blood with the horn can be likened to mixing sawdust with concrete – it weakens it considerably. This is particularly the case with the white line, which is an inherently weak structure, and at the sole ulcer site where there may be almost 'neat sawdust' because so much haemorrhage is present. The whole process is very similar to the changes which occur when your finger-nail is bruised (Plate 9.20B): the blood spot often starts at the corium of the skin–nail junction and then slowly grows to the tip of your nail over the next few months.

*Changes associated with the pedal bone*
In Plate 9.3 we saw that the inner border of the pedal bone is arched in shape. The pedal bone is suspended within the hoof by the laminae, with a much stronger attachment to the outer wall than to the inner one. When weight is transmitted down the leg the bone rotates slightly inwards, putting increased weight on the flexor tuberosity, which is the rear projection of the pedal bone (F in Figure 9.15 and Plate 9.3). Increased weightbearing at this point puts extra pressure on the corium and if it is already in a fragile state, then it is even more likely to become damaged. Pinching of the corium between the pedal bone above and the horn of the

sole beneath can lead to bruising, as shown in Figure 9.15 and Plate 9.20A. This bruising will appear on the surface of the sole one or two months later and may be seen as:

- yellow discolouration – if only serum was released
- haemorrhage – if the blood vessels ruptured
- a sole ulcer – if the damage to the corium was so severe that horn formation was totally disrupted

If there is a generalised inflammation of the corium, the suspension of the pedal bone within the foot is disrupted, allowing the bone to sink within the foot, as shown in Figure 9.16. This further complicates the situation by producing:

- both sole and toe ulcers
- permanent poor horn formation
- expansion and weakening of the white line
- swelling around the coronary band

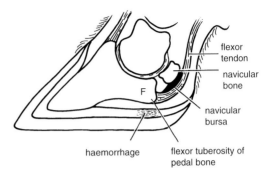

Figure 9.15. Sole ulcer formation. Pinching of the corium between the flexor tuberosity (F) of the pedal bone and the horn of the sole leads to release of blood into the horn.

As the pedal bone sinks within the hoof it displaces the corium out to the side, as shown in Figure 9.16. This produces a very wide, weak white line and a very large and flattened sole. Sometimes the corium is displaced so far to the side that the wall curves outwards. I find such feet particularly difficult to trim. On the one hand you want to bring the claw back to its correct shape, but in so doing it may be necessary to remove all the weightbearing wall. The sinking pedal bone may also displace part of the corium upwards. The upward displacement is seen as a thickened ring of swollen tissue, running around the hoof just above the coronary band, as in Plates 9.18 and 9.19.

As the pedal bone sinks onto the corium, sometimes the front part of the bone sinks before the rear, producing haemorrhage at the toe. This is clearly seen on the left claw in Plate 9.21 and is often referred to as a *toe ulcer* (A). Note how there is also haemorrhage (H) in the white line towards the heel on both claws, extensive yellow discolouration of the sole due to serum infiltration and an early sole ulcer (S).

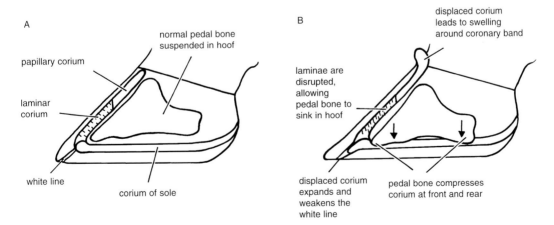

Figure 9.16. In the normal claw (left) the pedal bone is suspended within the hoof by the laminae. Coriosis/laminitis may disrupt this suspension (right), allowing the pedal bone to drop onto the sole, thereby further compressing the corium (courtesy Dr. P. Ossent).

However, it is more usual for the rear edge of the pedal bone to sink within the hoof, pinching the corium under the flexor tuberosity and producing the classic sole ulcer.

Continual compression of the corium of the sole can lead to generalised poor horn formation, sometimes seen in older cows where a sole ulcer fails to heal totally. A layer of very poor-quality horn may form over the ulcer site, and the tip of the flexor tuberosity of the pedal bone can sometimes be palpated as a hard lump just below. Once the pedal bone has sunk within the hoof, it is unlikely ever to regain its original position. This is why it is so important to prevent the development of sole ulcers in heifers.

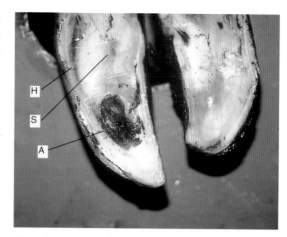

Plate 9.21. A toe ulcer is produced when the front tip of the pedal pinches the corium. (A – toe ulcer, S – sole ulcer, H – white line haemorrhage.)

## Sole Ulcers

A sole ulcer is formed when damage to the corium is so severe that there is total disruption of horn formation. If the foot is pared in the early stages, before the ulcer appears, removal of the surface layers of sole horn may expose a soft area of moist, damaged horn, and yellow/brown fluid will run out (Plate 9.22). This is serum. At this stage there is no infection present, just physical damage. When the damaged horn has worked its way to the surface, infection enters from the environment and the area turns black and necrotic, as in Plate 9.23.

A sole ulcer is a physical condition, caused by trauma, and treatment must be aimed at reducing this trauma. The main steps for treatment are:

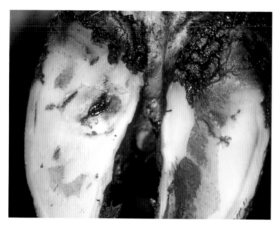

Plate 9.22. Sole ulcer, early stage. Note the discharge of fresh blood and serum at the ulcer site.

- Dish the sole ulcer site so that weightbearing is minimised.
- Remove any under-run horn around the ulcer, to eliminate pockets of necrotic horn and infection, thus allowing the formation of new horn.
- Remove any protruding granulation tissue (shown in Plate 9.24).
- Reduce the size of the affected claw as much as possible, so that weightbearing on the sound claw is maximised.

The use of blocks is an excellent treatment and is described on page 319.

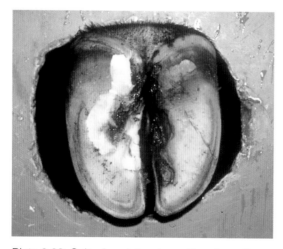

Plate 9.23. Sole ulcer, later stage. The ulcer site has turned black and necrotic.

On occasions, severe or neglected ulcers (or white line abscesses) may allow infection to

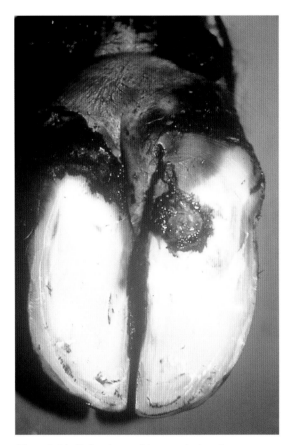

Plate 9.24. Sole ulcer, with granulation tissue protruding from the damaged corium.

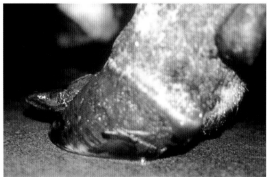

Plate 9.25. Sole ulcers which damage the attachment of the flexor tendon to the pedal bone result in a permanent upward rotation of the toe.

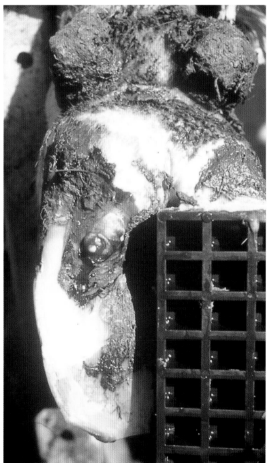

Plate 9.26. A swollen claw and pus discharging from the ulcer site are a clear indication that infection has penetrated deeper structures within the foot.

penetrate into some of the deeper structures within the foot. Examination of Figure 9.15 shows that a sole ulcer lies immediately beneath the point of attachment of the flexor tendon to the pedal bone. Small fragments of white, fibrous tissue can sometimes be seen protruding from deep ulcers. An example is shown in Plate 9.58. These are pieces of flexor tendon. If infection is allowed to progress, there may be total rupture of the tendon, to leave the toe permanently rotated, as in Plate 9.25. Penetration into the deeper structures, such as the navicular bursa or even the pedal joint itself, produces a very severe lameness, with a swollen claw and purulent discharge from the ulcer site, as in Plate 9.26.

Radical treatment is now needed, perhaps using a block (as in Plates 9.26 and 9.58), flushing the abscess, or possibly total amputation of the digit. A block, a very large drainage hole and a long course

The internal changes within the foot which lead to sole ulcers and white line diseases are:

- pinching of the corium between the pedal bone and the horn of the sole
- increased fragility of the corium
- disruption of the pedal bone suspension, allowing it to sink into the hoof
- lateral displacement of the corium of the sole into the white line area and dorsally to the coronary band

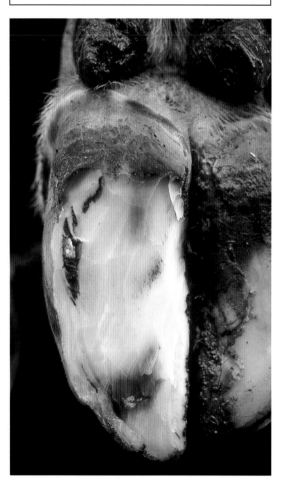

Plate 9.27. White line separation, with a penetrating stone. The stone may be shed by the normal growth of the hoof, or may penetrate deeper until it reaches the corium.

of injectable antibiotics at a high level (for example 7–10 days) will often be successful. Although digit amputation can work well, additional time and effort are needed for regular dressing of the foot, and considerable strain is imposed on the remaining claw.

## Heel and Toe Ulcers

Although sole ulcers are by far the most common, there can be areas of haemorrhage or even total perforation at other areas of the sole. Toe ulcers are thought to occur when the pedal bone sinks within the hoof 'bows first', that is the front of the pedal bone drops before the flexor tuberosity at the rear (Plate 9.21). Heel ulcers (sometimes referred to as 'necrotic heel tracts') are seen as small dark red/black marks in the central sole area towards the heel. Some simply track down to the corium and fade to nothing. Others lead to under-running of horn at the sole–heel junction and can produce a marked lameness. The cause of these heel ulcers is not known, although one theory is that they are produced by a pinching of the corium under the rear edge of the pedal bone.

## White Line Diseases

Weakening of the white line, brought about by the inflammation associated with laminitis/coriosis, can result in a range of white line disorders. The most common of these are:

- sterile abscessation
- white line separation
- white line penetration and abscess

Sometimes the internal inflammation within the foot is so severe that pockets of necrotic tissue are formed. These can produce a sterile internal abscess and as there may be no obvious tracks running from the outside, they may be quite difficult to locate and treat. In severe forms of coriosis the whole sole becomes separated by an accumulation of inflammatory fluid. When foot trimming you may have seen a total layer of sole separated from the new sole underneath. This is known as a *false sole*.

More commonly the weakened white line starts to open up, a process known as white line separation. This occurs especially if the cows are walking over rough or stony ground, or when they make sudden turning movements, as when escaping from an aggressive cow. Small stones may then become impacted, as in Plate 9.27, and with continued walking these may eventually penetrate the corium.

The most common point for white line separation and penetration is on the outer wall, near to the heel, as in Plate 9.27 or point 3 in Figure 9.13B. During locomotion this is where there are the greatest sheer forces between the rigid hoof wall, the suspended pedal bone and the movements of the flexible heel. Once the corium has been penetrated, the invading foreign body (usually a stone or grit) introduces infection. The bacteria multiply to produce pus and the expanding pus then has to find the easiest way of escape.

For white line abscesses near to the heel, this escape route is usually through the soft horn of the heel, as in Plate 9.28. White line abscesses close to the toe do not have such an easy escape route and often infection tracks upwards through the laminae, to discharge at the coronary band, as in Plate 9.29. This produces a more severe lameness because, as shown in Figure 9.1, the pedal bone is tightly attached to the hoof towards the toe and there is therefore very little room for the pus to expand.

Whereas a sole ulcer results in damage to the underlying corium, the majority of uncomplicated white line lesions only produce separation of the horn from the underlying horn-forming corium. (Note: the word 'lesion' means any pathological change in a tissue. In this instance 'lesion' could be separation, haemorrhage, abscess etc.). White line lesions normally heal much more quickly, therefore, than sole ulcers. In Plate 9.28 you can see how pulling back the flap of sole horn with a hoof knife exposes a pink tissue. This is corium covered by epidermis and it will soon form another good layer of protective horn.

The treatment of a white line abscess is very similar to that for a sole ulcer, namely:

- Remove all under-run horn, even if this means removing the wall from the sole to the coronary band (as in Plate 9.30), or the whole of an under-run sole.
- Reduce the size of the affected claw, to minimise weightbearing, and leave the sound claw as large as possible.

Blocks and dressings are discussed on page 319.

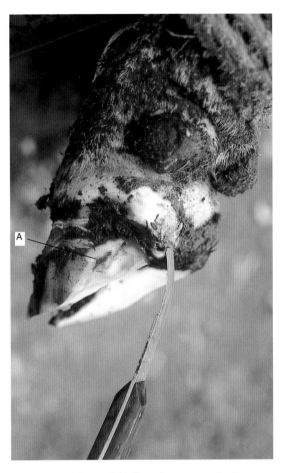

Plate 9.28. Many white line abscesses discharge at the heel. The original point of entry of infection is at A.

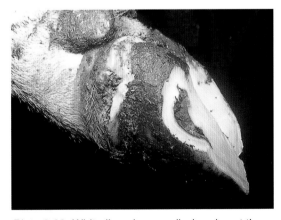

Plate 9.29. White line abscess discharging at the coronary band.

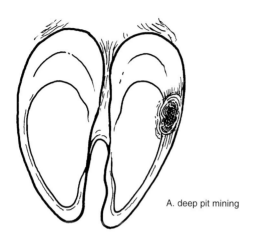

A. deep pit mining

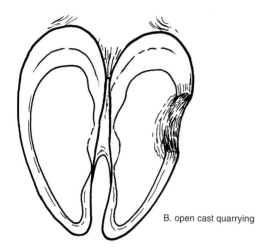

B. open cast quarrying

Figure 9.17. When searching for white line abscesses the technique should be one of 'open cast quarrying' (B), not 'deep pit mining' (A).

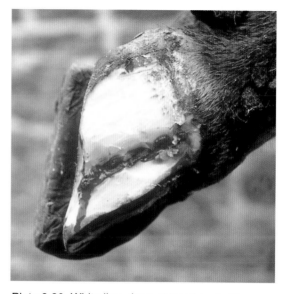

Plate 9.30. White line abscess treatment. All under-run horn must be removed.

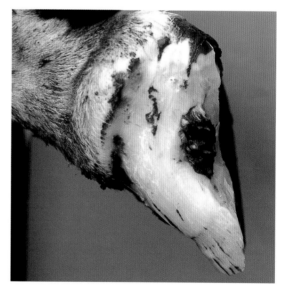

Plate 9.31. Protrusion of granulation tissue from the original white line abscess site probably means that there is further under-run horn. The coronary band is also swollen, suggesting infection of the deeper tissue.

When using a hoof knife to drain infection from the white line, the approach should be one of 'open cast quarrying' rather than 'deep pit mining'. This difference is shown in Figure 9.17. Digging a deep pit with the curved point of the hoof knife has two disadvantages, namely:

- It leaves a pit which can easily become impacted with stones or dirt, thereby impeding drainage and pre-disposing to further white line impaction.
- By digging a pit you are much more likely to miss areas of under-run horn and pockets of infection.

If a small area of adjacent wall is removed, it is much easier to expose and drain the affected area. Complications can occur with white line abscesses, particularly those which track up the wall (e.g. Plate 9.30). Plate 9.31 is a typical example. Note the granulation tissue protruding from the original site of white line penetration and how the coronary band area is enlarged and inflamed.

Protruding granulation tissue is often an indication that there is adjacent under-run horn which needs to be removed. The swollen coronary band is probably caused by infection tracking into deeper structures such as the navicular bursa or tendon sheaths. A similar change is produced when the pedal bone 'sinks' onto the corium of the sole in acute coriosis (see Figure 9.16).

## Causes and Control of Sole Ulcers and White Line Diseases

This is a huge subject, enough to fill a whole textbook on its own, and the reader must appreciate that only an outline can be given in this section. The internal changes within the foot leading to sole ulcers and white line disease were described on page 293. In the following the many environmental, managemental and nutritional factors which cause these changes is given. These could be listed in a variety of ways, but the system I have chosen, namely relating aetiology to pathogenesis, will, I hope, give a clearer understanding of how lameness is best controlled.

Earlier in the chapter I said that increased fragility of the corium predisposed to both sole ulcers and white line disease. So what causes increased fragility of the corium and what predisposes to damage? This will be covered under the following headings:

- calving
- excessive standing
- nutrition
- general management

### Calving

There can be no doubt that calving (or maybe the start of lactation) is a major stressor on horn formation. We only have to look at the rings on a cow's horns to see this. Plate 9.32 is a picture of Pinky, a thirteen-year-old cow from Figtree, Zimbabwe. She had only six calves in her thirteen years – not exactly a stressful life! – but note the six rings on her horns. There is one ring for each calving (although it is accepted that disease or periods of severe undernutrition can sometimes produce the same effect). Look at the bull's horns shown in Plate 9.5: you will not see any rings present, irrespective of his age. There is something about calving which produces a disruption in horn formation and this occurs in both the horns and the feet. It also explains why the peak incidence of lameness occurs one or two months after calving: this is because it takes this length of time for the horn produced at calving to work its way down to the surface of the sole.

The natural decrease in rumination at the time of calving, leading to periods of rumen atony and potential acidosis, was discussed in Chapter 6, Figure 6.8. The importance of feeding long straw at this time to stimulate rumen contractions after

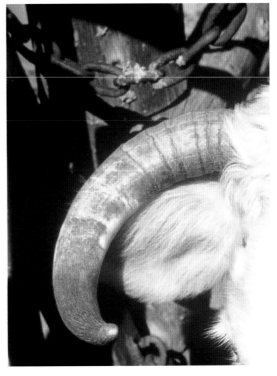

Plate 9.32. There are rings on a cow's horn, one for each calving. Disruption of horn formation also occurs in the claw. (Courtesy M. Conolly)

calving was also described. It is still not known why acidosis produces coriosis/laminitis, but bacterial endotoxins, leading to damage of the minute blood vessels (capillaries) within the foot, could be a factor.

Acute phase proteins are most commonly produced in response to disease. It is therefore interesting that the cow also experiences a marked rise in acute phase proteins at calving, especially as in the immediate post-partum period she is particularly susceptible to infection. Severe inflammation, caused by any disease, can

> It is not yet known why there is such a marked disruption in horn formation at calving. Suggested causes include:
>
> - reduced rumination times
> - an increase in acute phase proteins (for example, haptoglobulins)
> - repartition of sulphur amino acids towards milk production
> - cows (and especially heifers) spend longer standing immediately after calving
> - the greater susceptibility of the cow to illness around the time of calving

disrupt horn formation and lead to horizontal fissures (page 312), so could calving simply be an extension of this process? We know that administration of cortisone to horses can induce laminitis/coriosis and also that the 'signal' to initiate the process of calving is cortisone produced by the developing foetus (Chapter 5). Could these processes be connected with lameness?

Calving also sees the start of lactation. As milk production rapidly rises there is an enormous increase in the demand for sulphur-containing amino acids, because many are essential for lactation. Recent work has shown that horn produced at the time of calving has a lower sulphur content. Sulphur is an important ingredient of keratin, the protein which leads to hardening of horn; therefore an inadequate supply of sulphur will lead to soft horn. This in itself would not be sufficient to cause the enormous damage seen in the feet of some heifers, but it could be a contributory factor.

Even if they calve outside in a field, for a few days after calving, cows and especially heifers will spend far more time standing and their lying times will be decreased. There is therefore more weight on the corium and a greater potential for bruising. It is not known whether the decreased lying times are due to nursing behaviour (attending to the calf), discomfort from the perineum (vulva or vagina), an enlarged udder or some other factor.

Diseases such as mastitis and metritis are certainly more common immediately after calving and as we know from hooves with horizontal fissures (page 312), acute illness affects horn formation. However, this will only involve individual animals.

*Excessive standing*

Anything which leads to a decrease in lying times, especially in the immediate post calving period when the corium is in its most fragile state, will increase the incidence of sole ulcers and white line disease. Heifers are likely to be the most greatly affected, and the worst case scenario of heifers entering a dairy herd which was described in the section on stress in Chapter 8 (page 268) should be read in conjunction with the following.

> Increased lying times can be achieved by:
>
> - maximising cubicle comfort, or using straw yards for the first few weeks after calving
> - encouraging animals to enter cubicle houses
> - training heifers to use cubicles during rearing
> - minimising the time animals spend waiting to be milked and fed
> - providing ample loafing and exercise areas
> - avoiding overcrowding

One experiment deliberately housed heifers in an overstocked cubicle building (17 cubicles for 35 heifers) immediately after calving. Although the average lying time of the heifers was ten hours, some animals lay down for as little as five hours each day. This group showed the highest incidence of lameness, and quite severe haemorrhage persisted in the sole horn for up to four months after calving. In most dairy systems the heifers are forced to spend longer on their feet after calving. They will be waiting to be milked, they spend longer standing and feeding because they are often last to feed, and they need to eat more as lactation proceeds. They have recently been mixed with the main herd and are now having to compete with older cows. Fear may restrict their entry into a cubicle shed, especially if they are of low social dominance and have had no previous cubicle training.

Excessive standing may be bad for the immediate post-partum cow, but standing still is even worse. If the animal does not move around enough, the pumping mechanisms of the heel and digital cushion will be impaired, the blood will become 'stale', due to a lack of nutrients (particularly oxygen), and tissue damage, with poor horn formation, will result. It is essential that there are adequate loafing areas to allow the cows to walk around freely. Overcrowding should be avoided, even in collecting yards. Animals which are packed tightly together have little option but to stand still. Adequate loafing areas also help to improve fertility.

In summary, the incidence of sole ulcers and white line disease will be markedly reduced if animals are encouraged to maximise lying times in the immediate post calving period, for example, for the first two to six weeks.

**Post calving comfort** Of all the above factors, cubicle comfort is probably the most important. Cubicles may make the management of cows easy, but they are not always ideal in terms of cow comfort and lameness. For example, in a survey of dairy herds carried out by Edinburgh University, the incidence of lameness in cows housed in straw yards was only 5%, compared with 25% for cubicles. This must point to cubicles being less than ideal, especially for the immediately post calving cow. In fact a small but increasing proportion of farms are now housing their freshly calved cows in straw yards for the first two to six weeks after calving and then transferring them to cubicles. Experience from such systems suggests that in heifers especially, a post calving period of straw yard housing leads to:

- increased yields
- a decreased incidence of lameness
- improved cubicle acceptance when the heifers are eventually transferred from the straw yard to the cubicles

The third factor is perhaps the most surprising. One might have expected that cows and heifers which had got used to a straw yard would be very difficult to retrain to use cubicles. The fact that the reverse is true probably tells us that calving is a much more stressful experience than we think and that it is only when the cows have fully recovered that they are able to withstand the rigours of the cubicle system.

**Cubicle design** Cubicle comfort is obviously all-important. Ideally, cubicles should be long enough and wide enough (1.15 m wide and 2.4 m long) to accommodate the larger Holstein cows and with sufficient space at the front to allow the cow to lunge forwards 1–1.5 m as she stands up. If there are two facing rows of cubicles, a length of 2.2 m is adequate.

A good design is shown in Figure 9.18; there is a wide range of other designs which may be equally comfortable. This has a 100 mm fall from front to rear, a step of not more

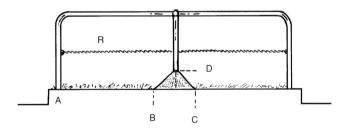

Figure 9.18. Cubicle design is important for comfort. They should be 1.15 m wide. A central concrete triangle BCD helps to position the cow correctly. A flexible rope R improves acceptance. (Courtesy John Hughes)

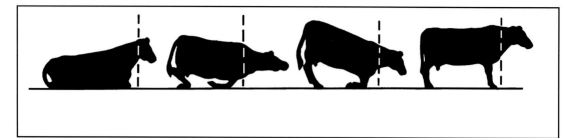

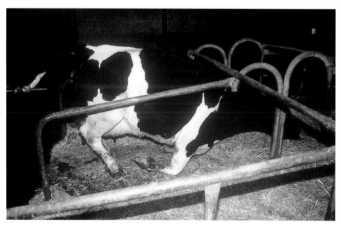

Plate 9.33. As a cow lunges forward to stand, she places enormous weight on her knees. The front of the cubicle therefore needs to be very well bedded.

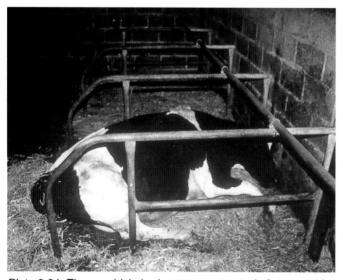

Plate 9.34. These cubicle beds were constructed of stone and only a thin layer of straw. In trying to get comfortable, this cow shuffled so far forward to the front wall that she was unable to stand up.

Figure 9.19. When rising, a cow lunges forward 1–1.5 m and puts enormous weight on her knees.

than 130 mm down into the dunging channel and an interesting concrete pyramid at the front. This pyramid prevents the cow from shuffling too far forwards, but at the same time provides ample space for lunging as she stands up. When rising she may place one foot on the slope of the concrete, to push herself up, but when fully standing she will have to keep her feet behind B and will then defaecate in the dunging channel. A neck rail is often not necessary and this may further increase cubicle comfort. The flexible rope division (R) eliminates pelvic damage which could occur with a solid central rail and it also avoids compression of the rumen.

If sitting in the cubicle means that the cow's rumen is excessively compressed, or if there is insufficient space for her to extend her neck whilst regurgitating the cud, the cow is more likely to stand up to chew the cud, rather than do it lying down. Again, this will increase trauma to the feet. Cubicles with a high step (greater than 130 mm) from the dunging passage, with low bottom rails and with limited lunging space, have all been associated with increased lameness.

When attempting to stand, the cow lunges forwards 1–1.5 m and lifts herself first on to her hind feet, then up on to her front feet (Figure 9.19 and Plate 9.33). When she is lying down or half standing, therefore, much of her weight is taken on her knees. If the floor surface is hard under her knees and particularly if it is also rough, cubicle acceptance will be low. The worst possible cubicle floor is a stone base, poorly compacted and with insufficient straw. This was provided for the cow in Plate 9.34. In an attempt to get comfortable she kept shuffling forwards – until she was so far forwards and so close to the wall that she was unable to stand. In the struggling, her back legs came forwards under her and by the time she was found in the morning such severe muscle damage had developed that she never stood up again. A cow lost, simply because the cubicle was uncomfortable. (There was also a very high incidence of lameness in this herd.) If you are finding a proportion of your cows stuck too far forward in the cubicles, re-examine cubicle comfort.

Most cubicle bases are made of concrete. This is fine provided the cubicle is *deeply* bedded, although it is often difficult to get the straw to stay in. If this is the case, first put a 150 mm layer of rotted muck (for example, from the calf shed) onto the bare concrete at the *front* of the cubicle and then put clean straw on top of it. 'Composted' bedding from a straw yard does not have a particularly high *E. coli* level and its use does not pre-dispose to mastitis, provided that plenty of clean straw is added to the top. It dries quickly and forms a good bed which adheres to the base of the cubicle. A variety of mats are available and these are certainly much better than concrete alone. However, some bedding should be used, even with mats; otherwise hock sores will develop (Plate 9.64). A disadvantage of mats is that it is difficult to get large amounts of straw bedding to adhere to them, although the cows enjoy standing on them.

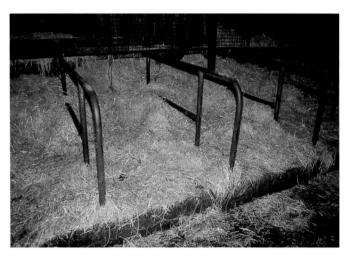

Plate 9.35. Luxury cubicle bedding. Although the cubicles are not ideal dimensions, the use of large quantities of straw made them very comfortable. (Courtesy M. Boynton.)

The best cubicles are comfortable cubicles and if you can make them like mini-straw yards, so much the better. While design and dimensions may be important, I am convinced that comfort is of even greater significance. The cubicles illustrated in Plate 9.35 are an example. Although these cubicles measured only 1.07 m by 2.05 m and housed large Friesian/Holstein cross cows, they were regularly bedded as shown, with straw 380 mm deep, up to the bottom rail! Needless to say, they were extremely comfortable and as a result, the incidence of lameness was minimal. Another design of high comfort cubicles, deeply bedded and having a highly flexible division, is shown in Plate 9.36.

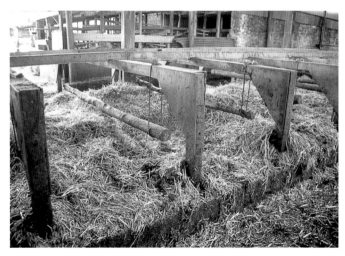

Plate 9.36. Luxury cubicle bedding with flexible dimensions for even greater comfort. (Courtesy R. Troughton.)

*Nutrition*

Although it is not easy to prove experimentally, diets which lead to acidosis undoubtedly predispose to coriosis/laminitis and subsequent lameness. The type of diet likely to cause acidosis and the prevention of dietary problems in general was discussed in Chapter 6.

Concentrate intakes should be built up slowly after calving, to reach a peak no earlier than two weeks post calving for average yielding cows and probably three weeks for higher yielding animals, which peak later. If there is a sudden change in diet to high concentrate feeding at calving, then problems may occur. For example, when the heifer whose foot is depicted in Plate 9.21 calved, her diet was immediately changed from an all forage (grazing) pre calving ration to a high fat, low forage out of parlour mix, together with 7 kg concentrate in the parlour. The resulting coriosis/laminitis produced severe lameness with both toe and sole ulcers and white line haemorrhage. Ideally no more than 4.5 kg of feed should be given in the parlour. The inclusion of 1–3 kg of long-chop straw, well mixed with the ration, helps enormously, in that it stimulates rumination, thereby promoting a good flow of saliva and decreasing acidosis. There is evidence that maintaining an ideal dietary cation–anion balance (DCAB, Chapter 6) may also help.

It is the composition of the ration and not its overall energy content which seems to affect the incidence of lameness. Table 9.1 shows two groups of cows, one of which (A) was fed a high fibre diet and the other (B) a low fibre and high concentrate ration. Both rations had the same overall crude protein (CP) content and both achieved the same energy (ME) intake, although the high fibre group clearly needed a higher dry matter intake to do so. The high

> The most common dietary faults associated with lameness are:
>
> ● a sudden increase in concentrates after calving
> ● too much concentrate fed in a single feed in the parlour
> ● insufficient long fibre
> ● high starch and high oil

incidence of coriosis/laminitis and sole ulcers in the low fibre group is striking. Despite regular foot trimming, group B also had a higher incidence of solar overgrowths (as in Plate 9.7). Although high protein diets have occasionally been suggested as a cause of coriosis, most people consider protein to be of less importance than other factors. High intakes of poorly fermented grass silage have been implicated, although this could be due to toxic amines rather than high protein.

Even feeding during rearing influences the incidence of sole haemorrhage, with heifers fed high levels of concentrate being the worst affected. As discussed in Chapter 4, high fibre diets are now recommended for rearing dairy heifers.

Many attempts have been made to improve hoof condition by mineral, vitamin and trace element supplementation. The use of zinc, particularly zinc methionine, is often promoted as a feed supplement having beneficial effects. If one of the reasons for the production of

Table 9.1. Two groups of cows having the same total daily protein energy intake, but Group A was fed a high fibre diet and Group B a low fibre diet.

| | ME (MJ/kg) | CP (g/kg) | No. showing clinical coriosis/ laminitis | No. showing sole ulcers |
|---|---|---|---|---|
| Group A: | | | | |
| 26 cows fed a high fibre diet | 10.8 | 158 | 2 (8%) | 2 (8%) |
| Group B: | | | | |
| 25 cows fed a low fibre diet | 11.1 | 157 | 17 (68%) | 16 (64%) |

Livesey & Flemming (1984), *Vet. Rec.* 114 510.

poor-quality horn at calving is a temporary deficit of sulphur amino acids, then it is logical to think that supplementation with zinc methionine might be beneficial at this time, since methionine is a sulphur amino acid and zinc promotes healing.

Biotin has been shown to improve horn quality in both pigs and horses and a recent two year detailed study in Canada demonstrated that supplementation with biotin significantly reduced the incidence of vertical fissures (sandcracks) in beef suckler cows. Cows which received a supplement of 10 mg biotin each day were 2.5 times less likely to develop vertical fissures than the control cows. Biotin has also been shown to improve the rate of healing of sole ulcers and white line lesions.

### General management

Many aspects of management have already been discussed in the housing and feeding sections above. This section will cover a few miscellaneous points relating to lameness and also place particular emphasis on those factors which might damage the corium, especially in the freshly calved or early lactation animal.

**Wet hooves** Wet hoof is softer than dry hoof and therefore the sole is more likely to become penetrated or bruised if the feet are damp. Cubicle passages should be scraped twice daily, and the addition of small quantities of slaked lime to the cubicle beds once a week (Plate 7.21) will help to dry the feet as well as control mastitis.

**Poor foot surfaces** Floor surfaces should not be too rough, stony or have broken concrete, all of which can damage the corium. On the other hand, very slippery surfaces can lead to leg damage.

One of the best demonstrations I have ever seen of the fact that cows do not like walking on concrete is shown in Plate 9.37. A strip of second-hand rubber belting, approximately 1.5 m wide, was laid along the centre of a concrete track which runs from a dirt yard to the milking parlour at a dairy in California. Although the cows can walk anywhere they wish on the track, note how they all prefer to walk on the rubber belt. This was particularly the case when it was raining, as you can see from the photograph.

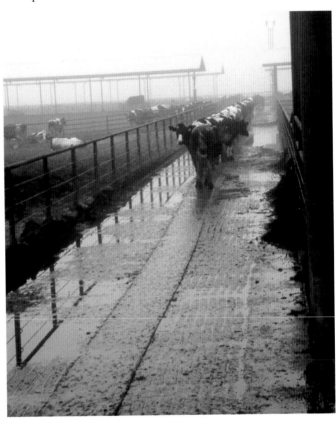

Plate 9.37. Proof that cows prefer to walk on a soft surface: they had the option of the whole width of concrete roadway, but preferred walking on the rubber belting in the centre. (Courtesy Karl Burgi.)

Management factors influencing lameness include:

- wet hooves, leading to soft horn
- poor foot surfaces
- rough handling
- inadequate or excessive hoof wear
- poor conformation
- routine foot trimming
- footbaths

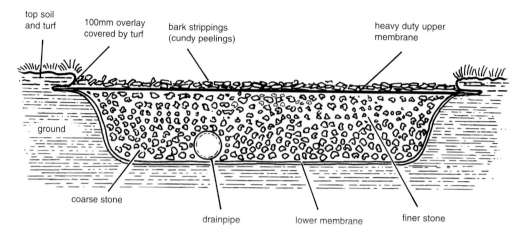

Figure 9.20. Construction of specific cow tracks provides a soft and comfortable walkway, helping to reduce lameness. (Courtesy John Hughes).

In the UK, if cows are allowed to amble out to a field at their own speed, they will usually choose to do so by walking on the soft earth of a grass verge, rather than on stones (Plate 9.38, right). They even place their feet in exactly the same spot each time, making holes in the ground. This preference for a softer surface has led to the development of specific cow tracks, as in Plate 9.38 (left) and Figure 9.20. The ground is excavated to 300 mm deep and 1–1.5 m wide and lined with a permeable geotextile membrane, a road construction membrane which prevents sinkage of the track. A drainage pipe runs along the base, surrounded by a large aggregate, perhaps having fine stone on the top. This is covered with a second special toughened membrane, which allows water to drain down through but will not allow mud to rise up through it. Finally a layer of bark strippings, sometimes

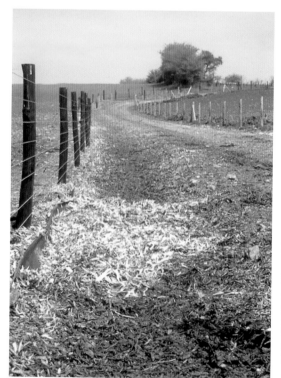

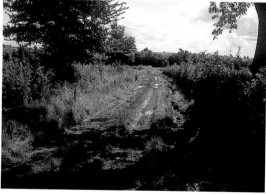

Plate 9.38. Specially constructed bark track will improve cow comfort and reduce lameness. (Courtesy Richard Cooke.)

known as cundy peelings, 100 mm deep, is placed on top of the upper membrane to provide a comfortable walking surface for the cows. It must not be used by tractors and other vehicles.

Similar tracks may be constructed in gateways and around water troughs and in other areas where the ground gets badly poached. Plate 9.38 (left) shows a track running from the dairy down to fields half a mile away. Although the cows walked in almost single file along the track, they came up much more quickly than when they could only walk on the stony roadway. On very well drained land some farmers have constructed a simple track by scraping away the top soil and then unrolling a large round straw bale onto the underlying stone. Wet bales too badly soiled for straw yards can be used. The straw needs replacing approximately every two or three weeks, depending on the weather, but it makes a good track and is certainly cheaper.

The influence of floor surface on white line disease is interesting. It is commonly stated that cows become lame because of a specific type of stone or gravel in a track, particularly if sharp flints are present. However, beef cattle could almost certainly walk along the same track without the stones penetrating their feet – which suggests that it is the softening of the hoof and the weakening of the white line which are the critical factors and not the sharpness of the stones!

**Rough handling** Rough handling also has an effect. A survey of farms showed that cows which were forcibly rushed along farm tracks by a herdsman, dog or tractor had a far higher incidence of lameness than farms where the cows were allowed to walk along at their own speed. This was presumably because in the latter case they chose their own footing, thus minimising bruising to the sole and corium.

**Hoof wear** Both inadequate and excessive hoof wear can cause problems. Heifers reared and housed in totally bedded areas (straw, shavings or sand) do not get sufficient hoof wear. The toes become overgrown, the foot rotates backwards and the corium becomes damaged. The provision of a lightly abrasive concrete feeding area is essential. At the other extreme, cows or heifers (and especially fresh calvers) which are made to walk long distances on gravel or even concrete roads can wear their soles so thin that they are easily compressed by thumb pressure.

A similar 'soft sole' syndrome is seen in young bulls introduced to work in a dairy herd, particularly if the bulls are large and do not use the cubicles. The soles of their hind feet can wear down to the corium. Ideally bulls in cubicle systems should be rested in a straw yard, for example cubicles by day and a straw yard by night, or alternate weeks in cubicles and straw yards. On a daily basis bulls soon learn which is to be their period of lying down and compensate for the cubicles by lying down for long periods in the straw yards.

**Conformation** Conformation affects the incidence of lameness, which is therefore influenced by genetics and breeding. Bulls should be chosen to give a good depth of heel and a good upright angle of the front wall, as in Figure 9.7.

**Foot trimming** The final management factor which influences the degree of bruising of the corium is routine foot trimming – and this brings the discussion almost round in a full circle! If calving is a major stress period for the development of coriosis/laminitis, then feet need to be in optimum shape at calving in order to minimise this effect. This means trimming at drying off, especially removing overgrown toes and overgrowth of the sole, both of which could damage the fragile corium of the freshly calved cow.

The use of footbaths is discussed on page 318.

## OTHER CAUSES OF FOOT LAMENESS

I have dealt extensively with sole ulcers and white line disorders because they are two of the most important causes of lameness and because their control is so complex. Other causes of foot lameness are:

**Hoof disorders**
　　foreign body penetration
　　slurry heel

haematoma in the heel
vertical fissures (sandcracks)
hardship lines and coriosis
horizontal fissures
broken toe

### Skin disorders
interdigital necrobacillosis (foul or
footrot)
digital dermatitis (hairy warts) and
interdigital dermatitis
interdigital skin hyperplasia (corns,
growths or tylomas)
mud fever

### Bone and joint disorders
pedal bone fracture
pedal bone tip necrosis
pedal arthritis

## Foreign Body Penetration of the Sole

Typical foreign bodies are stones (especially sharp flints), nails (particularly those with flat heads), fragments of wood, glass or tin, and occasionally even the sharp root of a cast tooth will penetrate the sole. Treatment is very similar to that for white line disease (page 299), namely remove the foreign body and then all under-run horn. In Plate 9.39 a nail has been removed but obviously there is still under-run horn towards the heel at A. This must be pared away to allow new horn formation on the underlying corium.

## Slurry Heel

The smooth, soft and pliable horn of a normal heel can be seen in Plates 9.23 and 9.24. In feet which have been exposed to slurry over a long period of time, the heel horn often becomes black and pitted and in more extreme cases totally eroded, as in the foot with digital dermatitis (Plate 9.47). Although per-

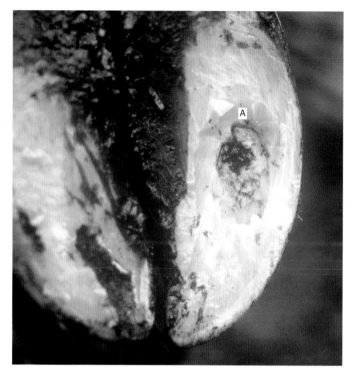

Plate 9.39. Puncture of the sole by a foreign body. The red area of corium is the initial point of penetration. There is still more under-run sole to be removed at A.

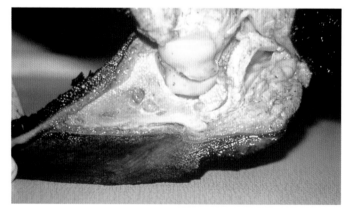

Plate 9.40. Advanced slurry heel removes support from the pedal bone which then pinches the underlying corium. An external view of slurry heel is shown in Plate 9.47.

haps not looking too serious from the outside, slurry heel causes important internal changes. Removal of weightbearing at the heel allows the foot to rotate backwards, thereby predisposing to sole ulcers, as explained in Figure 9.15. Plate 9.40 shows an advanced case in which the flexor tuberosity at the rear of the pedal bone no longer has adequate support and as a result is penetrating the horn of the sole. The corium at this point will be pinched every time the cow walks. Slurry heel is controlled by keeping the feet clean and dry, using lime in cubicles, frequent scraping of cubicle passages and footbaths (page 318).

## Haematoma in the Heel

A haematoma (blood blister) in the heel is almost certainly a result of trauma. Most cases occur in cows walking to and from grazing. Uncomplicated cases produce only a slight swelling of the heel bulb and mild lameness, and can be treated by incising the heel and draining the blood (as would be done for similar damage to a human finger-nail). In some cases the haematoma develops into an abscess or may even lead to necrosis and a total slough of heel tissue. More extensive drainage and use of a shoe on the sound claw are then required.

## Vertical Fissures (Sandcracks)

Vertical fissures occur as a result of damage to a small area of the periople and underlying coronary band. Horn formation is then disrupted at that point, although the adjacent horn continues to grow. This leaves a gap (the vertical fissure) running down the hoof wall from the point of disrupted production (Plate 9.41). In North America vertical fissures are commonly seen in both grazing beef cattle and older dairy cows kept in sand lots, where the combination of age, sand, wind and dry weather removes the protective periople. Vertical fissures can also occur as a result of a digital dermatitis infection on the coronary band (Plate 9.50). Supplementation of the diet with biotin (10 mg per cow per day) may help to prevent fissures.

For treatment, pare out the fissure using the curved tip of the hoof knife. A small abscess may be found under the wall, as in Plate 9.42. If the fissure is large and runs full length, apply a block as in Plate 9.50.

## Hardship Lines

Any disruption in horn formation may leave a groove, sometimes referred to as

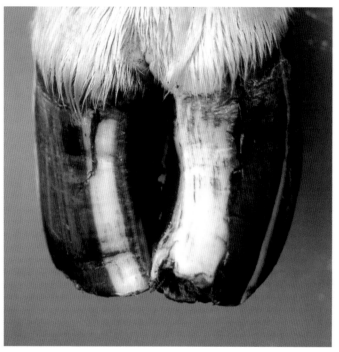

Plate 9.41. A vertical fissure is a split running down the front wall of the hoof.

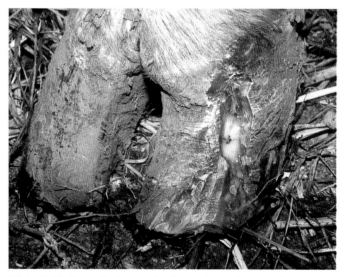

Plate 9.42. A small abscess in the laminae of the corium beneath a vertical fissure made this cow extremely lame.

a hardship groove, encircling the hoof wall. These are the result of coriosis/laminitis. Inflammation of the laminae leads to massive pressure under the hoof wall, causing the wall to push forward and the toe to lift, as in Figure 9.21. The eventual effect is a concave front wall with numerous hardship lines. In Plate 9.4 note the obvious bands of hardship lines running parallel to and just down from the coronary band.

## Horizontal Fissures

If an animal is severely ill, for example with mastitis, metritis or any toxic condition, there may be a total cessation of horn formation for a while. When horn production starts again, instead of there being a hardship groove, there may be a horizontal fissure completely encircling the hoof wall. Initially this may cause no problem, but as the defect grows down towards the toe it loses its support and attachment from the heel. The protruding 'thimble' of horn is then able to move on the underlying corium, causing pinching, pain and lameness. A typical example is shown in Plate 9.43. This cow had been badly affected by foot-and-mouth disease some three months previously and as a result had a horizontal fissure on the claws of all four feet. The date of the illness can be calculated by measuring the distance from the coronary band to the fissure (approximately 15 mm) and dividing this by the rate of horn growth, namely 5 mm per month: 15 divided by 5 = 3 months.

For treatment, remove the loose 'thimble' of horn. If the corium is extensively exposed, apply a block to the sound claw. However, beware: not all horizontal fissures lead to lameness. Some simply grow to the toe and are shed naturally. It is only necessary to trim the foot if the cow is lame. A cow with one long claw and one short, due to the horizontal fissure fragment having been shed from one claw only, is sometimes referred to as having a broken toe. This is shown in Plate 9.44.

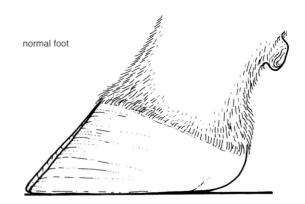

normal foot

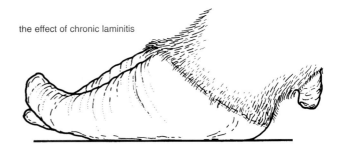

the effect of chronic laminitis

Figure 9.21. Laminitis distorts claw growth and may produce hardship lines, a concave front wall, an upward rotation of the toes and sinking of the heel.

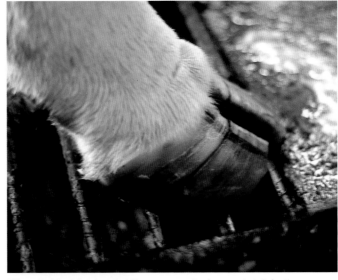

Plate 9.43. A horizontal fissure results from a total, but temporary, cessation of horn formation, usually caused by illness (in this case foot-and-mouth).

## Interdigital Necrobacillosis (Foul, Lewer, Foot Rot)

This is a bacterial infection of the interdigital cleft, caused by two organisms:

- *Bacteroides melaninogenicus* initially penetrates the skin surface and allows the entry of the secondary organism, namely:
- *Fusobacterium necrophorum* invades and its necrotising toxins destroy the deeper tissues of the dermis which causes the lameness.

Disease may be seen in both young calves and adult animals. Initially there is swelling of the foot, which typically pushes the claws apart. Soon after, the skin between the claws splits (Plate 9.45) to reveal pus, necrotic debris and sometimes blood. Some say that there is a characteristic smell. In untreated cases the infection may track up the tendon sheaths of the leg, or penetrate the pedal joint, both producing severe lameness.

Treatment is simply antibiotic by injection, but the foot should always be checked to ensure that there is no stick or stone present penetrating the interdigital skin. For control, ensure that cattle are not exposed to sticks, stones or thorns which might

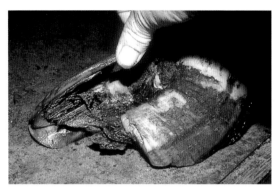

Plate 9.44. The thimble of loose horn beyond a horizontal fissure is sometimes referred to as a broken toe.

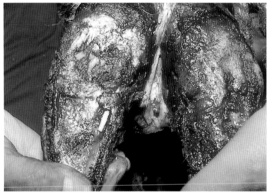

Plate 9.45. Interdigital necrobacillosis (foul, footrot, lewer) is recognised as a split in the skin between the claws.

damage the interdigital skin and make sure that areas around water and feed troughs are kept clean, as this is an area where infection can be transmitted from cow to cow. Footbaths (page 318) can also help.

In the UK a new and highly virulent form, colloquially termed 'super foul', sometimes occurs (Plate 9.46). The damage caused to the foot in as little as 24 hours is spectacular. No new strains of bacteria have been isolated, but most affected herds have a concurrent digital dermatitis infection which probably allows the entry of higher challenge doses of the 'foul' organisms. Prompt and prolonged antibiotic (for five to seven days or more) is needed for treatment. It has been suggested that strapping clindamycin or a similar antibiotic which is effective against anaerobic bacteria into the interdigital cleft may also help.

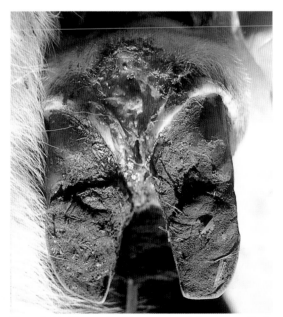

Plate 9.46. 'Super foul' is a colloquial term applied to an extremely virulent form of the disease which produces severe damage.

## Digital Dermatitis (Hairy Warts)

Digital dermatitis is another bacterial infection of the skin, but this time only the surface layer (the epidermis) is involved. It is caused by a spirochaete, probably a member of the *Treponema* family, but despite the worldwide incidence of the disease the organism has yet to be precisely identified.

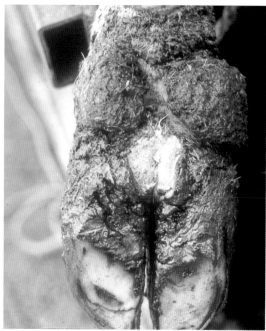

Early cases are typically seen as a moist, light greyish-brown area of exudate, with matted hairs, situated on the skin between the heel bulbs at the back of the foot (Plate 9.47). Cleaning the lesion reveals:

- a red, raw or necrotic area radiating out from the interdigital pouch. This pouch is at the rear of the interdigital cleft and often acts as a reservoir of infection
- a characteristic pungent, sulphur-like smell, thought to be caused by the Treponema bacteria decomposing the keratin within the skin
- intense pain, surprisingly so for what appears to be a relatively mild lesion

The above is a description of a typical acute lesion.

Chronic, longstanding cases produce the syndrome of hairy warts (Plate 9.48), common in North America but rarely seen in the UK. The filaments of these warts are in fact lengths of epidermis produced by the skin growing as fast as possible in an attempt to shed the organism from its surface. Because of their chronic nature, hairy warts are more difficult to treat than 'standard' digital dermatitis.

Although digital dermitis typically radiates from its reservoir in the interdigital pouch (as in

Plate 9.47. Digital dermatitis is seen as a moist, painful, smelly area, grey or red, radiating out from the interdigital pouch. Slurry heel is also present.

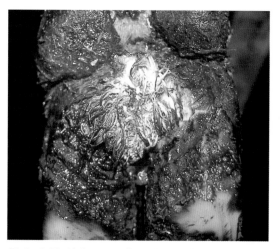

Plate 9.48. Hairy warts is a chronic form of digital dermatitis. The filaments of the warts are fronds of skin.

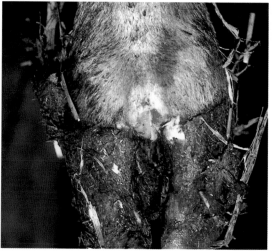

Plate 9.49. Digital dermatitis can also occur at other sites on the foot, including the coronary band.

Plate 9.47), lesions may be seen at many other places on the foot, for example:

- across one heel and spreading up towards the accessory digit
- under-running the sole from the heel
- at the front of the foot (Plate 9.49). Disease is particularly dangerous at this site. Involvement of the coronary band tissue can produce a total vertical fissure (Plate 9.50) leading to protracted lameness
- between the claws. Some books say that this is a separate condition, known as interdigital dermatitis, but its appearance, smell and response to topical antibiotics make it highly probable that it is digital dermatitis in a different site. Plate 9.51 shows digital dermatitis on the surface of a corn
- occasionally as a secondary infection to sole ulcers

Treatment of digital dermatitis consists of cleaning the lesion and applying topical antibiotics. Lincospectin and oxytetracycline are most commonly used and repeated topical applications are beneficial. With the more chronic form of hairy warts a dressing impregnated with antibiotics may have to be strapped in position for several days. For anterior lesions involving the coronary band, both injectable and topical treatments should be used.

Digital dermatitis is a disease associated with larger groups of cattle in conditions of close confinement, high stocking density, damp conditions and poor foot hygiene. Control measures are therefore based on the following:

- Scrape cubicle passages and feed areas at least twice a day, making sure that all stale slurry is removed from places like water troughs and feed areas.
- Keep feet as dry as possible. The use of lime in cubicle beds will help, as will the luxury straw levels depicted in Plates 9.35 and 9.36. Part of the straw will be pulled out into the cubicle passage, further reducing the exposure of feet to slurry.
- Give the whole herd antibiotic treatment. This can be applied either as a jet onto the heel of each cow, for example via a garden water sprayer, or by walking the cows through an antibiotic footbath (page 318). Usually once a month is sufficient.

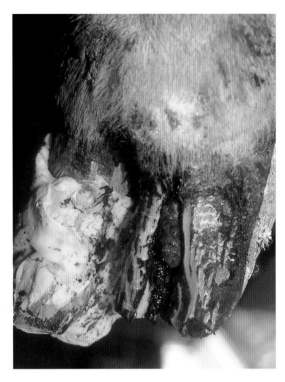

Plate 9.50. A vertical fissure may result from digital dermatitis affecting the coronary band.

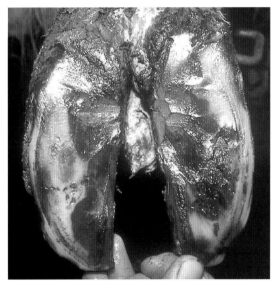

Plate 9.51. Interdigital skin hyperplasia (corns, tylomas) is caused by some factor irritating the skin between the claws. In this instance digital dermatitis is present on the surface.

Regular footbaths are even more important for the chronic form of hairy warts. Although they may not always cure affected cases, frequent baths will help to prevent the establishment of new and chronic cases. Over the course of two or three years of treatment of clinical cases and prevention of new cases by the use of a two- or four-weekly footbath, the syndrome should eventually come under control. A degree of immunity to digital dermatitis must develop, because in chronically infected herds the disease is most commonly seen in recently introduced heifers or in purchased cows two to six weeks after entry to a herd.

## Interdigital Skin Hyperplasia (Corns, Tylomas, Fibromas, Growths)

As its technical name suggests, this is an overgrowth of normal skin originating from a natural fold in the interdigital cleft (between the claws). A typical example is shown in Plate 9.51. In some cows, especially the heavier breeds, it can be hereditary. In others it is caused by chronic skin irritation, for example, from low-grade foul, digital dermatitis or simply impaction with dirt. Lameness is caused by the skin growth being squeezed by the claws during walking, or by the secondary infection of the growth with digital dermatitis or foul.

Mild cases can be treated by simply removing horn from the inner edges of the sole, adjacent to the sole ulcer site. This eliminates the pinching effect and the 'growth' then slowly disappears on its own. Larger lesions require surgical amputation.

## Mud Fever

Mud fever occurs following exposure to cold, wet and muddy conditions. The lower leg becomes slightly swollen, with dry, hard and flaking skin. There may be hair loss (Plate 9.52) and even bleeding if the skin cracks. For treatment, thoroughly wash the legs. Dry and then apply a greasy antiseptic ointment or a teat spray which contains a high level of emollient. As the organism *Dermatophilus* may be involved, three days of injectable antibiotic (penicillin) may also help.

## Fracture of the Pedal Bone

Bulling activity, with the mounting cow falling back heavily onto hard or rough concrete, is the most common cause of a fractured pedal bone (viz the bone inside the hoof – Figure 9.1).

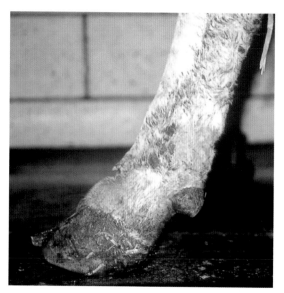

Plate 9.52. Mud fever occurs following prolonged exposure of the skin to wet and muddy conditions.

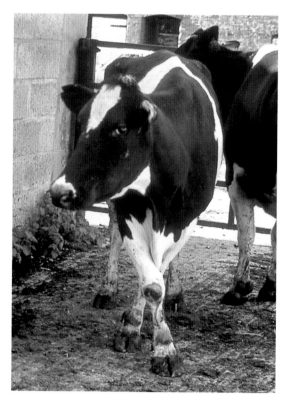

Plate 9.53. A cross-legged stance is said to be typical of a fractured pedal bone, but it can also occur if there are ulcers on both medial claws.

Bones weakened by age, fluorine poisoning or a foreign body penetrating the sole of the hoof may be more at risk of a fracture. Typically it is the inner claw of the front foot which is involved, and by adopting a cross-legged stance, as in Plate 9.53, the cow transfers her weight onto the sound lateral claw. However, the stance alone is not sufficient to diagnose fracture of the pedal bone. Cows with ulcers in both inner claws will adopt the same position. Most animals heal well if a block is applied to the sound claw.

## Pedal Bone Tip Necrosis

In a few cows, what initially appears to be a standard white line abscess at the toe sometimes fails to heal, even though it may have been treated thoroughly. At the second examination there will probably be a characteristic foul odour and even with further extensive removal of under-run tissues the toe fails to heal. A typical example is shown in Plate 9.54. Note how short the affected claw has become, compared to the normal claw on the left.

In such cases the front tip of the pedal bone has become infected (technically known as osteomyelitis) and unless the damaged and infected bone is all removed, the claw will never heal.

Each time you pare the toe, it seems to go back even further. This is because more of the tip of the pedal bone has been eroded. The only treatment for such cases is either total removal of the digit or, using a wire, sawing off the tip of the toe to remove all the necrotic bone.

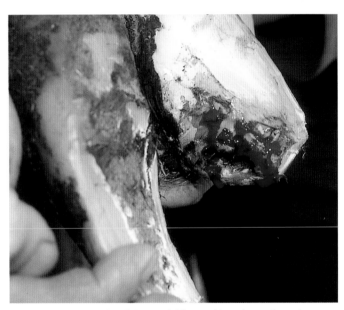

Plate 9.54. Necrosis of the pedal bone. Note how short the affected claw is compared to the normal one.

## Pedal Arthritis

Inflammation of the corium produces changes in the horn leading to disorders such as sole ulcers and white line disease. The corium also feeds the pedal bone and so an inflamed or infected corium, perhaps caused by a severe longstanding ulcer or white line infection, can also produce internal changes on the bone. The example shown in Plate 9.55 is quite mild, but imagine how the protruding spicules of bone (A) will impact on the joint surface to make walking uncomfortable. Cows which develop chronically enlarged claws following a longstanding sole ulcer will have much more severe changes than this. There is no treatment.

An infected pedal joint (purulent arthritis) is an even more serious condition. It is usually the result of a

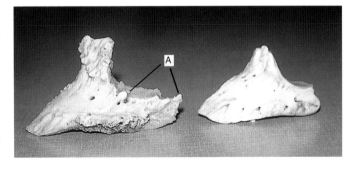

Plate 9.55. Mild pedal arthritis. Spicules of bone (A) protruding from the claw on the left will make weightbearing uncomfortable. A normal pedal bone is on the right.

severe or neglected case of foul, white line disease or sole ulcer. The foot becomes grossly swollen and infection may start to track up the tendon sheaths of the leg. The cow will be intensely lame, probably not using the leg at all. A typical example is shown in Plate 9.56. Radical treatment such as digit amputation and prolonged, aggressive antibiotic therapy may sometimes be effective. Many cases have to be culled.

## NURSING, FOOTBATHS, DRESSINGS AND BLOCKS

So far this chapter has dealt only superficially with treatments. The next section examines some of the general treatments in more detail and discusses the importance of nursing.

### Nursing

Lame cows obviously find walking difficult. They are much less able to compete with the rest of the herd, especially if they are at the lower end of the social dominance scale. In addition, they find it difficult to manoeuvre in and out of the cubicles. Cubicles are not easy to use at the best of times and if a cow is not fully mobile, they are even more difficult to negotiate. The result is that lame cows either spend longer standing up or, when down, they spend a long time lying and do not feed enough. This is one of the reasons for the marked

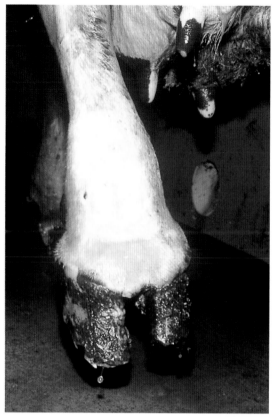

Plate 9.56. Severe pedal arthritis. This cow would not even put her foot to the ground. The degree of swelling indicates severe infection.

weight loss. Ideally lame cows should be transferred into a straw yard, where it is easier for them to lie down and get up again and where there is perhaps less competition for food. Herdsmen have commented that moving cows from cubicles into a straw yard results in an increase in yield in as little as 24 hours, especially in heifers.

### Footbaths

Footbaths are an excellent preventive measure for lameness, and cows should be walked through once a week during the winter housing period. Solutions of 5% formalin or 2.5% copper sulphate or zinc sulphate have been used, as have a variety of disinfectants. The main objective of a footbath is to clean and disinfect the foot and in so doing it should help to reduce the incidence of conditions such as:

● foul
● slurry heel
● growths or corns
● digital dermatitis

Formalin also has a drying action on the foot. However, it is unpleasant to handle and its use is not permitted in some countries. Similarly, copper sulphate baths may not be permitted by some environmental authorities because of the risk of pollution. Often two baths are used, the first containing water to wash and clean the feet.

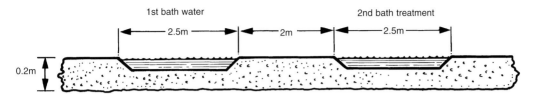

Figure 9.22. Two footbaths are sometimes used, the first to wash the feet and the second containing the active ingredient.

The cows next walk over a concrete strip to drain off excess water before walking into the second bath containing the active chemical, as shown in Figure 9.22. The liquid in the bath should be only 80–100 mm deep, as only the claws need to be immersed. Too great a depth, particularly if formalin is being used, can lead to damaged skin on both feet and teats.

Antibiotic footbaths are needed for the control of digital dermatitis. The frequency is dependent on the severity of disease but once a month is usually adequate. Many antibiotics will work, with the most commonly used being lincomycin (1 g/litre), lincospectin 150 (1.0g/litre) or oxytetracycline (6 g/litre). Lincomycin is totally degraded in the environment within 12 hours. Other treatments used include tylosin, erythomycin, or tiamulin, or twice weekly through a mixture of 40 g/litre copper sulphate plus 60 g/litre salt .

For best effects cows should have their heels cleaned by spraying them with water as they enter the parlour. Excess water then drains off during milking, after which the cows should exit through a footbath and into a clean environment, with the whole herd being bathed on the same day to avoid cross-contamination. If done carefully, a single passage through an antibiotic footbath will dramatically reduce the incidence of lameness due to digital dermatitis in as little as 24 hours. Unfortunately it does not eliminate infection from a herd.

## Foot Dressings and Blocks

Opinions vary on the need to apply a bandage and dressing to an exposed corium, for example following the trimming out of a sole ulcer or a white line lesion and under-run sole. There appears to be a minimal risk of infection from the environment penetrating the corium, even if cows with extensively under-run soles are allowed to walk back out into the slurry. It is surprising how quickly the exposed corium becomes covered by a layer of new horn. On the other hand, there are several potential disadvantages of applying a dressing, any of which may retard healing. These include:

- Unless changed almost daily, the dressing will impede drainage. Pus and infection may spread, producing further under-run horn.
- Dressings prevent exposure to air, and air often promotes healing.
- The presence of a bulky dressing on the sole means that the affected sole becomes weightbearing. This could make sole ulcers worse and certainly cannot be beneficial to the production of new horn.
- Astringents, sometimes used to 'burn back' proud flesh on a sole ulcer, discourage the formation of the new horn which is so badly needed to cover the sole.

At one stage I almost always applied a dressing. Now I rarely do so. Dressings may be used to control haemorrhage, or on the stump of an amputated digit, but otherwise I doubt if the extra cost of a dressing produces any additional benefits.

On the other hand, the use of a block applied to the sound claw is an excellent practice, as it both promotes healing and considerably improves the welfare of the cow. There are a variety of devices available, for example:

- tie-on shoes and boots
- nail-on blocks
- blocks and shoes which are glued on

Tie-on shoes are the least popular. They are difficult to fix and by encasing the whole foot keep it damp and can retard healing.

Nail-on blocks are used successfully in skilled hands, although the sole of the claw to be blocked needs to be flat. They are cheap and fast to apply. Personally I am not keen on making nail holes through the wall of the sound claw and although I have used them, I prefer the glue-on blocks.

Wooden blocks, rubber blocks and PVC shoes are all available and can be glued onto the sound claw. All have their advantages and disadvantages. At the time of writing I find the PVC shoe ('Cowslip', Giltspur UK) the best to use in most cases. It is easy to apply, the glue sets quickly even on a cold winter's day and because the shoe is attached to the wall and not just the sole, it gives better support and durability.

For all the glue-on blocks, the sound claw should be scraped totally clean and dry using a hoof knife, making sure that you do not touch it with your fingers. Access to the inner wall can be improved by forcing the claws apart with a small roll of paper towel. With the PVC shoe the glue is mixed in the shoe until it forms a paste, as in Plate 9.57. Wait until it is just starting to set and then push the shoe as far back towards the heel as possible (Plate 9.58). It is very important that the shoe or block supports the heel; otherwise the cow rotates backwards on the sound claw, leading to discomfort and very rapid wearing of the block. Cows with large claws should be trimmed in advance to ensure a good fit, or if this is not possible, use a wooden block (Demotec Ltd). Glue-on blocks should stay on for two or three months, by which time most foot problems have healed. The PVC shoes can easily be removed by clipping around their outer wall with hoof clippers.

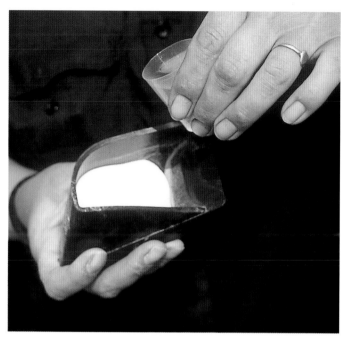

Plate 9.57. Liquid being added to powder in a PVC shoe ('Cowslip', Giltspur UK Ltd).

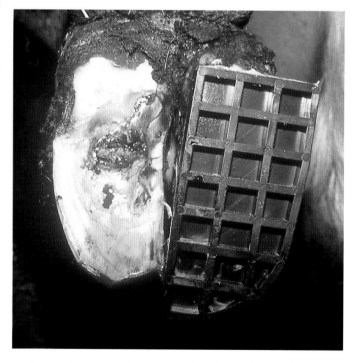

Plate 9.58. The Cowslip shoe needs to be pushed well back to provide adequate support for the heel.

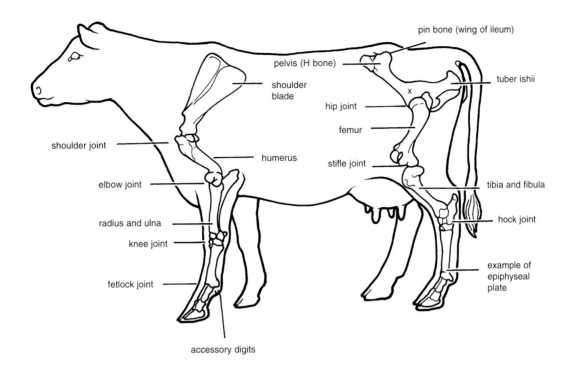

Figure 9.23. The bones and joints of the limbs.

## LAMENESS DUE TO LEG DISORDERS

One of my professors at veterinary school used to say that even if you thought an animal was lame in its head, you should always examine its foot, and I think this is an excellent piece of advice to pass on. Leg injuries do occur, however, and as you are moving the cow up to the crush to examine her foot, watch the way she walks: if the whole leg is stiff, or being carried, or if it is hanging completely limp, then you may well be dealing with a leg injury.

Figure 9.23 shows the names of the bones and joints in the front and hind legs. The correct technical terms will be used throughout this chapter, so be prepared to keep referring back to this diagram. The common leg, pelvis and muscle disorders causing lameness are listed in the following:

**Pelvic injuries**
   knocked down pin bone
   split H bone
   dislocation of the pelvis (Chapter 5)

**Leg and spine injuries**
   dislocated hip
   fractures
   spinal abscess and osteomyelitis

**Joint problems**
   arthritis (hip and stifle)

joint ill (Chapter 2)
capped knees and hocks
cellulitis
copper deficiency (Chapter 12)
and rickets (Chapter 12)

## Muscle, nerve and tendon injuries

obturator and peroneal nerve
paralysis (Chapter 5)
radial nerve paralysis
spastic paresis
(string halt, Elsoe heel)
muscle necrosis
(white muscle – Chapter 3)
muscle tearing
(downer cow, Chapter 5)
rupture of the stifle ligaments
rupture of the gastrocnemious
tendon (Chapter 5)
contracted tendons
overstretched tendons (Chapter 3)
popliteal abscess (Chapter 10)

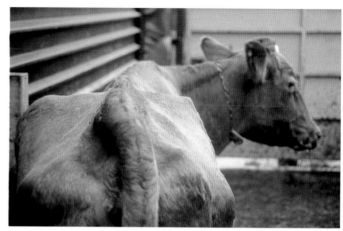

Plate 9.59. Fracture of the wing of the pelvis. Although it looks peculiar, it causes few problems.

For those conditions which have been covered elsewhere in this book, a page reference has been given and no further mention will be made in the following text. Calving injuries and the handling of downer cows are discussed in Chapter 5, which should be read in conjunction with this section.

## Knocked Down Pin Bone (Fracture of the Wing of the Pelvis)

The pin bone is the front wing of the pelvis (Figure 9.23 and Plate 5.7). It can be broken by cows pushing through doorways and other narrow entrances. The cow in Plate 9.59 looks peculiar with one side much lower than the other, but the condition rarely causes any lameness and if the skin is not broken, no treatment is necessary. She will continue to lead a normal productive life. However, if the skin splits and infection enters, as in Plate 9.60, the damage can be very slow to heal. This is especially the case if the bone becomes infected. Removal of all broken fragments of bone and thoroughly cleaning the wound help healing.

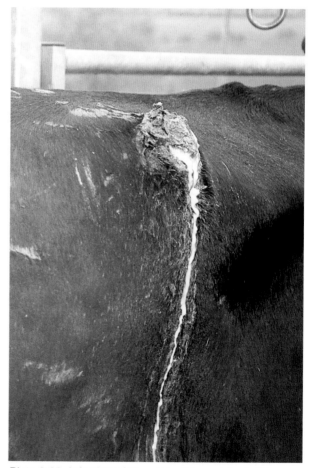

Plate 9.60. Infection of the wing of the pelvis. In this instance it may take several months for the skin to grow back.

## Split H Bones

The H bone (sometimes written as 'aitch' bone) is the name given to the pelvis and so a cow which has 'split her Hs' has a broken pelvis. It occurs as a result of a cow 'doing the splits', either because she lost her grip on slippery concrete, or because of an injury when she was bulling, or perhaps following obturator nerve paralysis at calving (see Chapter 5).

## Dislocated Hip

The normal position of the hip joint is shown in Figure 9.23. Dislocation (sometimes called luxation or subluxation) means that the ball of the upper end of the femur has been forced out of its socket in the pelvis. The head of the femur then pushes forwards, and the ball normally rests on the edge of the pelvis, at the point marked X in Figure 9.23, although occasionally it moves into other positions. It occurs as the result of a severe sprain or twisting of the leg and it is especially common in cows which have been bulling and have fallen on slippery concrete while trying to mount other cows. This is exactly what happened to the cow in Plate 9.61 and if you look carefully you can see the dislocated hip on her left side, producing a swelling under the skin. I find that the best way to appreciate this is to stand behind the cow with one hand over each hip joint and then let her walk slowly forwards.

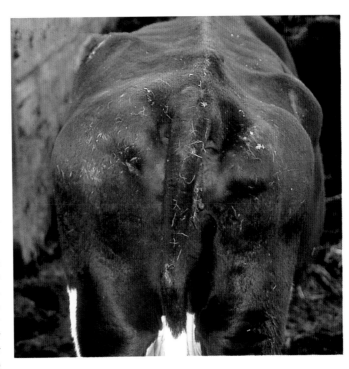

Plate 9.61. Dislocated hip. A swelling can be seen on the left side of the pelvis.

Very little movement is felt in the normal hip, whereas the dislocated end of the femur will force your hand out and slightly forwards as the cow tries to take weight on the affected leg.

If treatment is to be successful, it must be carried out soon after the injury, before the socket gets filled with blood and the joint becomes too loose. Your vet will sedate the cow and cast her onto her side; then he will extend the affected leg with ropes and pulleys as he tries to push the ball back into the socket. I have had a few successful cases, but many do not respond, or the hip dislocates again as soon as the cow stands up. This probably occurs when the ligaments holding the joint in place have also been totally ruptured. Affected cows may milk on for a while, but if they are already well past peak lactation, it may be better to sell them immediately, before excessive weight loss occurs.

## Fractures

Broken legs occur most commonly as a result of cows falling on slippery concrete, again often associated with oestrus. Younger calves may be stood on by cows or get their legs caught in gates. A fracture is diagnosed by moving the leg around, feeling for abnormal movement and listening for the grating sound of bone against bone. It always surprises me that this seems to elicit relatively little pain response from the animal, although weightbearing will probably be zero.

In older animals fracture of the femur is most common and in the majority of cases the cow is recumbent and unable to move. Treatment of adult fractures is hopeless. In calves, the lower leg is more commonly affected and if a plaster cast or even splints and elastoplast are applied, most will recover well. Fractures through the growth plate of the bone (the epiphyseal plate E) as in Plate 9.62 are the exception to this. A proportion of these fail to heal, or heal very slowly.

## Spinal Abscess and Osteomyelitis

Spinal abscesses, collapsed vertebrae and general spinal inflammation (osteomyelitis) are all difficult conditions to diagnose. The clinical signs will depend on the position of the lesion in the spine and the tissues

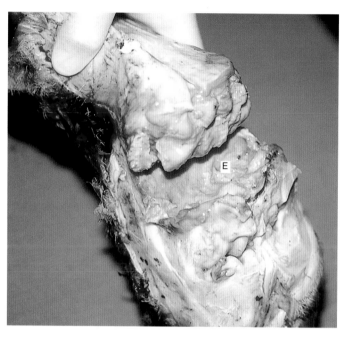

Plate 9.62. Fractures through the epiphyseal plate (E) (growth point of the bone) can be much slower to heal.

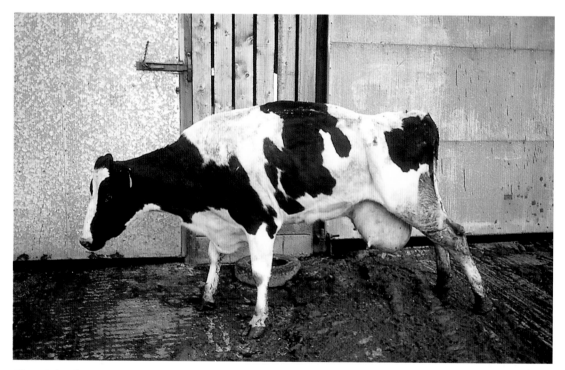

Plate 9.63. Osteomyelitis of the spine. This cow walked with extreme difficulty. A spinal abscess was found on post-mortem.

involved. Some cows walk very slowly and stiffly, with an arched back (Plate 9.63), others may lose the function of their hind legs, while one cow I dealt with who had an abscess in her cervical (neck) spine was unable to bend her neck and had to kneel down to graze!

## Arthritis and Stifle Ligament Rupture

The word means inflammation of the joint. The inflammation could be caused by degeneration due to age, by an infection (for example joint ill), by pedal arthritis (page 297) or by excessive movement within the joint. The latter occasionally occurs in the stifle joint (Figure 9.23) of adult cows, which is held together by ligaments. If the ligaments rupture, the two bone surfaces rub across each other and this leads to thickening and new bone formation. The condition is difficult to diagnose in the early stages: the cow has a low-grade lameness and no cause can be found. Later the hard, bony enlargement of one stifle joint becomes obvious. Rupture of the stifle ligament is a common injury in dogs.

A cow with arthritis will have little spicules of jagged bone (see Plate 9.55) protruding from the joint surface and you can imagine the pain caused as the surfaces rub across one another, especially with the weight of the cow pressing on them. Arthritis is most common in older cows, especially in winter. There is no long-term cure, but your vet may be able to suggest anti-inflammatory drugs which will reduce the pain and inflammation in the joint. Moving the cow out of cubicles and into loose housing where it is easier to get up and down will also help.

## Capped Knees and Hocks

Soft, fluctuating and painless fluid swellings over the front of the knee and at the side of the hock (Plate 10.25) are quite common, especially in cubicle-housed cows. Plate 9.64 shows an extreme example. The swelling is caused by continual bruising leading to excessive fluid production in the bursa, which is the name given to a type of shock absorber on the outside of the joint. The lesion is not painful and in the majority of cases it is best left alone. Most will slowly disappear after turnout in the spring or after moving the cow into a straw yard.

Sometimes you may wish to drain off the excess fluid. To do this, clip the hair over the centre of the swelling, clean off the area very thoroughly, then insert a sterile needle. A light straw-coloured or sometimes reddish-brown liquid will flow out through the needle. Great care is needed, however, because of the risk of introducing infection and creating an abscess. If the swelling is large and gets damaged it may develop into an abscess

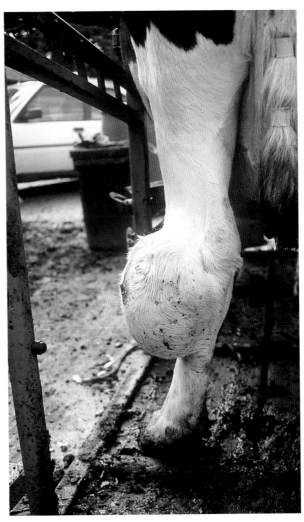

Plate 9.64. A capped hock (hock bursitis) is caused by continual trauma, usually the result of lying on inadequately bedded cubicles.

and then discharge on its own. This will need flushing out with water and antiseptic ointment infused into the hole to keep it open and promote drainage.

## Cellulitis (Infected Knees and Hocks)

This condition is also seen in cubicle-housed animals, and it is due to infection penetrating through the skin or even into the bursa over the joint. Rather than forming a localised swelling, which we would call an abscess, the infection tracks up and down the leg and causes a more generalised enlargement. This is known as *cellulitis* and is clearly shown in the right leg of the cow in Plate 9.65. The affected animal will be holding its leg in pain, and there will be some rise in temperature. Treatment consists of giving antibiotics to eliminate the infection and anti-inflammatory drugs to reduce the pain and swelling. In severe cases this may have to be continued for a week or more.

Both capped knees and infections are caused by the same factors; that is, poor housing. Cubicle beds which are rough and have inadequate bedding, or where there is an excessively large or sharp lip at the rear, all predispose to bruising. In some cubicles, the design is such that the hock is knocked on a sharp edge of a wooden division when the cow stands up. This leads to the type of

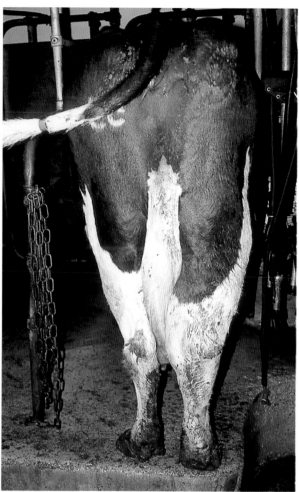

Plate 9.65. Cellulitis is a diffuse infection of the leg tissues. It can make the cow quite ill as well as lame.

injury shown in Plate 9.64. Cows which are lame from other causes also have difficulty getting up, and capped knees or infected hocks may develop secondary to the primary lameness.

## Radial Nerve Paralysis

The radial nerve runs from the spine across the chest and into the front leg. Its function is to contract the extensor muscles, thereby extending the leg

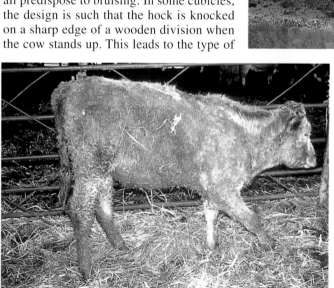

Plate 9.66. Animals with radial paralysis are unable to extend the front leg for weightbearing.

forwards and stiffening it for weightbearing. An animal with radial paralysis (Plate 9.66) is unable to extend its front leg and cannot bear any weight on it. There is no pain, just the discomfort of finding it difficult to move around. Many animals eventually learn to throw the leg forward at the shoulder and are then able to achieve a degree of weightbearing. The Charolais heifer shown in Plate 9.66 eventually recovered, but took four or five months to do so. Damage to the radial nerve occurs most commonly as a result of the leg being pulled away from the side of the chest, for example getting it caught in a gate or dismounting from a bulling cow.

## Spastic Paresis (String Halt, Elsoe Heel)

This is an inherited condition which leads to spasm of the gastrocnemious muscle, and it is most commonly seen in calves aged three to nine months. The leg goes very stiff, is extended backwards (Plate 9.67) and cannot be used for walking. The condition can be corrected surgically by cutting through either the nerve or the gastrocnemious tendon, just above the hock. If the tendon is cut, the leg initially collapses to the ground, like rupture of the gastrocnemious tendon in cows (Plate 5.34), but over a period of two or three months it will return to the upright position.

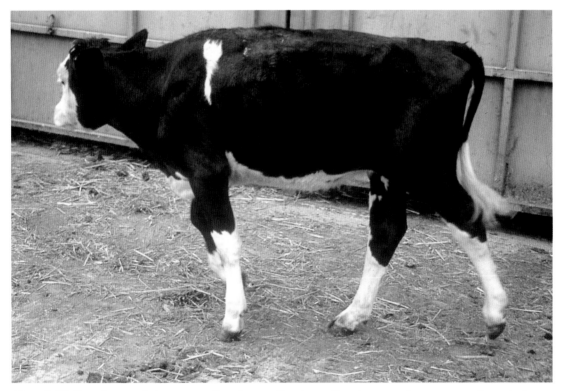

Plate 9.67. Spastic paresis is a nerve disorder resulting in continual spasm of one or sometimes both hind legs.

## Contracted Tendons

A proportion of calves are unable to stand at birth because their front legs are buckled over. Figure 9.23 shows the normal position for a front leg and Plate 9.68 shows a calf which cannot straighten its fetlock joint because the flexor tendons running up the back of the leg are too short. The majority of calves slowly improve over two to three weeks and you can help them by providing plenty of room for movement and by lifting them up onto their front feet as often as possible. I knew of one calf which could not stand on its own until it was 14 weeks old, but it eventually recovered. For more severe cases, keeping the leg extended with splints and elastoplast will help, and occasionally your vet may even have to cut one of the tendons to be able to extend the leg.

If the knee is also bent, the chances of recovery are much less. The calf in Plate 9.69 never fully recovered and even when sold at 15 months old it was still slightly unsteady on its front legs.

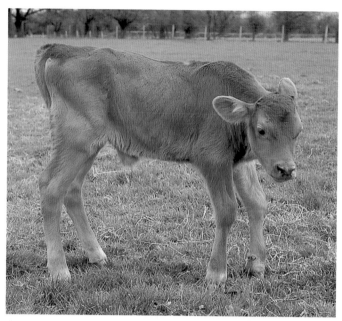

Plate 9.68. Most calves with mild contracted tendons recover with treatment.

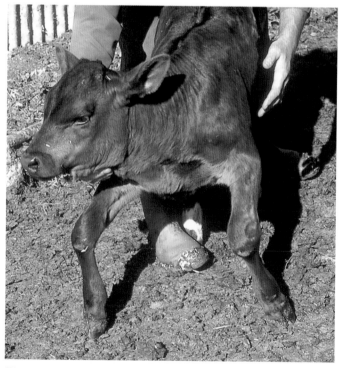

Plate 9.69. If the legs are also flexed at the knee, the chances of recovery are much less.

*Chapter 10*

# DISEASES OF THE SKIN

Skin diseases are commonly recognised in all ages of cattle. This is partly because they are easily seen and partly because close confinement, especially in the winter, leads to parasitic conditions being easily spread. In the summer, thinner hair cover, more air flow through the skin, reduced humidity and the effects of ultra-violet from sunlight generally reduce skin parasite infestations. The skin is, of course, the largest organ in the body. It has a wide range of functions which include physical protection, heat regulation (by sweating and insulation) and the synthesis of vitamin D via ultra-violet light.

The common skin conditions encountered are:

| **Parasitic** | **Infectious** | **Toxic** | **Trauma** |
|---|---|---|---|
| ringworm | lumpy jaw | photosensitisation | cuts and injuries |
| lice | wooden tongue | urticaria (blaine) | haematomas (blood |
| mange | jaw abscesses | septicaemia | blisters) |
| warble fly | malignant oedema | scouring | bursitis |
| fly strike | warts | poorly mixed milk | abscesses |
| | skin tumours | substitute | sterile abscesses |
| | skin TB | alopecia | cellulitis |
| | | | ingrowing horns |
| | | | burns |
| | | | tail injuries |

There are other conditions, for example PPH (Chapter 13) and severe dehydration (Chapter 2), where the skin shows secondary changes which are not included in the above list.

## PARASITIC CAUSES

### Ringworm

This is a fungal infection caused by *Trichophyton verrucosum*, although occasionally other species of ring-worm (e.g. *Microsporum*) may be involved. The fungus grows on the skin and penetrates the hair follicle (Figure 10.1). Affected hairs become very brittle and they break off at the surface of the skin, producing circular bald patches. The presence of the fungus also leads to thickening and flaking of the skin, and grey-brown debris can be easily picked off. The head and neck are the most commonly affected areas (Plate 10.1), especially around the eyes, nose and

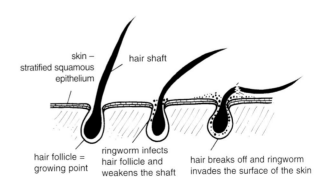

Figure 10.1. Ringworm infection. This leads to loss of hair and a crusty scaling over the skin surface.

ears, although lesions may occur over the whole body. Occasionally secondary bacterial infection occurs and the lesions become moist and discharge pus.

Ringworm can cause irritation. Affected calves may rub their heads on troughs and hayracks and these act as a source of infection for other animals. The spread from one calf to another is especially common at feeding time.

*Treatment*
Traditionally, affected skin was painted with creosote, diesel oil or other chemicals which would physically kill the ringworm. Aerosol cans of copper-based chemicals achieve a

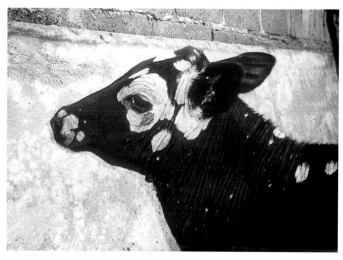

Plate 10.1. Dry crusty areas of skin are typical of ringworm.

similar effect and are often used. While these treatments are not without merit, they can be dangerous to the calves' eyes and they have been largely superseded by more modern drugs, the two most important being:

1. **Griseofulvin** This is an antibiotic-based drug which is given by mouth daily for seven days. The drug is incorporated into the growing hair and skin, so that by the end of a week's treatment the whole animal is covered by a protective layer of griseofulvin, and this persists for four to six weeks. Griseofulvin does not actually kill ringworm: it only prevents its growth. (It is fungistatic, not fungicidal – see Chapter 1.) The calf's own immune defences are left to destroy the fungus, and this has two important practical considerations. Firstly, healthy calves in good condition respond to treatment better than do poor and unthrifty animals, which may have concurrent pneumonia or salmonella infections. Secondly, although the lesions may start to resolve by the end of the first week, the calf remains infectious to others for a further two to three weeks.

Treatment should be given to the whole affected group. Since the incubation period of ringworm is approximately three weeks, attempts to separate and treat individual affected calves are generally unsuccessful, because further cases will probably continue to appear in the non-affected group. Occasionally higher doses for longer periods are required.

2. **Natamycin** This is administered as a spray and it is essential that all parts of the animal are thoroughly soaked at the rate recommended by the manufacturer. It is simply not sufficient to spray across the top of the calves at random. As with griseofulvin, the whole group should be treated and it is also worthwhile applying any remaining spray to troughs and fittings, since it will also counteract infection at these sites.

*Prevention*
The only sure way of prevention is to avoid contact with other animals and infective material. Ringworm seems to occur even in a closed herd, however. Often it affects successive crops of calves for two or three years, and then it is not seen again for a further few years. The spores produced are very resistant and may persist for up to four years if they are in a dry place. Elimination of infection from a building is therefore very difficult and is usually attempted either by a flame-gun or by painting with creosote or a 4% sodium carbonate (washing soda) solution.

Calves in poor condition are often the worst affected and maintaining a high standard of general health and nutrition will help to reduce the effects of ringworm. Sometimes an injection of vitamins A, D and E aids recovery. Ringworm is killed by ultra-violet light and many cases resolve spontaneously when calves are turned out in the spring. This is probably a combination of the effects of the sun and improved nutrition. Ringworm can also occur in outdoor cattle however, especially in the autumn, and if they are then housed under rather cramped conditions the disease can spread rapidly.

All species of animal ringworm are infectious to man, especially younger children, and care should be taken when handling affected animals.

## Lice

Although there are many cheap and effective treatments available, it never ceases to surprise me how many farms suffer reduced growth rates from heavy lice infestations. There are two separate types of lice:

**Sucking lice**
    *Haematopinus eurysternus*
    *Linognathus vituli*
**Biting lice**
    *Damalinia (Bovicola) bovis*

Lice live on the surface of the skin and can just be seen with the naked eye. They are dark grey/brown in colour and approximately the size of a flattened pin-head. To see them, it may be necessary to look in several places, pulling aside the hair with both hands and looking for movement at the base of the hair. The other sign of infestation is the presence of lice eggs which are glued to the hair shaft and are seen as small white dots (Plate 10.2).

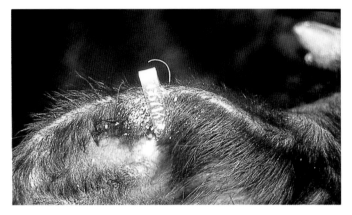

Plate 10.2. The small particles sticking to the hairs around the ear tag are lice eggs.

The life cycle is very simple: adult females lay eggs which hatch after ten to fourteen days into 'nymphs' or immature lice, and these take two weeks to mature. Adult egg-laying females may then live for a further four weeks, during which time they will lay several hundred eggs.

*Clinical signs*
The first sign of infestation is irritation. Affected animals rub their necks and backs, or there may be patches of hair loss where calves have been biting at their skin (Plate 10.3). This is especially true for biting lice, which can be intensely irritating. The shoulders, neck and back are usually

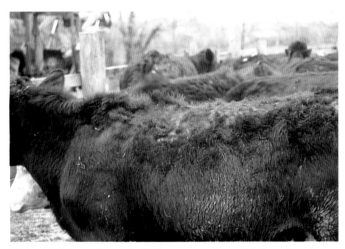

Plate 10.3. Lice. Irregular hair cover such as this in calves is a sign that they have been biting at their coat.

the worst areas, and the belly may also be affected. A common site is in the inguinal region, on the scrotum and in the groin (Plate 10.4). On a louse-infested neck, the coat is often arranged in lines running from top to bottom (Plate 10.5) and this makes diagnosis easy. Biting lice produce a crusty scurf on the surface of the skin, while sucking lice can produce a severe anaemia.

Calves of poor nutritional status are far more susceptible to lice. I have often seen instances where calves are so badly run down with a heavy louse infestation that they lose weight and are much more prone to ringworm, pneumonia and other diseases. The heaviest louse burdens are seen in calves eight to twelve weeks old.

Both lice and mange (see next section) cause a surprising amount of damage to the skins of cattle and in so doing reduce the value of the hide. *It takes at least 12 weeks for a hide which has been significantly damaged by lice to recover.* Even if cattle are treated well in advance of slaughter, it is possible that they will get reinfected.

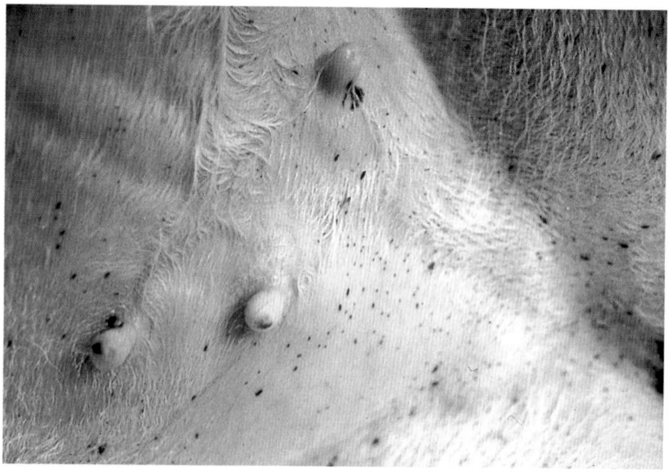

Plate 10.4. Lice can be seen as small dark brown dots around the teats.

*Treatment*

The traditional louse powder, 0.6–1.0% gamma benzene hexachloride (BHC) is effective, provided that it is thoroughly worked into the coat. Pyrethroid compounds can also be used and these are often available in the form of pour-on fly repellents. There are many brands and provided that they are well applied, they should give a persistency of two to eight weeks, although it is sometimes diffi-cult to get the full recommended dose to stay on the animal.

Pour-on organo-phosphorus warble fly treatments (Chapter 11) kill sucking lice very effectively. Normally only half the warble dose is sufficient, but many products are not recommended for use on calves less than two to three months old. You should check the manufacturer's instructions.

Avermectin anthelmintics (iver-mectin, moxidectin and doramectin) can be given by subcutaneous injection or as pour-ons. They are also

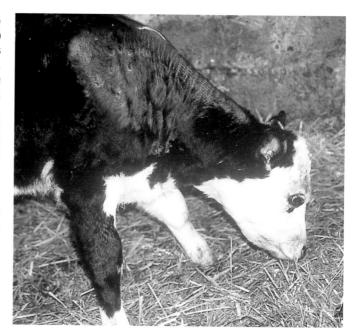

Plate 10.5. Lines running down the neck are typical of lice infestation. Ringworm and lice often occur together.

effective against sucking lice, mange and warbles. The small-volume dosage means that avermectins are very easy to administer, although they are more expensive than some other treatments, and are probably used mainly in the autumn when the whole range of their anthelmintic actions is needed. They are less effective against biting lice.

Only fly repellents and possibly avermectins have any persistency against lice and none of the products mentioned have any effect against their eggs. A repeat treatment should therefore be given after two weeks to kill any lice which have recently hatched from eggs which were present at the time of the first treatment. Avermectins persist in the body for two to three weeks, and repeat treatments are therefore not needed.

Infestations drop to a low level in the summer. This is probably because the animals' coats are cleaner, they are less tightly confined, their nutrition is better and the high temperatures of direct sunlight, ultra-violet light and dry skin conditions are all less favourable for growth of lice.

## Mange

Mange is most common in adult cattle. The mange mites are much smaller than lice and cannot be seen with the naked eye. They are closely related to the mites which cause scabies in man, canker in dogs' ears and scab in sheep. There are two types of mites in cattle, surface feeders and burrowing mites.

### Surface feeders
*Chorioptes bovis*
*Psoroptes ovis*

### Burrowing mites
*Sarcoptes scabei*
*Demodex bovis*

Although they are only surface feeders, *Chorioptes* and *Psoroptes* both cause intense irritation and thickening of the skin. The common site for infestation with *Chorioptes* is in the fold of the skin beside the tail head (Plate 10.6), although in neglected cases the mite can spread almost anywhere over the body. *Psoroptes* commonly occurs over the perineum (Plate 10.7), that is the skin extending from the base of the tail to the udder. *Sarcoptes* is also seen around the perineum, but often extends over the sides of the neck and along the belly and flanks. *Demodex* is less common.

The life cycle of all mange mites is direct. Adult females lay eggs on the skin (or in skin tunnels, like the burrowing mites such as *Sarcoptes*). Eggs hatch to form nymphs which mature to become adults in one to two weeks. Females may lay around 100 eggs in their lifetime and an adult may live for five to six weeks. Mite infestation is intensely irritant. Cattle rub and scratch against walls and posts, which damages buildings as well as leaving eggs on the wall. These eggs can

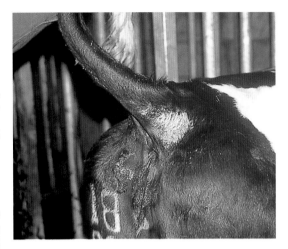

Plate 10.6. Chorioptic mange. Thick, scabby and sometimes moist areas are seen beside the tail.

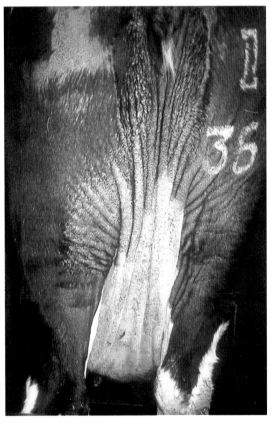

Plate 10.7. Psoroptic mange produces an inflammation and more generalised thickening of the skin from the tail to the udder. This could also be sarcoptic mange.

survive for three to four weeks and therefore can be picked up by other animals rubbing past at a later date. Continual irritation is a stress factor, reducing food intake and production.

During the 1980s very little mange was seen in the UK. This was associated with the compulsory warble fly dressing which was being applied at that time. Now that warbles have been eradicated, mange seems to be common. A routine treatment in December/January is a wise precaution for every dairy herd and is certainly not expensive. The treatments commonly used are organo-phosphorus pour-on products or avermectins, avermectins being especially used in younger cattle at housing. Most pyrethroids and other fly repellents are not effective against mange.

## Warble Fly

Warble flies have been eradicated from the UK. They are a notifiable disease and are discussed in Chapter 11.

## Fly Strike

Maggot infestations of cattle are not common in the UK, although in other parts of the world screw-worm is a major problem. Fly strike occurs in hot, humid weather, with the eggs being laid on warm, moist and dirty parts of an animal's body. The maggot infestation on a dehorning wound of the calf in Plate 10.8 is a typical example. Maggots may also be seen invading infected feet. In this site they will be removing debris from the wound and are often of benefit to the healing process. Sometimes infestations occur around the tailhead of recumbent cattle, especially if they are lying on soiled bedding. Provided that the animal is turned regularly, so that the skin is kept dry, this should not be a problem, even in a hot summer.

For treatment, physically scrape all the maggots from the affected area, clean the wound with a warm, dilute solution of antiseptic and then apply a fly repellent. Do not apply concentrated sheep dip, as this might be absorbed through the open wound and be toxic to the animal. An injection of an avermectin type wormer will also help in control.

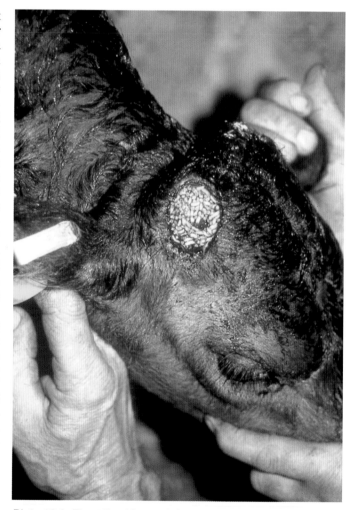

Plate 10.8. Fly strike. Maggot infestation following disbudding in a calf.

## INFECTIOUS CAUSES

Skin diseases can be produced by bacterial or viral infections. Sometimes the skin changes are only part of the overall disease syndrome, for example calf diphtheria (Chapter 2), which may produce a swelling on the face and/or on the tongue, and similarly for wooden tongue in older animals.

### Lumpy Jaw

This is an infection of the jaw bone caused by the bacterium *Actinomyces bovis*. The lower jaw on one side may very slowly develop a swelling. If you examine it carefully you can feel that the swelling is extremely hard and that it is firmly attached to, and even part of, the bone. Some say that injecting antibiotics (penicillin and streptomycin) into the lump in the

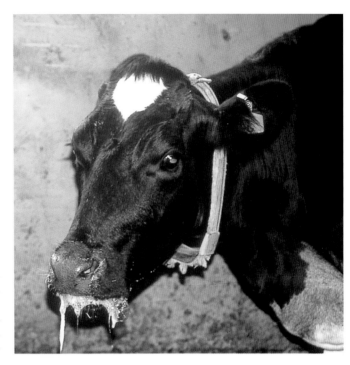

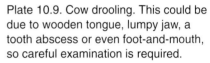

Plate 10.9. Cow drooling. This could be due to wooden tongue, lumpy jaw, a tooth abscess or even foot-and-mouth, so careful examination is required.

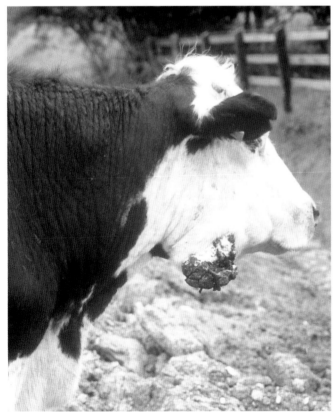

early stages may effect a cure. As the condition progresses, the roots of the molar tooth become displaced, eating and chewing the cud are painful and the cow begins to drool (Plate 10.9) and lose weight. The Hereford steer in Plate 10.10 is an advanced case. At this stage treatment is hopeless.

Severe knocks and bruising can cause a similar reaction in the jaw bone, but these will eventually heal, so you need to get your vet to examine it carefully before deciding to cull the animal.

Prevention is described under wooden tongue.

Plate 10.10. Lumpy jaw. This neglected case is unlikely to recover.

## Wooden Tongue

This is sometimes confused with lumpy jaw. It is caused by a different organism, the bacterium *Actino-bacillus lignieresii* which invades the soft tissues of the mouth. The tongue is the favourite site, although some-times the cheek or oesophagus may be affected, and I knew one farm where animals developed large, discharging lumps in their skin at sites all over the body.

This is a disease which is often easier to feel than to see. The hardening is on the raised portion at the back of the tongue (Plate 10.11), but you *must* use a mouth gag (Chapter 14) before putting your hand that far into the mouth; otherwise you might lose your fingers – as I almost did once (Figure 9.20B)!

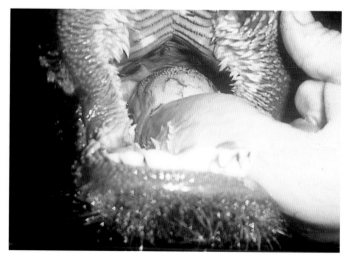

Plate 10.11. Wooden tongue. The back of the tongue is hard and thickened. This is best appreciated by palpation.

As the infection progresses, the tongue becomes hard and swollen. The animal is reluctant to eat, it drools and loses weight and often there is a secondary swelling in the throat as shown in Plate 10.12. If the oesopha-gus is affected, chronic bloat or cud regurgitation (Plate 6.6) may occur due to interference with rumination.

### Treatment

Unlike lumpy jaw, wooden tongue responds to treatment very well. Tra-ditionally iodine was used, giving an initial 'loading' dose of sodium iodide intravenously, followed by potassium iodide by mouth. Antibiotics are now the treatment of choice, and the treat-ment may need to be prolonged, e.g. penicillin and streptomycin injection daily for seven to ten days.

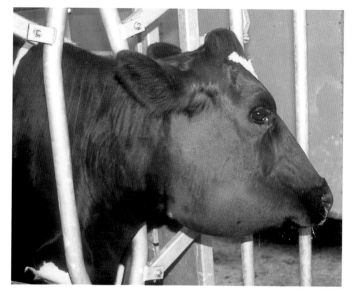

Plate 10.12. A swelling beneath the jaw, as in this animal, could be an indication of wooden tongue.

### Prevention

Both lumpy jaw and wooden tongue gain entry via abrasions in the mouth, lumpy jaw perhaps beside a loose tooth. Both organisms are found in the soil and outbreaks of disease may be associated with feeding potatoes or other foods heavily contaminated with earth and small stones, the stones leading to the abrasions which allow the entry of infection.

## Jaw Abscesses

This is a common condition in cattle of all ages, and leads to a hard swelling at the angle of the jaw bone. The lesion is clearly seen in the cow in Plate 10.13. Infection most probably originated from a penetration wound at the back of the pharynx (Figure 2.1), in other words from inside the mouth, but the pus then accumulates under the skin. Sometimes the abscess bursts on its own, but usually it has to be lanced, drained and flushed with antiseptic solution. Antibiotic cover may be needed.

## Malignant Oedema (Necrotic Cellulitis)

This is another disease which leads to a swelling of the face, but it is much more serious and unless treatment is

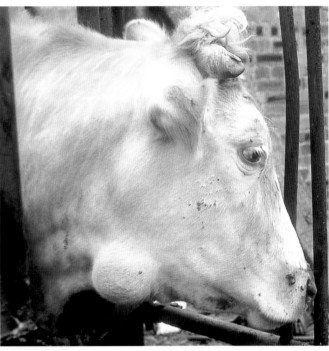

Plate 10.13. Jaw abscesses commonly result from penetration of the inside of the mouth (the pharynx) by sticks or other sharp objects.

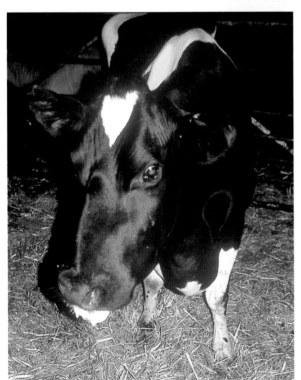

Plate 10.14. Malignant oedema (necrotic cellulitis) is an acute clostridial infection of tissues under the skin.

given quickly the animal may die. The cause is an infection under the skin and hence its alternative name of necrotic cellulitis. The disease is produced by a bacterial infection, *Clostridium septicum*, and is caused by any skin damage, such as sticks or stones in the feed, drenching gun injury or external trauma, which allows entry of the infection. Other species of *Clostridia* are also sometimes involved.

Care must be taken not to confuse this with wooden tongue or blaine. With necrotic cellulitis cows are much more seriously ill. They have a high temperature (41–42°C) and often only one side of the face is swollen. Plate 10.14 shows an advanced case, with swelling of the face, drooling and swelling of the brisket. Penicillins are the treatment of choice, but although this cow was dosed at a continuous high level for seven to ten days, infection spread down the front legs and she had to be culled. Anti-inflammatory drugs help counteract concurrent toxaemia.

## Warts

Warts are skin tumours caused by a virus infection. They most commonly affect the head, neck (Plate 10.15), belly and teats (Plate 7.45). They may also be found on the penis of young bulls (Plate 10.16). Young animals, one to two years old, are most commonly affected, especially when they are group housed and in close confinement. Flies have been implicated in the spread of infection. When neck warts are large and pendulous like those in Plate 10.15, they often develop a secondary bacterial infection and start to smell.

Some animals are so badly affected that the warts have to be removed surgically. Removal of a wart to prepare a vaccine may help, partly from the vaccine itself and partly because pulling off the wart may release some virus into the blood, generate immunity and result in a self-cure. (In some countries a licence may be required for a vaccine.) In most animals which are only mildly affected, the warts will eventually fall off without causing any problems. Teat warts are discussed in Chapter 7.

## Skin Tumours

Occasionally younger cattle develop small lumpy swellings of the skin over the whole body. This could be a cancer (tumour) known as a lymphosarcoma, as shown in Plate 10.17. There is no treatment and the animal should be culled.

## Skin TB

If you live in an area where TB is a problem and annual testing is a regular feature, you will have already seen skin TB. A typical example is shown in Plate 10.18. The small hard lumps are *under* the skin, whereas the TB test reaction occurs in the skin, as it is an intra-dermal test. The swellings of skin TB are enlarged lymph nodes and that is why they are often found in lines. They may also be seen on the legs (especially the front legs) and chest. Skin TB may be produced by non-pathogenic bacteria which are from the same family as TB. In this instance they can

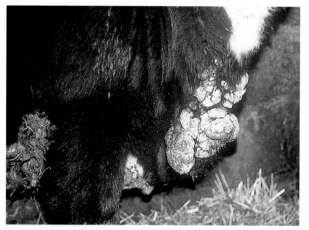

Plate 10.15. Skin warts are caused by a virus infection and are most commonly seen in younger animals.

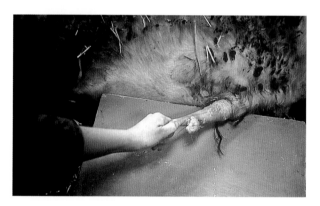

Plate 10.16. Warts on the penis, a common problem in younger group-housed bulls.

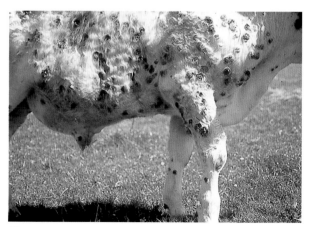

Plate 10.17. Lymphosarcoma – multiple small skin tumours. (Courtesy J. Gallagher)

influence the development of the skin reaction in the TB test and as such interfere with its interpretation. However, other causes are possible and in the United States similar lymph node enlargement (i.e. skin TB) is associated with bovine immunodeficiency virus (BIV) (see Chapter 13).

## TOXIC CAUSES

### Photosensitisation

This is a condition seen in grazing animals, and it is equally as common in adult cows as in young stock. It is caused by an accumulation of light-reactive pigment in the skin. When the skin is exposed to sunlight, the pigment absorbs radiant energy and this triggers off a chemical reaction which eventually leads to the release of histamine and causes extensive skin damage. Photosensitisation can be either primary or secondary:

- *Primary* This is caused by the animal actually eating the photosensitising compound. Examples include the chemicals contained in such plants as St John's wort and buckweed and also lantana, which is common in southern Africa.
- *Secondary* In this instance there is a dysfunction in the liver and chemicals which

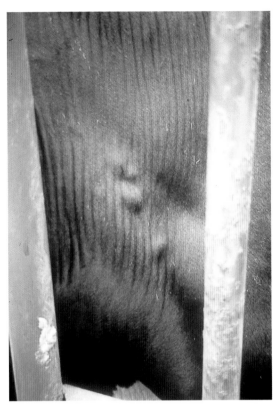

Plate 10.18. Skin tuberculosis (skin TB) is typically seen as a row of nodules under the skin of the neck.

are normally detoxified in the liver accumulate in the body. The best example of this is facial eczema, which is caused by ingestion of toxins produced by *Pithomyces*, a fungus which grows on ryegrass in New Zealand.

An obstructed bile duct can also lead to the accumulation of toxic products. The most common of these is phylloerythrin, a breakdown product of chlorophyll, the green pigment found in plants.

*Clinical signs*
In the very early stages of the acute disease the animal may simply be showing signs of liver failure, e.g. depression, off food and incoordination. Skin lesions are first detected

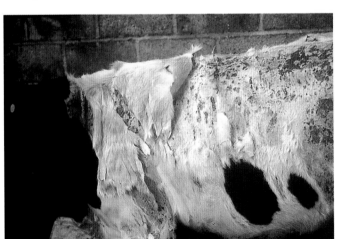

Plate 10.19. Photosensitisation. The initial insult probably occurred 3–4 weeks previously and by this stage the damaged skin is virtually painless and flaking off, with new (pink) skin forming underneath.

as a thickening of the white skin and, if you run your hand from black to white pigmented areas, the distinction can be easily felt. The skin over the back and sides is the worst affected, these being the areas most directly exposed to sunlight, although sometimes in severe cases the teats are so badly inflamed that the cow is impossible to milk for a few days. The thickened skin is very painful to touch during the first few days but later it forms a dry, leathery crust. This eventually drops off, leaving red, raw tissue exposed underneath. The animal shown in Plate 10.19 had reached this healing phase before she was noticed and this was probably one to two weeks or more after the initial histamine release and skin damage. In time new skin forms, but this may take several months. If the liver was badly damaged in the initial stages, poor growth and severe coriosis/laminitis may develop as secondary features.

*Treatment*

In the early stages the aim is to minimise the effects of the photoreactive chemical. If you suspect the condition, take the animal away from direct sunlight as soon as possible and shut it in a loose-box. Your vet will probably prescribe antihistamines and/or anti-inflammatory drugs to counteract the effects of the histamine and reduce any further skin damage. Antibiotic cover may be given to prevent skin infection and vitamins (especially A and D) to promote healing. While the skin is very raw, that is immediately after the initial 'peeling', fly repellents are useful to reduce irritation and to prevent fly strike and subsequent maggot infestation. Keeping the skin supple with a bland emollient cream also helps healing.

It can easily take a whole summer for the skin to completely heal and during this time the animal should be allowed out to graze at night only. There is no reason why photosensitisation should recur the following year, although the skin may be permanently damaged, similar to the scarring left after severe burns.

## Urticaria (Blaine)

This is an allergic or hypersensitivity condition with a sudden onset. The chemical which causes the allergy is often not identified. Animals of all ages can be affected, but most cases are seen in cows and heifers over 12 months old. The face, eyelids, lips and sometimes the vulva become swollen, with oedema or dropsy fluid accumulating under the skin. A good test for this is to squeeze the tissue gently between your forefinger and thumb. You can make quite a significant depression and when you remove your hand the finger marks remain. Sometimes the allergy is so severe that the whole head and neck are affected and this may interfere with breathing. In addition to swollen eyes and face, the cow in Plate 10.20 also had raised lumps on her skin. She recovered rapidly with treatment.

Mild cases disperse without treatment, but if severe, antihistamines and anti-inflammatories can be used to alleviate the symptoms, and diuretics, drugs which remove fluid from the body, may help to decrease the swelling. The syndrome is also known colloquially as ting.

## Septicaemia

Calves which have been severely ill due to septicaemia may lose their hair, especially around the head and face.

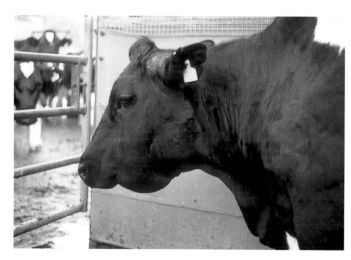

Plate 10.20. Blaine. Note the swollen eyes and face and the lumps on the skin over her shoulder.

## Scouring

Calves which scour badly often lose the hair over their hind legs, as seen in Plate 2.22. This is thought to be due to undigested fat and other substances in the diarrhoeic faeces reacting with the skin. Multivitamins may assist recovery, but most calves eventually recover naturally.

## Poorly Mixed Milk Substitute

Poorly mixed milk substitute, in which the fat rises to the top of the milk, can produce hair loss around the muzzle. A typical example is shown in Plate 2.18. Details of milk substitute problems are given in Chapter 2.

## Alopecia

Alopecia simply means hair loss, and a few calves seem to lose their hair for no obvious reason. They have neither scoured nor been ill and yet they may suffer from total hair loss over the whole body. Apart from giving an injection of vitamins A, D and E to improve skin condition, there is little that can be done for treatment. All the cases I have seen have recovered, although it may take two to three months.

# TRAUMATIC INJURIES

Because the skin is in such an exposed position it regularly suffers from trauma. This may be due to physical injury, burns or chemicals. An example of the latter is tank cleaner inadvertently used as a teat dip.

## Haematomas (Blood Blisters)

Haematomas most commonly occur on areas of the body where the skin covers bone. It is the pinching of the skin between bone and a hard object (e.g. a cubicle rail or narrow doorway) which leads to rupture of the blood vessel. The blood vessel continues to bleed, producing a large, soft, fluctuating swelling of blood under the skin. In areas where the skin covers muscle (e.g. on the 'thick' of the hind limb) there is a cushioning effect and haematomas are much less likely to occur. The common sites for haematomas are:

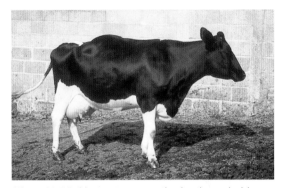

Plate 10.21. Haematoma on the back, probably damage by a cubicle rail.

- the back, often caused by trauma from a cubicle rail (Plate 10.21)
- the ribs (from squeezing through doorways)
- the point of the shoulder
- the pelvis, especially beside the tail (Plate 10.22)
- over the hind leg, at the point of the stifle (Plate 10.23)

If left alone, the majority of haematomas will slowly disperse, although this may take several

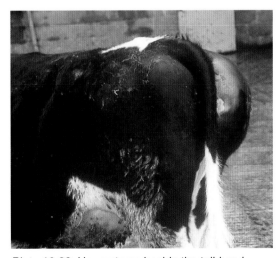

Plate 10.22. Haematoma beside the tail-head.

weeks. The problem with trying to lance and drain haematomas is that:

- The blood is not totally contained in a single 'pocket', so even if you open a large haematoma at one point, only a small area of it may drain.
- They may continue to bleed. This is especially the case if drainage is attempted only a few days after the haematoma has formed.
- Once opened, they can become infected and form an abscess. In some cases this secondary infection can make the cow quite sick.

For these reasons I would open a haematoma only if circumstances left no other option. The cow in Plate 10.22 is a good example. Blood from the haematoma had pushed through to the *inside* of the pelvis, putting considerable pressure on internal organs such as the rectum, vagina and urethra. This led to a cystitis and the cow was in considerable pain because she was unable to urinate.

In occasional herds 'outbreaks' of haematomas

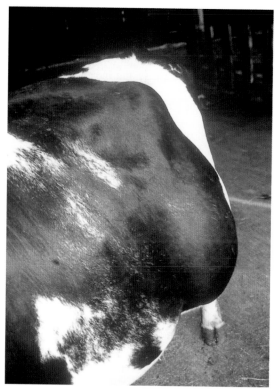

Plate 10.23. Haematoma on flank.

occur, where even normal everyday knocks will produce a haematoma, and large numbers of cows may be affected over a three or four week period. This is thought to be due to some factor interfering with the normal platelet aggregation process, thereby leading to increased bleeding, but no single factor has yet been implicated. I saw one herd where the syndrome appeared following a dietary upset which had led to severe ruminal acidosis. Others have suggested that it is a form of PPH (Chapter 13).

Haematomas should be carefully differentiated from abscesses and flank ruptures:

- Abscesses form slowly, gradually increase in size and are hard and often hot and painful. Haematomas are soft, fluctuating, painless swellings, which appear suddenly.
- Ruptures occur on the flank and may be differentiated (but not easily!) by feeling the tight edge of muscle which has torn to allow the intestine to pass through and lie under the skin. The Jersey cow in Plate 10.24 has a large rupture on her right flank.

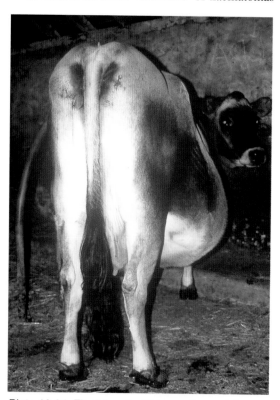

Plate 10.24. Flank hernia. This needs careful differentiation from a haematoma.

# Bursitis

A bursa is a small cushion of tissue acting as protection where skin covers bone and is often in an area where there is a considerable movement of the bone. The best example is on the outside of the hock. If there is excessive and repeated pressure on a bursa (for example cows lying in hard cubicles with insufficient bedding), then fluid accumulates in the bursa to form a *bursitis*. The most common points of bursitis are over the hock (Plate 10.25) and on the neck (Plate 10.26). Neck bursitis is usually associated with cows continually pushing against a rail over the feed manger. Like haematomas, swollen bursae are best not drained; otherwise they may become infected. Ideally remove the cow from the continual trauma; for example take the cubicle housed cow into a straw yard, and the swelling will eventually disappear. Often this is not possible. Continual trauma will erode through the skin, resulting in an abscess (Plate 10.27).

# Abscesses

Abscesses can occur on any part of the body, although they are more common at points which project or can become damaged. Most abscesses are the result of infection penetrating the skin. The bacteria multiply and pus forms. The natural defence mechanism of the body is to stop the infection spreading, so it tries to encase the infection in a thick, fibrous capsule. This retains the infection in one place, but as the bacteria

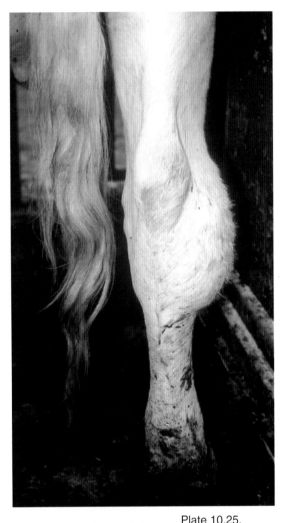

Plate 10.25. Bursitis of the hock ('cubicle hock'). At this stage the swelling contains only fluid and is not infected.

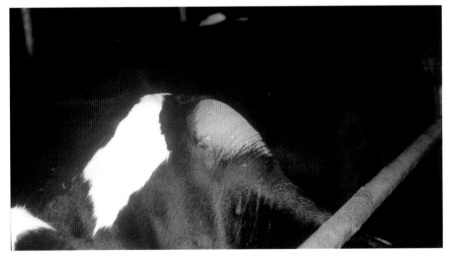

Plate 10.26. Bursitis of the neck, caused by the cow pushing against a feed rail.

continue to multiply, pressure builds up within the abscess. Eventually the abscess capsule starts to weaken at one point – and this is where it eventually bursts.

The best treatment for an abscess is:

- Wait until it is close to bursting (you should be able to feel a soft point).
- Enlarge the hole from the 'soft point' downwards, thus allowing pus to drain from the bottom of the cavity.
- Wash out the abscess cavity daily. The easiest way of doing this is to insert a cold water hosepipe. Obviously do not use excessive pressure as this will be both painful and dangerous. If you do not flush an abscess regularly, there is a risk that it will heal with some infection left inside and then form again.
- Antibiotics by injection are not normally needed unless the cut through the skin was quite deep.

Although abscesses can occur at any point on the body, the most common sites are:

- the angle of the jaw (Plate 10.13)
- over the hock, often secondary to a bursitis
- secondary to neck bursitis, as in Plate 10.27. These are very difficult to treat, because they do not drain properly. Regular flushing with warm antiseptic solution is ideal, but even then expect it to take at least one to two months to heal
- in the muscle of the hind leg (Plate 10.28). These are known as popliteal abscesses. They originate from very deep within the muscle and are thought to be the result of infection from a previous foot or lower leg infection, draining via the lymphatic system. They must be left for a long time, probably one to two months, before drainage is attempted; otherwise the muscle incision needed will be so deep that the abscess will not drain properly.

### Sterile Abscesses

Not all abscesses are caused by infection. Some result from inflammation caused by the injection of irritant liquids under the skin. The best example of this is the sterile abscess caused by the

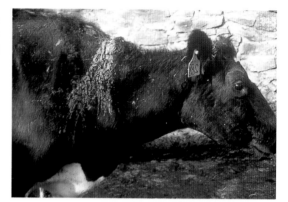

Plate 10.27. Neck abscess following bursitis. These do not drain well and so are very slow to heal. Regular flushing is essential.

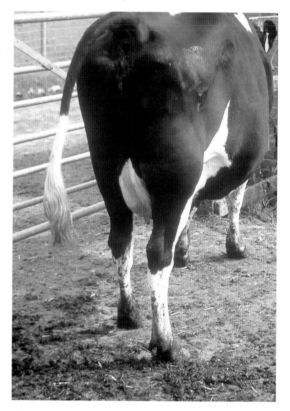

Plate 10.28. Popliteal abscess. Note the gross swelling of the right hind leg. The abscess must be left for one to two months before drainage; otherwise the incision through the muscle will be too deep.

subcutaneous injection of a 40% calcium solution. By no means all cows react to 40% calcium in this way, although it is more common if the whole bottle is injected into one site and the calcium is not dispersed (i.e. the site is not thoroughly massaged afterwards). Ideally, only 20% calcium solutions should be injected under the skin and the site should also be rubbed well after administration. Not only does the cow in Plate 10.29 have an unpleasant swelling on her side, but clearly the calcium was of no value to her, as it was not absorbed. Perhaps that is why she is having to be lifted on a hoist!

## Cellulitis

If infection fails to localise, i.e. fails to form an abscess, then bacteria may spread through the tissues, usually just under the skin. This is known as *cellulitis*. Cellulitis occurs most commonly on the legs, often extending upwards from the hock and causing severe lameness (Plate 9.65). It also occurs around the face, where it may be part of the malignant oedema syndrome (Plate 10.14). Affected cows will have a high temperature and will need several days of treatment with injectable antibiotics.

## Ingrowing Horns

Cows which have been badly dehorned, or where the horn has been damaged during growth, may develop an ingrowing horn. It is very easy to overlook the way the horn starts pushing into the skin beside the eye, especially when you see the cow every day and the change is slow. Plate 10.30 shows a typical example. The point of the horn can be removed using a wire or hacksaw. No anaesthetic is needed, because the 'quick' only comes about two-thirds of the way along the horn (see Plate 9.5).

## Burns

Burns are relatively rare in cattle, although when they do occur they can cause quite severe damage. The cow in Plate 10.31 was one of a group of 30 dry cows, most of which were badly burnt when a large barn of straw adjacent to their shed caught fire and they were unable to escape. Badly damaged skin leads to shock due to pain and fluid loss. In the healing process the skin scars badly and contracts and often the hair never regrows. If the teats or vulva are damaged this may produce permanent problems with calving and milking. Although the cow in Plate 10.31 was retained until after she calved, she proved impossible to milk and

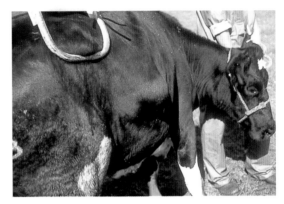

Plate 10.29. Sterile abscess caused by unabsorbed 40% calcium solution.

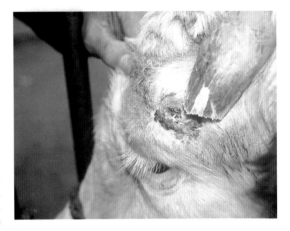

Plate 10.30. Ingrowing horn. This must be very painful, although unfortunately it is often unnoticed.

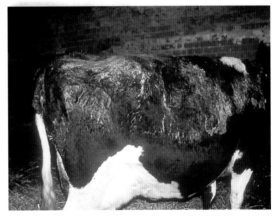

Plate 10.31. Severe burns caused by a straw fire in the adjoining building.

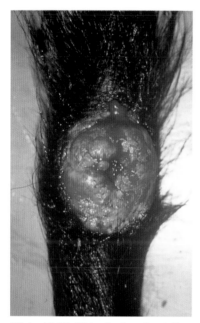

Plate 10.32. This discharging tail sinus is probably caused by a residual fragment of broken bone.

had to be culled. It is interesting that even quite badly burnt cattle can be sent for emergency slaughter and in my opinion this is the best option, especially if they are insured.

For those animals which are retained, ensure that they are put onto a high-quality, high protein diet to restore the lost body protein. For younger calves, this often means putting them back onto a milk diet.

## Tail Injuries

Tails commonly get broken. This may occur when cows are standing in overcrowded yards or cubicles; when the tail is caught in the diagonal of a gate; or unfortunately sometimes in association with rough handling. A simple break can be left untreated, but if an abscess or discharging sinus develops (Plate 10.32), or the tail tip is bleeding (Plate 10.33), intervention is needed. It can be quite difficult to stop bleeding from the tip of the tail by bandaging, probably because the blood vessel is held open by the bone of the tail. By far the best approach is to get your vet to give an epidural anaesthetic, remove the broken or infected fragment and suture across the tail tip.

**Faecoliths** are accumulations of faeces surrounding the tail. A typical example is shown in Plate 10.34. They should always be removed because the weight makes it uncomfortable for the cow to lift her tail when passing dung, so the hind quarters and the udder get badly soiled. If left they gradually dry out, contract and erode into the tail. The bottom part of the tail may even drop off.

Tail marker tape (for parlour concentrate allocation etc.) can cause similar problems if it is left on for too long, or applied too tightly.

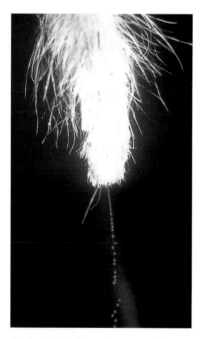

Plate 10.33. It can be very difficult to stop bleeding from the tip of the tail. This tail has been clipped ready for suturing.

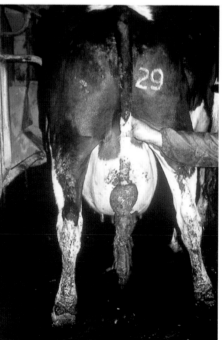

Plate 10.34. A faecolith, an accumulation of dry faeces around the tail.

# Chapter 11

# NOTIFIABLE DISEASES, SALMONELLOSIS AND ZOONOSES

## NOTIFIABLE DISEASES

In the UK most of the legal powers conferred onto the Ministry of Agriculture are contained in the *Diseases of Animals Act, 1950*, which has now been incorporated into the *Animal Health Act, 1981*. This enables the Ministry to record and control the movements of livestock, to regulate imports, to enforce quarantine and to establish and finance national disease eradication programmes. It is the Orders made under this Act which make it a legal requirement for all owners of livestock to keep detailed records of the movements of their animals, to identify cattle by means of an ear-tag, to report all cases of abortion and sudden death in cattle, and to dip their sheep when there is evidence of scab (mange). There are many other regulations of a similar nature.

The Act also states that any person in charge of an animal suspected of suffering from a *notifiable disease* must report it immediately to the police or to an inspector of the Ministry. Diseases are classed as notifiable when regulations have been made to control their entry into the country or to eradicate them. Current examples include:

Anthrax
Brucellosis
BSE (bovine spongiform encephalopathy)
Enzootic bovine leucosis
Foot-and-mouth
Tuberculosis
Warble fly

There are other exotic notifiable diseases of cattle, for example, rinderpest (cattle plague) and contagious bovine pleuropneumonia, which are not described in this book. Rinderpest was eradicated from the UK in 1877 by a quarantine and slaughter policy and pleuropneumonia in 1898.

### Anthrax

Anthrax is an infection caused by the bacterium *Bacillus anthracis*. In cattle it causes an acute septicaemic illness, resulting in very rapid death. I have only once been called to a live affected animal. It was extremely ill, swaying on its legs and died before I could treat it. In the typical case, after death, dark blood often runs from the nose, mouth and possibly the anus and vulva.

In the UK any animal found dead without an obvious cause must be reported to the Ministry of Agriculture. At no expense to the owner of the animal, the Ministry will send a local veterinary inspector to take samples and test for anthrax. A small cut is made in an ear vein (Plate 11.1), a swab is taken and one side of a microscope slide is coated with a film of blood. This is taken back to the laboratory, a special stain is added to the blood film and the slide is examined microscopically for the presence of anthrax bacteria. The carcase must not be moved or interfered with in any way until the results of the tests are available. With the use of McFadyean's old methylene blue stain, anthrax will be recognised as large blue square-ended rods (bacilli) surrounded by a pink-staining capsule.

The spores of anthrax are extremely resistant (see Chapter 1) and they are infectious to man and other animals. If anthrax is confirmed, the carcase must be destroyed on the farm by burning it together with any soil, bedding or any other material contaminated with the animal's blood or faeces.

The disease is now relatively rare, with the total confirmed cases in the UK numbering approximately ten to twelve per year. The most common source of anthrax was imported meat and bone meal which used to be incorporated into animal feedingstuffs. In 1977 there was a minor epidemic (139 cases) originating from this source.

Disease can occur in man, either as 'boils' arising from an infected scratch, or as pneumonia if the spores are inhaled. The latter used to be known as 'Wool-sorter's Disease', because dockers unloading hides and fleeces were occasionally exposed to skins which had been taken from anthrax carcases. Anyone at risk is now treated with penicillin or given anthrax vaccine.

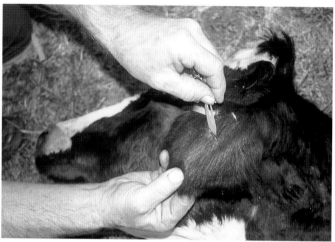

Plate 11.1. Testing for anthrax: a blood sample is collected from a small cut in the ear vein, stained and examined under the microscope.

## Foot-and-mouth Disease

This is a highly infectious virus disease which can spread very rapidly to other cloven-hoofed animals (pigs, sheep and goats) and to adjacent farms. Once infection has entered a herd, the incubation period can be as little as two days, that is to say there may be only two days between exposure to the virus and clinical signs being seen, and this accounts for the very rapid spread of the disease. An infected cow excretes virus in her urine, faeces, milk, saliva and even on her breath! The virus can survive on the ground for up to 30 days in winter, but only three to five days in summer.

One of the first signs in an affected herd is that a significant number of cows show a dramatic drop in yield

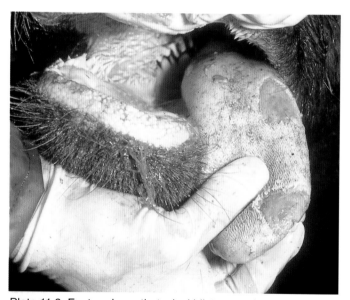

Plate 11.2. Foot-and-mouth: typical blisters on the tongue.

together with a high temperature. Within 24 hours the virus produces large 'vesicles', that is fluid-filled blisters, some 20–40 mm in diameter. These are most commonly seen on the tongue (Plate 11.2) and between the claws of the feet (Plate 11.3), although they may also occur on the teats. The blisters soon burst, leading to areas of exposed raw and painful tissue. You should imprint these pictures carefully in your mind in case you are unfortunate enough to see such cases in the future. There may be so many vesicles present that if the tongue is grasped almost all of its covering falls off in your hand (as shown in Plate 11.4). This makes affected animals drool (Plate 11.5) and they also become very uncomfortable on their feet, stepping from one to the other, and possibly kicking or shaking their legs.

If the disease is allowed to progress, affected animals will lose weight rapidly and milk production will suffer. Most adult animals will survive and develop a degree of immunity – although many of them

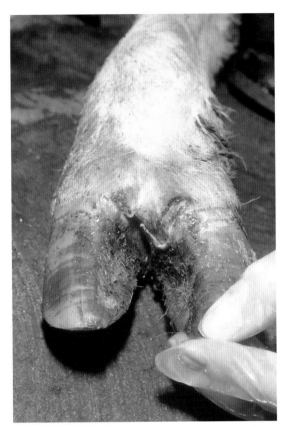

Plate 11.3. Foot-and-mouth: blisters between the claws.

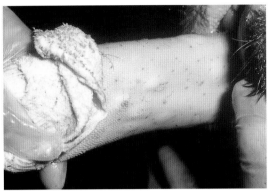

Plate 11.4. Foot-and-mouth: so many blisters may be present in the early stages that the skin of the tongue simply falls off in your hand.

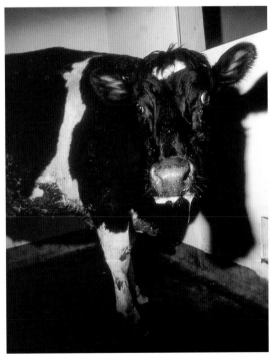

Plate 11.5. Foot-and-mouth: affected animals drool, are off their food and are uncomfortable on their feet.

will remain permanently infected and will be a risk to other animals. Mortality may be very high in younger animals (50–60%) due to heart lesions. There is no specific treatment.

Fortunately there are few other diseases in cattle which show similar classic signs, although the recent increase in 'soda grain' feeding has led to a few false alarms! Whole (i.e. uncrushed) grain can be mixed with solid sodium hydroxide and some water to achieve predigestion of the grain husk. If it is not mixed thoroughly, large lumps of sodium hydroxide may be eaten and this can lead to severe mouth ulcers and a very sick animal. However, usually only one or two animals are affected, there are no lesions on the feet and affected cattle do not have a high temperature. If sufficient sodium hydroxide is eaten, the whole of the inside of the mouth may slough off, and because of the changes within the rumen, death may occur due to shock. It is interesting to note that one of the local 'treatments' for foot-and-mouth disease in southern Africa is to smear the inside of the animal's mouth with sodium hydroxide or salt. This is said to reduce the rate of virus shedding and to speed recovery.

*Sources of infection*

Because Great Britain has an eradication policy for the control of the disease, determining possible sources of infection is extremely important. Imported live animals represent the greatest potential danger and so countries of origin are strictly monitored to confirm that they are totally free from any risk of foot-and-mouth. After arrival, animals may be quarantined and submitted to regular veterinary inspections. Imported carcases and other animal products can also carry infection. Again, the countries of origin are carefully monitored, as is the hygiene at their processing plants. For example, only boneless meat may be imported from infected countries, because if any infected animals were slaughtered the virus is most likely to die in meat which has 'set', whereas it can survive for much longer periods in bones. Infected countries may also have restrictions specifying that meat may only be imported from zones within the country that are free of foot-and-mouth. Infection from imported meat can reach farms via waste foods being fed to pigs, and there are strict regulations relating to the storage of swill and to ensure that it is cooked in approved equipment for at least one hour prior to feeding.

The virus is so infectious that air-borne spread is also a possibility. Many of the outbreaks of foot-and-mouth have started along the south and east coasts of England where migrating birds may have carried infection from the Continent. The outbreak which occurred on the Isle of Wight in 1981 was shown to have been carried by the wind alone and there is considerable meteorological data to support this. By a careful examination of the direction and speed of the wind, and of the prevailing temperature and humidity, it is now possible to predict mathematically the climatic conditions which might enable foot-and-mouth virus to blow across from Europe. This provides a useful forecast for times when extra vigilance is required.

At the time of writing the countries of the European Union are all considered free from foot-and-mouth, so there is relatively free movement of cattle from these countries into the UK. However, the movement of cattle from Eastern Europe into the EU and increasing EU membership from Eastern European countries represent a real threat.

*Control of foot-and-mouth*

Control is based on identification and slaughter of infected herds, plus restrictions on the movement of all livestock within a 10 mile radius, known as the *infected area*. Much larger *controlled areas* may be established if the disease is thought to be spreading. Slaughtered carcases, plus bedding and other infected material, must either be burnt or buried under six feet of earth. The farm must be thoroughly disinfected and cannot be restocked for a further six weeks.

Because of the rapid spread of infection, early identification of disease is vital and I would remind readers that it is their *legal obligation* to report even *suspected* cases of foot-and-mouth to the Divisional Veterinary Officer immediately. Failure to do so has in the past resulted in prosecution of stock owners, with quite heavy penalties being imposed.

Following the 1967–1968 outbreak of foot-and-mouth in Cheshire, one of the worst on record when 400,000 animals were slaughtered over nine months, stocks of vaccine were accumulated to carry out a 'ring vaccination' of animals around an infected area, should the disease ever get totally out of control. There are at least four good reasons why it is hoped that these measures will never be used.

- First, once Britain becomes an infected country, it will lose many of its export markets.
- Second, because there are a variety of different strains of foot-and-mouth, the vaccine in use may not be totally effective.
- Third, vaccinated animals can become carriers, shedding infection to other stock.
- Finally, and by no means least important, to give full protection, vaccination would have to be carried out each year, and in the long term this would be much more expensive than the current slaughter policy.

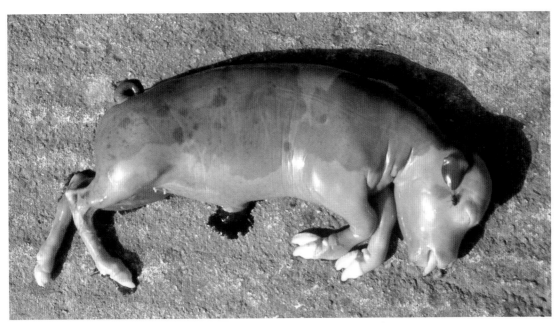

Plate 11.6. An aborted calf. This was at approximately the sixth month of pregnancy.

## Brucellosis

Brucellosis is caused by an infection by the bacterium *Brucella abortus*. Its preferred sites in the body for growth are the uterus, udder, testicles and joints, although the uterus is by far the most important. Infection can only become established in animals of breeding age and although it is usually contracted by licking aborted calves or eating contaminated pasture, it can also be spread by an infected cow swishing her contaminated tail and flicking droplets of *Brucella* bacteria onto the eyes or noses of 'clean' animals.

Inside the cow *Brucella* grows in the placenta, especially on the cotyledons, leading to damage and loss of function. This then causes death of the calf and subsequent abortion, most commonly at the seventh or eighth month of pregnancy (Plate 11.6 shows a foetus aborted at about six months of pregnancy). Most cows abort once only, although they often shed infection for two weeks or more after subsequent normal calvings. Following abortion, infected cows frequently develop a chronic uterine infection. This endometritis leads to difficulties and delays in getting them back into calf. It also causes a uterine discharge, so that aborted cows may remain important sources of infection for several weeks.

Disease can spread very rapidly in a non-infected herd, and abortion 'storms', with a major part of the herd aborting, were once common. This led to a tremendous loss of calves and of milk in the first year and to production problems in the future because of the difficulty of getting cows back into calf again. The financial consequences were often disastrous. As dry cows are usually run together in a group, if one animal aborts there is a strong chance that infection will quickly spread to the others. This is because of the inquisitive nature of cows and the likelihood of their licking or sniffing the aborted foetus.

*Other forms of brucellosis*
In man, the infection is known as *undulant fever*, because it causes intermittent bouts of flu-like symptoms, with aching joints, severe lethargy and psychological depression. Because the *Brucella* bacteria grow *inside* the body cells (most bacteria live in the tissue fluid between cells) they are very difficult to kill with antibiotics and a course of treatment for six to twelve months may be necessary. (*Pseudomonas*, Chapter 7, and tuberculosis also grow inside cells.) Farmers, vets and slaughtermen are most at risk. Although milk can carry *Brucella*, it is not a common feature of infected cows and in any

case the bacteria are destroyed by pasteurisation. Humans are usually infected by splashes from handling contaminated cows, the classic case being a heavily infected retained placenta following abortion.

Brucellosis can also occur in horses and dogs where it may cause chronic joint or tendon infections, for example fistulous withers in horses. Bulls may develop brucellosis in the testicles and could spread infection during service, although most infected bulls become sterile and would therefore be culled.

*Control of brucellosis*
In 1967 a voluntary register of non-infected herds was started in the UK and eradication began in 1971. Initially all calves between three and six months old were vaccinated free of charge with a live 'Strain 19' vaccine and in more severely affected herds the killed '45/20' product was used in adult animals. Although a few carriers persisted, vaccination dramatically reduced the incidence of abortion storms and therefore decreased the spread of infection within herds. This policy was combined with a 'test and remove' regime. All breeding stock were subjected to blood tests at intervals of four months. Infected animals were identified and removed on each occasion. Milk ring tests on bulk milk supplies from each farm gave further assistance in detecting infected herds.

Current testing involves a monthly milk ring test on bulk milk, biennial blood testing of all bulls and of female cattle over two years old which are not in the milking herd, and abortion investigations. On 1 October 1985 the whole UK was designated as being Officially Brucellosis Free (OBF). This meant that 99.8% of all the herds in the country were free, but since then sporadic cases have occurred. For example, in 1985 there were still 69 herds from which *Brucella* had been cultured, the majority of these being associated with an outbreak in Somerset. Extensive movement of cattle, especially through dealers' premises, is thought to be a major factor in the spread of the disease. The last cultural isolation of *Brucella* in the UK was from an imported heifer in Anglesey in October 1993. Blood-test-positive animals occur from time to time, but these are subsequently shown to be false positives.

The early identification of infected cows is vital, especially as vaccination was discontinued on 1 November 1978. This means that the national herd is now highly susceptible. For this reason, farmers have a *legal obligation* to report all cases of abortion or premature calving to their local Divisional Veterinary Officer. Affected animals should be isolated to prevent possible spread of infection to others and samples of blood, milk and placenta and/or uterine discharge may be taken and tested for brucellosis. If you wish the laboratory to check for other causes of abortion, including leptospirosis, then ideally the whole foetus and part of the placenta should be submitted as fresh as possible. Other causes of abortion are listed in Appendix 2 and discussed in Chapter 8.

## Warble Flies

There are two species of warble fly, *Hypoderma bovis* and *H. lineatum*. They have very similar life cycles which are shown in Figures 11.1 and 11.2. Adult flies lay their eggs on the skin of the animal's abdomen and legs during May to August, with *H. lineatum* attacking primarily the front legs and *H. bovis* the hindquarters of the animal. The eggs hatch into small larvae which burrow through the skin and into the tissues. They then migrate upwards through the other organs, some having a 'rest' stage in the oesophagus (*H. lineatum*) or around the spine (*H. bovis*) before arriving under the skin of the back from January onwards. There they make small breathing holes through the skin and the larva stays in one place, feeds and begins its slow transition towards the pupa stage. From the end of March to May the warbles may be seen as lumps under the skin of the back (Plate 11.7). Eventually they emerge as large white fleshy grubs, falling to the ground to pupate, that is to finish their development into adult flies in four to six weeks.

*Damage caused by warbles*
This is of four kinds. Firstly the noise of the adult fly frightens cattle, and herds of dairy cows may become restless and start 'gadding'. This obviously depresses milk production and growth and can lead to physical injury, especially to the udder and teats. Secondly the presence of large numbers of warbles under the skin in the spring is very uncomfortable and this also reduces production. Third the air holes made by the warbles render this part of the hide useless for leather and the back is the most valuable part

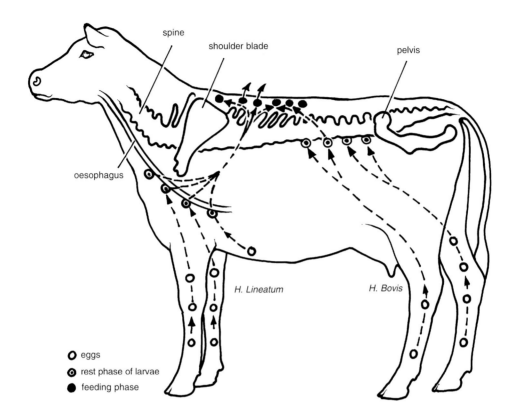

Figure 11.1. Life cycle of warble fly. Hypoderma lineatum lays its eggs on the animal's front legs and its larvae have a rest phase in the oesophagus, whereas H. bovis lays its eggs on the hindquarters and the larvae 'rest' adjacent to the spine. Both types of larvae arrive under the skin of the back from January onwards where they undergo a feeding phase before falling to the ground to pupate.

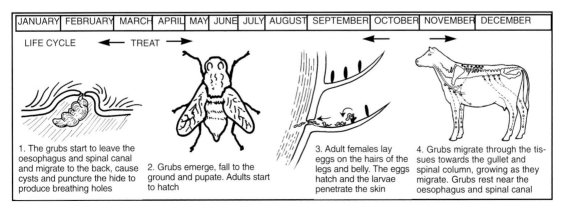

Figure 11.2. Warble fly migration and treatment period.

of the hide. Finally, occasional larvae migrating through the body enter the spine and cause paralysis, although this is more common when treatment is applied incorrectly.

*Treatment and control*
Traditionally the animal's back was scrubbed with derris to kill the emerging larvae; this has now been superseded by organo-phosphorus pour-on preparations such as 20% phosmet, and by the avermectins. The OPs are about 98% effective if applied during the autumn (Figure 11.2) but less efficient for spring treatments. Organo-phosphorus preparations cannot be used between 20 November and 15 March. Although the vast majority of larvae migrating through

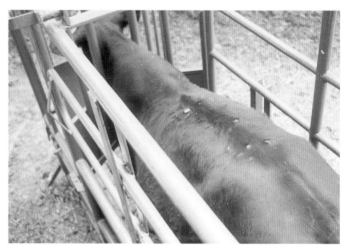

Plate 11.7. Warble fly larvae emerging from the back at the end of their feeding phase in March/April. They now fall to the ground and pupate into adult flies.

the spine cause no damage, if they are killed by organo-phosphorus compounds when at this site, they can stimulate a hypersensitivity reaction by the animal. This causes inflammation, swelling and pressure on the spine and may lead to paralysis of the hind legs. Several cases of treatment outside the recommended time periods have resulted in animals having to be sent for slaughter. It is interesting to note that the avermectin group (ivermectin, moxidectin etc) can be used at *any time* during the winter and as such is an extremely useful drug to administer to cattle which are being housed later in the year, for example in December, because it kills lice, mange, warbles, lungworms and intestinal worms, including the inhibited stages of type II *Ostertagia* larvae.

In 1978 legislation was introduced in the UK to make it compulsory to dress all obvious warble-infested cattle in the spring and this was accompanied by a vigorous advertising campaign to encourage voluntary autumn treatments, since these are more effective. There is now a *legal obligation* for stock-owners and others to report all *suspected* cases of warble-fly infestation. There are movement restrictions and compulsory treatment regulations for infected and adjacent herds and a compulsory herd inspection and treatment at the owner's expense if these regulations are infringed.

In the first five years of eradication, the incidence of infested cattle was reduced from 34% (1979) to 0.02% (1983) with Anglesey having a significant pocket of infection. From 1983 most of the infection was in the south-west of England, and the percentage of herds affected decreased rapidly each year:

| Year | % of herds infected | Number of affected cattle |
|---|---|---|
| 1978 | 40 | – |
| 1979 | 34 | – |
| 1982 | 0.02 | 705 |
| 1984 | 0.01 | – |
| 1986 | 0.0009 | 34 |
| 1989 | – | 2 |

No live warble larvae have been found on British cattle since 1990 and the final stages of eradication were carried out by means of serological surveys (blood testing). In 1991 there were four blood-test-positive animals from 300,000 examined, and by 1993 this had fallen to zero. The UK is now declared officially free from warbles. All imported cattle must be treated on arrival.

## Enzootic Bovine Leucosis (EBL)

This is a virus infection of cattle which produces tumours in the lymph nodes. Affected animals develop hard swellings under the skin, approximately the size of a flattened grapefruit, and the skin moves freely over them. Weight loss is quite marked. Other clinical signs may be seen, for example chronic bloat due to an enlarged lymph node in the chest compressing the oesophagus, or roaring breathing from pressure on the trachea. There is no treatment and affected animals slowly die.

A word of caution, however. There are other causes of tumour development in the lymph nodes and other organs, for example sporadic bovine leucosis. This is a different viral condition, and blood samples need to be taken to confirm the diagnosis. A skin form of lymphosarcoma is shown in Plate 10.17.

*Transmission of infection*
Calves are born free of disease but become infected via the colostrum during the first few hours of life. In infected animals the virus is found only in the lymphocytes. Lymphocytes are one of the types of white blood cells and are the main constituent of lymph nodes. The DNA of the virus actually becomes incorporated into the nucleus of the lymphocyte cell, and in so doing it alters its chromosome pattern and therefore the genetic content of the lymphocyte. This is a 'natural' form of genetic engineering.

Transmission to in-contact animals can only occur following transfer of infected blood cells and this can be via colostrum, blood-sucking insects, contaminated injection needles or even sputum, as sputum contains white blood cells. Only 0.0005 ml of blood is needed, an amount far too small to be seen with the naked eye. Even so, the risk of spread from one animal to another by physical contact is very low and by far the most important method of transmission is from the cow to the calf by colostrum. This means that provided infected animals can be identified and removed, control and eradication should be easy.

*Control of EBL*
The disease was made notifiable in the UK in 1977 and in the following year imported cattle and their progeny, a total of 9000 animals, were blood sampled. Evidence of infection was found in 67 Canadian Holstein animals and in two others but even then only 20% of the calves from the infected cows were carrying EBL. A register of EBL-free herds was established in January 1982, based on two consecutive clear blood tests, and this became a self-financing part of the Government Cattle Health Scheme in 1987. All cattle tumours found at meat inspection or at post-mortem must be reported to the Ministry of Agriculture and tested for EBL. Because of the low rate of transmission of infection and the accuracy of the blood test, it is likely that EBL will soon be eradicated from Great Britain. In 1995 there were only seven animals from seven herds, and in 1996 six animals from five herds.

## Tuberculosis

This is a bacterial infection caused by *Mycobacterium bovis* and was once one of the major diseases of cattle, especially when milking cows were tied in byres (shippons) in close contact with one another. It was estimated that well over 40% of all such animals were infected. Many developed tuberculosis in the udder. This led to infected milk and hence to human tuberculosis, known as *consumption*. Tuberculosis in man, especially children, was extremely common. In the UK in the 1930s some 15,000 people each year were said to be infected, with over 2000 dying and others remaining debilitated for life. Although animal reservoirs of infection did play a part, tuberculosis in man was due primarily to the poor standards of housing and hygiene at the time which permitted a greater spread of infection within the community. Pasteurisation of milk prior to sale was a major measure which reduced the spread of TB from animals to man.

It is now very unlikely that clinical tuberculosis will ever be seen, although it should always be considered in cows with gross thickening of the udder, or in cows which progressively go thin and cough up blood and pus (Plate 11.11).

*Eradication of tuberculosis*

A voluntary scheme to establish a register of free herds was started in 1935 and by 1950 there was a sufficient pool of clean stock to introduce compulsory eradication. This was generally very successful and by 1960 the whole country had reached the Attested Herd status. Testing is based on the comparative intradermal test. Two sites, one above the other, are located on the side of the neck by means of a scissor mark. The skin thickness at each point is measured using a pair of special calipers (Plate 11.8) and then a small volume (0.1 ml) of tuberculin is injected (Plate 11.9). The injection is made into the skin and not under it, that is intradermally and not subcutaneously. Tuberculin is an extract of tuberculosis bacteria and if an animal has been previously exposed to TB it reacts to tuberculin by producing a nodule at that point.

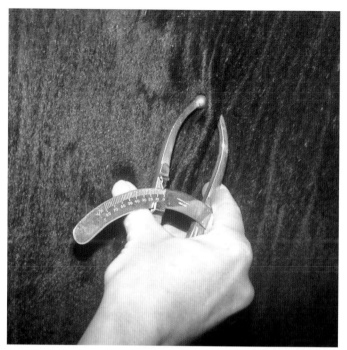

Plate 11.8. Tuberculosis testing. Two sites are identified by means of scissor marks and the skin thickness measured.

The test is a 'comparative' measurement, with injections of avian and bovine tuberculin being necessary. This is because there are conditions other than bovine tuberculosis which can occasionally give a reaction to bovine tuberculin. These include avian TB and skin TB, neither of which is harmful to cattle or man, and *Mycobacterium phlei* (an infection found on certain grasses), *M. kanasii* and Johne's disease (*M. johnei*, Chapter 13). Only *M. johnei* produces disease in cattle. Skin TB nodules are most commonly seen on the neck (Plate 10.18), legs or chest. The nodules are under the skin, not in it. It has been suggested that they may also be a sign of bovine immunodeficiency virus (BIV) (see Chapter 14), but as they are so common in the UK, this seems unlikely. Since the introduction of purified protein derivatives (PPD) of tuberculin, these cross-reactions have become much less important.

Plate 11.10 shows a beef cow which has reacted to the TB test. Note how the swelling at the bovine injection

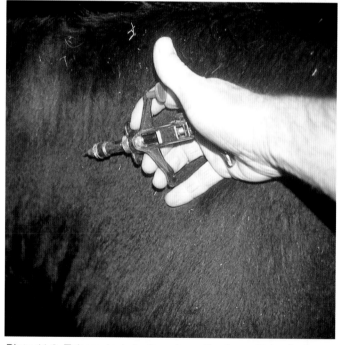

Plate 11.9. Tuberculosis testing. A small volume (0.1 ml) of tuberculin is injected into the skin, avian at the top and bovine at the bottom site.

site (the lower one) is considerably larger than at the avian, indicating a positive reaction to the test. This animal is classified as a reactor. After the test the cow was isolated and when slaughtered, small caseous nodular lesions were found within the carcase, from which TB was cultured. The whole herd then had to be retested at intervals of 60 days until two clear tests were achieved.

Of the cattle which are classified as inconclusive reactors (IRs) at the initial skin test, only 1.0% have TB. The majority pass when retested after 60 days.

Although the skin test has its imperfections, it is rapid, cheap and easy to carry out and is likely to be used for the foreseeable future. Its major problems are:

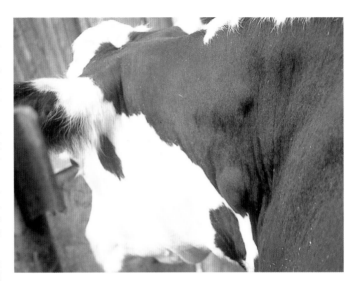

Plate 11.10. Tuberculosis testing. This animal is a reactor and TB lesions were seen at post-mortem. Note how the bovine (lower) reaction is much greater than the avian.

**False negatives** In the advanced stages of TB the cow becomes desensitised by a heavy challenge of infection. This is known as the anergic state and is typified by the cow shown in Plate 11.11. Because she was in a herd under movement restrictions, she was tested for TB to allow casualty slaughter on account of her chronic nasal haemorrhage. She passed the intradermal TB test – but was found to be heavily infected with TB two days later at the abattoir!

It is also possible that cattle slaughtered very soon after infection (especially lung infection) may have small lesions at post-mortem, but do not react to the intradermal test.

**False positives** In a proportion of animals which fail the test (viz they are classified as reactors), no TB is found at post-mortem. These are known as no visible lesion (NVL) reactors.

There are two possible reasons for false positives, namely:

- TB is present in the carcase, but is not found at post-mortem.

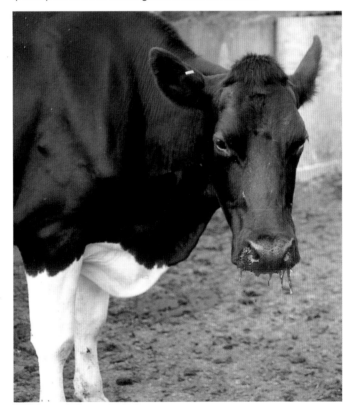

Plate 11.11. Tuberculosis testing – an anergic animal. Because she was so heavily infected with TB in her lungs (leading to bleeding from the nose), the intradermal TB test did not work.

Detailed dissections of such reactor carcases have shown that the TB nodule present might be as small as a pinhead, but even this is enough for a few of them to be shedding infection to other cows.

● The animal has been exposed to TB but has since recovered. She will continue to give a positive reaction to the test for a considerable period of time. This probably accounts for 70% of the NVL reactors.

As in the UK only 50 cattle each year are found to have TB at the abattoir, the skin test must be reasonably effective!

*Tuberculosis in badgers*

In 1970, despite the falling incidence of cattle reactors in most areas of the country, the level of infection in parts of Gloucestershire, Avon and a few other counties in the UK remained unchanged at around 0.1%. This was associated with the high incidence of TB in badgers in these areas. It may well be that cattle infected the badgers initially, but in areas of heavy badger density, and where they are living in close confinement, tuberculosis in badgers is rife. The Cotswold hills provided an ideal habitat and in the mid 1970s 27% of badgers examined in this area were found to be infected, rising to 33% in 1996! Compared with cattle, badgers have relatively little resistance to TB. Once infected, disease spreads rapidly and especially in the final stages, badgers excrete large numbers of bacteria in their urine, faeces and saliva. Unfortunately, because of their different immune system, the intradermal (= tuberculin) test used in cattle does not work in badgers and even blood samples are not particularly accurate. Cultural examination of urine, faeces and sputum can be used, but isolation of TB from faeces is difficult because so many other bacteria are present and because all TB cultures have to be incubated for several weeks.

Badgers like to dig in sandy soil and prefer to have a rocky roof to their sett, so wooded escarpments form their favourite habitat (Plate 11.12). On the other hand, as 60% of their diet consists of earthworms, they like to forage over short grazed pasture, in other words, where cattle might graze. Dry summers used to reduce the number of available earthworms and consequently the number of badgers. However, the increase in the quantity of forage maize being grown now more than compensates for this.

There are thought to be two main methods of transmitting infection to cattle, pasture contamination and contamination of feedingstuffs. The former is especially common because badgers have a specific 'latrine' area on pasture some distance away from their woodland sett and of course cattle will sniff and lick any unusual objects including badger urine and faeces. Second, badly affected badgers become weak and are no longer able to dig and forage for their food. This drives them towards farm buildings for easier access to feedingstuffs and hence TB contamination of cattle feedingstuffs can occur.

As the incidence of TB in badgers is very much higher than in cattle, it seems most probable that infection flows from badgers to cattle and not cattle to badgers. In the long term the elimination of infected setts must be beneficial to badgers as well as to cattle and man. However, elimination also has its problems. Because infected setts can become repopulated quite quickly by other badgers and as TB can live in the soil for up to two months, there is a risk that a repopulated sett will become reinfected. Similarly if you have a sett on your farm and no TB in the cattle, then you are legally bound to leave that sett intact. In any

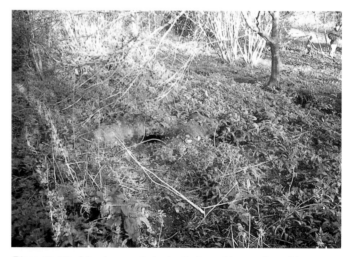

Plate 11.12. A badger sett, typically found in sandy soil in a wooded area.

case, eliminating could lead to repopulation – and possibly with infected badgers!

The motor vehicle is one of the main 'predators' of the badger. It has been estimated that 50,000 deaths each year are caused by road accidents. This represents 50% of all adult badger deaths – and should be compared with the 1000 badgers per annum eliminated by the culling of infected setts! In TB infected areas of the country road traffic deaths are commonly submitted for post-mortem and around 25% of badgers are infected with TB. This should be compared with the finding that in 1996 32% of all badgers trapped on the basis of being in contact with infected herds were positive. This must surely be further strong evidence supporting the link between TB in badgers and cattle.

From the mid 1970s control of TB in badgers was carried out by gassing infected setts with cyanide, but in 1982 trapping was introduced because it was said that death following exposure to cyanide was inhumane. Since then there have been numerous changes in badger trapping, testing and elimination policies, due primarily to political pressure from badger protection groups, who consider that the case against badgers is unproven.

After 1975, with the introduction of unrestricted gassing of those badger setts associated with TB-infected cattle, there was a sharp reduction in the number of new infected herds. For example, in the counties of Gloucestershire and Avon the number of new herds having 'reactors' to the intradermal tuber-culin test fell from 123 herds per annum in 1976 to around 40 per annum (range 36–48 over the years 1980–1988) by 1988 (Figure 11.3). Not all 'reactor' herds are confirmed by visible lesions or culture (although it is estimated that at least 70% of unconfirmed cases do have TB) and so the number of *confirmed* infected herds each year fell from 68 in 1976 to around 20 (range 17–26) by 1988.

Gassing of infected setts was banned in 1982 and was replaced by the 'clean ring' trapping and elimination strategy which eliminated all infected setts within a mile of infected cattle. In 1986 this was again changed and the Dunnet strategy was implemented which only permitted trapping and testing of badgers on the farm which had TB infected cattle. If the sett happened to be in an adjacent neighbour's field, trapping was not permitted! Since then there has been a steady increase in TB, with approximately 180 new reactor herds in 1997 and a further increase in 1998. This change in the inci-dence of reactor herds in Gloucestershire is shown in Figure 11.3.

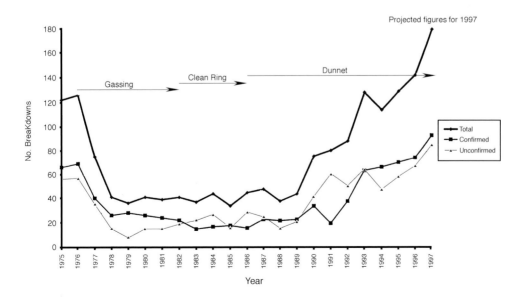

Figure 11.3. The incidence of new TB reactor herds in Gloucestershire and Avon from 1975 to 1997.

*The future*

Although there has been a limited trial of an oral administration system it will be many years before a vacine for badgers or cattle is available. Freedom from TB for cattle, badgers and man must be a logical long-term aim.

The massive increase in UK badger numbers (76% increase from 1985 to 1995) must have a contributory effect: as population densities increase, so will the rate of spread of infection to cattle. Some farms are already having to harvest their maize early in the autumn because of severe badger damage. Perhaps a limited cull will be permitted in the future.

In 1998 the report of the Krebs Committee in the UK proposed a field trial aimed at resolving the issue as to whether badgers are involved in the spread of TB to cattle. The trial, planned to last for at least five years, was to be carried out in TB 'hot spots'. Each trial area of 100 square kilometres (approximately 20,000 acres) would be subdivided into three treatments, namely

- in one area all the badgers would be totally eliminated for the five year period
- in the second area, badgers would only be eliminated if they were associated with farms where there is TB in cattle
- in the third area, only the badger numbers would be monitored. There would be no culling, irrespective of the incidence of TB in the cattle.

The results of this trial are awaited with interest.

In the interim the only practical steps are to reduce the amount of contact between badgers and cattle. This can be achieved by keeping cattle away from badger setts by means of electric fencing and perhaps using fencing 150 mm above ground level to redirect badger tracks away from pasture land. Any bedding discarded by badgers from their setts in the spring, as in Plate 11.13, should be burnt (wear gloves when handling it, as it may be infected). Submit all dead badgers for post-mortem examination to ascertain whether or not they are infected with TB (Plate 11.14). Finally, make sure that feed stores and cattle food and water troughs are not accessible to badgers. This means that they should be at least 800 mm high with smooth, solid walls, with perhaps a protruding

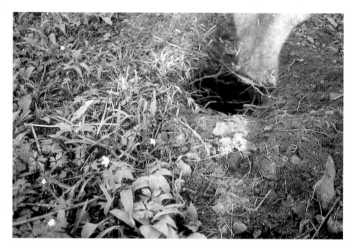

Plate 11.13. The bedding discarded from badger setts in the spring, as seen here, is best burnt, as it could be infected with TB.

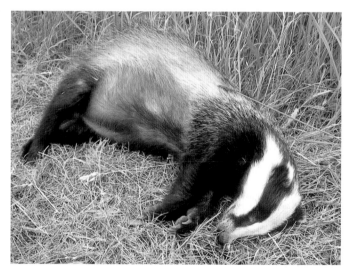

Plate 11.14. If you have TB in your herd, then it would be a wise precaution to submit any dead badgers found for a test for tuberculosis.

lip at the top. As mentioned previously, in the terminal stages badgers infected with TB are no longer able to forage for food and are therefore more likely to take the easy way out and eat cattle food, especially cereals. With even their saliva being infected, this represents a serious danger to the cattle and explains why young stock which have never been out to graze are sometimes infected with TB.

TB has been found in foxes, moles, ferrets and rats, but at a lower incidence and it is not known if these animals were shedding tuberculosis. If not, they are unlikely to act as a source of infection for cattle. Farmed deer have occasionally shown a high incidence TB, and there is concern this might spread to wild deer. Unfortunately for the badger, it is the only significant excretor of infection and as such, is likely to be a major reservoir for cattle. Until the problem has been resolved, TB in cattle may be controlled, but it will not be eliminated. In the longer term, it must be in the interests of man, cattle and the badger itself to have a healthy badger population.

> Attempt to minimise spread of TB from badgers to cattle by:
>
> * fencing cattle away from badger setts
> * burning potentially infected bedding discarded from the sett in the spring
> * ensuring cattle water and feed troughs are not accessible to badgers
> * submitting all dead badgers for post-mortem examination and testing

## Bovine Spongiform Encephalopathy (BSE)

First reported in 1986, BSE became one of the greatest issues ever to strike the British cattle industry, although it was the politics surrounding the disease, rather than the disease itself, which led to such massive economic losses. It was not until the end of 1998 that the world-wide export ban imposed by the EU on beef produced in the UK was lifted, and even then there were stringent restrictions, with only fully traceable animals under thirty months of age eligible for export. All the available evidence suggests that this epidemic will have virtually died out soon after the year 2004.

*Clinical signs*
The disease is seen primarily in mature dairy cows, three to six years old, with a variety of clinical signs including:

* weight loss, partly due to poor rumination
* incoordination: affected animals walk with stiff hind legs and may almost fall if rushed around a sharp bend
* excessive licking of the nostrils, first one side then the other, and sometimes biting the flanks and grinding the teeth
* ears flicking to and fro, and the skin over the chest and flanks twitching and fluttering repeatedly, as if flies were landing on it
* general apprehension, for example cows may appear nervous when entering a narrow doorway into the milking parlour; they may over-react with jumping and pricked ears at the sound of a hand-clap (Plate 11.15); and they occasionally kick violently and aggressively in the milking parlour. Aggression, such as attacking farm staff in the yard, is a rare feature and only occurs when the animal has been separated from the others and feels threatened
* in the terminal stages affected cows become recumbent with a characteristic 'dog-sitting' posture as shown in Plate 11.16.

If the condition were to progress, cows would be so uncoordinated that they would become recumbent and would eventually die from inability to eat and drink, and from self-inflicted injuries. There is no treatment.

No animal is ever allowed to progress to this stage in the UK, as it is a legal requirement that any animal showing any suspect signs of BSE is reported to the Ministry of Agriculture. The compensation paid to farmers is sufficient to encourage them to do so.

After a Ministry veterinary officer has confirmed the tentative diagnosis of BSE from clinical signs, the animal is destroyed by lethal injection and the head is taken away for examination.

Despite the quite characteristic clinical signs, there is as yet no test available in the live animal and confirmatory diagnosis can only be carried out by a microscopic examination of the brain at post- mortem.

*Causes*
BSE is one of a family of transmissible spongiform encephalopathies (TSEs), all of which are caused by closely related infections. The infectious agent has yet to be identified but it is most probably a prion, a subcellular protein particle, which replicates by becoming incorporated into the host cell. TSEs are not a new phenomenon: they have been in existence for many years. Examples (and the year in which they were first identified) include:

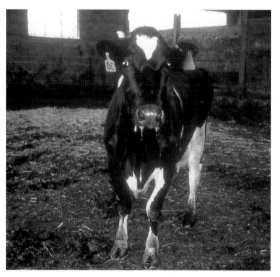

Plate 11.15. An animal with BSE over-reacts to a hand-clap, as in this cow. Note the startled look in her eyes and erect ears. She has also lost weight.

- Scrapie in sheep (1732)
- Kuru in man (1900)
- Creutzfeldt-Jakob disease (CJD) in man (1920)
- Transmissible mink encephalopathy (TME) (1947)
- Chronic wasting disease in eland and kudu (1967)
- Bovine spongiform encephalopathy (BSE) (1986)
- Feline spongiform encephalopathy (FSE) (1990)

All these diseases have a similar epidemiology, namely a very long incubation period of several years, after which 'spongy' vacuoles appear in specific areas of the brain (the brain stem) and lead to nervous signs. The average incubation period for BSE is around five years, although it can be as little

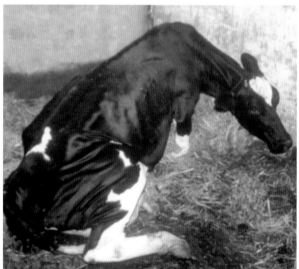

Plate 11.16. More advanced cases of BSE become recumbent and adopt a dog-sitting position.

as two or three years, with the youngest confirmed case being twenty months old.

All TSEs are progressive and always fatal. There is absolutely no treatment. Animals should be destroyed as soon as the diagnosis has been made. Death from TSEs in man is most unpleasant.

Epidemiological studies of the occurrence of BSE strongly indicate that it is associated with the feeding of meat and bone meal. Changes in the production of meat and bone meal in the early 1980s led to its being manufactured without the use of solvents and on a continuous production line, rather than on a batch basis. The lower incidence of BSE in Scotland is thought to be due to the fact that they continued with solvent and high temperature processing for much longer, although experimentally, solvents have had litle effect on the viability of the BSE agent. It is now known that temperatures probably in excess of 140°C are needed to destroy the agent, preferably under steam.

At the same time as these changes occurred in the rendering industry there was a considerable increase in sheep production, and therefore sheep slaughtering, in the UK and a switch towards the use of meat and bone meal because of high world soya prices. It remains unknown whether BSE is a mutation from scrapie in sheep or whether it is an infection which has always been present in cattle and the relaxation of offal processing in the early 1980s led to it recycling to produce very high levels of disease. Using mouse infectivity titrations, the BSE agent does not resemble any of the known strains of sheep scrapie and it would appear that there is only one strain of BSE.

### Control measures

In June 1988 BSE was made a notifiable disease. After this date all animals suspected of having the disease were incinerated and removed from the human food chain. In July 1988 a ban was imposed to prohibit the use of ruminant meat and bone meal (rM+BM) in ruminant rations. In June 1990 the use of certain bovine offals in human food was prohibited: brain, spinal cord, spleen and tonsils of animals over six months old, plus the thymus and intestine of calves less than six months old, all of which were termed specified bovine offals (SBOs). Then in September 1990 these SBOs were also banned from use in rM+BM for any livestock diets and had to be stained at the abattoir and then incinerated. Because such small quantities of brain (1.0 g) were found to be infective to cattle, later the whole head (excluding the tongue and lower jaw) became included and it was all known as specific bovine material (SBM). It had proved impossible for all traces of brain to be completely removed from the skull and there was concern that in attempting to remove it, nervous tissue might leak onto meat which would be used for human consumption.

These measures led to a dramatic reduction in the incidence of BSE from 1993 onwards (the average incubation period being 5 years). However, there were still far too many animals 'born after the ban', i.e. after July 1988, which developed BSE. At that stage it was realised that only a very low dose (1.0 g) of BSE infected brain tissue was needed to be ingested by a calf to cause disease. Despite the ban on feeding rM+BM it was found that some infective material was still getting into cattle diets. This was occurring because of:

- cross-contamination in feed mills. At this stage rM+BM was still being used in horse, pig and poultry food
- failure to keep SBOs totally separate at abattoirs, knacker yards and hunt kennels, so that even non-ruminant derived meat and bone meal (nrM+BM) was found to contain traces of ruminant SBOs

There was considerable tightening up of feed mill and abattoir practices to prevent this cross-contamination. Then in November 1994 a ban was imposed to prohibit the use of all mammalian (viz in addition to ruminant) M+BM to any ruminants. In March 1996 this was further strengthened by banning the feeding of any mammalian M+BM to any livestock species and it is now an offence even to leave it in the mill! This was monitored by careful checks on animal feed using an ELISA test, able to detect very low levels of mammalian M+BM. Consequently it was not until August 1996 that all traces of meat and bone meal were removed from all ruminant feeds and it will be the year 2000 and beyond before we can be sure if this was totally effective.

### Birth records and double tagging

A second part of the BSE control measures involves records of animal births and movements. All cattle born since 1 July 1996 have an individual passport which goes with them from farm to farm until they reach slaughter. It is illegal to trade in animals which do not have passports, none can be sold for human consumption, and to attempt to do so would result in a heavy penalty. Movement records had been a statutory requirement for many years, but as a result of the BSE episode, the following records have become mandatory for cattle in the UK:

- all movements to be recorded within 36 hours of the movement occurring

- births of dairy calves and their individual ear-tag to be recorded within seven days of birth
- births of beef calves and their individual ear-tag to be recorded within 30 days of birth
- the identity (ear number) of the dam to be recorded in each case
- deaths reported within seven days
- replacement of ear-tags to be recorded and reported within 36 hours
- all calves to be double-tagged, viz they must have a tag in each ear

The idea behind such comprehensive recording was to allow tracing of animals which had possibly been exposed to BSE and to confirm their age at slaughter for human consumption.

*Cohort and offspring cull*
In an attempt to reduce the incidence of BSE even faster, and in so doing win political approval to restart UK beef exports, it was decided to cull and incinerate those animals which were most likely to develop BSE later in life. This consisted of two groups, namely

- the birth cohorts. These were animals born on a farm at the same time (defined as within the same year) as a cow which later developed BSE. These animals were thought to be at special risk because, as calves, they would have eaten the same food as the BSE animal.
- the offspring cohorts. In 1998 it was decided to cull all offspring born to BSE cases after 1 August 1996. This represented a considerable tracing exercise, with approximately another 1000 animals found, culled and incinerated.

*Progress of control measures*
The incidence of BSE reached its peak in late 1992/early 1993, when 1000 cases were being reported each week. By October 1998 there had been over 172,500 confirmed cases of BSE slaughtered and incinerated, 37,187 of which had been born after the July 1988 meat and bone meal ban. By June 1997 67% of dairy herds and 15.8% of suckler beef herds had had at least one case. However, the weekly incidence had decreased by a factor of ten to less than 100 cases a week and by October 1998 the number of animals born after the ban was also showing a sharp decline:

| Year of birth | Number of cases to October 1998 |
|---|---|
| July–Dec 1988 & 1989 | 24,483 |
| 1990 | 5,524 |
| 1991 | 4,254 |
| 1992 | 2,350 |
| 1993 | 1,057 |
| 1994–95 | 110 |

Despite the characteristic clinical signs and the considerable experience of the veterinary personnel carrying out the clinical examinations, approximately 15% of all animals slaughtered as suspect BSE eventually proved to be negative, with listeriosis being one of the main diagnoses in negative cases. As the incidence of BSE fell, so the error rate of diagnosis increased, reaching almost 20% by 1997. By this time around 20,500 animals had been slaughtered as suspect BSE cases but were subsequently found to be negative at post-mortem.

It is impossible to explain why other European countries, supposedly virtually BSE-free, failed to identify similar numbers of suspect animals, that is animals which showed typical signs of BSE but which were found to be negative on post-mortem examination. After the UK, Switzerland reported the second highest number of confirmed cases (228) and Ireland the third (188), but in both cases the numbers are nothing to match the incidence (172,000) in the UK. Considerable concern was also raised about possible under-reporting in other European countries when a survey of cattle exported from the

UK prior to 1989 was published in 1997. This survey compared the actual numbers of BSE cases reported in cattle exported from the UK with the predicted incidence, that is the incidence that would have occurred in those cattle if they had remained within the UK. The figures reported were:

|  | Predicted incidence to Jan 1997 | Reported incidence |
|---|---|---|
| UK | n/c | 165,323 |
| Switzerland | n/c | 228 |
| Ireland | 911 | 188 |
| Portugal | 262 | 61 |
| France | 32 | 28 |
| Germany | 243 | 5 |
| Italy | 50 | 2 |
| Denmark | 29 | 1 |

n/c = not calculated

In addition, as many thousands of tons of both infected meat and bone meal and cattle concentrates were exported from the UK prior to 1989, it is impossible to speculate why this apparently did not produce BSE in any European country apart from Switzerland.

*Maternal transmission*
There is little firm evidence for significant maternal transmission. Studies of field cases of BSE show:

● the incidence of BSE in the offspring of BSE dams was not higher than the national average
● when one case had occurred, an individual farm was no more likely to get further cases of BSE than any other farm

A similar trend was found when offspring from BSE and non-BSE dams were purchased from farms and reared to seven years old. Most of these animals had been reared for several weeks on the farm of origin and had therefore been exposed to potentially BSE contaminated feed. Although initial results suggested a maternal transmission rate of around 10% when the calf was born within six months of the cow developing BSE, extrapolation to the field situation showed that if maternal transmission of BSE existed, it was at a very low level and certainly not sufficient to have a significant influence on the course of the epidemic.

*BSE and human health*
This was the aspect of BSE which had the least proof and yet politically produced the most devastating consequences for the cattle industry throughout Europe and even throughout the world. The concern was that tissues from BSE-infected cattle could enter the human food chain and lead to CJD in man. There was no definitive evidence that this was occurring, but near panic broke out when in March 1996 the CJD Surveillance Unit in Edinburgh announced that ten cases of a variant form of human CJD (nvCJD) had been identified in an age group under 45 years old. Because no other explanation was readily available it was assumed that these nvCJD cases were associated with the consumption of BSE-infected beef or beef products (Will R.G. & others (1996), *The Lancet*, vol 347, p. 921).

In March 1996 this caused the collapse of the beef industry in Europe and a considerable depression in beef consumption worldwide, brought about in no small part by EU governments grossly over-reacting and imposing a worldwide ban on the export of all UK beef and beef products. At the same time all animals over 30 months of age (both clean beef and barren cows) were considered to be unfit for human consumption and the Government paid compensation to the farmers for them to be slaughtered and rendered or incinerated. By October 1998 over 2.5 million animals had been destroyed in this way and at the same time the Government was paying farmers to slaughter male animals within the first few weeks of life.

It should be remembered that this took place despite the fact that almost all the available evidence suggested that by that stage of the epidemic there were so many controls in place that meat was quite safe to eat. For example:

- Even in *affected* animals the BSE agent had only ever been found in the brain and spinal cord, and all affected animals had been slaughtered and incinerated since June 1988.
- Even when meat and milk from animals clinically affected by BSE was injected into the brains of mice, no BSE was reproduced.
- From June 1990, all specified offal (bovine brain, spinal cord, thymus, spleen and intestine) had been removed from the food chain.
- From March 1996, no animal over 30 months old was permitted to enter the human food chain.
- In animals known to be incubating the disease following a very heavy (100 g) experimental challenge of infection, the agent had been identified only from the small intestine – which at this stage was being discarded – in all animals under 30 months old. All other tissues were 'safe', including the brain and spinal cord.
- From December 1997, it even became illegal to sell beef 'on the bone' because of the risk that, in animals incubating BSE, the dorsal root ganglia (part of the nervous system) might contain the BSE agent.

The latter measure was considered by many people to be an 'over-kill' in terms of food safety. It had been calculated that even if the beef was not deboned, there was only a 5% chance that one person in the UK *might* develop nvCJD. This equates to a risk of one in 600 million, and should be compared to other UK risks, for example being struck by lightning (1:10 million), murdered (1:100,000) or dying from a smoking related illness (1:200). Despite all these additional safeguards, the worldwide export ban on UK beef was retained until 1998.

Experiments did show a similarity between mice injected with BSE and nvCJD, whereas mice infected with classical CJD were different. This is by no means proof that BSE was the cause of nvCJD, however. If there had been any risk, ever, it had occurred prior to June 1988, at the time before BSE had been made a notifiable disease, or possibly before specified offal had been removed from the

| Summary of BSE legislation | |
|---|---|
| June 1988 | BSE made a notifiable disease and all animals showing clinical signs removed from the food chain and incinerated |
| July 1988 | Feeding of ruminant M+B to ruminants prohibited |
| June 1990 | SBO from all healthy cattle removed from the human food chain |
| September 1990 | SBO from all cattle banned from inclusion in any livestock diets |
| November 1994 | Ban on feeding ruminants mammalian M+B from any source |
| March 1996 | Total ban on feeding all livestock mammalian M+B from any source |
| July 1996 | Compulsory registration of all calf births, with passports issued |
| August 1996 | No further traces of M+B detected in routine compulsory screening of rations. |
| 1997–99 | Cull of cohorts from BSE farms:<br>– birth cohorts = animals born at the same time as BSE case.<br>– offspring cohorts = calves born to BSE dams |

food chain in June 1990. Transmission has never been shown possible in milk, even when milk from confirmed cases of BSE was injected into the brains of mice. Despite this, and as an additional safety precaution, milk from suspect BSE cows is always discarded.

In spite of these reassurances, there were still certain high profile pseudoscientists predicting that there would be a cataclysmic outbreak of nvCJD and that we were about to 'lose a generation of the nation's children'. It has to be accepted that this is a possibility and it will be ten to twenty years after publication of this book before we can be sure it did not happen. With only thirty-five cases of nvCJD having occurred at the time of writing (March 1999), which is more than ten years after BSE was made notifiable, this seems highly improbable. In fact nvCJD case number 20 occurred in a person who had been a strict vegetarian since 1985, i.e. one year before the first case of BSE had been reported. By this stage even the national press was starting to doubt whether there was any connection, and possibly part of the increase in nvCJD cases was simply due to more surveillance. Other suggestions included a genetic link (consistent DNA pattern found in many patients), surgical intervention (nvCJD prions had been found in an appendix following routine removal), blood transfusions (nvCJD present in white cells) and vaccines prepared from bovine products. If nvCJD *did* originate from cattle, it is much more likely to have been transmitted by injection – i.e. from vaccines or blood – than by ingestion of food.

## SALMONELLOSIS

Many aspects of disease caused by salmonella have been covered already, for example in the young, bucket-fed calf (Chapter 2) and in the weaned animal (Chapter 3). This section deals with the disease in the adult cow and discusses some of the possible sources and the human health aspects. Salmonellosis is not a notifiable disease, but must be reported under the Zoonosis order.

There are many different strains of salmonella (almost 2000 in total) called serotypes. In the 1960s the commonest serotype in cattle was *Salmonella dublin*, but from mid 1970 onwards *S. typhimurium* became much more common and, in addition, a whole range of 'exotic' strains were encountered, with names like:

| | | |
|---|---|---|
| *S. agona* | *S. newport* | *S. virchow* |
| *S. enteriditis* | *S. heidelberg* | *S. seftenburg* |

and many others. *S. dublin* is found almost entirely in cattle and the source of infection must therefore be direct or indirect contact with other cattle. *S. typhimurium* and the exotics, on the other hand, are much more widespread. Infection occurs in a whole range of animals, including man, which means that the possible sources of infection are much more variable.

### Clinical signs

Salmonella particularly affects the intestine and scouring is therefore the most frequent clinical sign in animals of all ages. Dysentery is often seen, viz a profuse diarrhoea sometimes with blood, and often mixed with large pieces of 'fleshy mucus'. This is the damaged lining of the gut being shed. Lactating cows completely stop milking, their eyes become dull and sunken due to dehydration, and they run a very high temperature. The dung will contain millions of salmonella bacteria and hence isolation is vital to reduce the risk of infecting other cows. Ideally use a loose-box with no drainage to the outside and particularly avoid surface drains which run across an open yard.

Infection with salmonella does not always cause scouring, however. Abortion, especially from mid pregnancy onwards, may be the only clinical sign seen, and salmonella can be recovered in very large numbers from the afterbirth. *S. dublin* especially may be involved and sometimes abortion may precede an attack of acute diarrhoea and death. *S. dublin* may also cause pneumonia, joint ill or even meningitis with nervous signs, and cattle of any age may be affected. I have also seen *S. typhimurium* isolated from an aborted cow showing no other symptoms and with no further cases occurring in the herd. This makes it very difficult when advising farmers what action they ought to take following the confirmation of salmonellosis in their herd. Even calvings induced with cortisone or prostaglandin may be sufficient stress to precipitate clinical salmonellosis in a carrier cow.

*Treatment*

Treatment is largely symptomatic, aimed as much at treating the symptoms as eliminating the disease. Kaolin and chlorodyne may physically help to control the scouring. Sick animals should be encouraged to drink by giving them warm water. Animals not drinking can be orally dosed with electrolyte, or given intravenous fluid therapy if severely dehydrated. Antishock treatments (such as the non-steroidal anti-inflammatory flunixin) help enormously and are certainly worth giving to very sick animals. Multivitamins may assist in the healing phase, especially if the rumen (the major source of B vitamins for the cow) is not working properly.

The use of antibiotics in the treatment of salmonellosis has been called into question on two counts: firstly because of the risk of antibiotic-resistant strains of salmonella spreading into the human population, and secondly because antibiotics may prolong excretion rates and produce more carrier animals. However, I consider that antibiotics are justified on both economic and welfare grounds. A septicaemic animal with a high temperature cannot be left to die and provided that an adequate dose of the correct antibiotic is administered for a reasonable period of time to a cow in isolation, personally I believe that the risk to the human population is extremely low. Although care should always be exercised, it has been suggested that most antibiotic resistance in man is likely to be due to the misuse of antibiotics in humans, rather than from any excessive use in animals.

*Progress of a herd outbreak*

Disease due to *S. typhimurium* and the exotics appears to be much more common in the autumn and this is thought to be because warmth and humidity predispose to the survival and spread of the organism. The isolation of salmonella from one cow, whether she is scouring or following an abortion, should certainly cause alarm and lead to increased vigilance, but possibly no other immediate action is needed, apart from treatment and separating her from the remainder of the herd. Ideally, faecal swabs should be taken from her until at least two consecutive negative results have been obtained. The cow can then be released from isolation.

However, if the disease starts to spread, careful control measures will be needed. The precise details will depend on the management and design of your unit, and the action necessary should be discussed with your vet. As a general rule, calves from infected cows should be given ample colostrum and then penned individually to prevent the spread of infection. Nutritional stress, for example a sudden change in diet for either the cows or calves, should be avoided, because stress can precipitate an outbreak of disease. Separation of the different age groups of cattle is important, and any possible measures to prevent faecal contamination of food should be taken.

Salmonellosis often strikes batch-calving herds, with disease being seen as a severe scouring just after calving or following abortion. In such herds control measures should include:

- Calve each animal in isolation in a clean box. With the stress of calving, a cow which has been carrying salmonella may start shedding infection in her dung. Ideally every cow should remain isolated until faecal swabs are negative, even if not scouring. This is unlikely to be feasible in most herds.
- Vaccinate. A dead vaccine given at six weeks and three weeks prior to calving will provide good protection against both the enteric (i.e. scouring) and abortion forms of the disease and, through the transfer of antibodies in the colostrum, it reduces the excretion of salmonella and thereby reduces salmonella problems in calves. In the event of an outbreak, the whole herd should be vaccinated, irrespective of their stage of lactation or pregnancy.
- Minimise faecal contamination of food. This might entail keeping dogs, chickens, pigeons etc. away from feed stores and troughs and reducing the contamination of food by tractor wheels, e.g. by scraping passages more thoroughly. Do not walk on cattle food with dirty boots.
- Do not use dirty water from yard drains etc. for the irrigation of land currently being grazed.
- Feed diets which will not produce digestive upsets and which will lead to firm dung. The latter helps to reduce faecal contamination of feed.
- Minimise overcrowding and keep buildings well ventilated. Infection is more likely to spread if cattle are tightly packed into humid buildings.

- If possible, get the dry cows well away from the milking cows to minimise any chance of faecal contamination between the two groups. As it is the cow at calving who is most susceptible to salmonella, reducing her risk of contracting and spreading infection is all important.
- Dose for liver fluke in areas where fluke infection is a possibility, since even quite low fluke infestations appear to increase the likelihood of disease from *S. dublin*.

*Sources of infection*

From the early 1990s a specific strain of *S. typhimurium*, DT104, has become increasingly important both in man and in all species of farmed livestock. For example, in 1995 it accounted for over 30% of all salmonella incidents in cattle and was second in importance to *S. enteritidis*, PT4, in man. The DT104 strain is characteristically resistant to the antibiotics ampicillin, chloramphenicol, streptomycin, sulphonamides and tetracyclines, and a few strains are also resistant to trimethoprim. It is more pathogenic (i.e. causes more severe symptoms) than most other strains, with deaths occurring in around 40% of clinically affected cows and almost 50% of calves. This strain is also a greater risk to man and so careful hygiene measures are required.

By means of extensive swabbing, infected farms have been shown to have a widespread distribution of the organism. For example, it may be found in cubicles, feed passages, on tractors, cars, boots, drains, in rats and mice and often household pets. Sheep and pigs may also be carriers. With such an extensive reservoir it is difficult to instigate any effective control measures apart from vaccination.

The most common source of infection in calves is undoubtedly other calves which have been obtained via markets or through dealers' premises. The reasons for this are given in Chapter 2 and clearly calves which repeatedly pass through such premises present an even greater risk. However, disease outbreaks in dairy herds are often not associated with recent purchases and other sources of infection need to be identified.

Exotic salmonella species may be found in imported feedstuffs, especially fishmeal. Current importations are routinely screened at the docks. Unfortunately no legislation exists for impounding such imports and by the time that the laboratory culture results are available, many consignments will already have been incorporated into feedingstuffs and are being fed to livestock. At least the monitoring is able to identify commonly infected sources, however. For example one type of South American fishmeal once featured prominently in the results. Pelleting and other heat treatments destroy many of the salmonellae during processing, so that the number of contaminated finished feeds will be very much lower.

Home-produced animal protein food, for example, from chicken offal, was also once a high risk, but the *Protein Processing Order* (1981) made it compulsory for all such material to be heat treated before its incorporation into feedingstuffs and this should no longer present any risk. The legislation would be considerably strengthened if compulsory powers of sampling were included, however.

Sewage is a further possible source of salmonella, from both human and animal origin. Human carriers are not uncommon and seagulls or other birds feeding on effluent discharged directly into estuaries, or from inadequately supervised septic outflows, have been shown to contaminate grazing land. Sewage sludge is a possible source, although there are strict codes of practice governing its use and the subsequent grazing of treated land, and most of the salmonellae die from desiccation within a week of being spread onto the pasture, especially in the summer. Some may persist for a considerable time, however, particularly those protected in the moist environment of a dung pat. Although survival periods of up to six months have been recorded for both *S. dublin* and *S. newport*, it is doubtful whether there would then be a sufficiently large dose to lead to disease, since experiments feeding 100,000 *S. dublin* bacteria daily to healthy cattle failed to produce any symptoms. It does indicate a further possible source, however, and pasture contamination may be important in producing carrier animals which can develop disease following stress at a later date. This is particularly the case for *S. typhimurium* DT104. During periods of flooding, salmonellae may be deposited directly onto pasture and be ingested by grazing animals. The importance of hygiene and disposal of faeces during an outbreak of disease cannot be overstressed.

Many wild animals have been shown to be carriers of salmonella and they can contaminate animal feed. Salmonella-infected rats, mice or birds can contaminate stored feedingstuffs and it would be impossible to tell if infection came in with the original imported fishmeal or whether it was due to subsequent contamination either on the farm or at the mill. Clearly vermin control is important in this context.

Dogs or foxes may also be involved. They could drag an aborted foetus or its placenta from an adjacent field, or they may simply carry infection on their feet. This is why the placenta and foetus should always be carefully disposed of by burning or burying. One of the major problems in trying to identify the source of salmonella during an outbreak is that exposure to infection may have occurred some considerable time in the past. It is only under subsequent stress that disease then develops, and by that stage the original source of infection may have long since gone.

*Salmonellosis in man*

With the increase in incidence in animals, there has been a corresponding rise in human infections of *S. typhimurium* and the exotics; human infection with *S. dublin* is very rare. Symptoms of salmonellosis are seen as food poisoning, with fever, severe abdominal pain, vomiting and diarrhoea. The elderly and very young children are particularly susceptible and deaths may occur. As with cattle, symptomless human carriers can develop and these people could be a risk to livestock, either directly or through inadequate sewage treatment.

The reverse, that is the spread of salmonella from animals to man, occurs most commonly through improperly cooked meat, improperly stored food or through drinking unpasteurised milk. For example, in Scotland, where consumption of unpasteurised milk was once common, there were 21 outbreaks with 1146 confirmed human cases (including 8 deaths) for the three year period 1980–82 inclusive. In 1983, legislation was introduced to enforce pasteurisation of all milk prior to sale and in the next three year period, 1983–85 inclusive, this reduced the human incidence of salmonellosis in Scotland to 15 outbreaks, but involving only 101 persons, all of whom were directly related to the farming community. It is expected that similar legislation will eventually follow in England.

The incidence of human cases from milk is relatively low, however. The dramatic increase of almost 300% in human *S. enteriditis* infection from 1987 to 1990 is well documented, and was of course associated with eggs and poultry meat. In the 1990s *S. typhimurium* DT104 became increasingly important and in 1994 there were 2500 human cases. As this organism has such a widespread distribution on infected farms, infection of farm personnel is almost impossible to avoid. However, clinical signs of disease are only likely to be seen in children and the elderly. Basic hygiene procedures are necessary to minimise the risks.

## ZOONOSES

A zoonosis is a disease which can be passed from animals to man – and of course from man back to animals. Many have already been mentioned in previous chapters, and the following is a list of the more important ones in cattle. Text page numbers for the discussion of each condition can be found in the index.

Anthrax
Brucellosis
BSE
Crytosporidia
Leptospirosis (*L. hardjo*)
Listeriosis
Pseudocowpox
Q fever
Ringworm
Salmonella, especially *S. typhimurium*
Tuberculosis

Readers should note that although BSE is now included in this list, there remains considerable dispute as to whether infection can in fact pass from cattle to man.

In the UK, the Zoonosis Order, 1975, requires that certain zoonotic diseases must be reported to the Ministry of Agriculture. At present this includes only salmonellosis.

# Chapter 12

# MINERALS, TRACE ELEMENTS, VITAMINS AND WATER

## MINERALS AND TRACE ELEMENTS

Cattle require a dietary supply of at least 15 different minerals for proper growth and production. Some, such as calcium, phosphorus, magnesium, potassium and sodium, are needed in quite large amounts and these are known as the major minerals. Others are required in only minute quantities, usually expressed as parts per million (ppm), and these are called the trace elements.

### Pasture levels and supplementation

Table 12.1 shows the average mineral content of samples of temporary leys analysed by ADAS laboratories over a three year period. This is compared to the requirements of an adult Friesian cow giving 20 litres per day.

It can be seen that an average pasture (first column in Table 12.1) contains insufficient phosphorus, zinc, copper and iodine to meet the needs of 20 litres production (expressed in the second column of Table 12.1). The *average* mineral content of pasture consists of the mean of a very wide range of individual values, however. Soil type and geographical location can have a marked effect. Very acid soils tend to reduce the availability and uptake of all minerals into plants. In addition, temporary leys tend to be lower in minerals than permanent pastures and this is especially so if they have been heavily fertilised and growth is lush – which is exactly the stage at which cows would be grazing without supplementary feeding. On the other hand, mixed swards, for example with clover or other legumes, generally have higher mineral contents.

All of these factors lead to an enormous variation in the mineral content of pastures and the third column in Table 12.1 shows the proportion of the pastures analysed which did not meet the cow's requirements. Taking calcium as an example, the table shows that although the average calcium content of the leys was 0.63% and this would satisfy the cow's requirements (0.52%), 33% of the individual samples contained less than 0.52% calcium and were therefore inadequate. In the case of phosphorus, the average mineral content (0.37%) was less than the cow's requirements (0.42%). This accounted for only 61% of the individual values, however; or put another way, 39% of pastures were adequate despite the fact that the average pasture level provided less than the requirements.

Table 12.1. The adequacy of mineral content of grazing for dairy cattle. All figures are given on a dry matter basis.

| Element | Average values in temporary leys | Dietary requirements for a cow giving 20 l/day | % of samples which were below requirements |
|---------|----------------------------------|------------------------------------------------|--------------------------------------------|
| Calcium | 0.63% | 0.52% | 33% < 0.50% |
| Phosphorus | 0.37% | 0.42% | 61% < 0.40% |
| Magnesium | 0.16% | 0.15% | 40% < 0.15% |
| Potassium | 2.75% | 0.70% | 1% < 1.00% |
| Sodium | 0.21% | 0.14% | 48% < 0.10% |
| Manganese | 85 ppm | 80 ppm | 58% < 80 ppm |
| Zinc | 38 ppm | 50 ppm | 93% < 50 ppm |
| Copper | 8 ppm | 10 ppm | 81% < 10 ppm |
| Cobalt | 0.12 ppm | 0.1 ppm | 52% < 0.1 ppm |
| Iodine | 0.20 ppm | 0.8 ppm | 100% < 0.8 ppm |
| Selenium | 0.07 ppm | 0.1 ppm | – |

Source: Mr G. Alderman, ADAS.

The table shows that there is a real need for mineral supplementation when the cows are grazing – and yet this is often not provided. Another survey looked at conserved forages in a similar manner. It was found that all the samples of hay analysed contained sufficient calcium for maintenance, but some 20% were deficient in magnesium and over 90% of hays and silage were deficient in phosphorus. The latter was especially common if the forage was very mature. Cereal-based rations, on the other hand, contain quite high levels of natural phosphorus and low levels of calcium and this helps to counteract the imbalance in the maintenance ration.

Of course, Table 12.1 can only give approximate values for the calcium requirements of a cow. Requirements will vary depending on the level of yield, total dry matter intake, levels of other minerals in the diet (especially sodium and magnesium) and stage of pregnancy. Therefore this table should only be used as an example of the complexity of mineral supplementation. For precise figures the reader would be advised to refer to detailed tests on nutrition such as Chamberlain and Wilkinson (1996) and ARC (1980). Full details are given in the Further Reading section.

Mineral and trace element supplements are of course added to proprietary 'cow cake' to try to ensure dietary adequacy over a wide range of basic rations. The manufacturers will be assuming that you are feeding concentrate for almost all production, however, and if the overall diet contains malt residue, brewers' grains, sugarbeet pulp or some other by-product, then additional minerals may be necessary. Although it can be a costly exercise to have each component of the ration checked for its mineral and trace element content every year, this would be the ideal situation and I would certainly recommend that at least the forage is analysed every few years. You will then build up a picture of the mineral status of your own farm and supplementation can be provided much more precisely. The money wasted from the haphazard and over-use of mineral supplements could well be equal to the loss of productivity due to inadequate supplementation! Avoiding excessive supplementation and providing each mineral at the correct level are almost as important as counteracting deficiencies.

I do not believe the theory that, when faced with a multiple choice, cows will only eat those minerals which they need. If this were the case, hypomagnesaemia would never occur. On a free access, free choice system, some cows will eat far more than their requirements of a mineral, simply because they enjoy its taste, while others will not bother to take any.

So far only deficiency has been mentioned. The classic signs and symptoms of deficiency may be fairly specific, and there is a tendency for farmers to think that if they cannot see any of these changes, then minerals are not a problem. This is a fallacy however, because mineral *imbalance* can also occur, when an excess of one element interferes with the action of another. Typical examples would be high levels of molybdenum, sulphur or iron interfering with copper metabolism, and the importance of the calcium : phosphorus ratio in the diet. The symptoms of such imbalances can be very vague, for example lack of thrift, depressed production or poor fertility, and the cause can be very difficult to diagnose. There could still be a significant economic effect however.

Because any one mineral may be involved in a variety of metabolic processes, deficiency signs can vary considerably from one animal to another and it is often difficult to recognise a deficiency on clinical grounds alone. Blood, liver or even bone samples will probably be needed for laboratory testing. In addition, many deficiencies render the animal more susceptible to disease, for example to ringworm or calf pneumonia, and there is always a danger that the secondary disease is treated but the primary mineral deficiency is overlooked.

Some of the more important mineral deficiencies have been covered already, for example magnesium in Chapter 6 and vitamin E/selenium in Chapter 3. This chapter discusses the animal's requirements and some of the deficiency symptoms which may be seen. The information is summarised in tabular form in Table 12.2.

## Calcium

Calcium accounts for one-third of the constituents of teeth and bones and in fact 99% of all the calcium in the body is found in the animal's skeleton. Calcium also has important metabolic functions in the soft tissues. For example, it is involved in blood-clotting mechanisms and in the transmission of nerve and

Table 12.2. A summary of the daily mineral, trace element and vitamin requirements of cattle, including the more important deficiency signs.

*Holstein/Friesian eating 19 kg DM*

| Element | Maintenance | Pregnancy (20 wks) | Milk/per litre | Deficiency signs | Comments |
|---|---|---|---|---|---|
| Calcium[1] | 24.3 g | 1.1 g | 1.8 g | Milk fever = short-term imbalance. Rickets | Short-term deficiencies occur in high-yielding cows at peak, but may cause no problems. |
| Phosphorus[1+7] | 28 g | 0.7 g | 1.4 g | When severe, licking bones & soil. Ca:P imbalance may impair fertility | Low levels in some pastures, and in maize silage. Supplementation required. |
| Magnesium[1] | 11.1 g | 0.4 g | 0.8 g | Grass staggers | Continual daily intake required. Falls in spring and autumn, and with high K fertilisers. |
| Sodium[1+2] | 4.2 g | 3.6 g | 0.6 g | Licking, drinking urine, then poor growth and production | Lush grazing and maize silage are deficient. Ample salt in minerals and concentrates. |
| Potassium | 3.g/kg DM | | | Never seen | All plants contain very high levels. |
| Copper | 10 mg/kg[3,4] 15 mg/kg DM for preg. and growth | | | Changes in coat colour, anaemia, poor growth, lameness in calves | May be primary soil deficiency or induced by excess Mo, S, or Fe. |
| Cobalt | 0.1 mg/kg DM | | | Anaemia and weight loss | Needed to form vitamin $B_{12}$. Some soils deficient. |
| Iodine | 0.2 mg/kg DM 0.8 mg/kg DM for preg. and lact. | | | Reduced milk production; stillborn calves; increased retained placenta | May be primary soil deficiency or induced by goitrogens, e.g. kale |
| Manganese | 80 mg/kg DM[5] | | | May lead to impaired fertility | Some pastures are low. |
| Zinc | 50 mg/kg DM | | | Dry scaly skin. Possibly poor hoof strength and lameness | Some pastures are low. |

| | | | |
|---|---|---|---|
| Iron | 35 mg/kg DM | Anaemia in milk-fed calves. Never seen in grazing animals | All plants contain very high levels. |
| Selenium | 0.1 mg/kg DM | Muscular dystrophy in calves, retained placenta. Reduced disease resistance | Many soils are deficient. |
| Vitamin E | Depends on Se intake | As for selenium | High intakes will partly compensate for selenium deficiency. |
| Vitamin A | 85 i.u./kg b.wt. | Night blindness, poor appetite, fainting, bone defects in calves | Seen with poor-quality feeds in winter. |
| Vitamin D | 10 i.u./kg b.wt. | Bone irregularities and other signs of rickets in growing calves | Problems in housed cattle only. Vitamin D is synthesised in the skin by sunlight. |
| B vitamins | Nil in healthy animal | See cobalt ($B_{12}$) and CCN[6] (thiamine) | All B vitamins are synthesised in the rumen. Deficiency can be induced. |
| Vitamin C | Nil | Not seen | Produced in the animal's tissues. |

1. Figures taken from Chamberlain and Wilkinson (1996), ARC (1980) and MAFF publication LGR21.
2. This is the sodium requirement. For salt, multiply by 2.5.
3. All levels are expressed as the amount required in the dry matter of the final ration. Units are mg/kg = ppm = g/ton.
4. If induced deficiencies are present (e.g. high Mo, S or Fe), minimum dietary requirements may be very much higher.
5. Some sources quote much lower requirements than this.
6. A full description of CCN is given in Chapter 3.
7. Requirements vary with forage quality.

muscle impulses. Blood levels of calcium normally remain very stable and are maintained in this state by an interaction of vitamin D and parathyroid hormone.

The general term of *homeostasis* is given to the sequence of processes which maintain the various body systems in equilibrium. Milk fever is due to a breakdown of homeostasis. The cow is not suffering from an overall deficiency in calcium, she simply cannot mobilise her reserves sufficiently rapidly to cope with the sudden increase in short-term demand. Older cows have fewer vitamin $D_3$ receptor sites in their bones and intestines and so they are even less able to cope with the sudden change in calcium requirements. Under the influence of $D_3$ and parathyroid hormone, a cow immediately after calving is usually able to increase the efficiency of absorption of calcium from the intestine quite rapidly, from approximately 35% to over 55%, and this then compensates for much of the increased demand. This concept is explained in more detail in Chapter 6. Blood calcium levels show very little variation with dietary intake and are therefore a poor indicator for the metabolic profile test (see Chapter 6).

Forages contain ample calcium for maintenance but as milk production has a very high requirement (1.8 g calcium per litre – Table 12.2), high-yielding cows on grazing alone may fall into 'negative calcium balance' (Table 12.1) and have to withdraw calcium from the reserves in their skeleton. Provided that this can be restored during later lactation and in the dry period, it is probably of limited importance and does not seem to harm the cow. Cereal grains are rich in phosphorus but low in calcium and if high-yielding cows are fed a diet based on maize silage, straw and grain, additional calcium supplementation will definitely be needed.

If young growing cattle are affected by a combined calcium and vitamin D deficiency, then symptoms of poor growth, lameness, stiffness, bone fractures and other signs of rickets will be seen. This can occur in the winter in calves which are on diets of very poor hay and unmineralised barley, and especially if they are housed in dimly lit buildings, because light is needed to produce vitamin D in their skin.

In dairy cows excess calcium may also present a problem. This can occur with over-enthusiastic mineral supplementation, or on diets involving large amounts of kale, sugarbeet, or delactosed whey, all of which are very high in calcium. Calcium interferes with the uptake of manganese, zinc and phosphorus from the intestine and if these elements were originally present in the diet at only marginal levels, increasing the calcium intake could produce a deficiency.

## Phosphorus

Phosphorus is the other major component of bones and the combined calcium (36%) and phosphorus (17%) contents account for over half (53%) of the total bone ash. Phosphorus is also an extremely important element in the soft tissues. It is involved in the structure of membranes, in the formation of a suitable framework for nuclear division and other cell functions, and in the all-important transfer of chemical energy for metabolic reactions.

Phosphorus deficiency occurs in many parts of the world and in the British Isles additional supplementation is usually provided at grazing. Milking cows on grazing alone could be deficient even if they were only producing 10–15 litres a day (see Tables 12.1 and 12.2) and blood phosphorus levels may fall because homeostatic mechanisms are less precise than for calcium. However, as with calcium, there are considerable reserves available in the skeleton and there is some doubt regarding the importance of a temporary shortfall of intake over requirements. Maize silage is very low in phosphorus (1.8 g/kg DM) and additional supplementation may be required. Other feeds, for example kale and lucerne silage, are very high in calcium (12.5 and 17.5 g/kg respectively) and although their phosphorus levels are not particularly low (4.0 and 3.0 g/kg respectively) their calcium:phosphorus ratios are quite wide (3:1 and 5.8:1).

The calcium and phosphorus requirements of the cow are roughly similar for maintenance (1:1) although calcium absorption is slightly more efficient if the ratio is 1:2. During lactation the requirement for calcium is higher than for phosphorus. Most diets contain calcium and phosphorus at 2:1 and few problems will be experienced with absorption until the ratio goes beyond 2.5:1. Most grass silages have a calcium : phosphorus ratio of 2:1. This can be balanced by feeding cereals and by-products such as brewers' grains which have higher levels of phosphorus than of calcium. Maize gluten feed is another good example, with 10.0 g/kg phosphorus and only 2.7 g/kg calcium. Clearly a carefully balanced ration, with adequate and balanced supplies of both calcium and phosphorus, is the best option. Alternatively you could feed a 'reverse ratio' mineral, that is one which contains a higher content of phosphorus than calcium to balance any excess calcium.

Symptoms of severe deficiency are similar to those of calcium rickets, although weight loss and lethargy are likely to be much more pronounced, and affected animals develop a craving (pica) for chewing bones and other phosphorus-rich materials. The temporary phosphorus deficit incurred by grazing or silage-fed cows may result in impaired fertility. Some experiments have suggested that phosphorus intakes below 18 g/day may reduce conception rates, and below 10 g/day fertility may be significantly impaired. However, other trials comparing, for example, 3.5 g phosphorus/kg DM (low) with 4.4 g/kg DM (high) over a three year period showed no effect on fertility. Opinions tend to be divided on this subject, and my own approach would be to say that when a herd fertility problem exists it is very difficult to be sure which factor or combination of factors is involved and it is therefore most logical to correct all dietary abnormalities when trying to improve the situation. This concept is discussed in greater detail in the section on nutrition and fertility in Chapter 8.

If possible, ask about the source of the phosphorus supplements being used. Certain types of rock phosphorus once contained high levels of *fluorine*, an element which can be toxic to cattle, leading to teeth and bone deformities. Sources are now carefully monitored, however, and it is unlikely that such products will find their way onto the market.

## Magnesium

Magnesium is the third of the major elements and, like calcium and phosphorus, it is important in the structure of the skeleton as well as having many metabolic functions. Magnesium deficiency and hypomagnesaemia are described in detail in Chapter 6.

## Sodium

Sodium is of major importance in maintaining the fluid balance of the body. This was referred to in Chapter 2. A scouring animal looses both fluid and sodium in the faeces, and oral electrolyte solutions which contain sodium are given for treatment, as these positively promote the uptake of water. Sodium is also involved in the absorption of other nutrients (for example, magnesium) from the gut and in the function of the nervous system. As discussed in Chapter 7, mastitic milk has high sodium levels (explaining its bitter taste) and cows with a persistent mastic discharge (as in a non-responsive case of *E. coli*) and chronic scour will often develop a craving for salt.

Table 12.1 shows that almost half of the spring leys analysed had inadequate sodium for cows producing 20 litres, and heavily fertilised leys can be particularly low because potassium blocks the uptake of sodium.

As most cows enjoy the taste of salt, it is commonly added to free access minerals to encourage increased intakes. A severe deficiency of sodium, leading to depressed growth, is unlikely in the UK, although periods of temporary deficiency may occur in grazing cows, especially towards the end of a dry summer. It is then that cravings for drinking urine and eating salt may develop. Trials in Wales have suggested that the addition of sodium to fertiliser improved pastures and increased both milk yield and milk quality. Maize silage is low in sodium and it is important that herds receiving significant intakes are given additional supplementation. In one herd fed on 100% maize silage the cows had become so seriously depleted that they started licking the sodium hypochlorite teat dip from their teats immediately after milking! Sodium may be involved with magnesium absorption, and there is some evidence that provision of salt licks in the spring and autumn helps to reduce the incidence of hypomagnesaemia.

Excess sodium intakes, most commonly seen when borehole water is used, can also be a problem. If salt levels are too high, water intakes are depressed and this has an effect on milk production. Borehole water may have to be desalinated prior to use. Total mineral levels above 1.0% will depress water intakes and cattle will always select 'soft' water if it is available.

## Potassium

Potassium is such an abundant element in plant material that deficiency will never occur. In fact the urine of cattle contains very high levels of excess potassium which is being excreted from the body. The main importance of potassium is that it interferes with magnesium uptake by plants. As there are high levels in slurry, cows should not be allowed to graze slurry-fertilised pastures in the spring because of the increased risk of hypomagnesaemia.

Cereal grains such as barley have a much lower potassium content than forages, and in the malting and brewing processes most of this potassium is leached out. Brewers' grains therefore have very low levels of potassium (for example 0.1% in DM compared to 2.5% in fresh and conserved forages), and potassium deficiency could occur in cattle on very high grain intakes.

## Copper

Copper deficiency is seen in many parts of the United Kingdom and is a widespread problem in the rest of the world. Table 12.1 shows that over three-quarters of leys contain insufficient copper for milk production. Copper deficiency may be either *primary*, that is the pasture simply does not contain sufficient copper, or *secondary*, that is some other element is interfering with copper uptake.

The best example of secondary copper deficiency is found in the teart pastures of Somerset, where high levels of molybdenum and/or sulphur interfere with copper absorption. Pasture levels of 2.0 mg/kg molybdenum can produce a deficiency, even though copper levels appear adequate, and sometimes levels up to 100 mg/kg molybdenum are found. A copper : molybdenum ratio of less than 3:1 is undesirable, and even at this ratio very high sulphur intakes (e.g. 3–5 g/kg DM) may still cause deficiency. Molybdenum and sulphur react with copper in the gut to form thiomolybdates which cannot be absorbed. The use of sulphuric acid as a silage additive significantly increases sulphur intakes. For example, 4 litres/ton of 50% sulphuric acid provides 70 g sulphur per tonne of silage and may be enough to induce copper deficiency. Sulphur forms an important linkage bond in the construction of protein molecules, and this is why protein feeds contain quite high levels of it. A more mature pasture with a lower protein content will therefore have a lower sulphur level, and this makes its copper more easily absorbed. On the other hand, lush spring leys not only have a lower initial copper level, but their high protein content gives them increased sulphur, and this interferes with their already marginal status. Other factors such as excess zinc, iron and lead and excessively low or high soil pH may also have a detrimental effect on copper absorption. Minerals very high in iron can be particularly counterproductive.

Recent experiments have shown that animals with a primary copper deficiency do not show any clinical signs. If a trace of molybdenum is added to their ration, however, deficiency signs (coat colour changes, loss of wool crimp in sheep etc.) appear very rapidly. This has led to the proposition that the function of copper is to prevent molybdenum poisoning. Elements such as sulphur and iron interfere with this action of copper, and hence if they are present in the ration in significant quantities, signs of molybdenum poisoning may be seen.

Copper is needed in the body for the formation of haemoglobin, in the processes of energy transfer, for hair and wool production and in the shaping of bones during growth. Deficiency signs are associated with these processes and are therefore very varied. They include:

- stunted growth, anaemia and general unthriftiness
- lameness in calves due to bone deformities, which are seen particularly as swellings around the fetlock
- changes in coat colour, leading to a 'rusty' rather than black coat, and classically a 'spectacled' appearance due to the loss of pigment around the eyes. But note that loss of coat colour is a difficult clinical sign to interpret, because it can be due to a number of other conditions, for example poor growth due to inadequate nutrition, some previous illness from which the animal is still recovering, or simply bleaching of the normal winter coat which is being shed in the spring (Plate 12.1). In my experience, copper deficiency is not the most common cause of lack of coat colour and rustiness.
- scouring and weight loss in adult animals having a molybdenum

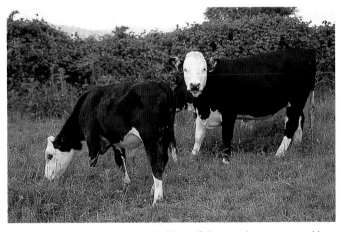

Plate 12.1. A rusty coat, as in this calf, is not always caused by a copper deficiency.

and/or sulphur induced copper deficiency. Sometimes simply bringing the animals indoors helps to control this

● possible reduction in milk production
● reduced conception rates and suppressed oestrous behaviour, particularly if the copper deficiency has been induced by excess molybdenum. There is some dispute over the importance of copper deficiency in relation to fertility under UK conditions, but if there is any doubt it seems sensible to ensure that copper status is adequate, thus ruling out copper deficiency as a potential cause.

*Diagnosis of copper deficiency*
Analysis of the ration for copper, molybdenum and sulphur levels will indicate if deficiency is a possibility and why it is occurring, but the best method is to take samples from the animal. Blood is most commonly used, although in the early stages of copper deficiency, blood levels remain high at the expense of liver stores and it is not until deficiency is quite well advanced and liver stores have been exhausted that blood copper values fall. The most reliable method of diagnosis is therefore to take liver samples from cull cows, animals being sold for slaughter, or even get your vet to take a biopsy, that is a small piece of liver from a live animal. Blood is best taken from late pregnant heifers which have not been receiving supplementary feeding, because the copper requirements for growth and pregnancy are higher than for maintenance and milk production (see Table 12.2). Another approach is to give additional copper and monitor the response. While this may be safe for adults, the increasing number of cases of copper poisoning indicates it is a potentially hazardous approach for younger cattle.

*Methods of supplementation*
Dairy cakes generally provide sufficient copper for milking cows, although circumstances exist when it is necessary to have a special 'high-copper' mix. You may need a veterinary prescription for this. Copper is stored in the liver, and this, plus the introduction of several slow release preparations, means that *copper injections* can be used. This is a very simple and positive way of ensuring that every animal gets its correct dose and there is no risk that molybdenum or other elements can interfere with copper absorption. Ideally give one injection three to four weeks before calving, so that calves are born stronger with better copper reserves. Copper deficient calves are more susceptible to scours and to infections generally, and hence adequate supplementation in late pregnant cows is very important. Although colostrum has a high copper content, levels rapidly fall and milk soon becomes insufficient to meet the needs of the growing calf, even though the young animal has an increased efficiency of absorption. This is why primary copper deficiency is more common in suckled calves than in calves fed milk substitute.

The frequency of copper injections and the amount given will obviously depend on the severity of the deficiency. Copper injections tend to release a large quantity initially and a reduced amount towards the end of their period of cover. There is therefore a risk of toxicity if too much is given in one dose. However, the absorption of oral copper is partly governed by requirements and although not so easy to administer as an injection, fragments of copper wire (known as 'needles') which are given orally in a gelatine capsule (Plate 12.2) are becoming popular. The capsule dissolves in the stomach,

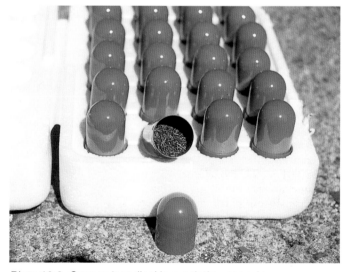

Plate 12.2. Copper 'needles' in a gelatine capsule.

liberating the copper needles. These then burrow into the wall of the abomasum where they slowly dissolve to provide a source of copper for up to 12 months. Ideally cows should be dosed between drying off and four weeks prior to calving. Not only does this then provide adequate copper for the calf, but it also covers the cow during the period of conception.

Other methods of supplementation include application of copper salts to pasture, the use of slow-dissolving pellets suspended in a container in the drinking water (Aquatrace, see Chapter 4), a

---

Copper absorption is influenced by:

- molybdenum
- sulphur (and hence dietary protein)
- iron, zinc and calcium
- sward composition and stage of maturity
- soil pH
- age of animal
- high concentrate diets

---

glass bolus containing copper, cobalt and selenium and a variety of other trace element boluses. A potential problem with multi-component boluses is that they are unlikely to contain the trace elements in the ratio needed by the cows in your herd and if, for example, enough is given to control the copper deficiency, excess selenium may also be supplied.

*Copper toxicity*

Copper is a cumulative poison. Excess intakes are stored in the liver, which eventually reaches the stage where no more can be accumulated and the liver literally 'bursts'. This leads to a severe haemolytic anaemia, blood in the urine, jaundice, abdominal pain and often sudden death. At post-mortem the liver is enlarged and golden yellow in colour, with jaundice throughout the carcase. Liver failure and death often occur following some form of stress, for example handling, transport or a sudden dietary change, especially if it results in acidosis. If one animal is affected by copper poisoning, it means that the others are at great risk and must be handled very gently.

Put the rest of the group on a copper deficient diet (for example using a low copper sheep ration) and hope that the copper will be withdrawn from the liver stores over a period of time. The procedure can be speeded up by adding 1.0 g sodium thiosulphate and 100–400 g (depending on bodyweight) of ammonium molybdate to the ration: this complexes with the copper in the gut to form thiomolybdate, which then increases the rate of faecal excretion of copper. Also ensure there is a high intake of vitamin E: this stabilises cell membranes and reduces the chances of liver cell rupture.

Copper poisoning usually occurs following a prolonged period of high intake, for example cattle grazing in an orchard where the trees have been sprayed with copper salts, or following over-enthusiastic supplementation of the ration with copper. In some cases the acute toxic episode may not occur until after the animals have been removed from the copper source, but are then stressed in some way.

Over the past few years there have been a few incidences of copper poisoning in animals which have been on diets not considered to be grossly excessive. This seems to be due to the combination of an increase in the amount of copper absorbed, plus some factor destabilising membranes and possibly a high copper status of the basic diet. Examples include:

- increased efficiency of copper absorption from the intestine
  - in young animals (50% absorption in a milk fed calf vs. 5–10% in an adult) and
  - in animals on high concentrate diets
- diets low in vitamin E and/or selenium
- diets high in polyunsaturated fatty acids (PUFAs), which have a dual effect. Firstly, they increase the animal's vitamin E requirement and secondly, if the diet is also high in calcium, calcium–PUFA 'soaps' are formed, which complex with and increase the absorption of copper. Spring grazing and brewers' grains are both very high in PUFAs (which also explains why both can also lead to low butterfat in milk)
- diets unusually high in copper, for example brewers' grains (which can be high in copper), when used as a replacement for forage
- diets low in molybdenum, sulphur, iron, cadmium and zinc, because all of these trace elements

would normally interfere with copper absorption. It also means that copper toxicity is more likely to be seen in housed cattle, because these are the animals which will be on high concentrate diets and because they will not be eating the amount of iron-rich soil ingested by grazing cattle (see page 382)

Recent UK food safety legislation has made the copper poisoning syndrome even more relevant, because animals with very high liver copper levels are put under restriction and may not be sold for human consumption. One word of warning: a high liver copper level at post-mortem does not necessarily indicate that copper poisoning was the cause of death. It may simply be a coincidental finding.

## Cobalt

Cobalt deficiency occurs in small but well-defined areas of the United Kingdom, particularly those associated with the old red sandstone and granite soils of Devon, Cornwall and Derbyshire. Deficiency is widespread in North and South America and Australia. Cobalt is a vital component of vitamin $B_{12}$, which is synthesised by the bacteria in the rumen and which is needed by the micro-organisms to digest cellulose. The excess vitamin is then absorbed by the cow and it plays an essential role in her energy metabolism. The changes in cobalt deficiency are an inability of the animal to utilise the energy in its diet, a syndrome sometimes referred to as 'pine'.

Sheep seem to be more susceptible than cattle. In both species the symptoms are poor growth, anaemia and increased susceptibility to infection. There is some evidence that dairy cows suffer reduced milk yields and infertility. Clinical signs such as these can occur from a wide variety of causes however, including inadequate nutrition and parasitism, and cobalt deficiency should never be diagnosed on the basis of clinical signs alone. Occasionally vitamin $B_{12}$ deficiency arises from chronic digestive upsets, leading to depressed ruminal synthesis.

Diagnosis of cobalt deficiency is usually made by blood sampling or simply monitoring the response to supplementation with oral cobalt or by injection of vitamin $B_{12}$ (injection of cobalt itself is not effective). Because of the differences in 'active' and 'complexed' forms of vitamin $B_{12}$, blood values are difficult to interpret. Hence the trial supplementation route is often used. Supplements are very similar to those given for copper, i.e. cobalt sulphate onto the soil or added to the drinking water, specially designed pellets for the drinking water and cobalt 'bullets' and glass boluses.

The amount needed each day (see Tables 12.1 and 12.2) is extremely small – only 2 mg for an adult cow – and provided that cobalt minerals are available, deficiency is unlikely. Cobalt is an expensive element however, and may not be present in some of the cheaper products. The analysis of a mineral should always be checked before purchase. Improving marginal hill pasture by the application of lime tends to reduce the availability of cobalt to the plants and can worsen a deficiency.

## Iodine

Iodine is required by the cow to produce the thyroid hormone, thyroxine $T_4$, which acts as a general metabolic stimulator for all body processes. Iodine deficiency thus leads to a lack of thyroxine, and normal body functions simply proceed more slowly. For example:

- Milk production and growth rates may be retarded.
- Reproductive activity is suppressed, leading to failure to show oestrus and poor conception rates.
- Prolonged or 'lazy' calvings may lead to an increase in stillborn calves, retained placenta and endometritis.
- Calves born may be more susceptible to scour, pneumonia and other infections.

As with many other trace element deficiencies, some herds seem to exist with a low iodine status and to have few health problems, while others respond dramatically to supplementation. Probably the best-known sign of iodine deficiency is the 'stillbirth and perinatal weak calf' syndrome, which in some herds can produce up to a 30% stillbirth rate. The thyroid gland, situated around the trachea adjacent to the larynx (Plate 12.3), works hard to compensate for iodine deficiency, and this often leads to an increase in the size of the gland, a condition known as *goitre*. The diagnosis of iodine deficiency is confirmed by blood sampling the adults and dissecting out and weighing the thyroid gland from stillborn calves.

Whole blood iodine is the best indicator of iodine status, but the test is expensive and so sensitive that you have to stop iodine teat disinfection for at least four days before sampling. However, measurements of thyroxine $T_4$ can give misleading results, because factors other than iodine status can alter blood levels. For example, thyroxine levels are low in late pregnant and immediately post-partum cows, high in concentrate fed animals and they fall with increasing environmental temperatures. The normal thyroid weight (the combined weight of both thyroids) for a calf is 15 g, sometimes expressed as 0.0375% of bodyweight. If the thyroid of a stillborn calf weighs over 25 g, deficiency should be strongly suspected. Milk iodine is another excellent indicator of iodine status.

Iodine deficiency may be primary, when soil or plants are deficient in the element, or it may be secondary, as a consequence of feeding a *goitrogenous* diet. Examples of the latter include

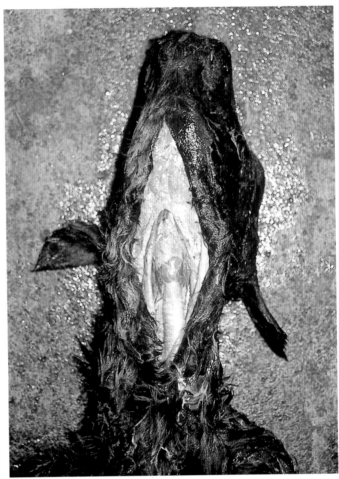

Plate 12.3. The thyroid gland, seen as the darker tissue surrounding the larynx in the neck, is much heavier in iodine deficient calves.

kale, turnips and white clover containing thioglycosides and thiocyanates which inhibit the uptake of iodine by the thyroid, and rapeseed meal and raw soya bean which contain thiourea and thiouracil, both of which are competitive inhibitors of thyroxine synthesis. All of these foods prevent thyroxine production and should only be fed in moderate amounts. For example kale intakes of greater than 20 kg/day fed for long periods have been shown to affect fertility. Some varieties of rape are now being grown which have a much lower gossypol content and hence a reduced goitrogenic effect and a less bitter taste.

Almost all pastures contain inadequate iodine for pregnant and lactating cows (see Tables 12.1 and 12.2) and therefore if they are on grazing or forage alone, additional supplementation will be required. Clovers may contain even less iodine, some being as low as 0.05 mg/kg DM, compared with the animal's maintenance requirement of 0.2 mg/kg DM. Iodine deficiency is particularly common in Ireland, where grazing constitutes a large part of the diet and where many herds are supplemented with 60 mg iodine per cow per day. Compound dairy concentrates should always contain ample iodine, and in many cases this may eliminate the need for additional supplementation.

Iodine is not stored very well in the body and so a regular daily intake is required: if the supplement is removed from a deficient herd, blood iodine levels may start to fall in as little as seven to ten days.

Supplementation is often added to the drinking water or it may be sprayed onto other feeds (for example, use 40 g of potassium iodide in 1 litre of water and give 2.0 ml per cow/day, i.e. 60 mg iodine cow/day). For dry cows some people recommend that approximately 10 ml of iodine solution is painted in a 15 cm long strip over the flanks every one or two weeks. The cow licks this off during her natural grooming processes.

*Do not supplement to excess* as this could lead to excessive levels in milk, with human health implications. Milk is a major source of iodine for man. As the daily human requirement is around 50–150 micrograms/day and this is contained in only 300 ml of average milk (containing 350 micrograms/litre), care should be taken not to over-supplement.

## Manganese

Manganese is an element which is often discussed in relation to reproductive problems in dairy herds, especially where poor conception rates and failure to show heat are involved. There is certainly a wide variation in the manganese contents of pasture in the UK and some people have produced results showing an improvement in fertility following manganese supplementation. Others would dispute this. Dairy concentrates normally contain sufficient additional manganese to make up any deficit, but in the spring and early summer, when no concentrates are being fed, over half of the diets are likely to be deficient (Table 12.1). Deficiency can also arise in the winter if the ration consists of a high proportion of by-products such as sugarbeet pulp or malt residue. It has been suggested that an overall content of 80 ppm manganese in the dry matter (see Table 12.2) is sufficient to avoid fertility problems, and as the mineral is very cheap it would be unwise not to provide this.

## Zinc

Zinc is similar to manganese in that many pastures do not contain sufficient to meet the requirements of lactating cows (Table 12.1). Deficiency in pigs causes skin problems, and a similar *parakeratosis* which responds to zinc treatment has been reported in calves. Affected animals have a dry, crusty, scaly skin, especially over the head and shoulders, but sometimes the whole body is affected. This should not be confused with ringworm or lice, where the scaling effect is much less. Zinc deficient parakeratosis is an inherited defect of Friesian calves, leading to poor intestinal zinc absorption, but is only likely to be seen in an individual animal. Dosing with 15 g zinc oxide once a week will help recovery.

It has been suggested that dietary zinc, and especially a zinc methionine complex, will reduce lameness in dairy cattle, and in some countries zinc injections are available. However, the evidence for its benefit is not conclusive. Hard horn has certainly been shown to have a higher zinc content than soft horn. For many years zinc ointment has been used to promote healing, and in human medicine low levels of zinc are added to intravenous infusions to promote the healing of skin ulcers. Zinc may not necessarily reduce the incidence of lameness, but it can perhaps increase the speed of recovery. Doses of 4.0 g zinc oxide per cow per day have been suggested. Do not over-supplement, as excessive zinc can induce a copper deficiency. With a large number of galvanised metal water troughs on farms, it seems unlikely that zinc deficiency will be a major problem in the UK.

## Iron

Iron, like potassium, is unlikely ever to be deficient in cattle diets. There are high levels in most plants, and as animals normally consume significant quantities of soil when grazing, overall intakes are boosted even further because soil is very rich in iron. For example, grazing cattle probably eat around 100 g soil each day, but this can increase ten-fold to 1 kg or more daily if grazing is very sparse, has been recently flooded, is dirty or has been trampled during wet weather. Dietary requirements for iron are around 35 mg/kg DM, and deficiency (which is sometimes seen in milk-fed calves) can result in anaemia and retarded growth. However, toxicity (depressed growth) can occur at intakes above 500 mg/kg DM (i.e. above 7.5 g/day for an animal consuming 15 kg of dry matter). It is not difficult to exceed these intakes.

For example,

- 10 kg DM pasture at 260 mg/kg iron contributes 0.26 g iron.
- 100 g soil at 50,000 mg/kg contributes 5 g iron.
- Free access minerals and compound rations supply further iron.

Iron is important in that if in excess, it reduces the availability of copper. This is an interesting point. At one time it was almost traditional that minerals should be either red or green and these colours were achieved by the addition of high levels of iron salts. Minerals with iron levels greater than 1000 ppm should be avoided. Heavy soil contamination of silage will lead to high iron, lead and zinc levels and may therefore induce copper deficiency. This can occur when silage is made over very rough ground, on inadequately rolled swards, during wet weather, or from pasture which has been recently flooded or trampled.

## Selenium

Selenium functions in association with vitamin E. Deficiency in the United Kingdom is quite common. The average value in pastures is insufficient for lactating cattle (Table 12.1), and high fat concentrates increase the overall requirements of the animal because vitamin E is involved in the metabolism of fat. Many of the clinical signs attributed to selenium deficiency have been described elsewhere in this book. They include:

- white muscle disease in calves (Chapter 3)
- increased incidence of retained placenta (Chapter 5)
- slow or 'lazy' calvings
- reduced fertility
- increased susceptibility to infection
- longer term effects such as retarded growth and anaemia

Selenium status is normally assessed by measuring blood levels of glutathione peroxidase, which is a selenium dependent enzyme. However, as is so often the case with trace element deficiencies, herds may be found with low glutathione peroxidase levels, yet show no clinical signs whatsoever.

## Ways of Improving Trace Element Status

Several different methods of supplementation have been described with the individual trace elements. The purpose of this section is to take an overall look at the advantages and disadvantages of the various supplementation systems. These can be divided into three categories, namely:

- altering the trace element content of the soil and herbage
- oral supplementation
- supplementation by parenteral methods, that is, by injection

*Soil and herbage*
The type of soil in a particular area affects not only its trace element content but also the type of plant which grows there and the rate of uptake of minerals and trace elements by those plants. It is for precisely these reasons that there is a wide geographical variation in the deficiency areas. Various treatments can affect the uptake of mineral by the plants. The influence of soil pH on mineral and trace element uptake by the plant is demonstrated in Figure 12.1. The uptake of all elements, apart from iron, is decreased in very acid soils and hence liming will invariably have a beneficial effect. Conversely, if the soil becomes too alkaline, uptakes of manganese, boron, copper and zinc are depressed.

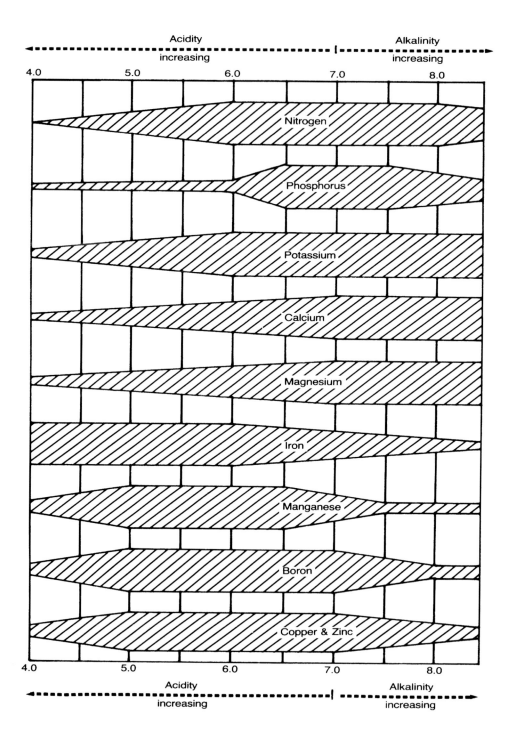

Figure 12.1. Effect of soil pH on plant nutrient availability.

Artificial fertilisers have three actions on this soil/plant relationship. First, some fertilisers, for example ammonium sulphate, will acidify the soil, and this leads to a reduced mineral uptake by the plants. Second, fertilisers produce faster plant growth, often with a higher protein level, and this tends to decrease its mineral and trace element contents. Third, the elements contained in the fertiliser either intentionally (for example, potassium or phosphate) or as contaminants (for example fluorine) may react with natural minerals and trace elements and reduce their uptake. Heavy use of artificial fertilisers therefore generally decreases the mineral and trace element levels of plants.

Trace elements can be applied directly to the soil in an attempt to boost levels in plants. This works well with cobalt, but for copper such large applications are needed that it is not economic. Manganese has been applied to soil and pasture and while it may boost herbage growth in deficient plants, it has little effect on the overall manganese content of the pasture and is therefore of no value for animal supplementation.

*Oral supplementation*

Giving trace elements by mouth is probably the cheapest and most efficient way of counteracting deficiency, especially if it is a primary rather than an induced deficiency, and this must be the method of choice if cereals or concentrates are being fed. Animals must either be given a regular daily supply, for example in the food or in drinking water, or a method of providing a single large dose in a slow release form must be found. Examples of the latter include 'bullets' for cobalt, selenium and magnesium supplementation, a glass bolus containing a mixture of copper, cobalt and selenium, and copper wire (see Plate 12.2) which lodges in the abomasum and is then slowly dissolved over the following six to twelve months. Magnesium can be dusted onto pasture to give a regular daily supply and although this works well, it entails a fairly high labour input.

Minerals can also be offered on a free access basis, and while this is a simple system, individual animal intakes can be very variable. For example, one trial showed that cow consumption ranged from 0 to 500 g/day of one particular mineral, with less than half the cows taking in sufficient to meet their requirements. Free access is therefore not a reliable method of supplementation.

*Parenteral supplementation*

The word 'parenteral' means that the trace element is injected or implanted directly into the animal's body ('parenteral' is also applied to drug administration). This is undoubtedly the preferred route for the treatment of animals clinically ill from deficiency, since it can produce an immediate improvement in trace element status. It also has the advantage that there are no interactions to consider which might compete with plant uptake or intestinal absorption and that a precise and controlled dose can be given to each animal. Unfortunately it is difficult to produce preparations which can give a single large dose, capable of slow release over a period of time. Injectable products for copper and selenium supplementation are now available and certainly for copper they provide a reasonably cheap and efficient preventive method. One disadvantage of parenteral administration is the risk of toxicity from overdose, since the animal cannot regulate its intake and absorption.

# VITAMINS

Only the fat-soluble vitamins A, D and E have any major importance in ruminant diseases. Vitamin E and selenium are discussed in Chapter 3.

## Vitamin A

Cattle obtain their vitamin A from carotene, which is the yellow pigment present in abundance in all green plants. Provided the animals are grazing or are receiving well-made forage, deficiency is unlikely to occur, although maize silage can be deficient in carotene. Drying, bleaching and weathering of grass will reduce carotene levels, however, and there is relatively little in cereal grains. Overheating of hay and prolonged storage also reduce the vitamin A content. Cattle fed on poor-quality hay in winter or on a straw and cereal diet will need additional supplementation, and levels of 10 million i.u./ton are usually recommended. Provided that the feeding of the dry cows is adequate, colostrum will be rich in vitamin A and give the calf the reserves it will need during its suckling period. This is often not the case, however, and winter-born calves may be deficient, leading to an increased susceptibility to scouring, pneumonia and other diseases. This is why many farms inject vitamins A, D and E to all winter-born calves and consider they get a response.

Deficiency of vitamin A produces a variety of symptoms. There is decreased appetite leading to reduced growth and, even in the early stages, night vision is impaired. Reproductive function may be affected and there may be an increase in the number of stillborn calves. This could be especially relevant when the dry cows are being fed only very poor-quality fodder. Fainting fits may also be seen: the calf collapses as if in a deep sleep, and a few minutes later it gets up and walks away quite normally. In the later stages of deficiency bone growth becomes affected. This can cause pressure on the nerve to the eye and eventually leads to total blindness. Most of the changes (apart from total blindness) are reversed when the deficient animal is injected with vitamin A. Vitamin A assists in maintaining the membranes of the body in a healthy state and deficient animals are more susceptible to diseases such as ringworm, calf pneumonia and scouring.

A diagnosis of vitamin A deficiency is made from an investigation of the history of the animal, especially the diet, from an analysis of blood and/or liver samples, and from response to treatment.

## Vitamin D

Vitamin D is involved with the absorption of calcium and phosphorus from the intestine, the absorption and deposition of minerals in bone and the maintenance of normal blood levels. Details of its action in conjunction with parathyroid hormone are discussed in the milk fever section in Chapter 6, which should be read in conjunction with the following.

There is relatively little vitamin D in plants, and cattle obtain the majority of their requirements by synthesising the vitamin in the skin under the influence of ultra-violet light from the sun. Milk contains only low levels, and calves fed solely on milk may develop a deficiency. However, deficiency is most likely to occur in young growing cattle in dimly lit buildings during the winter, especially when only poor-quality hay is being fed. A similar syndrome, involving non-specific lameness and multiple spontaneous fractures, has been seen in rapidly growing beef calves on a diet of maize silage and maize gluten which had no mineral or vitamin supplementation and has been referred to as metabolic demineralisation.

The symptoms are those of rickets: growth rates are reduced, the legs may be bent and have abnormal swellings and many animals show stiffness and lameness. The teeth may be pitted and out of line and the jawbone deformed. Treatment is by injecting vitamin D and by correcting the ration, which may include oral supplementation with vitamin D.

## Vitamin K

Vitamin K is involved in blood clotting mechanisms. It is synthesised by the ruminal micro-organisms and there are also ample supplies in leafy forages. Primary deficiency does not occur therefore, although deficiency may be induced by poisoning with dicoumarols, compounds which prevent the action of vitamin K. Sources of dicoumarol include warfarin rat poison and mouldy clover hay. The latter is sometimes known as sweet clover poisoning. Symptoms are caused by a failure of blood clotting and include bleeding excessively from cuts, the appearance of large red haemorrhagic areas on the membranes of the mouth, eyes or nose, abdominal pain and lameness. The latter is due to haemorrhage into the joints. The treatment is to give vitamin K by mouth or by injection and to try to identify and remove the source of the poison.

## B Vitamins

The B vitamins are all synthesised by the micro-organisms in the rumen and the excess is absorbed by the cow. They are also present in ample quantities in milk, so primary dietary deficiency is never seen. Induced deficiencies can occur however, for example with CCN (Chapter 3), where there is a factor preventing the action of thiamine (vitamin $B_1$), and with cobalt deficiency which leads to inadequate vitamin $B_{12}$. There is evidence that supplementation with biotin (vitamin $B_6$) will improve the quality of the hoof and reduce the incidence of sandcracks and of white line lesions.

Although all B vitamins are synthesised in the rumen, there is very little storage in the body. Temporary deficiencies can therefore occur during illness and anorexia, for example following a toxic mastitis, and particularly following severe ruminal upsets such as acidosis (Chapter 6) and overeating (Chapter 13). Injection of B vitamins would be a sensible supplementary therapy for such animals.

## Vitamin C

Vitamin C is produced in the tissues of all farm livestock. A dietary supply is therefore unnecessary and deficiency is never seen. Only man and guinea pigs are unable to synthesise vitamin C.

## DRINKING WATER

Without an adequate supply of drinking water, animals will not eat as much, the efficiency of utilisation of their food will be depressed and milk yields will fall. Water intakes and requirements vary enormously and depend on factors such as:

- the level of milk production: 0.9 litre of water is required for each litre of milk produced
- the dry matter content of the diet: cows eating dry foods need more water
- the total amount of dry matter eaten (which will also vary with milk yield)
- environmental temperature: water intakes increase in hot, dry and windy weather
- diets high in minerals, for example high salt intakes or caustic treated grain
- the palatability and temperature of the water. Cows prefer to drink warm water in the winter (the outflow from a plate cooler is ideal for this) and cold water in the summer. Brackish water with a high (0.75%) salt content depresses intakes and may need to be desalinated before use.

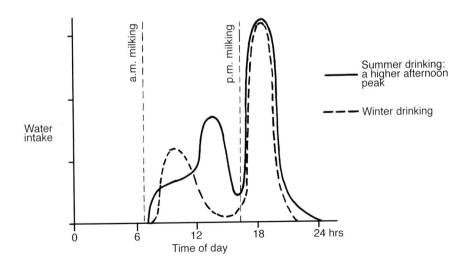

Figure 12.2. Daily drinking patterns of cows in summer and winter.

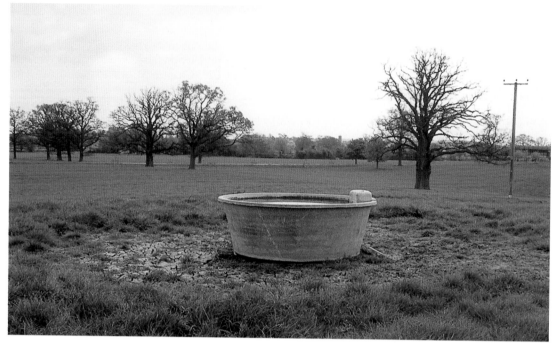

Plate 12.4. Free-standing water trough with good access.

Water intakes may vary between 20 and 100 litres daily for lactating dairy cows, with a figure of 55–65 litres per day being an approximate average value.

Despite these intakes, cows normally go to the trough to drink only four to six times each day and the daily pattern of drinking is surprisingly constant in both summer and winter. This is shown in Figure 12.2. There is a rise in intake around mid day and a considerably greater peak soon after evening milking, when up to 50% of the total daily intake may be drunk in three consecutive hours. This short peak of drinking activity has important implications in terms of the supply provided. Because all the cows want to drink at the same time, it is essential that you have sufficient space to allow adequate access, that there is ample reserve capacity in your trough and that the supply pipe is of sufficient bore to carry water at the rate at which the cows are drinking it.

As cows can drink at a rate of up to 20 litres per minute, and as there may be several cows drinking at any one time, an enormous rate of supply is needed, so a large-capacity tank is by far the best idea. Circular troughs holding 1600 litres, and which allow 15 cows to drink at any one time, are now available. As an approximate rule of thumb, allow sufficient space for at least 10% of the herd to drink at the same time, or allow 6 cm of trough space for each cow, which is equivalent to 6 m for 100 cows. Cow comfort, access and water intakes can all be improved by using a free-standing trough (Plate 12.4) rather than one which is sited in the corner of a field or building, and by constructing a concrete or even a bark-based apron similar to a cow track (Plate 9.38) around the outside to improve conditions underfoot. If the area around the water trough is a mixture of deep mud, surplus bricks and lumps of concrete, you should not be surprised if water intakes – and milk yields – are depressed.

As milk is 87% water, thirsty cows will have depressed yields. Thirst also reduces food intake and this can cause a further fall in milk production and even bodyweight loss.

Water can be a problem for sick animals. If they are too weak to reach the trough, or unable to compete with the other cattle when they get there, dehydration soon sets in. Even low levels of dehydration will make the animal feel lethargic and depress its appetite, and this is bound to retard recovery. Sick animals, cows or calves, are therefore best penned individually so that food and water can be made easily accessible and their intakes monitored.

*Chapter 13*

# MISCELLANEOUS DIGESTIVE, RESPIRATORY AND OTHER CONDITIONS

In the earlier chapters we dealt with diseases affecting one particular age group of cattle. These tended to be mainly of an infectious or metabolic nature. There are many other conditions which can occur on a 'one-off' basis however, affecting only an individual animal in an age group. Some of these conditions will be described below, starting with those associated with the digestive tract. The anatomy of the digestive system is shown in Figures 2.1, 2.2 and 2.6, and you may need to refer back to these diagrams.

## THE DIGESTIVE TRACT

### The Teeth

Cattle have front teeth, or incisors, only in their lower jaw (Figure 13.1). They pull grass into their mouth using their tongue and then cut it off by closing the incisors against the upper gums. Calves are born with eight temporary incisors and these are replaced at a later date by permanent teeth. As in children, the central pair of incisors is replaced first, and the number of permanent teeth present at any one time can be used to age the animal. The approximate ages of eruption are given in Table 13.1

Examination of dentition became very important following the UK BSE crisis in the 1990s, because animals over 30 months old were not allowed to enter the human food chain. However, this demonstrated the inaccuracy of ageing, because there were plenty of animals over 30 months old with only two teeth showing and, conversely, plenty under 30 months old with three or four teeth!

The teeth come into wear approximately three months after eruption, so that a heifer is almost four years old before she is using her full set of permanent incisors. The table also shows that a two year old calving heifer will have to change almost all her teeth

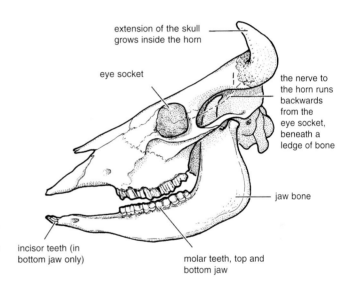

Figure 13.1. The skull of a cow. Note that there are front (incisor) teeth in the lower jaw only.

Table 13.1. The approximate age at which the permanent incisors erupt.

| Incisor teeth | Age of eruption |
|---|---|
| Central pair | 1 year 9 months (21 months) |
| Second pair | 2 years 6 months (30 months) |
| Third pair | 3 years (36 months) |
| Outer pair | 3 years 6 months (42 months) |

389

during her first lactation and this is bound to cause problems with feeding (Plate 13.1). For example if self-fed from a heavily compacted silage face 3 m high, young growing and finishing animals can be affected by weight loss, presumably because they are changing their teeth. One trial in Ireland showed a reduction in weight gain of 0.27 kg/day comparing self-feed silage with easy feed.

There are three temporary molars, or grinding teeth, on each side of the upper and lower jaws. These are replaced by six permanent molars, so that the adult cow has a total complement of 32 teeth (four sets of six molars plus eight incisors). The permanent teeth grow throughout adult life and the incisors change from a spade shape in a young cow to small square pegs in the aged animal (Figure 13.2).

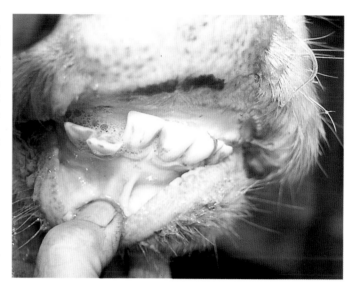

Plate 13.1. A heifer changing her teeth. While the teeth are loose like this she will find eating more difficult, especially from a compacted self-feed silage face.

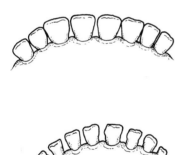

Figure 13.2. Incisors change with age from a spade shape to small pegs in the old cow.

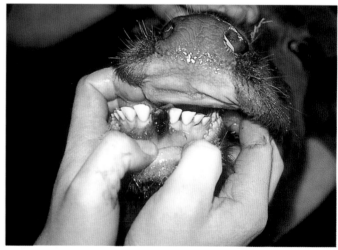

Plate 13.2. Fractured jaw in a calf. Put back onto milk, the calf healed without treatment.

*Tooth abscesses*

These are uncommon but should always be looked for in a drooling animal. The incisors are most commonly affected and often cause a swelling of the lower lip. Most respond to antibiotic treatment.

*Fracture of the jaw*

Provided that the fracture occurs at the symphysis, which is the natural join of the two jaw bones under the incisor teeth, most animals recover well without treatment. The calf in Plate 13.2 was put back onto milk, to make feeding easier, and made a full recovery.

*Misaligned molars*
This most commonly occurs as a result of a lumpy jaw bone infection (see Chapter 10). There is no useful treatment.

*Undershot jaw*
During feeding it is necessary for the teeth to make contact with the hard palate, in order to achieve a cutting action. If the bottom jaw is too short (Plate 13.3), the incisor teeth fail to make good contact with the gums and eating becomes difficult. The 18 month old heifer shown in Plate 13.3 was much smaller than the rest of her group. There is no treatment.

*Severe incisor wear*
In some cows the incisor teeth become so badly worn that it seriously affects their ability to eat. If the teeth are so badly eroded that the dentine (quick) is exposed, eating will be particularly painful. Food intake falls and weight loss occurs.

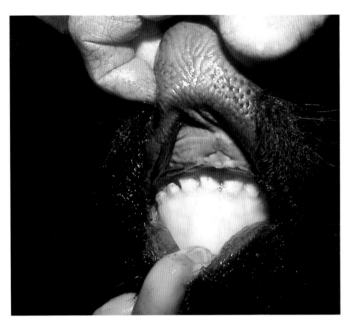

Plate 13.3. An undershot jaw. This 18-month-old heifer remained stunted because she was unable to feed properly.

Very acid silage has been suggested as a cause of severe incisor wear. However, although extracted teeth become pitted if exposed to very acid silage, the high pH of saliva in the mouth probably counteracts any effect of silage acid in the living animal.

Jaw abscesses, wooden tongue, lumpy jaw, malignant oedema and blaine are described in Chapter 10.

## Choke

Moving away from the mouth and down into the oesophagus, the main problem here is an obstruction and the animal is said to have *choke*. Potatoes and apples are most commonly involved and they are considered particularly dangerous if apples are eaten from trees or if potatoes are eaten from raised troughs. This is because when the animal eats food from the ground, it is more likely to be chewed into small pieces before it is swallowed.

*Clinical signs*
The first indication that there is something wrong may simply be that one animal is standing apart from the others, with its head stretched forwards and its mouth slightly open. It may go up to feed, but then turns away again. If the blockage is severe, saliva produced in the mouth cannot be swallowed and so the animal will be drooling. On the other hand, gas cannot escape from the rumen and bloat develops. If left untreated, there is a risk of death either from severe bloat or from infection due to an erosion of the oesophagus at the point of obstruction.

*Treatment*
Saliva and digestive juices from the mouth often dissolve enough of the potato or apple for the remainder of it to be swallowed and some people say that the best treatment is to insert a trocar and cannula (Plate 13.8 and Figure 3.2) into the rumen to alleviate bloat and then leave the animal to recover on its own. Drugs are available which help to relax and dilate the oesophagus, thereby making it easier for the foreign body to pass down into the rumen.

Alternatively you can try to push the obstruction down into the rumen using a probang. This is a long length of pliable nylon tubing with an enlarged metal lump at one end. The handle is attached to a long cane which runs through the centre of the tube to give added rigidity. The animal's mouth is held open using a metal gag (Plate 13.4) inserted between the teeth, and the probang is carefully pushed down the oesophagus. If you push too hard there is a danger that you will rupture the wall of the oesophagus, so this is a job which is best left to your vet.

The best treatment, but sometimes not possible, is to work the potato up the oesophagus from outside and then, with a gag in position, push your hand into the animal's mouth and pull the apple out. This was successfully achieved with the calf in Plates 13.5 and 13.6. Sometimes you have to wait for a few hours (or even days) for the oesophagus to relax sufficiently and/or for the apple to be digested enough to be able to achieve this.

*Never* put your hand into the back of an animal's mouth without using a gag (Plate 13.4). The molar teeth are strong enough to cut off your finger – a near miss is shown in Plate 9.20B!

## Vomiting

Cows rarely vomit. If they do, it could be due to:

- wooden tongue (Chapter 10) at the base of the oesophagus, that is where it enters the rumen. A five to seven day course of antibiotics by injection may help to resolve this
- acidosis, causing the cud to be regurgitated (see page 397)
- rhododendron poisoning (page 450)

## Bloat (Ruminal Tympany)

Gas is produced by the micro-organisms in the rumen as part of the normal fermentation of food; following a meal the rate of gas production may be as much as 30 litres per hour. If it cannot escape, it makes the rumen

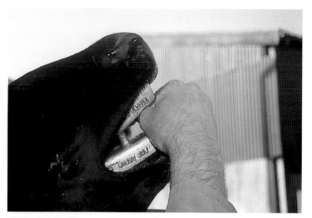

Plate 13.4. The mouth gag slots over the top and bottom molar teeth and in so doing holds the mouth open.

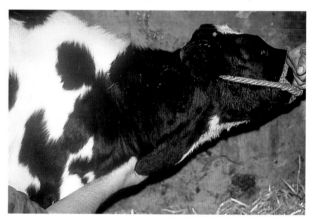

Plate 13.5. Choke: the foreign body in the oesophagus can be seen just above the operator's hand.

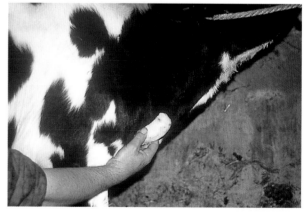

Plate 13.6. Choke: this was a fortunate case in which the apple could be squeezed up, into and out of the animal's mouth. Note how the outside of the apple has undergone digestion by the salivary enzymes.

swell and this we call bloat. The rumen is situated on the *left* side of the animal, so that bloat is first seen as a swelling in the left flank, as in the calf in Plate 2.15. In more advanced cases, however, both sides will be distended. The animal is obviously in discomfort by now and it stands stiffly, with its legs spread wide apart. A typical example is shown in the calf in Plate 13.7. It may be drooling or frothing at the mouth and if you examine it carefully you will find that the heart is beating extremely rapidly. Eventually the pressure inside the rumen becomes so great that the animal goes down onto its side and death soon follows, either from heart failure or because liquid rumen contents have been forced up into the throat and inhaled into the trachea.

To appreciate how bloat develops it is important to understand how the normal rumen functions. The ruminant has four stomachs as follows.

The *rumen* is a large fermentation vat (approximately 200 litres in an adult cow) where micro-organisms (bacteria and protozoa) ferment ingested food at around pH 6.5 and in the absence of air. The length of time the food stays in the rumen varies with the type of food and the amount eaten. It can take up to ten days for it to be broken down through fermentation and chewing the cud into small enough particles to pass on. However, this is an extreme example. An average forage will be retained in the rumen fibre mat (Figure 13.3) for around thirty hours, and concentrates, which are broken down quite rapidly, for as little as ten hours. Products of fermentation, absorbed from the rumen into the blood, are used as food by the cow.

The *reticulum* is really an additional part of the rumen. Contractions help to force small food particles into the omasum. The heavy autoworm (Figure 4.5) and trace element boluses are retained in the reticulum, as are other ingested metallic objects, some of which may later penetrate to produce the classic 'wire' (Figure 13.3).

The *omasum*'s main functions are the absorption of water (about half the total water drunk is absorbed here) and rumen fermentation products. It also prevents the reflux of food back from the abomasum into the rumen.

The *abomasum* is the 'true' stomach, with a very acid pH of 1–2. Its digestive enzymes and functions (see Chapter 2) are similar to those of the human stomach.

There are approximately two waves of rumen muscle contraction each minute. In the first wave

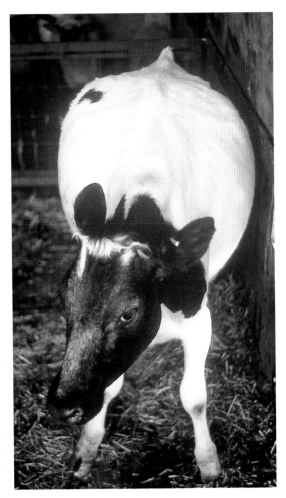

Plate 13.7. Severe bloat. Both sides of the abdomen are dilated. The heifer has her head down and legs apart, attempting to remain standing.

---

The four stomachs of the ruminant:

- the rumen
- the reticulum
- the omasum
- the abomasum

The rumen, reticulum and omasum together are sometimes referred to as the forestomachs.

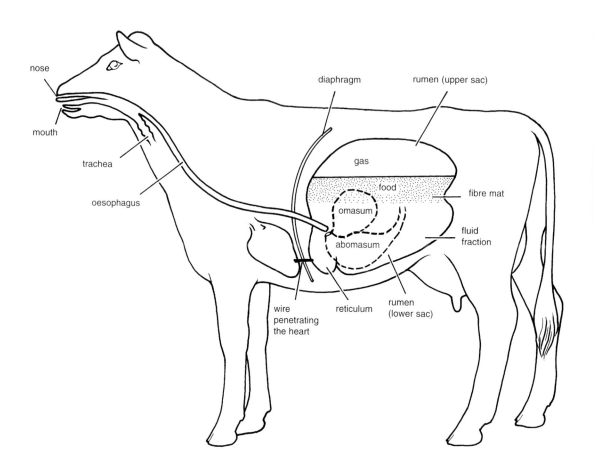

Figure 13.3. Upper digestive tract of the cow showing the point at which a wire penetrates the reticulum and its close proximity to the heart.

the lower sac of the rumen and the reticulum contract: this mixes the food, and any liquid sludge which has finished its digestion is transferred into the omasum, the third stomach (see Figure 13.3). During the second wave of muscular contraction, the upper sac of the rumen compresses the gas, forcing it down towards the reticular end of the oesophagus, which then opens to allow the gas to escape into the mouth.

Fibrous food is also transferred back to the mouth for further chewing by the same process, known as *eructation*, and we say that the cow is 'chewing her cud'. An essential part of any examination of a cow's health is to stand back and watch to see if her rumen is functioning correctly. It is easy to see the left flank moving in and out as the rumen contracts twice each minute, and eructation with regurgitation is clearly audible.

*Causes of bloat*
Bloat occurs when something interferes with the natural processes of gas release. This can occur in three ways: first a lack of ruminal contractions, second an obstruction in the oesophagus and third the presence of froth or foam in the rumen. Causes of bloat are listed in Appendix 2.

**Cessation of ruminal contractions** This is technically called ruminal 'atony'. It occurs most commonly in the weaned calf and the symptoms and treatment were discussed in Chapter 3. Atony is also seen as part of the vagus indigestion complex in adult cows, when the nerve supply to the rumen has been damaged; in association with acidosis, e.g. caused by grain overload, where it may be referred to as feedlot bloat (page 170); and secondary to other conditions such as a wire, overeating of potatoes and digestive upsets. Failure of rumen contractions can occur with tetanus (Chapter 4) or botulism (Chapter 4) and may also cause bloat.

**Obstruction in the oesophagus** Choke is the most common obstruction, although abscesses and occasionally tumours (for example EBL, Chapter 11) compressing the outside of the oesophagus can cause a blockage. Actinobacillosis infection (wooden tongue) of the lower end of oesophagus can cause bloat or regurgitation of food (vomiting): a five to seven day course of antibiotics should effect a cure.

**Frothy bloat** Normally free gas collects as a single bubble in the upper part of the rumen (Figure 13.3) until it is expelled. However, under certain conditions, as the gas is released from the semi-solid fermenting food in the bottom of the rumen it forms a froth or foam. This foam can be very stable, so much so that the gas it contains cannot be expelled by the normal mechanisms of ruminal contraction, so although the rumen is contracting and there is no obstruction in the oesophagus, a severe and often fatal bloat develops.

Certain pastures are particularly prone to producing frothy bloat. For example, alfalfa can be a problem and animals may become bloated and die only ten to fifteen minutes after they have started grazing. In Britain, clovers, lush leys and even kale are more commonly involved. It seems to be the stage of growth rather than the species of plant or weight of crop which is important. If you find that you are getting several blown cows in a particular field, simply take them away for two to three weeks. After this period the same pasture may be quite safe to graze again, even though the crop may then be even heavier.

*Treatment*
Whatever is causing the bloat, the prime objective of treatment must be to relieve the pressure of the gas before it leads to heart failure. You may not know which type of bloat you are dealing with, so, provided that the animal is only moderately affected, first take it out of the field if it is grazing, and give it a bloat drench. This is something which you should always have in stock, 'just in case'. If you do not have any, then 500 ml of linseed oil works well for a cow. If she is unable to swallow the drench, then you know you are dealing with an obstruction and you need to call for veterinary assistance. Bloat drenches (including linseed oil, poloxalene and other surfactants) act by dispersing the foam. Free gas can then be expelled in the normal way. You may even hear the cow belch within a few minutes of giving the drench and then you know that all is well.

The safest way of releasing the gas, provided the cow is still standing, is to pass a stomach tube. Hold the cow's teeth apart using a gag (Plate 13.4) and push a length of fairly soft 20 mm plastic tubing into the throat. As you feel her swallow, push the pipe slightly further and then down into the oesophagus. If this produces a cough, or if you can feel air rushing in and out of the end of the pipe as the animal breathes, you know that you are in the trachea and you must start again. I find stomach tubing works well in younger cattle, but it is less successful in adults, partly because the end of the pipe gets caught in the food and liquid at the bottom of the rumen (Figure 13.3) and so the gas is not released. If this happens, move the tube in and out of the rumen until you get to a position where gas flows. Sometimes it helps to blow down the tube: this will often remove the obstruction, more gas flows until it blocks and then you can blow again. Whether you are using a trocar and cannula or a stomach tube, if frothy bloat is present the foam will probably be so stable that it will not pass out and this is why a froth-dispersing drench should always be given first.

It is important to keep a bloated animal on its feet for as long as possible and this is why traditionally they were walked for long periods. Once the cow lies down you have an extreme emergency on your hands because death follows quite quickly. Try to get her to stand up again so that you can give her a bloat drench. If this is not possible, or if it has not worked, you must release the gas, preferably using a trocar and cannula. The trocar, which has a handle at one end and a sharp metal point at the other (Plate 13.8), fits inside the cannula. It will need to be held in both hands like a dagger and brought down with tremendous force to penetrate the skin of the cow. Once in the rumen, remove the trocar so that gas can escape through the cannula. Hold the cannula in position while the gas is escaping, then call for veterinary assistance to have it sutured in position. If the rumen slips off the end of the cannula while gas is escaping, rumen contents will be discharged into the abdomen and this could lead to severe peritonitis and even death.

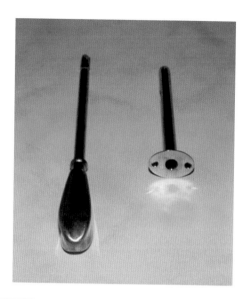

Plate 13.8. A trocar and cannula. The trocar has a sharp point to enable it to be forced through the skin and into the rumen. The holes in the collar around the base of the cannula allow it to be sutured into position when the trocar has been removed.

If you do not have a trocar and cannula, then in an *extreme* case a large carving knife with a wide blade can be used. Push the knife into the rumen, then turn the blade through 90 degrees and hold it transversely across the original cut, so that the gas can escape. The correct position to puncture and deflate a cow is shown in Figure 3.2 and Plate 13.9. It is on the *left* side, 5 cm behind the last rib and 15 cm down from the spine.

I should stress that releasing the gas in this way should only be done as an extreme measure and only when the cow is recumbent. There is a serious risk of peritonitis and other

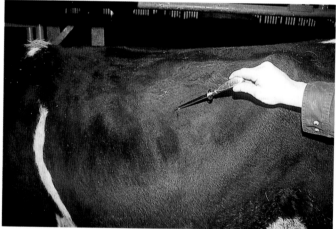

Plate 13.9. In severe bloat a trocar and cannula can be forced through the skin on the left flank.

complications which can be fatal to the cow, especially if a carving knife is used. In either case, you should call your vet to advise you on how to dress the wound and to give any other antibiotic treatment necessary to prevent peritonitis.

### Prevention

Cows grazing lush pasture should always be given access to mature silage, hay or palatable straw before turnout. Not only does this reduce the incidence of bloat, but it also helps to maintain butterfat (see Chapter 6), reduces the incidence of hypomagnesaemia and helps to prevent ruminal impaction and the 'cold cow' syndrome. If you are forced to graze bloat-producing pastures, they can either be sprayed daily with mineral oils, or a better alternative is to add the chemical poloxalene or other surfactants to the drinking water, using a proportioner similar to that shown in Figure 6.5, or include it in the concentrate. The drinking water route is preferred, because supplementation can be installed very quickly and all cows must drink, whereas many of them may not be receiving concentrate when they are grazing lush pasture. Poloxalene can also be used very effectively as a bloat drench, that is, for treatment.

## Overeating Syndrome (Acidosis)

Another condition which primarily involves the rumen and which can affect cattle of all ages is the overeating syndrome. This is most commonly seen when a door to a concentrate or grain store has been blown open, or possibly some sacks of concentrate have been left within reach of the cows. Sometimes a group of calves is accidentally given double their normal ration and a few gorge themselves.

Once in the rumen the grain is rapidly fermented by the bacteria. This produces very acid conditions (lactic acid) and, if severe, contractions cease and the whole of the contents of the rumen turn sour. The rumen wall then becomes inflamed (rumenitis) making it more easy for toxins to be absorbed. It is the effect of these toxins, producing liver damage, a generalised metabolic acidosis, and then shock which can eventually lead to the death of the animal. Plate 13.10 shows a red and inflamed rumen wall from a cow which died from overeating fresh sugarbeet roots. Even if such animals survive, the rumen wall may be permanently scarred (Figure 3.1), leading to poor absorption of nutrients, or infection may 'leak' through the rumen wall to produce liver abscesses and subsequent depressed performance. Liver abscesses can be quite a problem in barley beef or feedlot cattle.

The detailed rumen changes associated with acidosis are described in Chapter 6. The normal rumen pH is 6.0–6.5, whereas with acidosis it may fall to 4.5–5.0. At pH 4.0 death is almost certain. As the pH falls, the cellulose-digesting protozoa especially start to die, which further depresses feed (forage) intake.

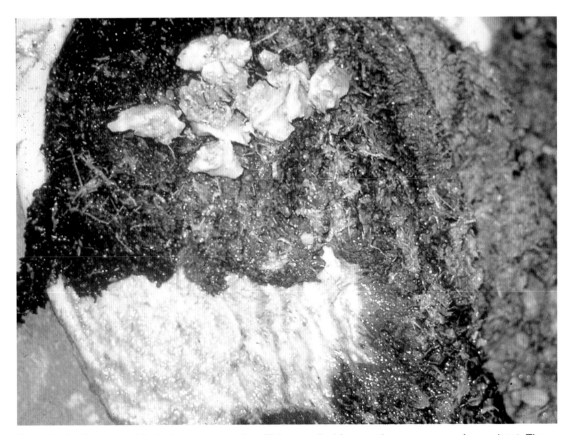

Plate 13.10. Rumen acidosis due to overeating. This cow died from eating an excess of sugarbeet. The rumen wall is very red and inflamed (rumenitis) and the normal black surface lining is peeled off far too easily.

*Clinical signs*

The clinical signs depend very much on the amount eaten and the time lapse since the animal gorged itself. If you are lucky, rumen contractions will continue and 18–24 hours after overeating the cow will develop a profuse, foul-smelling scour, containing whole particles of undigested grain. The beige-yellow colour, semi-solid consistency and foul smell of the faeces are almost diagnostic of overeating. There will be a drop in yield and the cow will be off her food for a few days, but apart from this there will be no other adverse effects.

If contractions cease and acidosis and toxaemia set in, then the syndrome is much more severe. The cow becomes very dull, her eyes sink and she may appear blind and start to stagger. In the early stages she may be almost constipated, although the faeces which are passed later will be typically foul-smelling and pale yellow in colour. When she becomes recumbent, stops drinking and grunts with every breath, the chances of recovery are very poor.

*Treatment*

Provided the rumen is still working, most cases can be treated medically. Sulphonamide by mouth (250 ml of a 33% solution) is very useful because not only does it stop the rapid bacterial fermentation, but being very caustic it also neutralises the acid in the rumen. One of the main groups of bacteria which proliferate are the lactobacilli, so penicillin can be used as an alternative to sulphonamides. Sodium bicarbonate (at least 250 g four times daily) can also be used as a neutralising agent, and large doses of water (10–15 litres or more three times daily), preferably given by stomach tube, help to reduce the concentration of lactic acid and thus prevent fluid from being withdrawn from the circulation. Calcium given intravenously or subcutaneously will stimulate ruminal contractions and both calcium and B vitamins assist the liver to metabolise the toxins absorbed from the rumen. Severely affected cows do in fact have a mild hypocalcaemia. Thiamine is a particularly important B vitamin to use, because there are often thiaminases present which destroy thiamine.

You must then watch your cow very carefully for the next 24 hours. If she deteriorates and no cudding or any other signs associated with ruminal movements can be detected, your vet will probably have to empty the rumen. This can be done surgically, by cutting a large hole in the left side (a rumenotomy) and removing the contents by hand. Alternatively, a large tight-fitting plastic tube can be passed into the rumen via the oesophagus, or through the skin, and the toxic products and concentrate 'sludge' washed out with water. This procedure is quite stressful to the animal, however, and she will need careful nursing afterwards. In beef cattle, casualty slaughter would be a better option.

Badly affected cows will have a metabolic acidosis as well as a ruminal acidosis and intravenous administration of calcium borogluconate and 300 ml of 5% sodium bicarbonate may help. However, care is needed because if an excess is given the cow develops alkalosis, which can be even worse. Oral administration of a 1:1 mix of magnesium hydroxide and magnesium carbonate helps to correct rumen pH. During the convalescent period supplement with B vitamins by injection, because as the rumen flora has been all but destroyed the cow could be short of B vitamins.

Cows which have overeaten high oil foods such as peanuts or precooked potato chips (waste products from the food industry) are much more difficult to treat. The oil coats both the bacteria and the food particles and seriously impedes rumen function. Casualty slaughter is then the best option.

## The Cold Cow Syndrome

Following turnout to lush spring grazing, some cows develop a digestive upset which leads to a type of shock reaction. The symptoms vary considerably, but usually include dullness, off food, oedema of the vulva and a drop in milk production. Ruminal movements are poor, the dung has a partially digested appearance and it will probably be rather loose. The nose and skin of the animal feel cold and hence the name cold cow syndrome. Some cows are unsteady in their movements, almost as if they are drunk, and with a high pasture intake you are bound to suspect hypomagnesaemia. Most cows recover following symptomatic treatment, but it may be a while before milk yield returns to normal.

Various theories have been put forward regarding the possible cause and these include fungal toxins in the grass and the rapid fermentation of pasture with a very high sugar content. Personally I think that a contributory factor may also be a sudden intake of cold and very wet grass reducing the rate of fermentation by the ruminal bacteria. The rumen contents then turn sour, leading to stomach pain, the absorption of toxic products and scouring due to the passage of only partially digested food.

## Rumen Impaction

In some ways impaction is similar to the cold cow syndrome. In this instance however the cow gorges itself on very dry or fibrous food, which becomes impacted as a hard, fibrous mass in the rumen. The symptoms are also similar, but generally much less severe. One dose of 500 g Epsom salts by mouth usually produces a cure, although on two occasions I have seen deaths from ruminal impaction, when very hungry animals had gained access to unlimited quantities of straw.

## Wire (Traumatic Reticulitis)

This is one of the classic causes of stomach pain in the cow and it can also lead to other complications. Fragments of metal wire, copper flex, pig netting or even sharp bristles from a broom, which are accidentally taken in with the food, tend to drop into the reticulum. The recent increase in cases of 'wire' has been associated with the use of car tyres to hold down the plastic sheeting covering silage clamps. Over the years the tyres degenerate in the sun and small fragments of wire may fall onto the silage. Any tyres with crumbling rubber should therefore be discarded.

As the reticulum contracts the sharp-pointed object may penetrate its wall and with further contractions the object can slowly work its way into the peritoneal cavity, where the infection it has carried with it sets up a localised peritonitis. The position the wire normally penetrates is shown in Figure 13.3. Affected cows usually suffer a sharp drop in yield, they are off their food, dull, stand with their back slightly arched and they may be reluctant to move. They will have a raised temperature and will be slightly blown. The heifer in Plate 13.11 shows the typical stance of a wire. She has her head and one ear forward and her back is arched, depicting pain. Her tail is held up, but it is painful to pass dung. Her eyes are sunken. However, she is not bloated. The next stage in diagnosis is to listen carefully for the reticular grunt.

Earlier (on page 393) we saw that there were two phases of ruminal movements, so stand back and watch your cow from the left side. The left flank will move slightly as the first wave of contraction passes through the rumen and the cow belches immediately afterwards. This is activity in the upper ruminal sac. You then see another ruminal contraction, but without a belch, and at the same time the cow may grunt with pain. This second contraction is the mixing phase, and as the contraction passes through the lower ruminal sac and then the reticulum, the wire moves slightly, causing pain, and the cow grunts. This is an excellent diagnostic feature and is known as the Williams reflex.

Another test for a wire is to squeeze her back. As you pinch the skin she dips her spine. This stretches the reticulum and causes pain, which

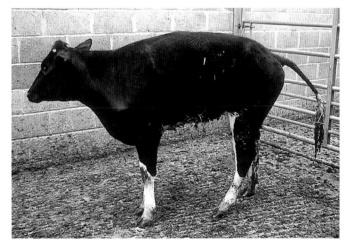

Plate 13.11. Typical stance of a heifer with a wire. Her back is arched, tail slightly lifted because dunging is painful and her eyes sunken.

again elicits a grunt. The next time you squeeze her back she knows what will happen and will probably remain with her spine horizontal. The 'pain grunt' can also be evoked by lifting the reticular area, either by raising your knee underneath her stomach or by a pole held by two people, one each side of the cow.

Diagnosing a wire is certainly not an easy task and you are bound to want veterinary advice. The best treatment is to remove the wire by surgery. An alternative is a magnet (Plate 13.12) covered by a plastic case, approximately 10 cm long and 3 cm in diameter, which can be given by mouth and which pulls the wire back into the reticulum. If left untreated there is a risk that the cow may die, either from a more generalised peritonitis, or because the wire works forward to penetrate the heart. The heart is very close to the reticulum (Figure 13.3) and a penetrating wire can easily cause a pericarditis (an infection of the pericardium, the heart sac, Plate 13.13). Whichever treatment is used, antibiotic therapy will be necessary to counteract peritonitis.

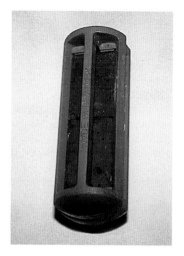

Plate 13.12. A rumen magnet for treating a wire. The plastic case ensures that once attached, lengths of wire are not rubbed off by the friction of rumen movements.

## Vagus Indigestion

The vagus is the main nerve running to the rumen and it was once thought that vagus indigestion was a primary defect of this nerve. In fact the syndrome is an obstruction either of the outlet of the abomasum, when it is termed *pyloric stenosis*, or of the outlet from the reticulum, when it is called *reticulo-omasal stenosis*. The obstruction leads to a massive dilation of the rumen with fluid. The cow slowly goes off her food, over the course of days or even weeks. In the advanced stages she produces very little dung, her abdomen is grossly enlarged, similar to bloat, and she will be in a good deal of pain. If the obstruction is at the pylorus (pyloric stenosis), she will be even more sick, because of greater fluid imbalance changes. There is no treatment: casualty slaughter is the only available option. Most affected cows seem to have a low-grade inflammation present, suggesting that the initial problem was possibly caused by a wire or some other form of localised peritonitis.

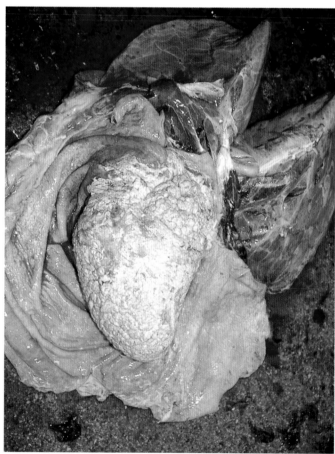

Plate 13.13. This cow died because the wire (which can be seen in the picture) passed through the diaphragm and into the heart sac, producing a pericarditis. The outer sac (the pericardium) and the heart itself are covered in pus.

## Forestomach Obstruction

Cows which develop an obstruction of the fore-stomachs (rumen, reticulum or omasum) often display a characteristic 'ten to four' appearance. This expression is used because when viewed from behind (Plate 13.14), the cow appears swollen at the top of the left flank ('ten to') and at the bottom of the right flank ('four o'clock'). Clinical signs are generally less acute and slower to develop than with intestinal torsion and it may be only after three to four days of low-grade illness that the rectum becomes empty. On rectal examination the rumen will feel grossly enlarged. There is no treatment and casualty slaughter is the best option.

## Left-sided Displaced Abomasum

The abomasum is the fourth and last stomach of the ruminant. It resembles the true stomach in man, in that it is the site of digestion by enzymes produced by the stomach wall. It normally lies along the right side of the cow, just under the abdominal wall, as shown in Figure 13.4, and it is held in this position by attachments to the duodenum at one end and to the omasum at the other. However sometimes the abomasum passes underneath the rumen and up to the left flank, and lies between the skin and the upper sac of the rumen. This is a displaced abomasum. Gas accumulates and cannot

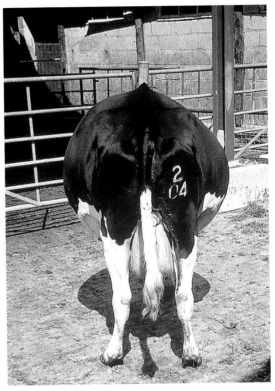

Plate 13.14. Forestomach obstruction, showing the typical 'ten to four' appearance: abdominal enlargement at the top of the left flank and the bottom of the right flank.

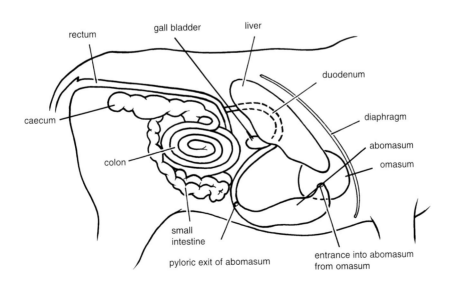

Figure 13.4. The normal position of the abomasum on the right flank.

escape because the duodenum is stretched under the rumen. If you listen carefully, you may be able to hear the gas and liquid making resonant splashing sounds under the *left* flank. It can be detected much more easily by flicking your finger onto the rib cage on the left side and listening for the resonance (described as a 'ping') with a stethoscope.

| Disorders of the abomasum include |
|---|
| ● left-sided displaced abomasum |
| ● right-sided abomasal dilation and torsion |
| ● abomasal ulcer |
| ● abomasal bloat in calves (see Chapter 2) |

*Clinical signs*
Probably the first thing you will see is a sudden drop in yield and the cow is off her food, especially her concentrates. In this respect the clinical signs are very similar to acetonaemia. After a few days a proportion of cows do in fact develop acetonaemia as a secondary symptom. Their dung tends to be very hard and they soon lose weight. The left flank over the rumen becomes distended due to the presence of the abomasum, and the cow may look slightly blown. It is not necessarily an acute condition, however, and some affected cows can live for several weeks. In mild cases the abomasum may even return to the correct position on its own, but the majority become displaced again a few days later. Acute cases occasionally occur, when the abomasum ulcerates or even ruptures and causes death, but this is rare.

*Treatment*
There are two main types of treatment and your vet will probably have his own preferences. By far the most successful is to open the cow surgically on her right flank and pull the abomasum back underneath the rumen into its correct position. It can then be sutured in place, thus preventing further displacement.

Surgery is expensive, however, and carries a degree of risk, so I like first to try to replace the abomasum

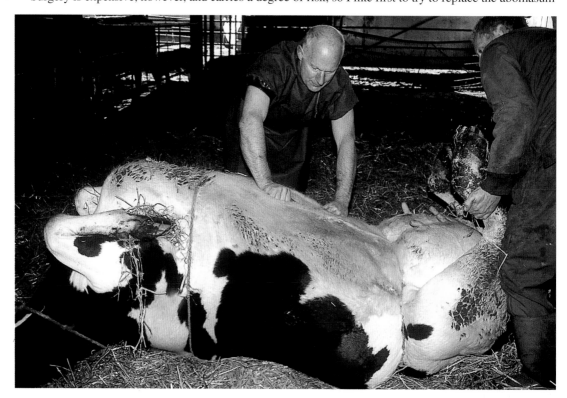

Plate 13.15. Correcting a displaced abomasum. If the cow is rolled onto her back, the abomasum can be pummelled across from left to right to return it to its original position.

by rolling the cow. If she is sedated and then laid on her back, the abomasum can be pushed from left to right over the top of the rumen by a pummelling action with the fists (Plate 13.15). It is almost always possible to replace the abomasum in this way, but unfortunately more than half the cases recur a few days later and still have to be treated surgically. Even so, I consider that this simple approach is worthwhile for the 30–40% of cows which do recover, and only a few days have been lost if the abomasum does displace again. After rolling, the cow should be put into the comfort of a straw yard and onto a high fibre:low concentrate diet, so that the rumen fills up and the abomasum is unable to displace underneath the rumen for a second time. Wait at least two weeks before bringing her back up to full rations.

*Causes and prevention*

The abomasum is suspended by attachments to the duodenum at one end and the omasum at the other (see Figure 13.4), so that as it contracts during normal digestion it pulls itself into the correct position. Displacement occurs when these abomasal contractions are weak or absent, or sometimes when a bubble of free gas accumulates. A displaced abomasum is most commonly seen in high-yielding cows in early to peak lactation. Potential causes include:

- high concentrate diets
- low fibre diets and especially diets with inadequate long fibre, both of which lead to poor rumination and acidosis. Adding hay, straw or big bale silage to the ration helps in prevention
- digestive upsets, which allow only partially digested food (especially starch) into the abomasum, where it may ferment to produce gas
- very high oil rations (those greater than 4.5% of the total diet), because excess oils suppress rumen fermentation
- a rumen that is not full, thus allowing the abomasum to pass underneath the rumen
- unsuitable precalving ration. All cows experience a reduction in appetite immediately before calving. An increase in nutrient density is needed to compensate; otherwise a degree of ketosis develops which can predispose to displaced abomasum.
- gross overfeeding, leading to overfat cows at calving and development of fatty liver (Chapter 6)
- an excessively rapid buildup of concentrates post calving can lead to acidosis (Chapter 6), which in turn predisposes to displaced abomasum
- stress. It has been shown that if some cows are simply taken out of the cubicles and put into the comfort and luxury of a straw yard, they will recover on their own
- intercurrent disease. A displaced abomasum often follows some other illness, for example recurrent milk fever, severe metritis, acidosis or fatty liver. It has been shown that cows with low blood calcium at calving are three to four times more likely to develop a displaced abomasum, even if they did not get clinical milk fever (see Table 6)
- sand accumulating in the abomasum (due to feeding dirty potatoes or fodder beet) may predispose, although one might expect this to hold the abomasum in position, rather than allowing it to displace
- there may be an hereditary predisposition – which could explain an increased incidence in some herds – associated with weak abomasal attachments

## Right-sided Abomasal Dilation and Torsion

Sometimes the abomasum remains on the right side, but either twists over on itself (torsion) or simply undergoes gross dilation. Instead of lying in its normal position on the floor of the abdomen, the dilated organ may occupy the whole area under the ribs on the right side, from belly to spine. A resonant 'ping' can be heard when the ribs are tapped with the fingers, sounding identical to left displacement (but obviously on the right-hand side). Cows with right-sided dilation and/or torsion tend to be more seriously ill than those with left displacement. Mild cases may be treated medically for a few days, using drugs such as metoclopramide, which contract the abomasum. More severe cases need to be surgically opened and drained. Most animals recover quite well. There has been an increase in incidence in the UK, perhaps associated with the increased feeding of maize silage.

## Abomasal Ulcer

Stomach ulcers are, of course, common in man and they also occur periodically in dairy cows. Many of the cases which I have seen have been in early spring or in the autumn, when the cows are grazing lush grass with a high nitrogen content. The initial symptoms are mild abdominal pain, a drop in yield and loss of appetite. There may or may not be a slight increase in temperature. Many ulcers bleed profusely, and when the blood is passed the dung turns to a dark, black, tar-like scour as in Plate 13.16. Badly affected cows will need a blood transfusion and some animals die, either from excessive blood loss or perforation of the ulcer leading to peritonitis. Blood transfusions may be difficult to justify economically. There is nothing to say that the ulcer has stopped bleeding, and giving blood will increase blood pressure and may even start further bleeding.

Less severe cases can be treated medically using kaolin and astringents (e.g. 20 g copper sulphate) given by mouth to try to arrest the bleeding, and iron injections to assist with re-forming blood. Dosing the cow with 60–100 ml of 10% sodium bicarbonate first may help to close the oesophageal groove (Chapter 2) and may allow the kaolin and copper sulphate to bypass the rumen and go straight to the abomasum.

High yields, high concentrate diets and stress have all been suggested as potential causes. Low-grade abomasal ulcers are common in young calves.

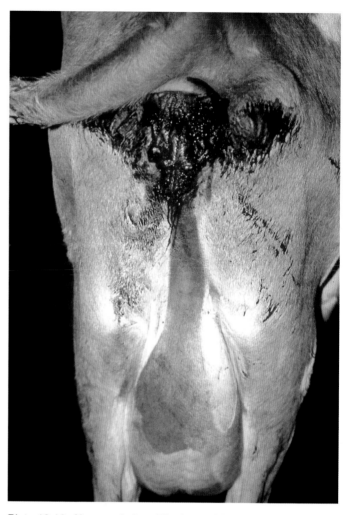

Plate 13.16. Abomasal ulcer. The loose, black, tarry faeces seen around the tail of this cow are typical of an abomasal ulcer.

## Intestinal Obstruction (Stoppage)

A blocked intestine can arise from a range of different causes, three of which are described in the following.

**Intestinal torsion (twisted gut)** The intestine is suspended from the animal's spine by the mesentery, and resembles a small piece of tubing running around the outside of a fan (Figure 13.4). Sometimes the whole mesentery twists over on itself (a twisted gut) or

---

Disorders of the intestines include

- Obstruction (stoppage) from
  - intestinal torsion (twisted gut)
  - intussusception
  - gut tie
- winter dysentery
- dilation and torsion of the caecum
- Johne's disease
- infectious and management causes (see Chapter 2)

perhaps only one segment of the intestine is twisted. This cuts off the blood supply to the intestine and causes a blockage (Plate 13.17).

**Intussusception** A length of intestine may telescope into an adjacent piece, as shown in Figure 13.5. This constricts the blood supply and leads to a swelling which in turn obstructs the flow of food material. The intestine below the obstruction will be empty but otherwise normal. The length above will be distended with accumulating intestinal contents. Very occasionally the constricted intestine sloughs off and is discharged in the faeces and the two opposing edges of the intestine heal naturally (A joins to B and C joins to D in Figure 13.5). However, this is rare.

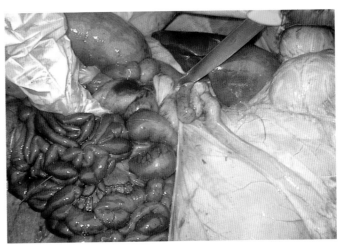

Plate 13.17. Intestinal torsion (twisted gut). The post-mortem knife marks the point of the torsion. The dark-red dilated loops of intestine on the left are degenerating and have a very different appearance to the normal cream-coloured intestine on the right.

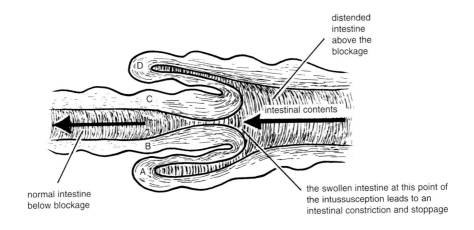

Figure 13.5. An intussusception: a segment of intestine telescopes into the piece behind. This constricts the blood flow and leads to a stoppage.

**Gut tie (pelvic hernia)** This can only occur in male calves which have been surgically castrated. A length of intestine prolapses through a small tear in the sheet of mesentery which originally carried the vas deferens. It then twists and becomes obstructed. This may occur several months after the castration, by which time the calf may be large enough for a rectal examination to be performed. The hole in the mesentery can then be enlarged manually, the loop of intestine is freed and the calf recovers rapidly. In other cases surgery may be needed.

*Clinical signs*

The clinical signs of a stoppage are similar, whatever the cause, although they will vary depending on the severity (partial or complete) and the position of the obstruction (whether near to the abomasum or near to the rectum). Initially the animal is dull. It picks at its food or stops eating altogether. It may show signs of colic, by kicking its flanks, looking at its sides or perhaps getting up and lying down repeatedly, in obvious discomfort. Some dry dung may be passed in the early stages, possibly covered with mucus, but later the rectum becomes sticky and empty. The animal's temperature will probably be below normal and its pulse very fast.

If left, most animals will develop peritonitis and die. In valuable animals an intussusception can be treated surgically by resecting the obstruction, and gut tie may be released by surgery or by rectal manipulation, as described above. However, for most cases prompt casualty slaughter is the best option.

A word of caution: cows and young stock can develop colic simply from a spasm in the gut, that is from excessive muscle contractions. This will give symptoms very similar to the initial stages of a stoppage, but it is a colic which responds rapidly to treatment with muscle relaxants, so make sure that you get your vet to examine the animal before sending her off. This temporary colic syndrome is particularly common in young stock.

## Winter Dysentery

Waves of scouring may pass through dairy herds, especially during the winter housing period, when the risk of faecal contamination is much greater. Some authorities consider that BVD is the primary agent of this so-called 'winter dysentery' of dairy cows, although others consider that a coronavirus infection is involved. In the first year that disease is seen, up to 80% of cows may be affected by this condition over a two to three month period, each animal running a temperature for a few days, scouring, off its food and with a sharp drop in milk production. Mouth and nose lesions are very rare. Occasional cases develop a very severe scour and die within a few days. However, the majority recover, although yield may be affected for the remainder of the lactation. During the second winter, further cases may be seen, but far fewer in number, and thereafter the disease becomes endemic in the herd, producing only occasional cases each winter, especially in heifers or purchased cows. Although winter scour is not too serious, it does cause a considerable nuisance and loss of milk.

## Dilation and Torsion of the Caecum

The caecum is a blind-ended sac which is part of the large bowel (Figure 13.4). It lies under the right flank high up towards the spine, and torsion and dilation can occur in the same way as with the abomasum. The symptoms are very variable: mild cases present as a low-grade digestive upset and can be treated medically or simply left to recover on their own. More severe cases often produce marked abdominal pain and need to be surgically drained and deflated.

## Johne's Disease

Johne's disease is an infection caused by *Mycobacterium johnei*. The bacterium is related to tuberculosis and this is why Johne's is sometimes called *paratuberculosis*. Infection is taken in by mouth and produces a thickening of the lower part of the small intestine and the upper large intestine, although lesions can sometimes extend down as far as the rectum. The thickening interferes with the function of the gut, particularly the absorption of water and nutrients. Disease is usually seen following the stress of calving. The cow develops a profuse watery diarrhoea which characteristically froths when it hits the ground. Symptomatic treatment with kaolin, chlorodyne or astringents such as sulphonamides or copper sulphate may temporarily alleviate the scour, but it soon returns.

The other prominent feature of Johne's disease is a massive weight loss. This continues until the cow is so thin and emaciated that she cannot stand and she dies from an inability to absorb the nutrients from her food. No animals should ever be allowed to reach this stage, of course, and once the diagnosis has been confirmed with a blood or dung sample, casualty slaughter is indicated. Johne's disease provides a good example of bacteria which live inside cells and are therefore protected from the action of antibiotics. Tuberculosis and brucellosis are similar.

Although typical Johne's disease is by no means as severe a problem as it used to be in the UK, the move towards larger herds has produced an increased incidence. There is evidence that it can persist in a subclinical form for eight to ten years or more, and may be a cause of chronic poor growth and disappointing production. These cows will be intermittent excretors of infection and will perpetuate the disease within a herd. They may transmit infection to their calves, both across the placenta and via colostrum. In one study around 30% of all calves born to clinically affected cows were positive to Johne's, and even 10% of calves born to subclinically affected cows were positive. All calves from Johne's cows should therefore be considered as suspect carriers. There is an additional danger in using pooled colostrum in an infected herd, because this could also be spreading infection.

*Control of Johne's*
Calves up to six months of age are the only animals in which infection can become established, but because the incubation period is *two years* or more, disease will not be seen until after the first or second calving at least. The stress of calving often precipitates the onset of scouring and at this stage the dung will contain massive numbers of Johne's bacteria. Important control measures are therefore to remove the calf from its mother immediately after birth, to isolate affected animals and thus to avoid further faecal contamination of the environment, to identify and cull infected animals as soon as possible, and to make sure that feed and drinking water have not been infected. Unfortunately there is no good test to positively identify carrier animals. Probably the two major reasons why Johne's is now less common are that calves are removed from their dams soon after birth and that clean water troughs have replaced drinking from dirty farm ponds.

In herds where Johne's is a problem, vaccination can be carried out. A special licence may be needed, because the vaccine can interfere with the interpretation of the tuberculosis test. Calves are vaccinated during the first four weeks of life, by means of a subcutaneous injection into the dewlap between the front legs. Check that a hard nodule has formed. This indicates that there has been a good vaccine 'take'. As two to three weeks are required for the vaccine to become effective and as it will not protect against a very heavy challenge of infection, vaccination should always be combined with the hygiene and management measures described above.

*Relationship to Crohn's Disease in man*
Johne's bacteria have also been isolated from a few cases of people suffering from a human intestinal malabsorption syndrome known as Crohn's disease. Although the link is by no means certain, the finding that pasteurisation did not fully remove all Johne's bacteria from milk, and that up to 5% of samples of milk tested were positive for Johne's, caused some concern in the UK. Pasteurisation times have now been increased, so the risk will be negligible. Even so, it is important to test all cases of chronic diarrhoea in adult cows, thereby removing any risk to both animals and man.

# Liver Fluke (Fascioliasis)

The liver plays a vital part in dealing with the products of digestion and so I have included liver fluke in this section. Fluke is caused by a small parasite called *Fasciola hepatica* and hence sometimes the disease is called fascioliasis. It is an important condition in both sheep and cattle and is especially common in areas that are warm and wet.

*Life cycle*
The life cycle of the fluke is shown in Figure 13.6. Taking the adult egg-laying fluke in the liver as our starting point, fluke eggs may be shed in the dung throughout the winter, but it is only when the weather becomes warm (above 10°C) and wet that they begin to hatch. Hatching releases the miracidia and these swim around in a film of moisture until they contact and penetrate the snail *Lymnaea truncatula*. There is

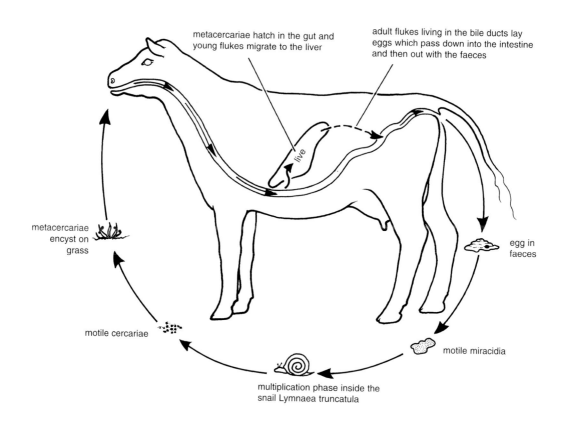

metacercariae hatch in the gut and young flukes migrate to the liver

adult flukes living in the bile ducts lay eggs which pass down into the intestine and then out with the faeces

live

metacercariae encyst on grass

egg in faeces

motile cercariae

motile miracidia

multiplication phase inside the snail Lymnaea truncatula

Figure 13.6. The life cycle of the liver fluke, Fasciola hepatica.

a multiplication phase inside the snail, so that one fluke miracidium entering the snail can lead to the release of over a thousand fluke cercariae from the snail. Cercariae swim onto blades of grass and encyst to form resistant structures, the metacercariae. After infected pasture has been eaten by cattle, the metacercariae hatch in the intestine to produce immature flukes. These migrate to and then burrow across the liver, continually feeding as they pass through its substance, until they reach the bile ducts. In the bile ducts they complete their final stage of development to adult egg-laying flukes. The eggs pass down to the gall-bladder, into the intestine and then out in the faeces, thus starting another cycle.

Compared with other parasites like husk or the stomach worm *Ostertagia*, liver fluke has a fairly long life cycle as shown in Table 13.2. The stage inside the cow, from eating the metacercariae until eggs are seen in the faeces, takes around three months, and even under favourable conditions, the stage outside the animal, that is the hatching of the eggs, development through the snail and production of metacercariae, takes at least another two months. By favourable conditions I mean a temperature above 10°C and plenty of wet weather. It is said that if there are eleven weeks of continuous wet weather, including the four weeks of June, this will produce ideal conditions for fluke. Hatching of the fluke eggs *and* the development of the snails are both stimulated by warmth and humidity, so if June and July are wet, all the fluke eggs which have been passed from December of the previous year onwards and which have overwintered on the pasture hatch at the same time as the snail population increases. This leads to a massive production of cercariae with a subsequent heavy infestation of metacercariae on the pasture. The metacercariae may be eaten by cattle from September onwards, but as adult flukes take three months to develop, there may be no significant disease seen until December or January. If, on the other hand, the summer months are either very dry or very cold, fewer fluke eggs hatch and there are fewer snails around anyway, so far fewer metacercariae encyst on the grass. This is the basis of the 'Fluke Forecast' issued by the Ministry of Agriculture in the UK. It is a very useful warning to farmers of when there is likely to be a high incidence of fluke and when treatments are necessary.

So far we have been talking about what is known as the 'summer infection' of snails. If September and October are warm and wet, then a second wave of fluke eggs may hatch and these weather conditions will also lead to an increase in the number of active available snails. By the time that the snail has become infected, however, the coldest weather will almost certainly have arrived and the snail then becomes dormant until the spring. As soon as spring weather conditions permit, snail activity starts again and metacercariae are deposited on the pasture. This is known as the 'winter infection' of snails. Clearly in the southern hemisphere winter and summer apply but the months will be different.

Summer infection of the snails is by far the most common, producing pasture infestation with metacercariae in the autumn, so that disease can be seen from December onwards, but usually not until January and February. However, as metacercariae can persist on grass over the winter and as snails can carry cercariae until the following year, it is possible to get outbreaks of fluke in the spring or even in the summer.

Cattle slowly build up an immunity

Table 13.2. Time spans in the fluke life cycle.

| | | |
|---|---|---|
| Ingested metacercariae to immature flukes in liver | = 4 weeks | |
| Immature flukes passes through liverfeeding | = 6 weeks | 3 months inside the animal |
| Flukes mature in bile ducts and produce eggs | = 2 weeks | |
| Egg to miracidium to snail to cercaria to metacercaria | = 2 months *minimum* outside the animal | |

Fluke populations survive the winter in three ways:

- as adult flukes in the livers of infected animals, which, if outwintered, will be continually passing fluke eggs which all hatch at approximately the same time to produce the summer infection of snails
- as resistant metacercariae on pasture
- as cercariae in dormant snails, the result of the winter infection

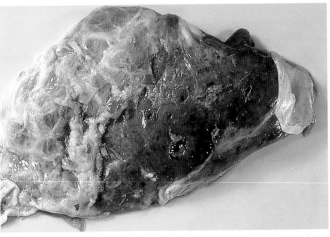

Plate 13.18. Liver fluke. The bile ducts are grossly thickened, giving a classic 'pipe-stem' appearance. Adult flukes can sometimes be squeezed out of the bile ducts. They are easily visible to the naked eye.

to fluke and they seal them off in their bile ducts by laying down a thick, fibrous barrier, reinforced with calcium. This produces the classic 'pipe-stem' liver seen on post-mortem (Plate 13.18). The immunity limits the life span of the adult flukes to approximately one and a half years, so continual reinfestation of dairy cows is needed to maintain fluke populations.

*Clinical signs*

Although immature flukes cause some damage during their migration, the main effect is due to the blood-sucking activities of the adult flukes in the bile ducts. There is no 'acute fluke' type of disease as is seen in sheep. The blood loss leads to anaemia, and affected cattle look in poor condition, with rough staring coats, and they are generally unthrifty. Occasionally they develop a 'bottle jaw' appearance, due to the accumulation of fluid (known as dropsy or oedema fluid) under the skin of the chin, although again this symptom is much more commonly seen in sheep. In dairy cows quite low fluke burdens will depress protein in milk, and heavier infestations can lead to reduced yields. I have seen beef suckler cows so badly infected that many went down after calving and never recovered. Scouring is not a common feature of fluke and outbreaks of scouring in animals in poor condition in February or March are more likely to be due to type II *Ostertagia* (see Chapter 4). Liver fluke may increase the susceptibility of cows to *Salmonella dublin* infection.

*Treatment and control*

Only the drug oxyclozanide is currently licensed for use in milking cows in the UK, and there is a milk withholding period. On fluke farms the dairy herd should ideally be drenched twice during the winter period; for example, once in late December and then again in early February. The second dosing needs to be at least two and a half months after housing, so that all the metacercariae which were eaten during the autumn have reached adult stage and are then susceptible to the drug. If there is only a low risk of infestation, the first dose can be omitted. Outwintered cows and heifers which could have been eating infected pasture throughout the winter ought to receive a further dose in March or April.

Some drugs such as nitroxynil, rafoxanide and triclabendazole kill flukes at a much earlier stage of their life cycle and are very good to use in young stock and non-lactating animals. A single dose four weeks after housing should be adequate in the majority of cases.

The other aspect of the control of liver fluke is either to remove the snail habitats by drainage, or simply to fence them off. Cattle can then neither graze in these areas and become infected, nor dung there to deposit fluke eggs to infect snails with miracidia. *Lymnaea truncatula* snails prefer to live in a moist environment. They like the puddles beside streams and ponds or even hoof-marks in the mud if the ground is very wet. They do not like very acid soils such as peat bogs, so the application of lime to increase soil pH may lead to an outbreak of liver fluke. Under adverse conditions such as the cold in winter, or a very dry summer, snails become dormant and do not allow flukes to multiply.

## RESPIRATORY DISEASES

Many of the major respiratory diseases have been described elsewhere in this book. Some affect calves, and others can affect all age groups. They include:

- calf pneumonia (Chapter 3)
- IBR (Chapter 4). This respiratory disease affects dairy herds, although the occular form (conjunctivitis) is also quite common without respiratory signs.
- lungworm (Chapter 4). 'Reinfection husk' is the name given to the syndrome where partially immune dairy cows are subjected to a high larval challenge from the pasture. Although the cows cough (perhaps causing the milking units to fall off) the partial immunity of the cow may prevent any larvae from being seen in the faeces. This makes the syndrome more difficult to diagnose.

The respiratory conditions described in this chapter include fog fever, pulmonary haemorrhage, allergic respiratory diseases and bovine influenza A (described on page 426).

### Fog Fever

Fog fever is the name given to a syndrome of severe respiratory distress in cattle. It is mainly seen in the autumn, especially in September and October, and affects cattle which are two years old or more.

Suckler cows are particularly prone, although I have also seen outbreaks in milking cows. Disease typically occurs zero to two weeks after the cattle have been moved onto a lush autumn aftermath and this is especially so if their previous grazing was a very sparse and dry pasture. Many theories were suggested as to a possible cause, for example an allergy to lungworm larvae or to fungal toxins on pasture, but it is now known that the syndrome is an *anaphylaxis*, sometimes called a *hypersensitivity* reaction. This is the name given to an overactivity of the normal immune defences of the animal, as described in Chapter 1. Lush autumn grazing, particularly if it has a high nitrogen content, contains increased levels of the amino-acid L-tryptophan. In the rumen this is converted to the chemical 3-methyl indole, a toxin which is absorbed into the bloodstream and leads to a hypersensitivity reaction, the most prominent effects of which are seen in the lungs.

*Clinical signs*
The syndrome is very sudden in onset. One or more cattle may be seen standing listlessly in the field, not grazing, and characteristically their breathing is accompanied by forced grunts. The toxin 3-methyl indole leads to congestion of the lungs and many of the small alveoli burst, leaving the animal 'broken winded', a condition known technically as pulmonary alveolar emphysema. (The alveoli are shown in Figure 4.7.) Although the cow can breathe in without any problems, the loss of elasticity in the broken alveoli means that she has great difficulty in breathing out, and if you stand and watch her carefully you will see that she grunts as her flanks and chest move inwards, trying to *expel* air from the lungs. In this respect fog fever resembles human asthma but it differs from cows with severe pneumonia which show difficulty both when breathing in (inspiration) and when breathing out (expiration). The burst alveoli allow air to infiltrate between the lung tissues and to pass deeper into the body, and in long-standing cases I have even seen cows with air crackling under the skin of their backs (subcutaneous emphysema). Although this looks peculiar, it is no cause for alarm and provided the animal recovers, the air will slowly disperse. Badly affected animals stand with their necks stretched forwards, mouths open and froth around their lips. They cannot eat or drink and eventually they die, simply because they cannot get sufficient air.

*Prevention and treatment*
Making a more gradual change from bare summer grazing to lush autumn aftermaths, for example by strip-grazing, is considered to help reduce the severity of outbreaks, and feeding hay or straw at this time may also be worthwhile. Treatment is quite complex, and the drugs used will depend on how bad the animal is and how long it has been affected. Non-steroidal anti-inflammatories, antihistamines, corticosteroids and other anti-inflammatory drugs may be used to try to reduce the toxic effects of 3-methyl indole, and antibiotics will help to prevent a secondary bacterial pneumonia developing in the congested lungs. Respiratory stimulants may be needed if the cow is very ill. One drug which is effective in both treatment and prevention is monensin. Monensin is also used as a growth promoter in beef rations and is effective against coccidiosis in chickens. Fed at the rate of 200 mg/cow/day this prevents the conversion of L-tryptophan into 3-methyl indole in the rumen, and if given at the start of an outbreak it will certainly stop the syndrome deteriorating and may prevent further cases from occurring. Even though only a few animals may be showing clinical symptoms, it is likely that the majority are subclinically affected. Fortunately the dose of 200 mg monensin/cow/day is the same as that recommended as a growth promoter for grazing cattle, so you can simply purchase a few sacks of standard ration and start feeding it following the normal gradual introductory period. For dairy cows check that no milk withholding period is necessary.

Even if all these treatments are given there will still be a proportion of animals in which the lung changes are so severe that death is inevitable. Affected cattle may have great difficulty in breathing, so it is important not to walk them too far or too quickly. It may even be necessary to pen them into the corner of the offending field and carry hay and water rather than risk moving them.

## Pulmonary Haemorrhage

Occasionally you may see a cow bleeding from the nose, as in Plate 11.11. Although it may not look particularly serious, in most cases the blood is coming from a ruptured pulmonary (= lung) artery or vein. The animal may have had pneumonia as a calf, and although it may have appeared to recover, a small abscess was left in the lung. Over time the abscess may slowly erode into a blood vessel, which then 'leaks', and the blood passes up the trachea and back down into the mouth and nose. In some cows the haemorrhage is so severe that the animal is simply found dead, sometimes with the coughed-up blood splashed all around its pen. Others, such as the cow in Plate 11.11, may survive for a few days, but they are best sent for casualty slaughter.

Pulmonary haemorrhage may also result from thromboembolism. An abscess anywhere within the body may start to 'leak' and allow clumps of blood and bacteria to float around in the blood vessels. These clumps are known as emboli. Some may localise in the lungs, or even in the major blood vessels within the lungs, and grow until they eventually lead to blood vessel rupture and haemorrhage.

## Allergic Respiratory Diseases

Cattle can become allergic to mouldy hay or straw and develop a syndrome which is effectively bovine farmer's lung, sometimes technically called interstitial pneumonia. The fungus *Micropolyspora faeni* is often involved and, as you would expect, disease is more common –

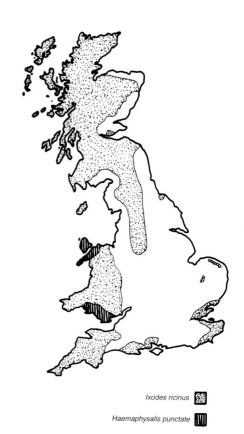

- in the winter, when cattle are housed, perhaps on damp and mouldy straw, or fed on mouldy hay
- in wetter areas of the country, which are the areas most likely to have damp hay and straw

The primary clinical sign is coughing. In severe cases, growth is affected and weight loss may occur. All ages of cattle can become affected, including milking cows. Dusty feed in itself can also cause coughing and/or sneezing, and as described in Chapter 3, dust will make cattle more susceptible to pneumonia.

There is no specific treatment. Anti-inflammatory drugs will help, but the most important thing is to remove the mouldy or dusty food and bedding.

## TICK-BORNE DISEASES

There are two major species of cattle ticks in the British Isles, namely *Ixodes ricinus* and *Haemaphysalis punctata*. *Ixodes* is by far the most common and it is found throughout Scotland, Wales, north and south-west England and in a few areas of Dorset and the south-east. Tick areas are shown on the map in Figure 13.7. *Haemaphysalis* is found only in coastal areas of Wales. Ticks prefer coarse, uncultivated pasture, because the tufts of grass provide them with moisture and protection.

*Ixodes ricinus*

*Haemaphysalis punctate*

Figure 13.7. The distribution of cattle ticks in the United Kingdom. From R. E. Purnell (1982), *Proc. Brit. Cattle Vet. Assoc.*, p. 103.

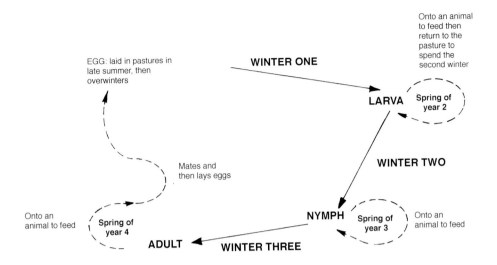

Figure 13.8. The three year life cycle of a spring-feeding tick.

Ticks and tick diseases are much more important in warmer parts of the world, for example in central and southern Africa and America.

*Life cycle of the tick*
Different ticks may have different life cycles and local texts should be consulted. The life cycle of *Ixodes ricinus* is spread over three years, as shown in Figure 13.8. An egg laid in the grass in year one slowly develops over the following winter to hatch as a larva in the spring of year two. The tick larva climbs to the top of the grass or a small bush, and waits there until an animal brushes past, whereupon it attaches itself to the animal and then slowly engorges itself with blood. This takes four to six days. When full it drops onto the ground and remains there over the summer and the second winter until the spring of the third year, when it moults and emerges as a nymph. The feeding process is repeated and the nymph returns to the ground until the spring of the fourth year, when a further moult occurs, and it emerges as an adult. The adults feed, then mating takes place, either on the animal or on the ground. The males die soon afterwards, but the females live slightly longer and lay their eggs into thick matted pasture.

There are two phases of tick activity, one in the spring (May and June) and the other in the autumn (September). Ticks which hatch as larvae in the spring continue as spring-feeding nymphs and adults, whereas those hatching in the autumn

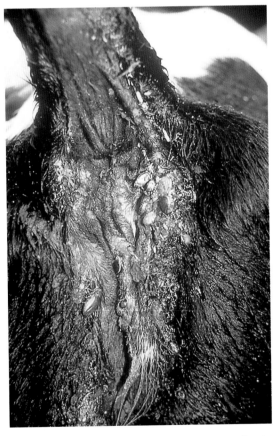

Plate 13.19. Ticks attach to an animal only to feed. The animal shown was from Zimbabwe. Whilst feeding, the ticks secreted a toxin which produced sweating sickness, which is not seen in the UK.

continue as autumn feeders. To feed, the tick inserts its mouthparts through the animal's skin, squirts in saliva to act as an anticoagulant and then begins to fill itself with blood (Plate 13.19). When fully engorged it drops back onto the pasture, where it remains in cracks and crevices, to complete the moult which is the next stage of its development. It takes three years for a tick egg to become an adult, therefore, and during this time it will have fed only once each year. Most of the tick's life is spent on the ground.

Ticks can feed on most animals including sheep, cattle, deer, rabbits, dogs and even man. However, although they may transmit sheep infections to cattle and vice versa, these infections only become established in the correct host species.

Disease caused by ticks is of two kinds, primary and secondary. Primary disease is related to the tick's feeding activities and consists of irritation and anaemia due to extensive blood loss. It is rare that tick burdens are ever high enough to produce significant anaemia under British conditions, but this can be a problem in some countries. Secondary disease is far more common and is due to the effects of the parasites carried by the ticks. In the UK the two main conditions in cattle are redwater and tick-borne fever, both of which are carried by *Ixodes*. *Haemaphysalis* carries a less important form of redwater and another blood parasite called *Theileria*. Ticks also carry the sheep disease louping-ill and cause tick pyaemia. Tick-transmitted diseases in southern Africa include heart water and gall sickness.

## Redwater

Redwater is caused by a small single-celled protozoan parasite called *Babesia divergens*. It is related to the parasite which causes malaria in man. *Babesia* is transmitted into cattle with the drop of saliva which is pushed down through the tick's mouthparts as an anticoagulant at the start of feeding. Once in the bloodstream *Babesia* starts to multiply in the red blood cells. Waves of infection occur, with the new crop of *Babesia* rupturing the red blood cells as they are released. Haemoglobin pigment is also liberated from the ruptured cells. It passes out in the urine and hence the name of redwater. Other causes of red urine are given in Appendix 2.

*Clinical signs*
In the early stages of the disease the animal will be standing apart from the others and running a very high temperature (41°C). This is the multiplication phase of *Babesia*. Within 24 hours and possibly sooner, the urine turns a deep port-wine red colour (Plate 13.20) and froths as it lands on the floor. The animal's pulse is very fast because of the anaemia associated with the rupturing of the red cells and often you can hear the very loud heartbeat if you stand quietly nearby. In the early stages, the dung is passed under pressure due to a spasm of the anus and this produces a 'pipe-stem' effect, almost as if the animal is scouring. As the effects of the anaemia develop, however, constipation sets in. If left untreated, death may occur. A proportion of animals will undoubtedly have less serious infections and some recover without treatment, possibly without having been noticeably ill.

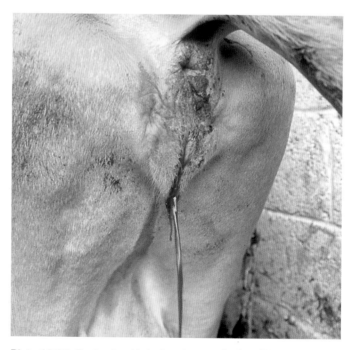

Plate 13.20. Redwater. Note the deep red urine. There are other causes of red urine apart from *Babesia*.

*Treatment*
Drugs such as imidocarb can specifically kill the *Babesia*. Quinuronium sulphate has also been used, although it must be given subcutaneously and not intramuscularly or intravenously. If the urine is still discoloured after 24 hours, a repeat treatment may be needed. Iron injections and vitamins will help re-form the red cells, although if the anaemia is severe a blood transfusion may be necessary.

*Immunity*
Young animals have an inherent immunity (sometimes called a premunity) against redwater, and the disease is unlikely to be seen in cattle less than nine months old. If they are then slowly exposed to low levels of infection they can build up their own true immunity.

However, as immunity is quite shortlived and as exposure to *Babesia* may be erratic, this may not be sufficient to give total protection. *Babesia* can persist in the pasture for prolonged periods, only occasionally infecting cattle because

- There are only two phases of tick activity each year, in spring and autumn, and cattle need to be grazing infested pasture during these periods to become exposed.
- By no means all parts of a farm will be tick infested.
- *Babesia* can survive inside the tick for three years as it passes from the egg through its larval, nymph and into the adult stages, despite the fact that the tick may not have fed on cattle blood over this period. It can even pass into the next generation of ticks via the ovary and tick egg. In this way pastures can remain infective for up to six years, even in the absence of cattle and certainly without cases of redwater being seen.

A vaccine, consisting of *Babesia*-infected blood which has been partly inactivated by radiation treatment, has been produced, and although it is not available in Great Britain it is used in other parts of the world where ticks are a much more serious problem.

*Control*
Prevention of redwater is based on reducing tick populations, promoting immunity (discussed above) and the strategic use of drugs.

**Reducing tick population** Ticks need thick cover and continuous moisture. If pastures are improved, for example by harvesting them very short, ploughing or tight grazing, this will reduce tick numbers. Ticks can *feed* on sheep, but they can only contract the redwater infection when they are feeding on cattle (or deer) during the *active* phase of *Babesia* multiplication. Consequently allowing dipped sheep to graze the pasture (dipping kills ticks) would help in tick control. Only if the land has been totally free of cattle and deer for six years or more will it be 'redwater free'.

**Strategic use of drugs** A large dose of imidocarb diproprionate (at 2.5 times the normal rate) can be given to cattle when they first enter a tick area, or when an increase in tick activity is suspected. The drug gives total protection for 28 days, and then as its effect slowly fades, it is hoped that exposure to *Babesia* will occur and immunity will develop without disease. This drug is only available under special licence in the UK.

## Tick-borne Fever

This is another important infection carried by ticks. It is caused by *Cytoecetes phagocytophilia*. This is a rickettsial parasite, an organism with size and characteristics partway between viruses and bacteria. Whereas *Babesia* attacks red blood cells, *Cytoecetes* destroys neutrophils, which are one of the types of white cells in the blood. Naturally, disease only occurs in tick areas and only during the periods of tick activity. Affected animals show stiffness in the joints, lethargy, a loss of appetite and they run a high temperature. Deaths are rare, although infection can cause weight loss or a drop in milk production, and the high temperature can often lead to abortion.

Treatment with the antibiotic oxytetracycline is usually very effective and a long-acting injection gives a four day cover. Infections are probably quite common, more so than with *Babesia*, but because the symptoms are mild and rather non-specific, the majority of attacks go unnoticed. With up to 50% of its white blood cells destroyed, however, an animal suffering or recovering from tick fever will have lost some of its defence mechanisms and so it will be more susceptible to other diseases for the next one to two weeks.

## Louping ill

This is a virus infection carried by the tick *Ixodes ricinus*, and although it mainly affects sheep (causing nervous signs and abortions) it can occasionally affect cattle and even man. Most infections in cattle are asymptomatic, which means that no clinical signs are seen because infection does not reach the brain. The animal is then left with lifelong immunity. However, if the virus reaches the brain clinical signs include trembling, staggering and a very stiff gait. Fortunately most heifers recover, although some may be left with a permanent mild twitching.

A killed vaccine is available for use in areas where the disease is a problem. Annual boosters are required. Do not use in the last month of pregnancy.

## DISORDERS OF THE HEART AND CIRCULATION

As with respiratory diseases, many conditions of the heart and general circulation have been discussed already, for example:

- degeneration of the heart muscle in white muscle disease (Chapter 3)
- pericarditis, an infection of the heart sac caused by a wire (page 400)
- pulmonary haemorrhage, redwater and tick fever, described in the previous section.

This section describes two other conditions.

### Endocarditis

The word endocarditis means inflammation of the inside of the heart and is normally used to describe infection of the heart valves. Plate 13.21 shows a typical example. The infection could have originated from any site in the body, for example a foot infection, mastitis or liver abscess, and travelling through the bloodstream it is by chance that it localises on the heart valve. If small abscesses have also developed in the liver, lungs and kidneys, the animal is said to have *pyaemia*. Pyaemia can only be diagnosed at post-mortem and may be a cause of carcase rejection at the abattoir. It could also be that the heart valve infection (i.e. endocarditis) was primary and pyaemia spread from there.

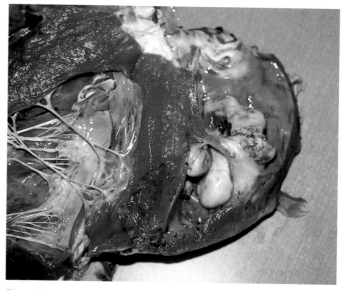

Plate 13.21 Endocarditis: large lumps of pus on the valves cause the heart to 'leak', producing an animal with poor circulation.

*Streptococcus uberis* is becoming an increasingly common cause of endocarditis. Infection is seen particularly in first lactation heifers in high stress housing situations.

In the early stages of endocarditis the animal will be a bit lethargic, with a drop in milk yield and a mild temperature. High level antibiotic for seven to ten days at this stage can sometimes produce a cure. However, when the general circulation starts to fail (see next section) casualty slaughter is usually the best option.

## Congestive Heart Failure

This occurs as a result of endocarditis, but can also be due to pericarditis (caused by a wire) or any other condition interfering with heart function. With endocarditis the valve fails to close properly and when the heart contracts to pump blood into the lungs, some of the blood is pushed back into the circulation again. This results in a swelling of blood vessels, particularly seen in the jugular vein in the neck (Plate 13.22) and an accumulation of fluid (dropsy) under the jaw (bottle jaw) and sternum. The Limousin steer in Plate 13.23 was so badly affected that the whole of his lower body, from brisket to belly, and all four legs were swollen. At post-mortem he was found to have pericarditis.

## DISORDERS OF THE UROGENITAL SYSTEM

The urogenital system includes the reproductive organs, kidneys and bladder. The majority of the problems affecting the uterus (endometritis, metritis, torsion, prolapse etc.) were dealt with in Chapters 5 and 8. This section includes a few more female and male reproductive disorders and diseases of the urinary system.

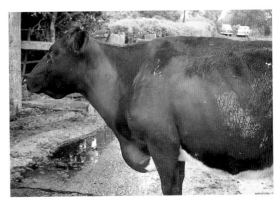

Plate 13.22. Heart failure: the thickened jugular vein is clearly seen running down the neck and there is oedema under the jaw and brisket.

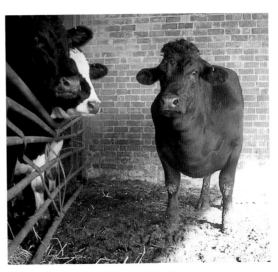

Plate 13.23. Heart failure. This Limousin steer was so badly affected that the whole of his lower body became enlarged.

## Hydrops of the Uterus

In the sixth to seventh month of pregnancy there is normally a marked increase in the production of allantoic fluid, but in some cows this becomes uncontrolled so that the uterus continues to accumulate fluid. Some 250–300 litres may be present. The cow's abdomen becomes massively dilated and she loses weight rapidly. Once she becomes recumbent, slaughter is necessary, although if the condition is recognised soon enough, termination of the pregnancy, for example with prostaglandin, cortisone or a caesarean section may be effective. Even then the sudden loss of fluid may lead to death from shock.

There was originally some confusion as to whether the fluid was accumulating in the allantoic or amniotic sacs (see Chapter 5 for explanation of these terms), and hence the condition is sometimes referred to as 'hydrops amnion' or 'hydramnios', rather than the correct name of 'hydrops allantois' or 'hydrallantois'. Hydrops amnion can occur, but is rare.

The cow in Plate 13.24 was a long time (six weeks!) overdue to calve and had been slowly getting bigger. Her abdomen was swollen on both sides, the skin was very tense and she was losing weight. She was induced to calve. A few days later a 'monster' calf (Chapter 5) was delivered, but she did not recover.

## Abscesses, Tumours and Polyps

Abscesses and tumours are occasionally found in the kidneys, and sometimes the bladder may turn itself inside out and is seen as a prolapse through the vagina. This is shown diagrammatically in Figure 13.9. It should not be confused with a *vaginal polyp* (Plate 13.25), which is a tumour attached to the vaginal wall by a long stalk and which may also be seen protruding through the lips of the vulva. When the cow stands up, polyps are often pulled back into the vagina. Tumours of the bladder wall (squamous cell carcinomas) can be induced by bracken poisoning (page 447). The only clinical signs are those of cystitis.

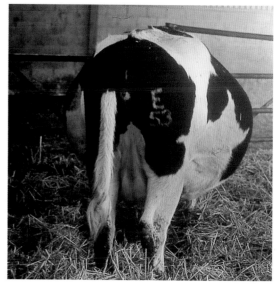

Plate 13.24. Hydrops of the uterus (hydrallantois). The cow was grossly enlarged, her abdomen very tense, and she had lost weight. After induction of abortion, an 11-month prolonged gestation 'monster' calf was delivered, but she did not recover.

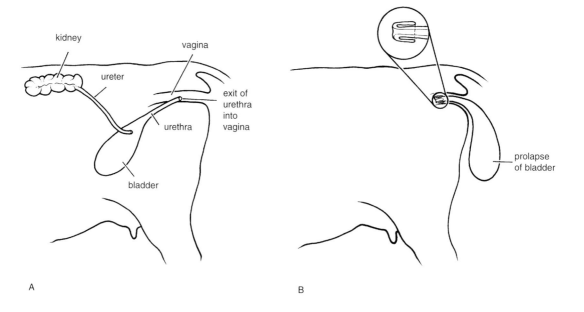

Figure 13.9. The positions of normal (a) and prolapsed (b) bladders.

## Cystitis and Pyelonephritis

The word cystitis means inflammation of the bladder and pyelonephritis means inflammation and pus in the kidney. One of the common causes is infection with the organism *Corynebacterium renale*. This is a condition seen chiefly in cows and heifers, as males are rarely affected. They run a moderate temperature, will be off their food for a few days and the urine may be a red colour, due to blood leaking from the inflamed surface of the bladder. This should not be confused with the darker purple-red urine of redwater, however.

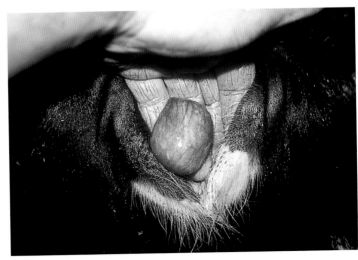

Plate 13.25. A vaginal polyp is often seen only when the cow is lying down.

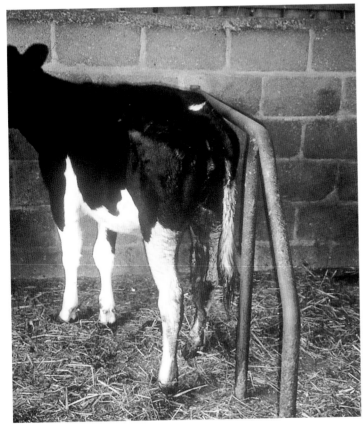

Plate 13.26. Cystitis. The strong smell of urine and grey-brown staining around the vulva are typical signs.

Provided that treatment is given fairly promptly, recovery rates are good. Your vet will probably use streptomycin, ampicillin, sulphonamides or some other antibacterial drug which is excreted via the urine, thus achieving a high concentration at the site of the bacterial attack. If the condition is allowed to progress, infection can track up the ureter towards the kidneys (see Figure 13.9 and note the unusual shape and structure of kidneys in cattle). Once the kidneys become badly infected and abscesses develop, treatment is unlikely to be successful. The animal loses weight rapidly and may become toxic and die.

Cystitis can also develop as a consequence of other diseases. The heifer in Plate 13.26 had scoured badly as a calf and then developed cystitis at three to four months old, presumably as a consequence of the scouring. Note the badly stained legs from frequent urination and urine dribbling down her thighs. Cystitis can also occur as a complication of navel ill, as discussed in Chapter 2.

# DISORDERS OF MALE REPRODUCTION

Three of the more common male disorders, namely tumours on the penis (fibropapilloma, Chapter 10), hermaphrodite/intersex (Chapter 5) and obstruction of the penis (urolithiasis, Chapter 3), have been described already.

## Damage to the Prepuce

Posthitis means inflammation of the prepuce and in most cases this is caused by physical injury followed by infection. The prepuce becomes swollen and hangs down from the belly. This further increases the risk of injury and infection. A typical example is seen in the Charolais bull in Plate 13.27. If the damaged prepuce is pushed back into the sheath and held in position with sutures, many cases heal without further problems. The sutures need to be left in place for at least three to four weeks to allow sufficient time for healing, and of course there must be a large enough gap to permit urine flow. Allow at least six weeks' rest from work, penning the bull well away from cows on heat. In non-responsive cases part of the prepuce has to be removed surgically.

## Balanoposthitis

This is an inflammation of the prepuce and penis. It occurs with IBR and is the male form of infective pustular vulvovaginitis, IPV.

## Orchitis and Testicular Swellings

Orchitis means inflammation of the testicle itself and can be caused by a range of bacterial infections including tuberculosis and brucellosis. The testicle(s) will be swollen and painful

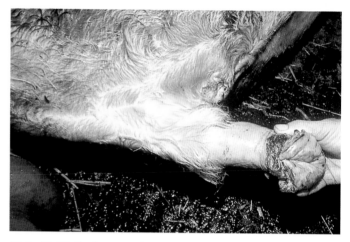

Plate 13.27. Prolapse and eversion of the prepuce (posthitis). Because the damaged prepuce hangs down from the belly, further damage is likely.

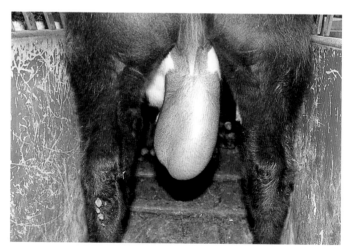

Plate 13.28. Most scrotal swellings are haematomas and can be left to resolve on their own.

and the animal may be off-colour. However, simple bruises and haematomas are more common. Although the swelling may look gross (Plate 13.28), most animals are unaffected by bruising and slowly recover or, as in Plate 13.28, may be sent for slaughter when fit. Necrosis of the scrotum may occur as a result of improper use of the Burdizzo bloodless castrator (page 438).

## Fracture of the Penis

Despite its name, the condition is not a true fracture but rather a rupture of the outer casing of the penis leading to a haematoma (blood blister) under the sheath. It occurs when a cow or heifer moves during service, or if the bull slips or is pushed off. A swelling beneath the skin is seen halfway between the scrotum and prepuce. Provided that the bull is rested for two to three months, many cases recover without treatment. Surgery can also be used.

## Corkscrew Penis (Spiral Deviation of the Penis)

In some bulls the penis deflects to one side or the other as it extrudes when they are attempting to serve, or goes so low that it is unable to enter the cow. This is usually associated with damage to the ligaments or the outer wall of the penis, for example as caused by warts (Plate 10.16). As some cases are inherited, they are best not treated.

# LEPTOSPIROSIS

Like IBR, leptospirosis can cause quite a wide range of clinical signs. These are:

- a mild and transient increase in temperature (pyrexia), which may well pass unnoticed, particularly in heifers
- mastitis and milk drop
- abortion
- reduced conception rates

It has been estimated that around one-third of all abortions in the UK are caused by leptospirosis (other causes are given in Chapter 8 and Appendix 2). The strain involved in cattle is *Leptospira interrogans var. hardjo.* By measuring antibody levels in the blood it has been shown that 60% of herds in the British Isles have been exposed to infection, although the actual clinical disease is much less commonly diagnosed. Cows are infected by urine splashing into their eyes, mouth or cuts in their skin.

The first stage of the disease is simply a raised temperature and a slight reduction in appetite, when the leptospires are multiplying in the liver. Such mild clinical signs may not be noticed in maiden heifers, many of which recover in one or two days without treatment. In higher-yielding dairy cows, however, the clinical signs can be much more pronounced and they are characterised by a sharp fall in milk production. The udder becomes flaccid, the milk is thick, almost like colostrum, and at first you may think that your cow has mastitis in all four quarters, but without any swelling, heat or hardness. This is why leptospirosis is sometimes referred to as 'milk drop' or 'flabby bag' syndrome.

The third clinical sign caused by leptospirosis is abortion. This usually occurs six to twelve weeks after the initial infection and temperature rise and is especially common if the cow is in the final third of pregnancy. It is quite possible that the earlier infection did not cause a significant milk drop and that abortion is the only clinical sign seen. There are two major problems in the diagnosis of leptospirosis from abortions:

- The organism does not live very long and it is difficult to grow in culture. The best method of diagnosis is to take a freshly aborted foetus (within 12 hours) straight to the laboratory to check its liver and kidneys for leptospires. Fluorescent antibody tests are also used.
- Antibody levels in the blood persist for only a short while. (Often called titres, antibody levels are a measure of the concentration of antibodies in the blood. See Chapter 1 for a full explanation.) Two weeks after the initial infection (and the 'milk drop', if seen), antibody titres will be high, for example 1:1600. However, they fall very rapidly, so that six to twelve weeks later (the time when abortion occurs), titres may be low (1:100) or (in approximately 30% of cows) no longer detectable.

If you think leptospirosis is a possibility in your herd, it is useful to blood sample 15–20 cows at random. Even then, I know of one case in which seven cows aborting over a short period all blood sampled negative for leptospirosis, a further 18 bloods at random were also negative and yet leptospirosis was eventually confirmed in a freshly aborted foetus! An alternative approach is to measure leptospira antibodies in bulk milk. This gives a useful estimate of the proportion of the herd infected.

The fourth clinical sign is reduced conception rates. Leptospirosis organisms can live in the reproductive tract for a considerable period of time, leading to both regular and irregular returns to service, the latter being due to early embryonic death. For example, in a survey of 529 animals in five infected herds, cows with blood titres of 1:100 or greater had a conception rate of 34%, whereas cows which were negative on blood test had a conception rate of almost 53%. Similarly, in another trial involving known infected herds, 200 cows which were vaccinated had a conception rate of 51%, whereas 215 unvaccinated cows only achieved 34%.

*Treatment and control*

If left untreated, affected cows will slowly recover on their own, although they will probably never regain their full milk potential for the present lactation. Antibiotics and vaccination can be used.

**Antibiotics** The use of antibiotics, especially streptomycin, will speed recovery. Following infection, some cows rid themselves of *Leptospira* and develop an immunity. However this lasts only one to two years, after which they are susceptible to further attacks. Other cows remain carriers with a focus of *Leptospira* infection in their kidneys which periodically bursts out and leads to intermittent excretion in the urine, and some of these animals will not even show a reaction (antibody titre) in their blood. This combination of carrier cows and waning immunity leads to repeated outbreaks of disease, even in a closed herd.

**Vaccination** There is a good killed vaccine available for cows and heifers. Two doses are given, four weeks apart, and a booster is needed each year. Most outbreaks of disease seem to occur during the grazing period, especially during a wet spell. This is because *L. hardjo* can survive for longer on pasture during warm, damp weather. The best time to vaccinate is therefore just before turnout in the spring, to prevent such outbreaks. Some people recommend only vaccinating heifers prior to their entry into the main herd and they rely on the normal spread of infection within the herd to provide immunity. Although this is clearly much cheaper, an on-farm vaccination trial suggested that it may not be correct. Four hundred and sixty-four heifers were monitored serologically (via the blood) for leptospirosis after they were introduced into 14 known infected herds. Half the heifers entering each herd were vaccinated and half were not. Vaccination reduced the incidence of abortion from 5% to 0.85%. The results are shown in Table 13.3. Overall the vaccinated cattle also produced 50 litres more milk per lactation than the non-vaccinates, although where there was clear serological evidence of infection, vaccinated heifers showed an advantage of 785 litres. This is despite the fact that no obvious cases of milk drop had been seen in either group. It is well known that cases of 'milk drop' are only sporadic and as such can easily pass unrecognised by the herdsman.

Unfortunately cows can still remain carriers of leptospirosis even after vaccination, so only if calves are vaccinated at six months old and then annually thereafter can you be fairly sure of avoiding the carrier status. In some countries the disease is considered to be so important that cows receive a booster vaccination every six months.

| | Number of pregnant heifers | Incidence of abortions Number | % |
|---|---|---|---|
| Vaccinated | 238 | 2 | 0.85 |
| Unvaccinated | 226 | 11 | 5.00 |

From ADAS.

Table 13.3. Heifers were introduced into 14 known infected herds, half entering each farm being vaccinated against leptospirosis and half left unvaccinated. The reduction in abortions during the first lactation was dramatic in vaccinated heifers, and vaccinated heifers also produced more milk.

*Prevention*
Preventing the entry of leptospirosis into an otherwise clean herd can be best discussed by examining the risk factors, that is those factors which have been associated with an increased incidence of disease. These are:

- purchased cattle (including bulls). This doubles the risk of a closed herd
- the use of natural service rather than AI, especially if the bull is hired or shared. This increases the risk four times
- grazing sheep with cattle. Because sheep carry leptospirosis, this increases the risk six times, *unless* the sheep are moved at least two months before the cattle graze. By then the majority of the leptospires will be dead
- access to water courses and streams (eight times risk), because *Leptospira* organisms excreted from one farm can be carried downstream to the next. Leptospires have been shown to survive for up to four months in fresh water and six months in urine-saturated soil. (Note that these are maximum persistence times.)

If purchased cattle or hire bulls are to enter a clean herd, they should ideally be injected on arrival with both antibiotic and vaccine and again three to four weeks later.

Some outbreaks of disease can be dramatic, for example causing up to 30% reduction in total milk sales. However, it is more common for infection to pass through the herd fairly slowly and in such cases leptospirosis is more difficult to recognise and diagnose. Herds with a chronically high abortion rate, for example 6–8% per year, should consider vaccination, and programmes are available for eradication following vaccination.

*Leptospirosis in man*
Although cattle are the main hosts of *L. hardjo*, other animals can become infected, including man. Anyone working in a milking parlour is especially at risk, because it is so easy to get splashed with urine from an infected cow. The symptoms in man include headaches, fever and aching joints, very similar to a severe attack of influenza, and occasional cases of meningitis. Cattle vaccination hence reduces the human health risk. *L. hardjo* is different from *L. icterohaemorrhagiae*. The latter is the classic Weil's disease, which causes liver failure and jaundice. It is spread from rats to man and is quite rare.

# MISCELLANEOUS CONDITIONS

## Listeriosis

This is an infection caused by the bacterium *Listeria monocytogenes*. In cattle it is mainly seen as a nervous disease, although it may also cause abortion or even sudden death. In the typical case you will see one side of the animal's face droop, due to paralysis of the facial muscles, and this leads to drooling (Plate 13.29). The ear and eyelids are also paralysed, leading to a dry eye surface and a glazed expression, with total blindness on the affected side only. Eating is difficult, appetite is

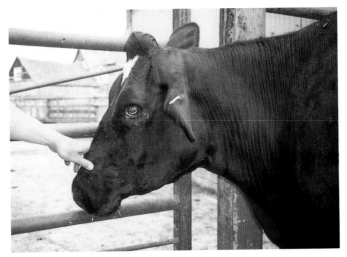

Plate 13.29. Listeriosis is a brain infection leading to paralysis of the muscles of the face (e.g. lips, eyelids and ears) on one side only.

depressed and weight loss occurs. There may also be nervous signs: initially walking around in circles, perhaps pushing the head against a wall, then in the terminal stages convulsions and eventually death. Listeriosis is the most common diagnosis in cows which are suspected of having BSE, but on slaughter are found to be negative. Provided that listeriosis is diagnosed early enough, very high levels of penicillin injection (probably twice daily), continued for seven to ten days, can produce a cure in a reasonable number of animals.

Do not confuse listeriosis with middle ear disease (Plate 13.30). Because of the pain, an animal with middle ear infection stands with its head on one side and may walk around in circles, but it is not blind and is much brighter and more alert, usually continuing to feed. Most middle ear infections respond well to antibiotics.

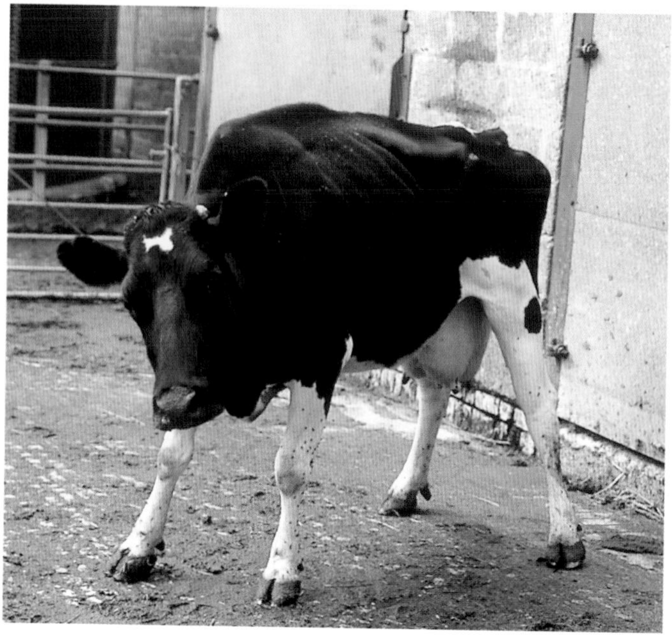

Plate 13.30. Although an animal with middle ear infection walks around in circles, similar to listeriosis, it will normally be more bright and alert and will not develop facial paralysis.

*Listeria* is an interesting organism. It can survive for many years in dung or soil, it is a common contaminant of silage and yet disease is relatively rare. Most cases occur in silage-fed cattle in late winter, and the stress of poor housing, unhygienic management and dietary changes increase the risk of disease. It has also been implicated as a possible cause of 'silage eye' or bovine iritis (Chapter 4). The organism is frequently found in man, and can occasionally cause food poisoning. High levels of human infection from sewage sludge can be a danger to animals.

## Blindness

Blindness may be present at birth, when we say that the calf has a congenital defect (Plate 1.13), or it may occur later in life, possibly as a result of an improperly treated New Forest eye (Plate 4.13). Some cows suddenly go blind, however, with no symptoms, and this can be due to a localised blood clot or an abscess in the brain. Sudden onset blindness may also be due to hyphaema (Plate 4.23).

In calves the most common defect is a lens opacity or cataract (Plate 1.12). If you look at an eye with a *cataract* you see that the circle filling the centre of the pupil is blue-grey in colour and light cannot enter. This is thought to be caused by toxins or infections (e.g. BVD virus) acting on the cow in early pregnancy, at the stage when the eyes are being formed. Cataracts can be treated by making cuts on the surface of the lens with a very small 'needling' knife. The fluid of the eyeball (the aqueous humour) then dissolves away the lens. Sight is slowly restored over one to two months, but for distant vision only. Some cataracts are of genetic origin, and occasionally groups of calves are affected but no cause is found.

Blindness can also be a symptom of some other condition, for example lead poisoning, meningitis, CCN or vitamin A deficiency (a full list is given in Appendix 2). Some calves are born without eyes (anophthalmia) or with very small, non-functional eyes (microphthalmia).

## Aujeszky's Disease

This is a virus infection which occurs mainly in pigs, where it causes nervous disease, pneumonia and reproductive failure. Cases in cattle are rare, but when they do occur there is excitement, drooling and intense itching. There is no treatment. Aujeszky's disease is also called pseudorabies, because the symptoms are indistinguishable from a true rabies infection of cattle. It is a notifiable disease in the UK.

## The PPH Syndrome

This is a disease of cattle which can cause intense itching. The letters PPH stand for pruritus (itching), pyrexia (raised temperature), and haemorrhage (bleeding from various sites in the body). It is a rare condition, seen only in dairy cows. The early signs are intense irritation of raised patches of skin on the head, neck, tail and udder, and in mild cases this is all you will see. In more severe cases, however, the cow runs a high temperature, goes off her food, may develop haemorrhagic areas inside the nose and mouth, and sometimes passes fresh blood with the dung. These cases do not recover and the animal is best slaughtered.

The cause of PPH is unclear, although the fungal toxin citronin, which leads to kidney damage, has been implicated. Citronin, which is produced by *Penicillium* and *Aspergillus* moulds, has been found in a range of foods including citrus pulp, and mouldy citrus pulp, containing 30 ppm of citronin, was suggested as the cause of one outbreak. The original theory, namely that PPH was associated with feeding silage having a sulphuric acid additive, has now been largely discounted.

## Bovine Immunodeficiency Virus (BIV)

BIV belongs to a family known as lentiviruses. Lentiviruses cause definite disease syndromes in many animals, for example equine infectious anaemia, maedi-visna in sheep, feline immunodeficiency virus (FIV) and the well-known human immunodeficiency virus (HIV), the cause of AIDS. Monitoring of antibody levels in blood samples has shown that the bovine form of the virus, BIV, is *present* in many countries in the world, but the evidence on whether it causes disease is much less conclusive. Those who believe that BIV causes *disease* say that it produces general ill-thrift, for example seen as cows which develop a high temperature and lose weight after calving, and calves which fail to grow. Skin lesions have also been reported. Numerous other secondary infections can be found (as happens with AIDS in man) but the underlying problem could be BIV, leading to an increased susceptibility to infection.

BIV is considered a definite disease entity by some in North America, with one of the classic features being enlargement of the lymph glands under the skin, identical to the skin TB lesions shown in Plate 10.18. However, skin TB is so widespread in the UK that if it is caused by BIV, then BIV is also widespread – and probably does not cause disease. The only herd in the UK suspected of having disease caused by BIV was in Cheshire in 1993/94 and even this was disputed by some investigators.

## Lightning Stroke and Electrocution

Death from electrocution and lightning is more common in cattle than in any other species, partly because of an inherent susceptibility, partly because their four feet placed firmly on the ground make a good earth and partly because they are often in milking parlours and other housing where free electricity can occur.

*Lightning stroke*
It is unlikely that you will see anything except a dead animal, or possibly a group of cattle lying together, although sometimes there are also one or two staggering around with concussion. Perhaps you will be able to see other evidence to substantiate your diagnosis, such as scorch marks on adjacent trees, broken branches, marks along the ground or burns on the animal itself, as in Plate 13.31. This is not necessarily the case, however. If lightning strikes damp ground, or if an overloaded power cable falls into a pool of

water, there may be sufficient ground current to be fatal and there are then no marks to be seen on the carcase.

*Electrocution*

Waterpumps, vacuum pumps and milking machines are the most common sources of free electricity and so milking cows are commonly affected. I have seen a case where four cows dropped dead during milking and, after they were released, others staggered around aimlessly, suffering from electrical concussion. They recovered eventually. In this instance there was a fault in the water heater, and the element had an earth which passed through the milking equipment. On another occasion the farmer thought that his cows had a low-grade grass staggers because they were

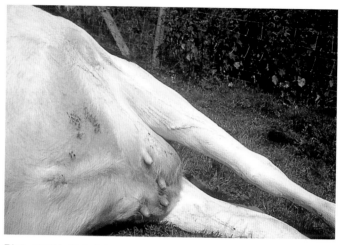

Plate 13.31. This late pregnant heifer was standing in a field, well away from trees or electricity, when she was struck by lightning. The scorch marks running down her legs confirm the diagnosis.

unusually nervous and jumpy in the parlour. The problem was eventually traced to a fault on the lift pump which gave the cows a shock as it switched on. The farmer felt nothing himself because he was wearing rubber boots.

Beef cattle can also be affected, and electrocution of animals inside a metal-framed building where the stanchions are standing in a damp area is not uncommon. I can remember seeing five from a group of ten finished beef cattle found dead from electrocution between two metal stanchions. The cause was traced to a short from a three-phase electric cable onto a metal pole some 20 metres away. The cattle had been killed by ground current: the electric cable blew against the metal pole and sent pulses of electricity along the ground to the cattle in the building.

If you wish to pursue an insurance claim for lightening or electrocution, it is most important that you do not move the cattle until your vet has arrived. He will want to see them in situ, looking for scorch marks and other electrical damage. He will also want to clear them for anthrax before carrying out a post-mortem examination to eliminate other causes of death.

## Bovine Influenza A

Many dairy herds have cows which experience a sudden drop in milk yield, an increase in temperature and show some respiratory signs such as drooling, increased respiratory rate, and coughing. In some cases there may also be a low-grade diarrhoea. Although there is a wide variety of causes, an influenza virus is known to be one possible factor. Being a virus infection there is no specific treatment, although if the cow is very sick, antibiotic cover will prevent secondary bacterial infection, and use of anti-inflammatory drugs such as flunixin will help to bring the temperature down and should hasten recovery. Diagnosis is based on blood sampling.

*Chapter 14*

# ROUTINE TASKS AND DEALING WITH POISONS

For many years there has been a marked decline in the number of dairy units in Britain. From 1960 to 1996 the number of holdings decreased from 151,000 holdings to 35,480 and the trend continues. Over the same period there was a much smaller reduction in the total number of cows, from 3.16 to 2.58 million. Yield per cow, on the other hand, rose from 3320 to 5500 litres. The effect of this was that the size of the average dairy herd increased from 21 to 73 cows, with many individual herds of over 200 cows. In turn this led to the need for a more specialised stockman. Many of the routine tasks and basic treatments which were once considered to be the province of the veterinary surgeon are now being carried out by stockmen and women, and it is likely that this trend will continue. The vet will do less routine work and instead will spend more time on preventive medicine programmes, training, monitoring performance and organising fertility control schemes.

Much of this book has been written with these changes in mind, that is to try to give the stockman a better understanding of the principles involved in disease control. It is more difficult to give a written description of practical techniques, however, and I would urge the reader to contact his local agricultural training group, for example ATB Landbase in the UK. They organise some excellent courses, where trainees are given the theory of the task as well as undertaking supervised practical training.

In the following I have tried to give guidelines and practical advice on some of the more basic procedures which the stockman may have to perform.

## Responsible Use, Storage and Disposal of Medicines

With increasing consumer concern about animal drug residues reaching the human food chain, it is extremely important that farm medicines are used and seen to be used responsibly. Legislation will vary in different countries and the reader must consult local regulations. For the UK the following are important areas of consideration.

Important aspects of the use of medicines:

● safe storage
● responsible use
● records of all treatments
● safe disposal of needles, bottles and unused medicines

**Safe storage** A special cupboard or room separate from the dairy is needed for medicine storage, and with increasing concern over drug abuse in man, needles and syringes should be equally as carefully controlled. Keep all medicines away from direct sunlight. Store all vaccines in a refrigerator. Read the labels on other drugs: some advise cool storage, others do not. A domestic fridge with a chain around it and running through the handle can be very conveniently locked with a padlock.

**Responsible use** Medicines should only be used when they are indicated. For example, in a lame cow which shows no swelling of the foot it is pointless injecting her with antibiotic without first lifting and examining the foot: there may be a nail penetrating the sole. Similarly, if a cow is slightly off-colour, but has no increase in temperature, you would need more than a diagnosis of 'off-food' to justify the use of antibiotics. (Of course the situation would be very difficult if, for example, you know you have leptospirosis circulating in the herd.)

SCHEDULE 2     Regulation 20(1)

VETERINARY MEDICINE ADMINISTRATION RECORD

THE ANIMALS, MEAT AND MEAT PRODUCTS (EXAMINATION FOR RESIDUES AND MAXIMUM RESIDUE LIMITS) REGULATIONS 1991

Name and full address of person keeping the record .................

| Date of purchase of veterinary medicine | Name of veterinary medicine and quantity purchased | Supplier of veterinary medicine | Identity of animal/group treated | Number treated | Date treatment finished | Date when withdrawal period ended | Total quantity of veterinary medicine used | Name of the person who administered veterinary medicine |
|---|---|---|---|---|---|---|---|---|
| | | | | | | | | |

Figure 14.1. Form for recording purchase and administration of animal medicines, a UK legal requirement from The Animals, Meat and Meat Products Regulations 1991. The legislation has now been simplified and so the reader should consult the specific requirements of the purchaser of his product or Farm Assurance Scheme.

You will get optimum value from medicines if they are used properly. Discard contaminated and out of date medicine bottles and use clean equipment for administration. It is important that your syringes and needles are rinsed through with clean water after use and that they are then boiled or soaked in alcohol to sterilise them. They should be stored, ready for use, in a clean, dry container with a lid. If a new needle and syringe are used for each course of injections, it is probably very little extra expense compared to the cost of the drug or the value of the animal being treated.

**Records of all treatments** It is a legal requirement in the UK to record all purchases and use of medicines (The Animals, Meat and Meat Products Regulations 1991). Many medicines will be purchased from the vet, although wormers, fly treatments, vitamins etc. may be purchased from a local merchant. All administrations must be recorded, whether they be oral, by injection, intramammary tubes or even intra-uterine pessaries, and the date, animal identity, amount used and withdrawal period, together with the name of the person administering the medicine, must also be given. The original form of the record required is shown in Figure 14.1.

**Safe disposal** Used needles are best disposed of in specially designed 'Sharps' containers, which can be taken away and incinerated when they are full. Do not put them in with normal household rubbish, as they can cause injury to refuse collection personnel. Empty and out of date medicine bottles can be conveniently dropped into a 25 litre plastic drum (most injection bottles fall through the neck quite easily) and the whole drum can be either incinerated or deeply buried when full.

## Giving an Injection

Injections can be given in four ways:

- intradermal (into the skin)
- subcutaneous (under the skin)
- intramuscular (into the muscle)
- intravenous (directly into the bloodstream)

Intradermal injections are used in the tuberculosis test (see Plate 11.9). The intravenous route gives the most prompt effect and it may have to be used for certain drugs which will cause irritation if given subcutaneously or intramuscularly. There are dangers in giving intravenous injections too fast, and some preparations, e.g. magnesium, are not suitable for intravenous use.

You should *always* read the instructions and consult your vet before administering any drug, and before giving the injection, make sure that the animal has been firmly restrained.

When giving an injection, you are administering chemicals directly into the body, and in so doing, many of the animal's normal defence mechanisms are being by-passed. If bacteria are introduced there is a risk of serious side-effects, so cleanliness and hygiene are essential.

Whatever the route of injection, make sure that the site chosen is clean. Ideally you should use a swab soaked in methylated spirits, but this is not usually done, and provided that the skin is not covered with mud or dung and that your needle is clean, the risk of abscess formation in cattle is low.

If you are repeatedly taking doses from the same pack *without* an automatic syringe, you *must* make sure that you leave one needle in the bottle to transfer the drug into the syringe and use a second needle to carry out the injections. For vaccines especially, if you use the same needle to inject the animal and then to draw the next dose from the bottle, there is a serious risk that you will introduce infection into the bottle. This not only risks abscesses in subsequent cattle, but can also inactivate the vaccine.

*To fill the syringe*
First shake the bottle to make sure that the contents are thoroughly mixed. Many antibiotics are in a suspension rather than fully dissolved and if you simply inject the liquid taken from the top of the sedimented drug you will be seriously underdosing. With the syringe plunger depressed and the bottle

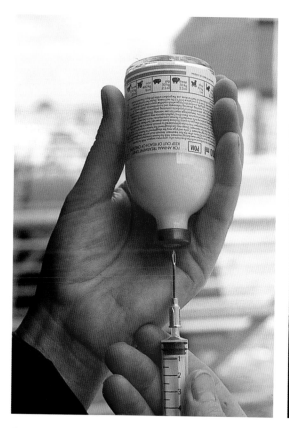

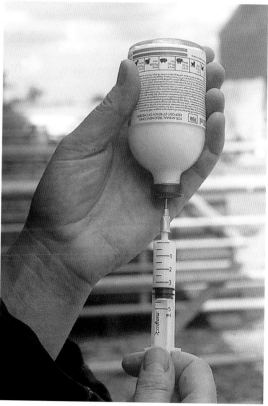

Plate 14.1. Filling a syringe: shake the bottle well, clean the rubber top, turn the bottle upside down and insert the needle.

Plate 14.2. Withdraw the correct dose. By keeping the syringe at eye-level, the dose is measured more accurately.

held upside down, insert the needle through the rubber bung (Plate 14.1). Then, holding the syringe at eye level, slowly pull the plunger back until you have the correct dose (Plate 14.2). If this creates an excessive vacuum in the bottle, simply disconnect the syringe from the needle (Plate 14.3). This allows air to enter and the filling process can then be continued. I do not like the more traditional method of first pumping in a volume of air equal to the volume of injection to be withdrawn. There is a greater risk of contaminating the drug, and it will put some bottles under so much pressure that the drug will be forced out through the rubber bung beside the needle.

*Subcutaneous injections*

I prefer to use the loose skin behind the shoulder. Catch hold of a fold between your finger and thumb, then push the needle forwards towards the shoulder (Plate 14.4). The cow's skin is very tough (after all, it is leather!) and you will be surprised how much force is needed, even with a sharp needle. If you are dosing large numbers of animals, for example blackleg vaccination or worming, then change the needle for a clean and sharper one every 15 to 20 animals, or immediately if you think it is dirty. The use of automatic syringes is discussed later in this section, and the special requirements needed with calcium injections in Chapter 6.

*Intramuscular injections*

In adult cattle I use the area of muscle covering the pelvis on either side of the tail. Firmly grasp the needle between your forefinger and thumb, and then stab it downwards with as much force as you can.

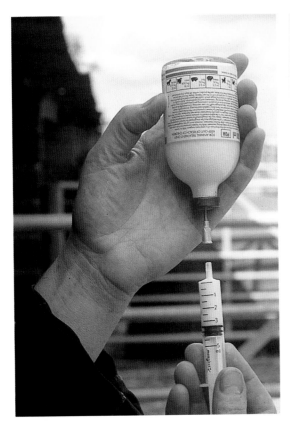

Plate 14.3. If a high vacuum in the bottle prevents further drug withdrawal, uncouple the syringe and allow air to enter.

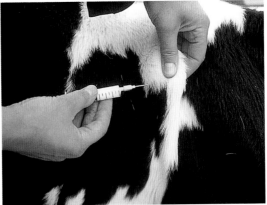

Plate 14.4. Subcutaneous injections are given by lifting a fold of skin behind the shoulder.

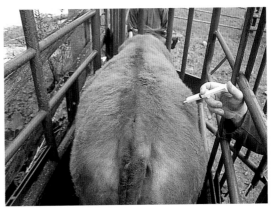

Plate 14.5. Intramuscular injections can be given into the pelvic gluteal muscles in adults.

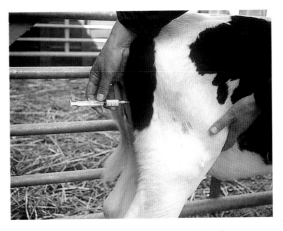

Plate 14.6. In calves, intramuscular injections are often given into the hind leg.

Connect the syringe and inject. A 25 mm needle should go in up to its butt, and in a fat cow a 40 mm needle will be needed. It is best to make the injection fairly well forward, towards the wing of the pelvis. It is often cleaner in this area, there is a good depth of muscle and the chances of injecting through into the pelvic cavity are minimised. Plate 5.7 shows that ligaments connect the sacral spine to the pelvis over the central pelvic area, and going too deep (e.g. using a very long needle on a thin cow) can result in the injection going through the ligament and even penetrating the rectum! If the injection is made further forwards, then an excessively long needle will impact on the pelvic bone – not ideal, but at least you would know and could start again!

In younger animals I use the fleshy part of the hind leg (Plate 14.6) and often hold the syringe in the palm of my hand, with the needle attached

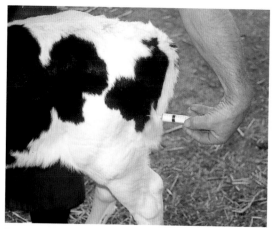

Plate 14.7. Holding the syringe like this permits rapid injection.

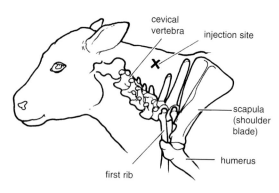

Figure 14.2. The neck is a useful intramuscular injection site, avoiding the more expensive cuts of the carcase.

(Plate 14.7). When the needle reaches its full depth in the muscle, the force from the palm of your hand propels the plunger forwards and the injection is given very quickly.

Although these are the 'traditional' sites for injection, they are also the most expensive cuts of the carcase and often the areas where the skin is most soiled with faeces. Even if infection is not introduced, an injection of a foreign substance can leave a scar in the muscle, especially if certain long-acting antibiotics, which tend to be irritants, are used. Because of this there has been a trend towards giving intramuscular injections into the neck muscle, as shown in Figure 14.2. The diagram shows that the spine, after leaving the base of the skull, dips down quite deeply towards the chest at the point where it is covered by the shoulder blade. This means that there is plenty of muscle, with no dangerous structure beneath, in the upper part of the neck. The ideal site for injection is at least one full hand-span back from the lower base of the ear, as shown in Figure 14.2.

*Intravenous injections*

These should always be given slowly and with great care. The jugular vein is found in a furrow which lies between the trachea and the muscle of the neck, shown as a white chalk mark in Plate 14.8. In this vein, blood is flowing from the head back to the heart, so if you obstruct the vein using finger pressure or a rope around the neck, you will see it swell up. I find it best to stab the needle into the centre of the vein first, slightly adjusting its position until blood flows. Then incline the butt of

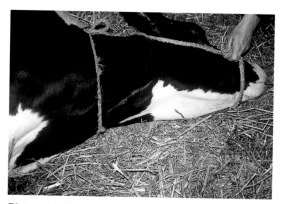

Plate 14.8. The chalk mark shows the position of the jugular vein.

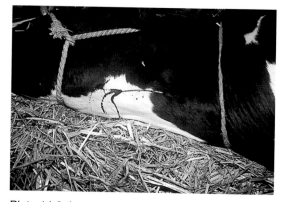

Plate 14.9. Intravenous injection. It is best to have the needle inserted to its full depth and with the tip pointing down the vein towards the heart.

the needle towards the cow's head and push the point *down* the vein until the butt is against the skin. This is shown in Plate 14.9. Once in this position the needle is far less likely to come out of the vein while the injection is being given.

*Collapsible packs and flutter valves*

Many large-volume injections are now prepared in plastic packs which collapse as the liquid runs out of them (Plate 14.10). These tend to be more expensive than the older-style bottles, but as there is no need to sterilise the 'giving set' each time, I think that the extra cost is well justified for on-farm use. Sometimes you have to use bottles, however, and the flutter valve is a device to allow air to enter the bottle as the injection liquid runs out.

It is used as follows. First attach the head of the flutter valve to the neck of the bottle, then turn the bottle upside down and check that air is entering through the air-bleed and that liquid is flowing through the tubing. Next insert the needle into the cow; then, making sure that there is no air left in the tubing by running through a drop more fluid, connect the tubing to the needle. Adjust the height of the bottle so that liquid runs in at the correct speed (Plate 14.11). You can check this by the rate at which bubbles are entering the bottle.

*Automatic syringes*

Many procedures, for example worming and vaccinating, are most easily carried out using automatic syringes. They have three great advantages: they are easy to use, the rubber seal on the top of the injection bottle is only punctured once and there is less risk of contaminating the drug. However, using the same needle repeatedly for a large number of animals can lead to the transmission of infection on a

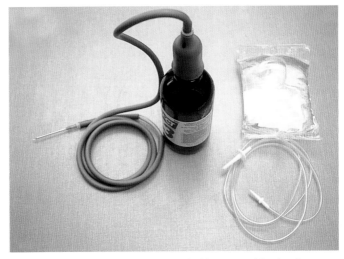

Plate 14.10. Rubber flutter valves (left) are used for bottles. Plastic dispensing packs (right) may be more convenient for on-farm use.

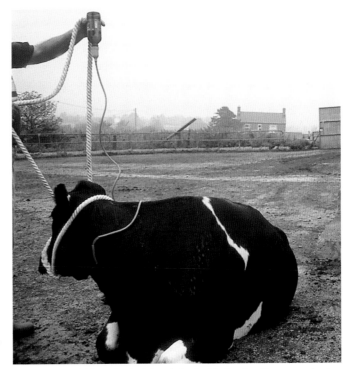

Plate 14.11. Adjust the height of the bottle to give the correct rate of flow – assessed by the rate of entry of air through the valve.

dirty needle. To overcome this, one manufacturer has produced a self-sterilising system, shown in Figure 14.3. The sterilising foam cap is held in a spring-loaded barrel, through which the needle must pass each time an injection is made. One cap will remain effective for three days or 100 injections and is relatively

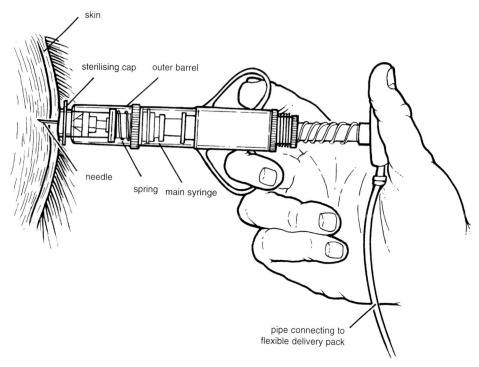

skin

sterilising cap     outer barrel

needle

spring    main syringe

pipe connecting to
flexible delivery pack

Figure 14.3. Mechanism of action of a self-sterilising multidose syringe. (Sterimatic Ltd)

cheap. This system certainly reduced the incidence of injection abscesses in sheep and it has the added advantage of protecting the needle when not in use, thus reducing considerably the risk of accidental self-injection. I find this particularly helpful. Self-sterilising attachments can be fitted to almost all existing multidose syringes, and the sterilising caps can also be fitted onto the top of glass bottles of injection.

## Giving a Drench

Drenches are best administered using a special dosing gun because the nozzle can deliver the liquid so far back over the tongue that it is virtually impossible for the animal to spit it out. Plate 14.12 shows the heifer's head being held well up, with the delivery pipe of the gun passing across the space between the incisor and molar teeth (Figure 13.1) and over onto the top of her tongue.

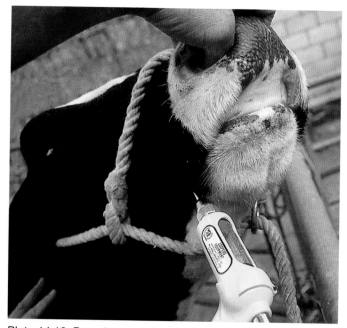

Plate 14.12. Drenches should be deposited on the back of the tongue so that they cannot be spat out.

## Disbudding Calves

A cow's horn consists of two parts, the outer casing of hoof-like material and a bone in the centre. In the calf the skin around the base of the horn becomes impregnated with an extremely hard material called keratin and this grows up over the horn to form the outer casing. An extension of the skull bone then occupies the space in the centre, as shown in Plate 9.5. The object of dehorning is to destroy the area of horn-forming skin. Unless chemical cauterisation is applied during the first week of life – and I would not recommend that method – the UK Protection of Animals Act 1911 states that calves must be given an anaesthetic before being dehorned or disbudded. The procedure is best carried out at around three to six weeks old, at an age when the horn bud can be clearly felt but before it gets so large that it cannot easily fit into the end of the disbudding iron.

The nerve to the horn runs out from behind the eye and underneath a small overhanging ledge of bone which is part of the skull. This is best seen in Figure 13.1. Using a short needle (25 mm or less), inject 3 ml of anaesthetic under this ridge on each side (Plate 14.13). You may find that blood flows from the injection site after you have withdrawn the needle. This is no cause for alarm. A vein and an artery run along beside the nerve and these can easily be punctured. It is sometimes recommended that you should slightly withdraw the plunger of the syringe before injecting the anaesthetic. If blood then appears in the syringe, you know you are in a blood vessel, and the position of the needle needs altering slightly, because intravenous injection of local anaesthetic can cause collapse.

Leave the calf for at least five to six minutes while the anaesthetic takes effect. Its action is almost immediate if you happen to have deposited it directly onto the nerve; however if you have just missed, some time must elapse before the drug can diffuse to its target. The speed of onset of anaesthesia also varies with the anaesthetic being used.

Clip the hair around the area; then, with the calf's head held firmly, place the hot iron over the horn so that the bud fits into the depression at the tip of the iron (Plate 14.14). Apply moderate pressure while you hold the iron in this position, count to ten and then angle the iron to scoop out the horn bud (Plate 14.15). Provided that the skin around the outside of the horn has been destroyed, it is not strictly necessary to remove the bud itself.

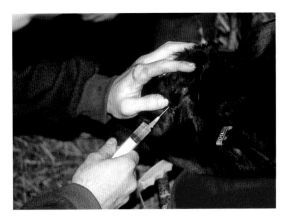

Plate 14.13. Dehorning. The correct anaesthetic site is under the ledge of bone halfway between the eye and the horn.

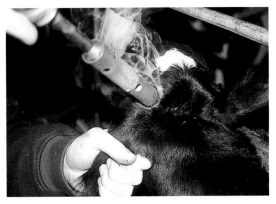

Plate 14.14. Dehorning. Make sure that the area of skin around the outside of the horn bud has been destroyed.

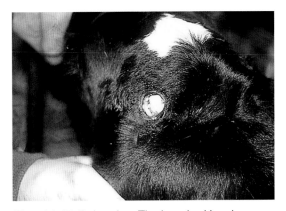

Plate 14.15. Dehorning. The horn bud has been enucleated.

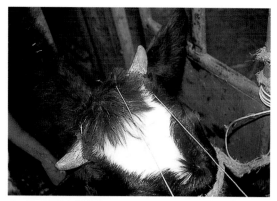

Plate 14.16. Dehorning larger cattle, using a cutting wire: make sure that the cut is deep enough.

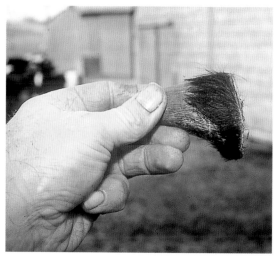

If the bud is too large to fit into the iron, first cut it off with scissors or even hoof clippers, and then proceed as before. When using hoof clippers or if

Plate 14.17. Removing the horn with a ring of hair around its base prevents regrowth.

removing larger horns, for example with a cutting wire (Plate 14.16), make sure the cut is deep enough to remove the horn with a small ring of hair around its base (Plate 14.17). This is the horn-forming tissue and there is then no risk of regrowth. Finally apply an antibiotic aerosol to dry the wound and promote healing.

## Removing Supernumerary Teats

As part of routine stockmanship you should always check for extra teats when disbudding calves which are to be retained for breeding. If left, spare teats may develop mastitis, or, even worse, when they are too close to a true teat they interfere with milking. By law in the UK you must use an anaesthetic in calves

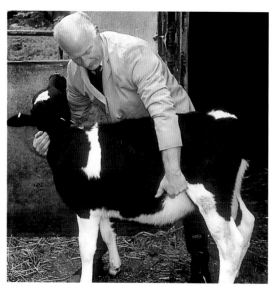

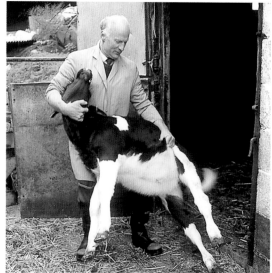

Plate 14.18. Turning a calf. Hold the calf by the flank and under the neck, lift and roll it across your knee (14.19), then use your legs to support it in a sitting position (14.20 [see facing page]).

over two months old, and if the calf is over three months old the operation may only be performed by a veterinary surgeon.

For calves between two and three months old, simply inject 2 ml of local anaesthetic into the base of the teat and disperse it by rubbing between your fingers.

In small calves it is best to hold the calf in a sitting position. To achieve this, put one arm around its neck, hold the base of its flank with your other hand (Plate 14.18) and put your knee into its opposite flank. Lift the calf slightly into the air, using a two hand hold, and roll it across your knee, with the knee as a pivot (Plate 14.19). With the calf sitting on its tail you can now hold it in position between your knees, leaving both hands free to examine the teats (Plate 14.20). There is also little risk of getting kicked in this position.

If an extra teat is found, put your finger underneath the skin to push the teat into a firm and accessible position (Plate 14.21); then amputate it flush with the skin using a pair of sharp curved scissors. The curved blades allow you to get closer and make a much neater finish. Finally, apply a topical antibiotic spray.

## Castration

There are three methods of castrating calves, namely rubber rings, the Burdizzo bloodless castrator and surgical removal of the testicles. Surgical removal is by far the most certain method, and provided that an anaesthetic is used, calves may be left entire until they are four to six months old or more to obtain improved growth rates and better conformation of the final carcase.

Since 1983 it has been a legal requirement in the UK that calves over two months old may only be castrated by a veterinary surgeon. I would suggest that stockmen never attempt surgical castration therefore, because at less than two months old the testicles are so small that the technique is quite difficult.

*Use of rubber rings*
These are only permitted in calves less than one

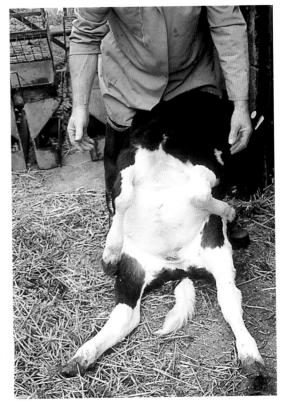

Plate 14.20. Examining the teats of a young calf.

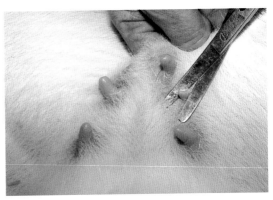

Plate 14.21. Supernumerary teats are best amputated at disbudding, when the calf is only a few weeks old.

week old. Hold the calf in a sitting position, make sure that both testicles are in the scrotum, then apply the ring to the base of the scrotum, as shown in Plate 14.22. Remove the applicator and check for a second time that both testicles are still in the scrotum.

Every year we are asked to examine groups of yearling heifers for pregnancy, because they have been running with a male which someone castrated without checking that both testicles were below the ring. If, at the time of castration, you still cannot find the second testicle, my advice would be to mark the calf

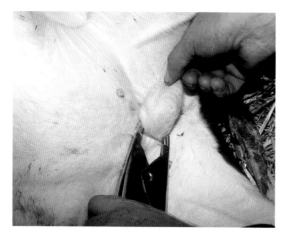

Plate 14.22. When applying an elastrator ring, make sure both testicles are in the scrotum.

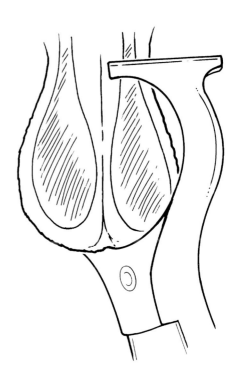

and get your vet to examine it at three to four months old or more. Do not apply a ring; otherwise you will overlook the possibility of a second testicle descending at a later date – possibly to the detriment of next year's heifers!

*Bloodless castration*
Burdizzo castration is based on the principle that crushing destroys the spermatic cord (which carries blood to the testicles) but that the skin of the scrotum remains intact. Approach the standing calf from behind and push one of the cords to the outside of the scrotum. Next apply the jaws of the Burdizzo, checking that the cord is held in one place by the cord-stops (Figure 14.4, position 1), and firmly close the handles. Count to five seconds. The procedure is best repeated just below the first crush (position 2) and then twice on the other cord (positions 3 and 4). You must make sure that the crush marks on each side do not join up to form a continuous line across the scrotum; otherwise there is a risk of the scrotum itself being destroyed. The second crush on each side should always be beneath the first, as shown in Figure 14.4.

## Taking a Temperature

A thermometer is a surprisingly difficult instrument to read and you ought to first practise holding it between your finger and thumb (Figure 14.5) and gently rolling it until you are quite sure that you can see the thick line of mercury. Before inserting the thermometer, hold it at the end away from the

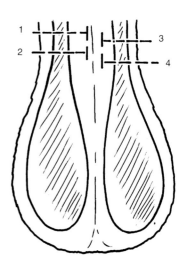

Figure 14.4. The sequence of Burdizzo castration crushing positions. Note that the first crush is always above the second, and that the crushes on each side must not be immediately opposite each other. The dotted line shows how the cord stop on the edge of one of the jaws makes sure that the cord cannot slip away.

mercury bulb and give it a few firm shakes. Now check that the mercury has returned towards the reservoir and that the thermometer registers 37°C or less. Apply some lubricant to the thermometer – I find saliva very effective and readily available! – hold the cow's tail up with one hand and insert the thermometer into its rectum with the other. You may find that the thermometer needs to be rolled to get it to pass through the anal sphincter. At least two-thirds of its total length should be inserted. Once it is in position, deflect the thermometer to one side (Figure 14.6) so that the mercury bulb is as close to the wall of the rectum as possible. If the thermometer is left in the centre of a lump of faeces, the temperature registered may be considerably lower than the cow's actual body temperature. This is particularly important when the cow is constipated, for example with milk fever.

Withdraw the thermometer after 30 seconds, gently wipe it clean, then take the reading by slowly rolling it between your finger and thumb until the thick line of mercury comes into view. If you are in any doubt, shake it back down and repeat the procedure.

A cow with a high temperature most probably has an infection, but this could be a viral, protozoal or bacterial infection and only the bacteria would respond to antibiotics. Temperature may also rise with excitement, for example in a cow

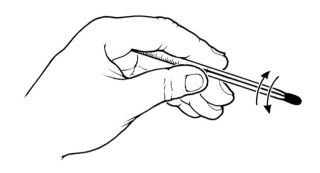

Figure 14.5. Roll the thermometer between finger and thumb until the thick line of mercury can be recognised.

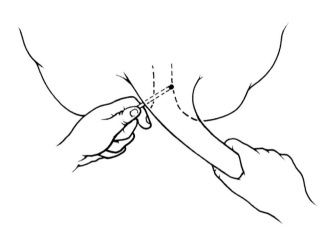

Figure 14.6. Taking a temperature: deflect the thermometer to one side so that the bulb is as close to the wall of the rectum as possible.

which has been in convulsions due to hypomagnesaemia. Unfortunately the reverse is not true, that is we cannot say that a cow with an infection will always have a raised temperature, or that a cow without a temperature definitely does not have an infection. The infection may be localised, for example an abscess or a mild mastitis, and although the infected area may feel hot to the touch, there may be no general rise in the whole body temperature. Another possibility is that the cow may initially have had a high temperature (for example in the early stages of *E. coli* mastitis) but as the condition progressed, toxaemia and shock set in and body temperature fell, often to below normal. A temperature below normal (that is less than 38.6°C) could be a bad sign – although it may simply mean that you did not have the thermometer positioned correctly in the rectum!

Normal values for temperature, pulse and respiration, and some of the factors affecting these values, are given in Appendix 1.

## Dealing with Wounds

There are many different types of wounds and often they need careful treatment. If you are in any doubt you should call in your vet. He can then suture it if necessary, apply the first dressing and leave you instructions for aftercare. The following gives a broad outline on the approach to wounds in general.

**Is it bleeding badly?** A steady drip, drip of blood generally does no harm and usually will stop on its own. If you can see a continual pulsating squirt of blood, however, this indicates that an artery has been severed and you must take action. If the legs or tail are involved it is quite easy to apply a tourniquet by using a loop of rope and twisting it tight with a stick. If there is bleeding following surgical castration, a tourniquet applied tightly to the top of the scrotum is very effective. In other areas often all you can do is to push a wad of cotton wool or a tea-towel hard against the wound until your vet arrives. Sometimes applying pressure for four to five minutes is in itself enough to stop the bleeding. A tourniquet should be applied just tight enough to arrest the bleeding and only for an hour or two. If too tight or if left on too long, it can lead to gangrene of the whole area. Dealing with post calving vaginal haemorrhage is discussed in Chapter 5.

**Does it need stitching?** Large skin wounds and cuts on teats are best sutured, *provided* that there is sufficient loose skin available and that the wound is fairly fresh. However, suturing a cut over the knee, for example, is not worth while because any sutures are likely to pull out as soon as the animal starts walking. If the edges of the wounds are dry and healing has already started, suturing may not be successful. Also if the skin flap is very thin, feels lifeless and is 'devitalised', that is it has no feeling, suturing is probably not worth while, and on teats it is best to simply amputate the flap with scissors to prevent further skin tearing during milking (see Plate 7.37).

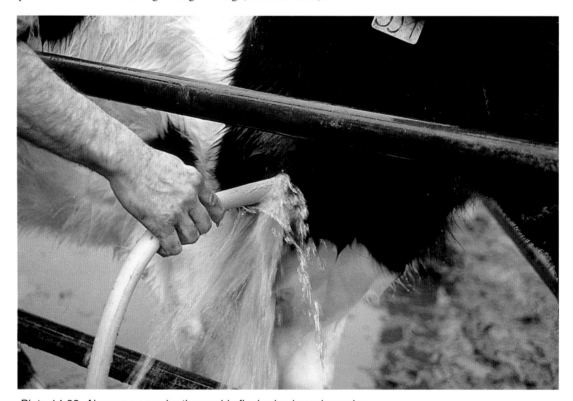

Plate 14.23. Abscesses can be thoroughly flushed using a hosepipe.

**Cleaning the wound** Infection, dirt and dead tissue seriously retard healing, so you must wash the area very carefully. If there is a skin flap, or if you are dealing with an abscess, do not be afraid to take a piece of cotton wool soaked in diluted disinfectant and wipe it deep under the skin. Repeat this with fresh swabs until they come out quite clean. Any dead tissue will have a creamy, pus-like appearance and this should also be rubbed away with your cotton wool. If the wound is an ulcer or some other lesion in the foot, then it can only be drained and cleaned by removing all the horn overlying the infected area. Abscesses may need to be lanced to allow the pus to drain, but first clean the skin, insert a needle and withdraw some of the contents of the swelling to make sure you obtain the characteristic off-white, thick, foul-smelling pus indicating that you are dealing with an abscess. If this is not found, leave the swelling alone and ask your vet to look when he next comes. Abscesses should be lanced at their lowest point, as this facilitates drainage. If possible, choose a place where the skin is softening and make a deep bold cut with a scalpel blade. Squeeze out all the pus, and then flush the abscess cavity with antiseptic solution.

This flushing process needs repeating every two to three days. It is most important that the initial cut does not heal over for at least a week; otherwise drainage will be inhibited and the abscess may re-form. One easy but very effective way of flushing out an abscess is simply to put a cold-water hosepipe into the cavity and then turn on the tap (Plate 14.23). The water pressure will help to remove all the pus and dead tissue present.

**Does it need a dressing?** Very large raw areas may be best covered but dressings must be regularly changed. Apply an antiseptic ointment, then a lint dressing, and cover this with cotton wool held in position with elastoplast. Abscesses are best left open for the pus to drain. Foot dressings, discussed in Chapter 9, are now rarely used. Burns are discussed in Chapter 10.

**Ointment or spray?** For many wounds, especially those on teats or other areas where the skin can crack, I prefer to use an emollient ointment, preferably one with antiseptic properties. This is especially important for severe teat chapping since teat skin lacks the sebaceous glands found on skin elsewhere in the body. Glycerine is an excellent treatment for chapped teats and for sores between the udder and thighs of freshly calved cows, as for example in Plate 7.41. Antibiotic aerosols containing coloured dyes tend to dry out wounds. They are therefore very good for superficial skin cuts and following dehorning, but if applied to teat skin they may lead to excessive cracking which would retard healing.

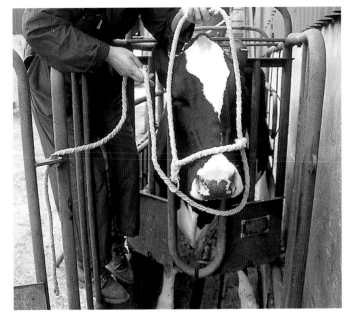

### Putting on a Halter

Perhaps this is hardly a veterinary task, but it surprises me how many people cannot apply a halter correctly. Lassoing a cow leads to unnecessary stress and does not restrain it particularly well because it can still move its head from side to side. The correct procedure is shown in Plate 14.24. There are essentially three pieces of the halter:

- the fixed length segment which fits over the animal's nose
- the lead rope which should come out from underneath the animal's chin
- an adjustable loop which fits behind the animal's ears

Plate 14.24. Applying a halter: the fixed length goes over the nose and the lead rope exits from under the chin.

If possible, apply the halter in one movement, by lifting the lower loop over the animal's nose and continuing to fit the upper loop behind its ears. Finally adjust the lead rope so that it is tight under its chin and check that the side pieces are not rubbing its eyes.

## Applying Nosegrips (Bulldogs)

Another method of restraint, which holds the animal even more securely for difficult procedures, is to apply nosegrips. These should be inserted behind the thick tissue of the nose and muzzle. Slide the metal clamps on the handle towards the nose, so that they cannot be pulled out (Plate 14.25). Within reason, the tighter they are, the less painful they are for the cow, because they are more firmly placed and less likely to pull out. In horses, pressure applied to the nose (for example by a twitch) leads to the release of endorphins, chemicals which specifically dull pain sensations throughout the body. The same probably applies to cattle.

## Casting a Cow – Reuff's Method

Although cattle are most commonly restrained in a crush, it is sometimes useful to be able to cast them. With the help of sedation, I use the Reuff's method of casting for rolling cows to correct a displaced abomasum and also for casting bulls for foot trimming when they are too large to go into a crush. Steady the cow with a halter, then tie a second rope around her neck, looping it behind her fore legs, and then in front of her udder, hind legs and pin bones, as shown in Plate 14.26. Tighten the chest loop, and then pull hard on the free end to tighten the abdominal loop. Provided sufficient tension can be applied, the animal will sink to the ground (Plate 14.27), and it will stay there while the rope remains tight. Although this

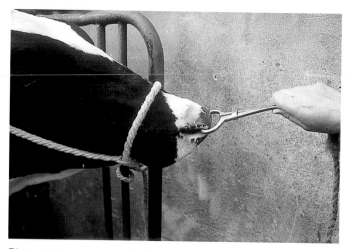

Plate 14.25. Nosegrips (bulldogs) permit additional restraint of the head.

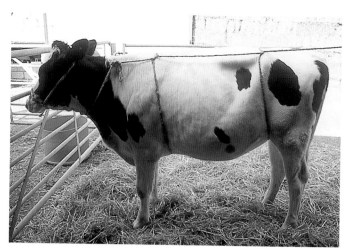

Plate 14.26. Casting a cow: a single length of rope is looped three times around the body.

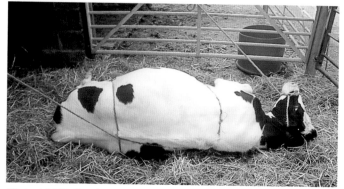

Plate 14.27. Casting a cow: by tightening all three loops, the heifer falls to the ground.

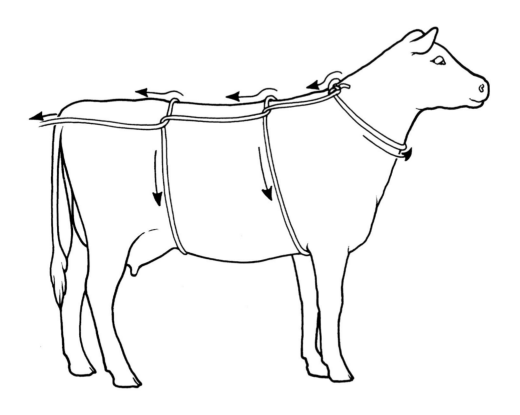

Figure 14.7. Position of rope to cast a cow by Reuff's method.

procedure will work with any cow, it is much easier if the cow has been sedated first. Take care
that the rear loop of rope is not catching on the
udder.

## Ringing a Bull

For ease of handling and for safety, I think it is
best to ring a bull soon after he is six months old,
and then make sure that he gets used to being led.
Holding the bull's head very firmly, inject a small
volume (1–2 ml) of anaesthetic into the soft tissue
dividing the nostrils before applying the nose
punch (Plate 14.28). The hole should be made as
far back from the nostrils as possible for added
strength, but it should not go through the harder
tissue of the cartilage of the nostrils. You can
easily feel this with your fingers. Having firmly
closed the punch, move it up and down a few times
to cut the hole through completely, and then insert

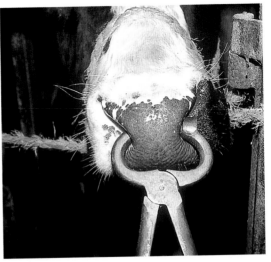

Plate 14.28. Bull ring nose punch: insert the ring
well back, but do not puncture the nasal cartilage.

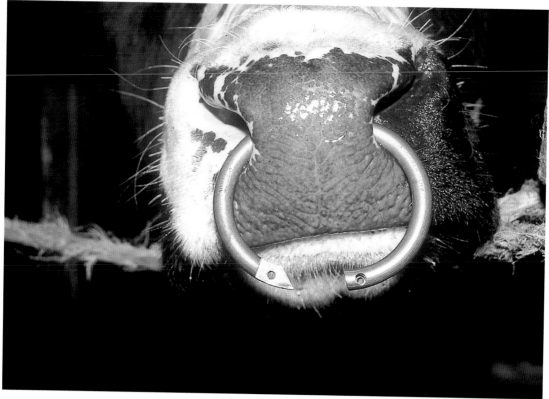

Plate 14.29. Ringing a bull: after being closed, the two ends of the ring are held together with a locking screw.

the ring (Plate 14.29). Carefully position the locking screw in the thread, screw it up as tight as possible, then break off the protruding segment. File away any rough edges. It is best to allow two to three weeks for the hole to heal before training the bull to lead.

## Hormone Implants and Growth Promoters

*Hormone implants*
During the early 1980s there was a marked increase in the number of hormone implants used for fattening cattle, and by 1986 well over 50% of all cattle slaughtered in the UK had been treated at some stage of their lives. However, following consumer pressure in 1988 the EU imposed a ban on all hormone implants even though the scientific committee which they had set up to investigate their safety had not at that time reported. A ban was also proposed for all other hormones used for non-therapeutic purposes in meat-producing animals.

At the time of writing, the hormone implant ban continues in the EU and, although zeranol has been cleared as 'safe' in North America, the EU prohibits the import of North American beef.

The rationale of hormone use was as follows:

● heifers and cows have ample female hormone so they can be implanted with male hormones
● steers have no hormones and can be implanted with male and female products
● bulls have ample male hormone and some female, and are given additional female hormones

The response to implantation is therefore greatest in steers, where a 30% increase in growth rate can be anticipated, with additional improvements in carcase quality and in feed conversion efficiency. Implanted heifers and cull cows become much more muscular and some may even develop a few male characteristics. As hormone implants affect growth rate it is clearly most advantageous to use them when the animal's natural rate of growth is already at a high level. For example, a 30% improvement in the growth rate of an animal growing at 0.3 kg per day is only 0.1 kg, whereas if the natural growth is already 1.5 kg per day, a 30% improvement would give 0.5 kg per day. The relationship is by no means as simple as this, but the example serves to illustrate the point very well.

The effects in entire bulls are much less dramatic, partly because of their natural rapid growth and good carcase conformation. Implants of female hormone should still give them a 5–10% increase in growth rate, however, and there may be additional benefits from reduced mounting behaviour and aggressiveness.

Implants were given under the skin of the ear, because this is the part of the carcase which is discarded and there is then no risk of large residual doses being eaten. The implanting technique is very similar to that for progesterone implants (Plate 8.5). The products used were either synthetic compounds (e.g. zeranol and trenbolone) or natural hormones (e.g. oestradiol, testosterone and progesterone). The natural hormones were equally as effective as the synthetic compounds, they had the advantage that no withdrawal period was necessary (that is, cattle could be slaughtered at any time after the hormone had been implanted), and it was hoped that they would be more acceptable to the consumer lobby.

BST, a hormone which increases milk production, may also become available as an implant. It is however not licensed for use in the EU. A full description of its function is given in Chapter 7.

*Growth promoters*
The growth promoters in use are primarily  substances which influence the growth of micro-organisms. Both avoparcin and zinc bacitracin were once widely used, but in 1997 avoparcin was banned in the EU due to concerns over possible carcinogenic activity and zinc bacitracin was banned in 1999. Growth promoters are totally non-absorbed from the gut and there is therefore no problem with meat and milk residues. They act by destroying certain gut micro-organisms and thus promoting a more efficient use of food.

The growth promoter monensin has a wide variety of uses. It is effective against coccidiosis in chickens and calves, it helps to prevent fog fever in cattle and it reduces the incidence of toxoplasma abortion in sheep. As a growth promoter, it acts in the rumen, altering the fermentation pattern to produce a higher proportion of propionic acid and hence to promote more efficient food utilisation and faster growth. Like bacitracin, it can be included in the concentrate portion of the ration. Animals over 160 kg bodyweight can be dosed at the start of the grazing period to provide a continual low dose of monensin for five months. Gains of around 15–20 kg would be expected, although there would not be the improvement in carcase conformation which is seen with hormone implants.

## Applying Eye Ointment

See Chapter 4.

## Using a Mastitis or Dry-Cow Intramammary Tube
See Chapter 7.

## Taking a Milk Sample

See Chapter 7.

## Foot Trimming

See Chapter 9.

## Handling a 'Downer' Cow

See Chapter 5.

## DEALING WITH POISONS

I find dealing with poisons a particularly frustrating area of veterinary medicine as there seem to be so many unknowns. For example:

- Many poisons give the same vague clinical symptoms of dullness, abdominal pain and nervous signs, so that you cannot diagnose on clinical grounds alone.
- Even if you suspect a poison, for example, from a history of possible access, it may be difficult and/or expensive to obtain confirmatory laboratory tests.
- If a laboratory test is available, the results are unlikely to be ready for several days and treatment usually has to be instigated immediately.
- Finally, even if you are convinced you know which poison is involved, there may be no specific antidote, and treatment is aimed at suppressing or alleviating the symptoms in the hope that the animal will recover on its own!

There are a few exceptions to this of course and lead poisoning is a good example. But even with lead the clinical signs can be variable, ranging from lethargy, dullness and blindness, to extreme excitement, racing around the pen, bellowing and trying to climb the walls. So, often, suspicions of poisoning must rest with a history of possible access to a known toxic substance, and this is why I have only listed some of the more common poisons in this chapter.

I have already said that clinical signs and treatment can be very variable and for this reason I have given very few details. If you suspect poisoning I would strongly recommend that you contact your vet for advice. Remember that for many poisons, small quantities are relatively harmless – they may even be beneficial. It is only when they are taken in excessive amounts – for example plants which are eaten because there is no other grazing available – that poisoning occurs.

### Acorns and oak leaves
Green acorns are particularly toxic if eaten in large quantities. The poison is called tannic acid, a chemical which was once used to preserve and harden hides in leather making. Initially cattle show dullness, abdominal pain and loss of appetite, but later there may be severe diarrhoea, the dung being black with blood, due to inflammation of the gut. Some cases are fatal. Drenching with chlorodyne (60 g) and linseed oil or liquid paraffin (500 ml) may help, and drugs can be given by injection to alleviate the intestinal spasm and pain.

### Antibiotics
Sometimes concentrates fed to cattle are contaminated with residues of antibiotics or other drugs which were perhaps being used as growth-promoters or medicants in pig or poultry rations. Although following the BSE crisis there is now a much stricter control at the feed mills when cleaning out between different mixes, mistakes can still occur. Most of the drugs involved destroy the normal rumen microflora. This makes the rumen go sour and the animal goes off its food.

Quite large quantities of some drugs, for example the tetracyclines and sulphonamides, can be eaten without any adverse effects, and both have been mentioned as a potential treatment earlier in this book. Oral penicillin is used for treatment of acidosis, when it is desirable to achieve a reduction in the activity of rumen bacteria, especially lactobacilli.

The antibiotic lincomycin, used in digital dermatitis footbaths, is potentially much more serious, probably because it destroys both bacteria and protozoa in the rumen. Even low levels of lincomycin in cattle food have caused quite severe reductions in yield and even death in dairy cattle. It is interesting to note that lincomycin can be given to cattle quite safely by injection, however: in fact it is a good treatment for joint ill.

### Arsenic
This was once a common constituent of sheep dips and potato sprays. It is now rarely used, but cattle may gain access to old cans and some seem to even like its taste! Arsenic causes severe inflammation of

the gut, leading to abdominal pain, colic and scouring. Badly affected animals become recumbent and die. Treatment is similar to that for acorn poisoning.

*Bracken*

Bracken poisoning occurs particularly in late summer when grazing is sparse, although clinical signs may not be seen until three weeks or more after the animals have been removed from the pasture. Although the green plant (Plate 14.30) is bitter, dried bracken may be readily eaten with hay, so bracken poisoning can occur indoors in winter. There are two types of clinical signs. The first is associated with gut inflammation caused by eating the fresh plant, and this leads to scouring with blood in the dung. The other syndrome is one of severe anaemia. Bracken affects the formation of certain cells, the thrombocytes (sometimes known as the blood platelets) in the bone marrow, and this produces a thrombocytopenia (a deficiency of thrombocytes) which interferes with blood clotting. You may see large red haemorrhagic areas in the mouth or vulva, the membranes of which will be very pale due to anaemia. Blood may accumulate in the eye to cause hyphaemia (Plate 4.23) and blood may also be passed in the urine, turning it red. This is sometimes called enzootic haematuria. Prolonged exposure to bracken can lead to polyps and tumours in the bladder, pharynx and oesophagus, and low grade bloat and vomiting may result.

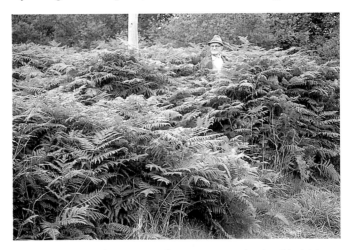

Plate 14.30. Bracken: some plants can grow to chest height.

*Caustic wheat*

Feeding caustic wheat which has been poorly mixed may lead to individual animals ingesting lumps of pure caustic soda (NaOH). This can produce severe mouth ulcers which have to be differentiated from foot-and-mouth disease (see Chapter 11.). The rumen also becomes very alkaline, shock develops and some animals die. Symptomatic treatment includes oral vinegar, to neutralise the rumen, fluid therapy and other measures to counteract shock, and B vitamins to compensate for lack of rumen function.

*Copper*

Copper toxicity is described in detail in Chapter 12.

*Creosote*

It is surprising what cattle will drink, and cases of creosote, diesel, paraffin and petrol poisoning are by no means uncommon. The early signs of poisoning are dullness, loss of appetite and abdominal pain, and these become more intense, leading to nervous signs and convulsions as the effects of severe liver damage become apparent. Often diagnosis is helped by the smell of creosote or diesel in the dung or even in the milk. At lower levels diesel may simply affect growth rate and hair formation.

*Fluorine*

Fluorine was once emitted from a large number of industrial processes and unless precautions are taken it can contaminate the surrounding grassland. It may also be present in certain types of rock phosphate. Most of the fluorine eaten is deposited in the animal's bones and teeth, and symptoms are unlikely to be seen until there has been a continuous exposure for several months. One of its main effects is lameness, which can be due to either a fracture of the bone in the hoof (see also Chapter 9) or to exostoses, which are small sharp lumps projecting from the surface of the bone as seen in Plate 9.55. If exostoses occur on the joints, lameness is particularly severe. Teeth abnormalities may also occur, especially in younger animals, with cracks in and pitting of the enamel. Many of the symptoms of fluorosis are similar to those of rickets. Very small doses of fluorine are beneficial to the bones and teeth, as we all know from dentistry advertisements. The only treatment for poisoning is to remove the cattle from the contaminated pasture, give vitamins A and D and wait for the fluorine to be slowly excreted.

*Insecticides*
There are three main groups of insecticides, the organochlorines (or chlorinated hydrocarbons), organo-phosphorus compounds and the pythrethroids which are not toxic.

**Organochlorines** The organochlorines include DDT (dichlorodiphenyltrichloroethane), BHC (benzene hexachloride, a common constituent of louse powder) and dieldrin, once used in sheep dips, but now banned from the EU and many other parts of the world because of its strong cumulative effects, particularly in wildlife.
    Poisoning results from a gradual build-up of the organochlorines in the animal's tissues, especially in the fat, although the onset of the clinical signs of excitability and muscle spasms can be quite sudden. Treatment is symptomatic only and consists of giving sedatives and muscle relaxants to control the convulsions.

**Organo-phosphates** Poisoning with organo-phosphorus compounds is far more common. This is because they are more widely used, because they can be absorbed through the skin and because they are inherently more toxic. Cattle may be exposed to sprays drifting from an adjacent field and I have seen several cases of poisoning when animals were allowed to graze orchards immediately after spraying. Although the spray may remain on the outside of the foliage for only a few days, it can take several weeks for the organo-phosphorus compounds absorbed by the plants to lose their toxicity. The main clinical signs of poisoning are salivation, colic, diarrhoea, difficulty in breathing and apparent blindness. Badly affected animals develop convulsions and die. Your vet will probably use atropine for treatment. This is a drug derived from deadly nightshade, which is in itself a poisonous plant. Atropine only counteracts some of the clinical signs however and recovery will be very slow.
    Organo-phosphorus compounds include pour-on warble dressings, fly repellants and some anthelmintics, as well as insecticides and sheep dips. Thirsty cattle should not be allowed access to sheep dips or water from run-off areas.

*Kale*
Overeating kale has been mentioned elsewhere in the book. There are three possible toxic syndromes. First, large intakes of kale over a short period may lead to a breakdown of the red blood cells. This is caused by a chemical in the kale called S-methyl cysteine sulphoxide, and it is seen clinically as blood in the urine and anaemia. Frosted kale is considered to be especially dangerous. Secondly, lower intakes of kale for prolonged periods may cause problems of depressed blood formation and anaemia. Thirdly, kale interferes with thyroid function, leading to goitre. Intakes above 20 kg per day for long periods should be avoided. Cabbage, rape and other members of the brassica family can cause similar problems if fed in excess. If in doubt, ensure ample supplementation with iodine, as discussed in Chapter 12.

*Laburnum*
Laburnum is one of the most dangerous trees grown in Britain, and you would be well advised to make sure that you can recognise it (Plate 14.31). All parts are poisonous, but the pods and seeds are especially toxic and produce nervous signs of excitement, incoordination, convulsions and death. There is no specific antidote, although your vet could give sedatives such as barbiturates to help control the nervous signs until the animal overcomes and excretes the toxin itself.

*Lead*

This was discussed in detail in Chapter 3.

*Mycotoxins*

When feedingstuffs are stored under unsatisfactory conditions, especially high humidity and warmth, moulds (a type of fungus) may grow. The majority of moulds are quite harmless and although they may reduce nutritional content and palatability, the affected food can still be fed to cattle. However, some moulds produce toxic byproducts, known as *mycotoxins*, and if eaten by cattle they can produce poisoning. The clinical signs seen depend on the type of mycotoxin present and this in turn depends on the species of mould which was originally growing on the food.

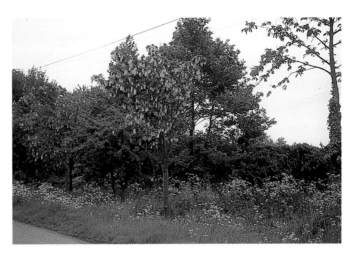

Plate 14.31. Laburnum: the pods and dry leaves are the most dangerous part of the plant.

Examples of mycotoxins include sterigmatocystin, ochratoxin A (causes kidney damage), citronin (causing PPH, Chapter 13), trichothecene (a gut irritant) and tremorgens (pasture moulds e.g. ryegrass staggers, Chapter 4). The most common however is called aflatoxin, which is a contaminant of imported groundnut and cottonseed cakes. In 1980, over 20% of the imports tested were found to contain aflatoxin, although many were below the level likely to cause symptoms. Some feedingstuff manufacturers have now stopped using groundnut and cottonseed, and legislation exists to prohibit the incorporation of materials containing more than 50 parts per billion of aflatoxin. Feed which is improperly stored, for example in an outside food bunker, or in a bin which leaks, may also grow moulds which produce aflotoxin. Levels greater than 100 ppb are said to be dangerous, causing liver damage, reduced yields and depressed growth, or in more severe cases sudden death due to haemorrhages into the abomasum and intestines. There is some concern that a breakdown product of aflatoxin which appears in the milk may cause liver tumours in man. Such tumours are very rare, however, and aflatoxin is not the only cause.

*Nitrates*

In the rumen, nitrates are converted into nitrites. These are absorbed into the blood where they combine with haemoglobin to produce methaemoglobin, which is incapable of carrying oxygen. Clinical signs of poisoning therefore include a marked blue discolouration (cyanosis) of the membranes of the eyes, mouth and vagina, followed by panting, gasping, trembling and eventual collapse. Death may occur in as little as half an hour from the clinical signs first being seen, and the blood of affected animals is very dark. In cows which recover, abortions and stillbirths may occur. It is not an easy condition to diagnose in the live animal, although the treatment, which consists of giving a 5% solution of methylene blue intravenously, is quite successful.

Many plants can accumulate dangerous levels of nitrates, and grazing itself may become toxic if there have been very heavy applications of slurry and artificial fertiliser. This is especially so during periods of drought when there has been no rain to wash nitrates from the soil, or during warm, overcast weather, when nitrates accumulate in the plant but there is insufficient sunlight to complete their conversion to protein. Other sources of nitrate include effluent from silage clamps or bags of compound fertiliser which cattle sometimes tear open and eat. There is some evidence that conserved forage is more dangerous than fresh grazing and deaths have been reported within one or two hours after giving cattle a particular bale of hay. Some weed sprays lead to increased levels of plant nitrate, so always read the manufacturer's instructions before reintroducing cattle to the grazing.

*Ragwort*

Ragwort (Plate 14.32) can cause permanent and irreversible changes in the liver and although clinical signs often appear quite suddenly, it is likely that the plant has been eaten in small amounts over several months. It is particularly dangerous in hay and silage, because then its bitter taste is not so obvious to the cattle. The onset of clinical signs may be triggered by some form of stress. For example, suckler cows have been reported to die at calving and/or peak lactation, even though the ragwort was ingested several months previously. Clinical signs include diarrhoea, jaundice, photosensitisation (Chapter 10) and nervous signs. The abdomen may become enlarged and swollen with excess fluid and the animal blindly wanders around appearing very dull and often bumping into things. There is no treatment and cases should be slaughtered before they lose excessive weight. Ragwort grows on marginal pastures and so cultivation and application of nitrogen are the best methods of controlling the plant. Sprays are also available.

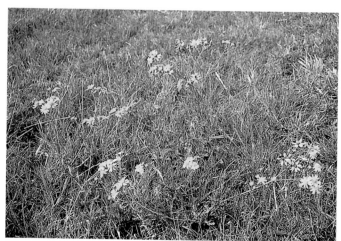

Plate 14.32. Ragwort is a cumulative poison causing liver damage.

*Rhododendron*

This is an interesting poison because it is one of the few occasions when you may see cattle vomiting. Other clinical signs include colic, drooling, nervous signs and difficulty with breathing. Stimulants such as ephedrine are said to be useful for treatment, and purgatives help to remove any rhododendron remaining in the gut, though the animal may still remain ill for several days during which warmth and nursing are vital.

*Slug bait*

I suspect that this is one of the more common poisons affecting both dogs and farm livestock, and I have had to treat several cases. The active chemical is metaldehyde and it is made attractive to slugs (and cattle!) by incorporating it into a cereal base. It is extensively used in crop husbandry. Metaldehyde causes dullness, depression, incoordination, staggering, shivering and colic. Eventually the animal becomes recumbent and death occurs from respiratory failure. There is also liver damage. Treatment is largely symptomatic, using respiratory and liver stimulants, with saline or calcium borogluconate intravenously. Barbiturates help to control convulsions.

*St John's wort*

The toxic chemical in this plant is called hypericin. It persists even when the plant has been dried and so remains poisonous in hay. The clinical signs are those of photosensitisation, and this was described in Chapter 10.

*Strychnine*

Strychnine is still used on farms for the control of moles. Poisoning leads to severe muscle spasms, with the whole animal going rigid and in this respect it resembles the final stages of tetanus. Muscle relaxants are used in treatment. Fortunately cattle are relatively resistant and in fact strychnine is used in low doses, in the form of nux vomica, as an appetite stimulant.

*Urea*

Urea-based feedingstuffs were once very common and they are still used in fattening and rearing rations. Although cattle can tolerate quite high levels of urea, they must be slowly introduced and they must continue to receive a constant intake. Even a gap of a few days can be dangerous. Ammonium sulphate fertilisers cause a similar poisoning syndrome, since most of the urea is converted into ammonia in the rumen. The clinical signs are dullness and rapid breathing in early or mild cases, although nervous signs and staggering can develop and death may be accompanied by violent struggling and bellowing. Increasing the acidity of the rumen reduces the conversion of urea to free ammonia, and also decreases the rate of absorption of ammonia from the rumen, so drenching a cow with 2–3 litres of vinegar will undoubtedly help. Moderate urea intakes have been associated with depressed fertility and embryo death.

*Warfarin*

This is a dicoumarol derivative and it is a commonly used rat poison. It prevents the action of vitamin K in the animal and thus interferes with blood clotting mechanisms. This was described in Chapter 12. Poisoning in cattle is not common, although calves sometimes gain access to large quantities of rat bait. The clinical signs are colic, dullness and sometimes stiffness due to bleeding into the joints. There may be bleeding from the nose or blood in the dung. Vitamin K and iron are used for treatment.

*Water dropwort (hemlock, dead man's fingers)*

Hemlock has been a well-known human poison for thousands of years. The species which causes most problems in cattle is water dropwort, which grows in wetland areas. Cattle gain access to its sweet-tasting root (known as dead man's fingers, Plate 14.33) when ditches have been cleaned out and the spoil is left on the bank within easy reach of the animals. These roots may also come to the surface and cause poisoning when cattle scramble down into ditches in dry summers in search of food or water.

The roots have a higher concentration of toxin than the rest of the plant, particularly in the winter and early spring. Most animals are simply found dead. Clinical signs, when seen, are non-specific and may include diarrhoea, trembling and convulsions. Treatment is symptomatic only.

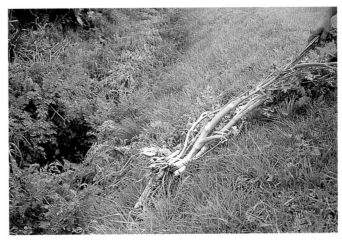

Plate 14.33. Water dropwort: the sweet-tasting roots, often called dead man's fingers, are sometimes left within easy reach of cattle after a ditch has been cleaned out.

*Yew*

The yew is the most poisonous British tree known to cattle, and I suggest you carefully study Plate 14.34 so that you can recognise the characteristic leaves and red berries. Branches from this tree led to the death of beef cattle that broke into a field and ate some yew not totally burnt in a bonfire.

All parts of the tree, the leaves and the berries, are toxic, except for the red flesh of the berries. Yew is therefore not toxic to birds as they are only able to digest the flesh of the berries and the seeds are passed out untouched. The active chemicals are taxine, a substance which stops the heart, plus cyanogenetic glycosides, which ferment in the rumen to produce hydrocyanic acid (i.e. cyanide). It could be either the slow release of taxine from the seeds of the fruit or the production of cyanide which accounts for some animals dying as late as one or two days after ingestion. By the time you realise that the cattle have eaten yew, those which are going to be affected have often already died. However, there are reports of clinically affected cattle surviving after being treated with hydroxycobalamin (5000 μg of vitamin B$_{12}$ intravenously and 2500 μg intramuscularly) and sugar (1 kg orally).

The logic of the treatment is that the cyanide released from the yew is as toxic as the taxine if not more so. Sugar reduces the rate of release of cyanide in the rumen and vitamin B$_{12}$ combines with the cyanide already produced to form cyanocobalamin, which is non-toxic. This may not be a well-recognised treatment, but it is cheap and certainly worth trying.

A rumenotony, to open the rumen and remove the yew, is an expensive procedure, difficult to carry out on a large number of animals and in any case many of them may not have eaten any yew. Unless the rumen is totally emptied, it is almost impossible to remove all fragments of yew from it.

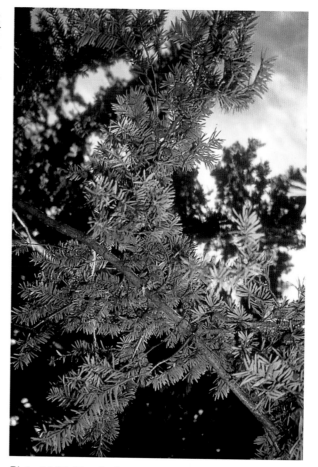

Plate 14.34. Yew is the most poisonous plant to affect cattle.

# APPENDICES

## Appendix 1 – Normal Values

| | |
|---|---|
| *Temperature* | 101.5°F   38.6°C |
| *Pulse rate* | 45–50 per minute |
| *Respiratory rate* | 15–20 per minute |

The figures apply to normal healthy adult animals at rest. Higher values will be obtained:

- from younger animals
- after exercise
- following excitement, e.g. handling or stress
- during very hot conditions
- in fevered animals, e.g. from infection and toxaemia
- immediately post-partum and in very early lactation

*Rumen contractions*

Twice per minute on high-fibre diets. The first contraction is the upper sac, and leads to regurgitation of food into the mouth for further chewing (cudding) or to release of gas (eructation or belching). The second contraction involves the lower rumen sac: small particles of digested food are pushed through into the omasum and abomasum.
Reduced rumen contractions occur

- with high concentrate diets which cause acidosis
- with diets with inadequate long fibre (= inadequate rumen 'scratch factor')
- with rumen impaction, e.g. from over-eating straw
- at the time of calving
- in cows with ketosis
- with any toxaemia or illness

*Sleep*

Cattle have two types of sleep, deep sleep and drowsy sleep. The total amount of deep sleep required is very little, around thirty to sixty minutes per day and individual periods last for approximately five minutes only. Rumination ceases and brain activity is reduced, but the animal remains sitting. Drowsy sleep accounts for about one-third of the total day and can take place when the animal is standing or sitting. Rumination continues, but at a reduced rate. Younger animals need more sleep than adults.

## Appendix 2 – Lists of Clinical Signs

Some of the more common clinical signs of disease have been selected, and a list of possible causes of each clinical sign has been given. Each cause may be referred to in more detail by consulting the index. The lists are by no means exhaustive and other diseases, apart from those mentioned, could be involved.

| | |
|---|---|
| *Abortion* | Aspergillosis |
| | *Bacillus licheniformis* |
| | brucellosis |
| | BVD |
| | coxiella burnetii (Q fever) |
| | fever/very high temperature |
| | IBR |
| | leptospirosis |
| | listeriosis |
| | Neospora |
| | nitrate poisoning |
| | salmonellosis (especially *S. dublin and S. typhimurium*) |
| | summer mastitis |
| *Anaemia* | abomasal ulcer |
| | bracken poisoning |
| | coccidiosis |
| | copper deficiency |
| | EBL |
| | fluke |
| | haemorrhage e.g. into uterus |
| | kale poisoning |
| | lice |
| | red water (*Babesia*) |
| | ticks |
| *Blindness* | anophthalmia/microphthalmia |
| | bovine iritis |
| | cataract |
| | CCN |
| | hyphaema |
| | lead poisoning |
| | listeriosis |
| | meningitis |
| | nervous acetonaemia |
| | New Forest eye |
| | overeating syndrome/acidosis |
| | spontaneous |
| | vitamin A deficiency |
| *Bloat* | abomasal displacement/abomasal torsion |
| | acidosis |
| | choke |

forestomach obstruction
frothy bloat
overeating
rumenal atony
tetanus
vagus indigestion
wire = traumatic reticulitis

*Blood in Faeces*    acorn, aflotoxin or bracken poisoning
*(melaena)*    abomasal ulcer
    acute BVD
    coccidiosis
    salmonella
    toxaemia

*Blood in Urine*    bracken poisoning
    copper poisoning
    cystitis
    kale poisoning
    muscular dystrophy (vitamin E deficiency)
    pyelonephritis
    red water (*Babesia*)

*Coughing*    calf pneumonia
    dust
    lungworm

*Downer Cow*    acute mastitis
    acute metritis
    debilitation and weakness
    fracture of pelvis or leg
    hypomagnesaemia
    milk fever
    muscle damage
    obturator paralysis
    scouring
    selenium/vitamin E deficiency
    severe haemorrhage

*Drooling*    BVD
    choke
    diptheria
    Foot and Mouth
    IBR
    lumpy jaw
    malignant oedema
    MCF
    mucosal disease
    tooth abscess
    toxaemia
    wooden tongue

| | |
|---|---|
| *Eye Discharge* | bovine iritis |
| | conjunctivitis |
| | enzootic pneumonia |
| | foreign body – e.g. barley awn |
| | fly irritation |
| | IBR |
| | MCF |
| | New Forest eye |
| | scratch on surface of eye |
| | tumour of third eyelid |
| | ultra-violet light damage |
| | |
| *Jaundice* | copper poisoning |
| | red water (*Babesia*) |
| | acute liver fluke |
| | ragwort poisoning |
| | |
| *Nervous Signs* | acetonaemia |
| | botulism |
| | BSE |
| | CCN |
| | hypomagnesaemia |
| | lead poisoning |
| | listeriosis |
| | meningitis |
| | middle ear infection |
| | over-eating barley or concentrates |
| | poisoning – by many substances |
| | tetanus |
| | toxaemia |
| | vitamin A deficiency |
| | |
| *Panting* | acetonaemia |
| | acidosis/over-eating |
| | anaemia |
| | excitement |
| | fever |
| | fog fever |
| | haemorrhage/blood loss |
| | heart defect |
| | hypersensitivity reactions |
| | hypomagnesaemia |
| | lungworm |
| | pneumonia |
| | poisoning |
| | scouring |
| | |
| *Red water* | see Blood in Urine |

*Scouring*                BVD
                         coccidiosis
                         coronavirus
                         cryptosporidia
                         digestive upsets (including acidosis)
                         *E. coli*
                         Johne's disease
                         mucosal disease
                         nutritional
                         ostertagia
                         over-eating
                         rotavirus
                         salmonellosis
                         toxic mastitis

*Straining (raised tail and abdominal contractions = tenesmus)*
                         abortion
                         calving difficulty
                         coccidiosis
                         cystitis
                         intestinal obstruction
                         intussusception
                         ragwort poisoning
                         urolithiasis
                         vaginal infection

*Sudden Death*           abomasal ulcer
                         bloat
                         copper poisoning
                         heart failure
                         hypomagnesaemia
                         internal haemorrhage
                         intestinal torsion
                         mastitis
                         muscular dystrophy
                         poisoning (especially yew + water dropwort)
                         wire (= traumatic reticulitis)

# INDEX

458

# Old Pond Publishing

Below is a sample of the wide range of agricultural books and videos/DVDs we publish. For more information or a free illustrated catalogue of all our publications please contact:

**Old Pond Publishing**
**Dencora Business Centre**
**36 White House Road, Ipswich, IP1 5LT, United Kingdom**

Website: **www.oldpond.com**

**Tel: 01473 238200**
**Fax: 01473 238201**
**Email: enquiries@oldpond.com**

## Mastitis Control in Dairy Herds

*Roger Blowey and Peter Edmondson*

Starts with the structure of the teats and udder and their defences against mastitis, then deals with the causes, epidemiology and control of the disease. Practical chapters cover the milking routine, teat disinfection, environmental factors, the somatic cell count and TBC/Bactoscan. Finally: targets and monitoring, mastitis treatments and dry cow therapy, summer mastitis and other diseases of the udder and teat. Hardback book.

## Cattle Lameness and Hoofcare 2nd Edition

*Roger Blowey*

Deals first with the structure of the foot, laminitis and the weight-bearing surfaces and hoof overgrowth. This leads on to a full description of best practice in hoof trimming. The book covers the common diseases of the foot, with detailed descriptions and clear colour photographs. Finally Roger explains the causes and prevention of lameness. Hardback book.

## Footcare in Cattle: hoof structure and trimming

*Roger Blowey*

Using laboratory specimens, Roger Blowey shows the anatomy of cattle feet and what happens when the hoof overgrows. He next visits a dairy farm to demonstrate hoof trimming to a novice dairy farmer who has a chance to trim under Roger's supervision. The perfect combination of theory and practice. Video/DVD.

## The Veterinary Book for Sheep Farmers

*David C Henderson*

The world's leading veterinary manual for sheep farmers, emphasising preventive medicine. Wide-ranging contents broadly follow the life-cycle of the sheep and contain guidance for health care of the animal throughout its life. Includes fertility and breeding, along with common problems such as skin parasites, lameness and respiratory diseases. Hardback book.

## The Goatkeeper's Veterinary Book 4th edition

*Peter Dunn*

Practical and easy to use, this updated book is the standard veterinary reference work for all goatkeepers, containing information on the symptoms and control of the major goat diseases. A sequence of colour photographs shows a normal kidding, and a calendar will assist in planning preventive medicine. Hardback book.

## Poultry at Home

*Victoria Roberts*

In this beginner's guide to poultry health and management, Victoria Roberts uses over 50 pure breeds to illustrate the various points to consider when choosing birds. She goes on to discuss handling, housing, feed, common ailments, breeding, candling eggs and rearing chicks. Video/DVD.